AAEVT's Eq
for Veterinary Technicians

AAEVT's Equine Manual for Veterinary Technicians

Deborah Reeder, RVT

Sheri Miller, LVT

DeeAnn Wilfong, BS, CVT

Midge Leitch, VMD, DAVCS

Dana Zimmel, DVM, DACVIM, DABVP (Equine Practice)

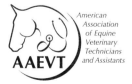

American Association of Equine Veterinary Technicians and Assistants

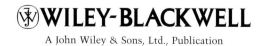

WILEY-BLACKWELL

A John Wiley & Sons, Ltd., Publication

Edition first published 2009
© 2009 Wiley-Blackwell

Blackwell Publishing was acquired by John Wiley & Sons in February 2007. Blackwell's publishing program has been merged with Wiley's global Scientific, Technical, and Medical business to form Wiley-Blackwell.

Editorial Office
2121 State Avenue, Ames, Iowa 50014-8300, USA

For details of our global editorial offices, for customer services, and for information about how to apply for permission to reuse the copyright material in this book, please see our website at www.wiley.com/wiley-blackwell.

Authorization to photocopy items for internal or personal use, or the internal or personal use of specific clients, is granted by Blackwell Publishing, provided that the base fee is paid directly to the Copyright Clearance Center, 222 Rosewood Drive, Danvers, MA 01923. For those organizations that have been granted a photocopy license by CCC, a separate system of payments has been arranged. The fee codes for users of the Transactional Reporting Service are ISBN-13: 978-0-8138-2971-5/2009.

Library of Congress Cataloguing-in-Publication Data

Zimmel, Dana.
    AAEVT's equine manual for veterinary technicians / Dana Zimmel, Deborah Reeder.
        p. cm.
    Includes bibliographical references and index.
    ISBN 978-0-8138-2971-5 (alk. paper)
    1. Horses–Diseases–Handbooks, manuals, etc.   2. Animal health technicians–Handbooks, manuals, etc.
I. Reeder, Deborah, 1952– II. Title.   III. Title: Equine manual for veterinary technicians.
    SF951.Z56 2009
    636.1'089–dc22

                                    2008044518

A catalog record for this book is available from the U.S. Library of Congress.

Set in 9/12 pt Palatino by SNP Best-set Typesetter Ltd., Hong Kong
Printed and Bound in Singapore by Fabulous Printers Pte Ltd

Disclaimer
The contents of this work are intended to further general scientific research, understanding, and discussion only and are not intended and should not be relied upon as recommending or promoting a specific method, diagnosis, or treatment by practitioners for any particular patient. The publisher and the author make no representations or warranties with respect to the accuracy or completeness of the contents of this work and specifically disclaim all warranties, including without limitation any implied warranties of fitness for a particular purpose. In view of ongoing research, equipment modifications, changes in governmental regulations, and the constant flow of information relating to the use of medicines, equipment, and devices, the reader is urged to review and evaluate the information provided in the package insert or instructions for each medicine, equipment, or device for, among other things, any changes in the instructions or indication of usage and for added warnings and precautions. Readers should consult with a specialist where appropriate. The fact that an organization or Website is referred to in this work as a citation and/or a potential source of further information does not mean that the author or the publisher endorses the information the organization or Website may provide or recommendations it may make. Further, readers should be aware that Internet Websites listed in this work may have changed or disappeared between when this work was written and when it is read. No warranty may be created or extended by any promotional statements for this work. Neither the publisher nor the author shall be liable for any damages arising herefrom.

Contents

Preface

The American Association of Equine Veterinary Technicians (AAEVT) took its first breath 4 short years ago and is now 1,200 members strong, with enthusiasm and energy far surpassing the anticipation of the American Association of Equine Practitioners' (AAEP) Task Force, which gave substance to the vision of Deb Reeder, RVT. She served on the task force and became the first president and executive director of the association, supported by an executive board of committed technicians and veterinary assistants, who saw the need for an organization that was dedicated to providing a means of continuing education for, and communication among, all who were employed in the field of equine veterinary medicine.

In keeping with its mission "to promote the health and welfare of the horse through the education and professional enrichment of the equine veterinary technician and assistant," the AAEVT proposed the creation of a reference specifically directed toward the tasks of these individuals. No other reference of this type and magnitude, which addresses the role of the technician or assistant in equine veterinary medicine in the United States, is available. The differences in the practice of equine veterinary medicine between the United Kingdom and the United States make a similar reference published in England less than ideal for individuals employed in this field in the United States.

Because of the spectrum of topics included in this manual, its use in the classroom is preordained. Veterinary technician programs will find it the ideal supplemental reference text for those students pursuing a career in equine practice. The list of authors is lengthy and drawn from both academia and practice, with multiple board-certified veterinary specialists and credentialed technicians included.

This manual is a salute to the vast number of faithful trusted assistants who have literally shouldered much of the day-to-day responsibility for work that includes client communications, preparation for the day's wide variety of tasks, patient care and handling, paperwork, and last but not least, care and feeding of the equine clinician! It is my honor and privilege to write this preface and to give recognition to the patient, tireless, hardworking, and caring individuals who have made veterinary medicine not only fun for many like myself, but also have made it possible.

Thank you.

Midge Leitch, VMD, DAVCS
September 1, 2008

Acknowledgments

This resource is dedicated to all the equine veterinary technicians, assistants, support staff, and students, who dedicate themselves day in and day out to this wonderful profession. The equine veterinary industry is indebted to you for your tireless, caring, attention to each patient, your compassion with each client, your commitment to education, and to providing the absolute highest standard of veterinary nursing care and medical treatment. Without you, equine veterinary care and this profession would not be where it is today and its future not nearly so bright.

I want to acknowledge first of all the equine technicians in the state of Texas, who fought for many years for official recognition of our profession. And to that special group (Joni, Kristi, Linda, Debbie, Ky, Lisa, Charly to name a few) who gave birth to the vision of an association for equine technicians and assistants and whose dedication and friendship have inspired me to turn that vision into a reality, I am forever indebted.

I would like to acknowledge my colleagues on the Executive Organizing Committee of the AAEVT, who eventually became its first board of directors: Sheri Miller, LVT, DeeAnn Wilfong, CVT, Kelly Fleming, CPA, Mandy Walton, LVT, and Jane Tyrie and Paul Vrotsos, CVT. Each of you has contributed to the path of the AAEVT, its foundation, its vision, and its future. I applaud you for the many hours you volunteered to steer this association, the commitment you made (unaware of the time it would require!), and for the incredible contribution you have made to the equine veterinary profession. I know you are not done, you are here continuing to contribute and will be the mentors for those that follow in our footsteps.

I also acknowledge the AAEP Board of Directors, David Foley, Executive Director and the staff, and the AAEVT Task Force members and original Advisory Council: Drs. Rick Lessor, Brad Jackman, Midge Leitch, Susan White, Dana Zimmel, Reynolds Cowles, and Bob Magnus for their support, guidance, and wisdom.

The AAEVT would like to acknowledge and thank the many contributors to this manual, without whom this outstanding resource for equine technicians, assistants, support staff, and the many aspiring students would not have become a reality. We want to also acknowledge those programs accredited by the American Veterinary Medical Association (AVMA) that are striving to incorporate equine courses into their programs. Here is your long-awaited text book. We thank Erica Judisch, Editor for Blackwell Publishing, for your patient guidance and encouragement. We made it!

I thank the other editors as well, for your tireless reviews, soliciting of authors, and organization of this manual. When DeeAnn Wilfong and I met with Wiley-Blackwell to discuss the idea of creating and publishing this manual, I am sure we had no idea of the magnitude of the task ahead of us; we simply believed that such a reference was dearly needed. With everyone's support, commitment, and teamwork, the words, the chapters, the illustrations, and the charts are now bound by the glue of that vision.

Deborah Reeder, RVT
AAEVT Executive Director

Contributors

Tanya M. Balaam-Morgan, DVM
Madrid, Iowa

Bonnie S. Barr, VMD, DACVIM
Department of Internal Medicine
Rood and Riddle Equine Hospital
Lexington, Kentucky

Dennis Brooks, DVM, PhD, DACVO
College of Veterinary Medicine
University of Florida
Gainesville, Florida

Gail Broussard
Texas A&M University College of Veterinary Medicine
College Station, Texas

Jennifer L. Davis, DVM, PhD, DACVIM, DACVCP
Assistant Professor of Equine Medicine
College of Veterinary Medicine
Raleigh, North Carolina

K. E. Davison, PhD
Land O' Lakes Purina Feed
Longview Animal Nutrition Center
Gray Summit, Missouri

Kira Epstein, DVM, DACVS
Clinical Assistant Professor
Department of Large Animal Medicine
University of Georgia College of Veterinary Medicine
Athens, Georgia

Katherine Garrett
Rood and Riddle Equine Hospital
Lexington, Kentucky

Mary Beth Gordon, PhD
Land O' Lakes Purina Feed
Longview Animal Nutrition Center
Gray Summit, Missouri

Kelsey A. Hart, DVM
Department of Large Animal Medicine
University of Georgia College of Veterinary Medicine
Athens, Georgia

Elizabeth Hinton
Texas A&M University College of Veterinary Medicine
College Station, Texas

Amanda M. House, DVM, DACVIM
Assistant Professor
Large Animal Clinical Sciences
University of Florida College of Veterinary Medicine
Gainesville, Florida

Laura Javsicas, VMD
College of Veterinary Medicine
University of Florida
Gainesville, Florida

Audrey Kelleman, DVM, Dip ACT
New Bolton Center
University of Pennsylvania, School of Veterinary Medicine Department of Clinical Studies, Section of Reproductive Studies
Philadelphia, Pennsylvania

Michelle LeBlanc, DVM, Dip ACT
Rood and Riddle Equine Hospital
Lexington, Kentucky

Midge Leitch, VMD, DAVCS
New Bolton Center
University of Pennsylvania
School of Veterinary Medicine
Philadelphia, Pennsylvania

Tracy McArthur
Texas A&M University College of Veterinary Medicine
College Station, Texas

Erin M. McNally, DVM
University of Florida
College of Veterinary Medicine
Gainesville, Florida

Sheri Miller, LVT
Lexington, Kentucky

Luisito S. Pablo, DVM, MS, DACVA
University of Florida
College of Veterinary Medicine
Gainesville, Florida

Contributors

Michael B. Porter, DVM, PhD, DACVIM
College of Veterinary Medicine
University of Florida
Gainesville, Florida

R. H. Raub, PhD
Land O' Lakes Purina Feed
Longview Animal Nutrition Center
Gray Summit, Missouri

Deborah Reeder, RVT
AAEVT Executive Director
San Marcos, California

Laura Riggs, DVM, PhD, DACVS
Assistant Professor
Department of Clinical Sciences
Louisiana State University School of Veterinary Medicine
Baton Rouge, Louisiana

Craig F. Shoemaker, DVM, MS
Manager
Equine Professional Services
IDEXX Pharmaeuticals, Inc.
Greenboro, North Carolina

Bryan Waldridge, DVM, DACVIM, DABVP
Rood and Riddle Equine Hospital
Lexington, Kentucky

DeeAnn Wilfong, BS, CVT
Littleton Equine Medical Center
Littleton Large Animal Clinic
Littleton, Colorado

J. K. Young, PhD
Land O' Lakes Purina Feed
Longview Animal Nutrition Center
Gray Summit, Missouri

Dana Zimmel, DVM, DACVIM, DABVP (Equine Practice)
College of Veterinary Medicine
University of Florida
Gainesville, Florida

Medical Acronyms and Abbreviations

Deborah Reeder and Sheri Miller

Acronym/ Abbreviation	Description
AAEP	American Association of Equine Practitioners
AAEVT	American Association of Equine Veterinary Technicians
ab, Ab	antibody
ACTH	adrenocorticotropic hormone
ag, Ag	antigen
AGID	agar immunodiffusion
AI	artificial insemination
ALP	alkaline phosphatase
APHIS	Animal and Plant Health Inspection Service (USDA)
AST	aspartate aminotransferase
Ax	anesthesia
BID	twice a day
BAR	bright, alert, responsive
BP	blood pressure
bpm	beats per minute
BEVA	British Equine Veterinary Association
BUN	blood urea nitrogen
BW	body weight
Bx	biopsy
C-1, C-2 . . .	the cervical vertebrae
C. diff.	*Clostridium difficile*
C. perf.	*Clostridium perfringens*
CAT scan or CT	computerized axial tomography; computed tomography
CBC	complete blood count
CC	cranial to caudal *or* caudal to cranial
CEM	contagious equine metritis
CF or CFT	complement fixation; complement fixation test
CK	creatine kinase
CL	corpus luteum

Acronym/ Abbreviation	Description
CN1, CN2, . . .	the cranial nerves
CNS	central nervous system
COPD	chronic obstructive pulmonary disease
CPK	creatine phosphokinase
CRT	capillary refill time
CSF	cerebrospinal fluid
CV	cardiovascular
CVP	central venous pressure
CVT	Certified Veterinary Technician
DDFT	deep digital flexor tendon
DDSP	dorsal displacement of the soft palate
DEA	Drug Enforcement Administration
DIRT	distal intermediate ridge of the tibia
DIT	distal intertarsal joint
DJD	degenerative joint disease
DLPMO	dorsolateral to palmar/plantar medial oblique
DMPLO	dorsomedial to palmar/plantar lateral oblique
DMSO	dimethyl sulfoxide
DNA	deoxyribonucleic acid
DP	dorsal to palmar/plantar
DSS	dioctyl sodium sulfosuccinate
DV	dorsal to ventral
DVM	doctor of veterinary medicine
Dx	diagnosis
ECF	extracelluar fluid
ECG	equine chorionic gonadotrophin
ECG	electrocardiogram
EDTA	ethylenediaminetetraacetic acid
EE	equine encephalomyelitis
EEE	eastern equine encephalomyelitis

Acronym/ Abbreviation	Description	Acronym/ Abbreviation	Description
EHV	equine herpes virus	MAP	mean arterial pressure
EIA	equine infectious anemia	MCH	mean corpuscular hemoglobin
EIPH	exercise-induced pulmonary hemorrhage	MCHC	mean corpuscular hemoglobin concentration
ELISA	enzyme-linked immunosorbent assay	MCII/MTII	second metacarpal or metatarsal bone (splint bone)
EMG	electromyogram	MCIII/MTIII	third metacarpal or metatarsal bone (cannon bone)
EPM	equine protozoal myeloencephalitis	MCIV/MTIV	fourth metacarpal or metatarsal bone (splint bone)
ET	embryo transfer	MCV	mean corpuscular volume
EVA	equine viral arteritis	mm	mucous membranes
Ex	examination	MRI	magnetic resonance imaging
EVR	equine viral rhinopneumonitis	NI	neonatal isoerythrolysis
FEI	Federation Equestre International	NIBC	noninvasive blood pressure
FFD	focal film distance	NPO	nothing per os (nothing by mouth)
FSH	follicle-stimulating hormone	NS	normal saline
fx	fracture	NSAID	nonsteroidal anti-inflammatory drug
GG	guaifenesin		
GGT	gamma-glutamyl transferase	O.D.	right eye
GI	gastrointestinal	O.S.	left eye
GKX	guaifenesin, ketamine, xylazine	OA	osteoarthritis
GnRH	gonadotropin-releasing hormone	OCD	osteochondrosis dissecans
HA	hyaluronic acid	P1	first phalanx (long pastern bone)
Hb or Hgb	hemoglobin concentration		
HBOT	hyperbaric oxygen treatment	P2	second phalanx (short pastern bone)
HCG	human chorionic gonadotropin		
Hct	hematocrit	P3	coffin bone
HR	heart rate	PaO_2	partial pressure of oxygen in arterial blood
HYPP	hyperkalemic periodic paralysis		
IBP	invasive blood pressure	PCV	packed cell volume
IgG	immunoglobulin G	PHF	Potomac horse fever
IM	intramuscular	PIT	proximal intertarsal joint
IN	intranasal	PPE	prepurchase examination
IV	intravenous	PPG	procaine penicillin g
kV	kilovolt	PPN	partial parenteral nutrition
LDH	lactate dehydrogenase	PRN	as needed
LH	luteinizing hormone	PSGAG	polysulfated glycosaminoglycan
LRS	lactated Ringer's solution	q	each
LVT	licensed veterinary technician	QID	four times a day
mA	milliamperes	q1h	every hour
MAC	minimum alveolar concentration	QAR	quiet, alert, responsive
		qd	every day

Acronym/ Abbreviation	Description
QNS	quantity not sufficient
qod	every other day
RBC	red blood cell
RJB	Robert Jones bandage
RR	respiratory rate
RV	rabies vaccine
RVT	Registered Veterinary Technician
SID	once a day
SQ	subcutaneously
SDFT	superficial digital flexor tendon
SDH	sorbitol dehydrogenase
SL	suspensory ligament
SMZ	sulfamethazine
sx	surgery
TAT	tetanus antitoxin
TID	three times a day
TDL	therapeutic drug level

Acronym/ Abbreviation	Description
TL	tracheal lavage
TMS	trimethoprim sulfa
TMT	tarsometatarsal joint
TP	total protein
TPN	total parenteral nutrition
TPR	temperature, pulse, respiration
TS	tendon sheath
TSH	thyroid stimulating hormone
TT	tetanus toxoid
VMD	veterinary medical doctor
VEE	Venezuelan equine encephalomyelitis
VS	vesicular stomatitis
WB	western blot (test)
WBC	white blood cell
WEE	western equine encephalomyelitis
WNL	within normal limits

AAEVT's Equine Manual for Veterinary Technicians

CHAPTER 1

General Horse Management

Dana Zimmel

Facilities

Stable Management

The design of an equine facility should consider positioning of the stables to maximize the health of the horse and to provide easy access in case of an emergency. Stables should be designed to enhance ventilation to minimize respiratory disease. The average stall size is 12′ × 12′. Foaling stalls and stallion stalls are even larger. The floor of all stalls should be designed to drain effectively. Each stall should be equipped with two water buckets and a feed bucket. The water buckets should be washed daily and refilled frequently. Some farms with a large numbers of horses will choose to use automatic watering systems in which the horse will drink out of a small bowl of water that will continuously refill. Although this system is convenient, it does not allow monitoring of the horse's water consumption. The use of hay racks is controversial because they create an abnormal eating posture for the horse, increasing the amount of dust it will inhale when chewing hay. However, if a horse has a painful neck and cannot bend to eat off the floor, a hay rack or hay net is a good option.

Grain should always be stored in a secured room to prevent any loose horses from eating large quantities of it because grain overload can result in severe endotoxemia and death. Grain transported in wheel barrows should be secured in a safe place for the same reason. The grain should be stored in airtight containers to minimize rodent contamina-

tion. In warm climates, the grain should be stored in air-conditioned spaces to prevent the formation of mold. Consumption of moldy corn can result in a severe neurologic condition called *leukoencephalomalacia*, which is often fatal.

Hay should be stored in a separate building rather than the stable. Studies have shown that stabling horses in close proximity to hay increases respiratory disease, and it is also a fire hazard. Hay should be stored in an area where it can be stacked off the floor on palettes, kept dry from blowing rain, and have minimal sun exposure. To eliminate the chance of spontaneous combustion, hay must be properly cured before placing it the barn. It is advisable to store tractors and other gasoline-powered equipment in a separate area to decrease the risk of fire.

Bedding should be stored in a separate facility to minimize dust and reduce the risk of fire. Common types of bedding are wood shavings, straw, and occasionally shredded paper. Wood shavings from Black Walnut trees should never be used because they can cause severe laminitis. Shredded paper has the least amount of dust and is preferred for horses with respiratory disease. Stalls are cleaned on a daily basis and the removal of all urine and feces are common practice. Accumulation of ammonia from poor sanitation is detrimental to the respiratory tract. Many stall products have been developed to absorb ammonia in excessively wet areas within the stall. Removal of manure waste should be considered in the design plans of any facility. The manure can be composted or taken off site to a disposal area. Good hygiene is essential to minimize

3

the spread of diseases, control flies, and prevent the spread of intestinal parasites.

Equine Hospitals

Equine hospitals should be designed with all the basic principles previously stated plus consideration for the type of patients that it will house. For example, when treating critical care neonates, it is helpful to have a divided stall in an environment that is climate controlled. This type of stall will allow the mare to stay with her sick foal but provide adequate space for nursing care. There should also be plenty of lighting and electrical outlets and a ready supply of oxygen. Stalls that have fully padded walls and a hoist are helpful when caring for recumbent horses. Most facilities will use a 2-ton hoist for lifting neurologic horses.

The stall floor and walls should be composed of a surface that can be appropriately disinfected between patients. Concrete walls and rubber floors are typically used in large animal hospital settings. Each stall should be fitted with a fluid hanger that can be used to hold at least 10 to 20 L of fluid at a time (Figure 1.1).

Each hospital should have an area that is appropriate for working up cases. Stocks are ideal for managing critical patients. The stocks keep the horse stationary while multiple staff members attend to the horse at the same time. Rectal examinations and diagnostic procedures are easy to accomplish in stocks. The floor should be non-slip and easy to disinfect. The workup area should be in a quite area away from mainstream traffic yet convenient to supplies and diagnostic equipment (Figure 1.2).

Isolation Facilities

To minimize the risk of spreading contagious diseases, every hospital and farm should have an isolation area and a corresponding protocol (Figure 1.3). The common contagious diseases are listed in Table 1.1. Contagious diseases can be spread between horses through contact with feces, aerosolization, or indirect contact with fomites such as water buckets, manure forks, and contaminated tack or brushes. It is important to be able to distinguish between con-

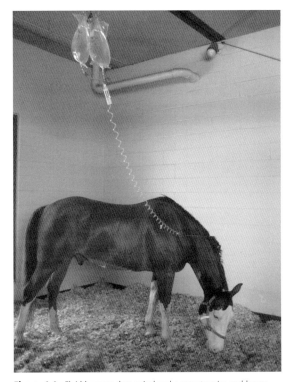

Figure 1.1. Fluid hangers that swivel and a rope to raise and lower them as needed should be placed in the center of the stall. Courtesy Dr. Dana Zimmel.

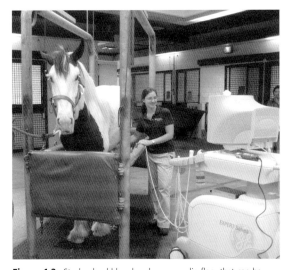

Figure 1.2. Stocks should be placed on a nonslip floor that can be disinfected. Notice the sides of the stocks can be raised or lowered or completely removed as needed to perform procedures. Courtesy Dr. Dana Zimmel.

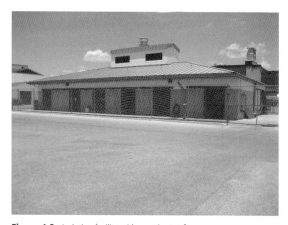

Figure 1.3. Isolation facility with a perimeter fence. Courtesy Dr. Dana Zimmel.

Table 1.1. Common contagious diseases.

Gastrointestinal	Salmonellosis
	Rotavirus
	Cryptosporidia
Respiratory	Strangles *(Streptococcus equi equi)*
	Equine influenza
	Equine herpesvirus (EHV-1 and EHV-4)
	Equine viral arteritis
Neurologic	Equine herpesvirus (EHV-1)
Reproduction/Abortion	Equine herpesvirus
	Equine viral arteritis
	Leptospirosis
	Contagious equine metritis (CEM)
Dermatologic	Dermatophytosis (ringworm)
	Dermatophilus
Blood	Equine infectious anemia (EIA)

had exploratory abdominal surgery. The criteria for housing horses in the isolation unit may vary between hospitals but usually includes the combination of fever, diarrhea, and a low white blood cell count. Fecal cultures for Salmonella are used to confirm a positive case. Because the organism is intermittently shed, five fecal samples collected 12 to 24 hours apart are required to rule out the disease.

The protocol for isolating horses that may have contracted the neurologic form of EHV is more challenging. This form of herpes can be spread through nasal secretions. If horses are coming from a location where a horse has tested positive for EHV, the horse in question should be isolated until testing is complete. Nasal swabs and blood samples are used to test for the presence of the virus. Likewise, if any horse has developed sudden onset of fever and neurologic signs, it is best to place the horse in isolation if its clinical signs are consistent with EHV. Common neurologic signs for EHV include ataxia, poor tail tone, poor anal tone, and urinary incontinence.

Isolation stalls should be self-contained with water and electricity and connected to an anteroom that serves as a boundary area for supplies and equipment. The stalls should be composed of a nonporous surface that is easy to clean. Typical isolation protocol requires the use of plastic booties, barrier clothing, and gloves (Figure 1.4). All materials are discarded after each use. Foot baths should be strategically placed to dip feet at least twice between the contaminated area and the clean area. Special red garbage bags are used to signify contagious waste. Manure and stall waste should be disposed according to state regulations. Each stall should have its own veterinary equipment, brushes, buckets, and stall cleaning equipment.

The stall and all of the equipment is disinfected between patients. All organic debris must be removed first, and then the surface may be scrubbed with the appropriate disinfectant. Chlorine compounds (bleach) can be used by adding three-quarters cup of bleach to 1 gallon of water. Bleach is inactivated in the presence of organic debris, so it is imperative that all the surfaces be cleaned first. Phenolic compounds are used in a hospital setting

tagious diseases and infectious diseases. A contagious disease is spread between horses, and an infectious disease is caused by a specific agent such as a bacteria, virus, or parasite.

In hospitalized settings, an isolation facility is required when dealing with horses that may have the neurologic form of equine herpesvirus (EHV) or *Salmonella*. These two contagious diseases can cause life-threatening illness and can be spread to other patients within the hospital.

Horses at risk of developing Salmonella infections are horses with colic, diarrhea, or who have

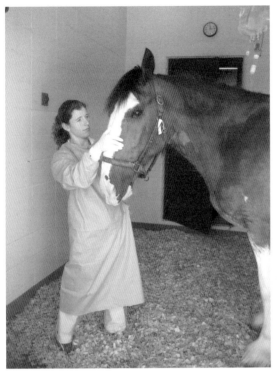

Figure 1.4. Horses in isolation should be handled with gloves, barrier clothing, and plastic foot covers.
Courtesy Dr. Dana Zimmel.

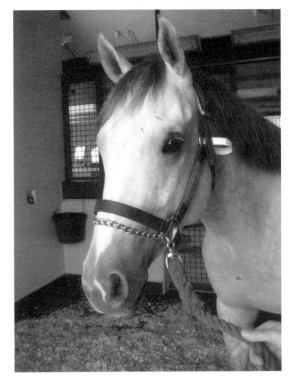

Figure 1.5. Figure A lead shank with a nose chain is used to control excitable horses.
Courtesy Dr. Dana Zimmel.

because they are effective against both rotavirus and Salmonella organisms. Iodophors and alcohol are commonly used for handwashing.

Restraint of Horses

Horses are trained to be handled from the left side. A halter and lead rope should always be used when working with a horse. The lead rope should never be wrapped around the hand or arm of the handler. Some horses may resist to being tied and will panic. For this reason, horses should not be tied unless the handler is sure the horse has received appropriate training. A horse should always be tied with a cotton lead rope with no chain attached and a quick release knot in case the horse needs to be released suddenly. For veterinary procedures, it is best to hold the horse rather than tie them to a wall or post.

The most common methods of restraint include a lead shank with a nose chain, lip chain, and nose twitch. The lead shank with a nose chain is an appropriate method to lead horses that are fractious (Figure 1.5). A lip chain is a method of significant restraint and is commonly used to control young racehorse or stallions. The chain portion of the lead shank is placed under the upper lip of the horse. Constant steady pressure is applied, and the handler should never jerk the rope suddenly (Figure 1.6).

A nose twitch is a good method of restraint for veterinary procedures because it will immobilize the horse. There are three types of twitches: one made of metal called a humane twitch and two with a wooden handle that has either a chain or rope loop at the end. The humane twitch is useful for weanlings because it is small and the pressure is fairly mild. The wooden handle of a rope or chain twitch is approximately 45 to 50 cm long. The small rope loop is placed around the upper lip, and the handle is twisted until the rope is tight (Figure 1.7). The handler should hold the twitch firmly and use

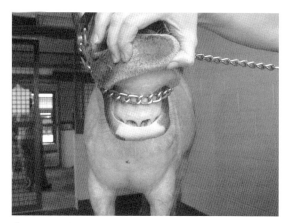

Figure 1.6. A lead shank with chain applied under the upper lip is a method of restraint used commonly in the breeding shed or to perform veterinary procedures on excitable horses.
Courtesy Dr. Dana Zimmel.

Table 1.2. Benefits of a national equine identification plan.

- The plan may reduce the potential effects and enhance control of equine disease outbreaks by identifying the contagious animals and isolating them quickly.
- Maintain freedom of transport in cases of disease outbreaks, such as of vesicular stomatitis, equine herpesvirus, or strangles.
- Assist horse shows, rodeos, and races in securing a healthy environment for participating athletes.
- Aid in recovery of horses when lost as a result of natural disasters, theft, or accidents. The identification system may be able to link the horse to a premise.
- Improve import and export of horses into the United States each year by providing a standard method of identification.
- Uphold the equine industry as a responsible member of the livestock community and counter bioterrorism.

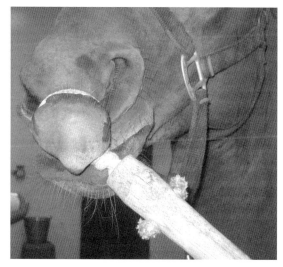

Figure 1.7. The rope twitch is common method of restraint for passing a nasogastric tube or doing a rectal examination.
Courtesy Dr. Dana Zimmel.

the lead rope to stabilize the head. The handler should be positioned on the side of the horse by the shoulder and should never stand in front of the horse. A nose twitch is used commonly to restrain the horse to pass a nasogastric tube, perform a rectal examination, or suture a wound. A twitch may be applied for short procedures and is often combined with chemical restraint. A skin twitch is another method of restraint that requires the handler

to grab a fold of skin along the neck and roll it until snug. This technique is appropriate to keep a horse still when administering an injection.

Methods of Identification

There are a variety of methods used to identify horses. In the United States, all horses must have a negative Coggins test, which tests for equine infectious anemia (EIA). The Coggins test form includes a hand-drawn picture depicting the white marks on the head, legs, and body. This form is often used as a legal document of identification for the owner. In some states the Coggins test results are printed on a laminated card with the horse's photo in color similar to a driver's license photo.

In the Thoroughbred industry, horses are identified by a tattoo placed on their upper lip. Freeze brands are common under the mane or hindquarters. The brand may be the registration number or signify the horse's breed.

The implantation of a microchip is easy and practical method for identification. A small chip encapsulated in biocompatible glass vial (about the size of a grain of rice) is inserted into the ligament of the neck 1 inch below the crest on the left side. A 12-gauge needle is used to implant the device. The device is inexpensive ranging from $25 to $100 to implant. The American Horse Council has identified several potential benefits of using microchips as part of a national identification plan (Table 1.2).

Hoof Care

Daily foot care is important in maintaining a healthy hoof. The feet should be cleaned each day with a hoof pick and stiff brush. The foot should be inspected for the presence of gravel along the hoof wall if the horse is barefoot. Mud and debris should be removed to keep the foot dry. If the horse is shod, the shoe should be inspected for fit and tightness. If the shoe becomes loose, the horse may lose it during exercise and damage the hoof wall. As the hoof grows, the shoe may shift and fail to provide the proper support resulting in lameness.

The hoof will grow 0.6 inches per month in a foal, 0.5 inches per month in a yearling, and 0.25 to 0.35 inches per month in an adult. The toe grows faster than heel. The feet should be trimmed every 6 to 9 weeks. If the horse is shod, the shoes will need to be reset every 6 weeks.

Shoes are used for a variety of reasons such as to protect the feet when the horse is worked on hard surfaces or to correct defects in hoof structure and growth. Shoes can assist in correcting the gait and can aid in gripping slick ground.

To remove a shoe, the clenches must be raised and each nail individually removed with a nail puller. This is an important skill for the veterinary technician to be comfortable performing. Removing shoes are necessary to evaluate the hoof, take radiographs of the feet, or to place a horse in the magnetic resonance imaging (MRI) unit (Table 1.3).

The hooves should be monitored for excessive moisture or extreme dryness. Excessive moisture from standing in mud or wet bedding can result in thrush. The loss of moisture, standing in urine and feces, and some astringent hoof dressings damage the protective layer of the hoof and may reduce the quality of the horn, thereby predisposing it to cracks.

Transportation of Horses

Health Concerns for Long Distance Travel

Many horses travel long distances via road, train, or air without complications. In human athletes, traveling can directly impact performance. Horses that travel long distances may encounter impaired respiratory health, fatigue, and stress resulting in decreased performance. A small percentage of horses will become severely ill developing shipping fever and subsequent pneumonia.

Studies have confirmed that mucociliary clearance is decreased when horses maintain an elevated head and neck position for as little as 6 hours. This is a common position for horses cross-tied during transport. The decrease in mucociliary clearance results in increased mucus, bacteria, and neutrophils in the trachea, predisposing the horse to pneumonia. Shipping horses in a box stall, which allows them to put their head and neck down, is a better option to reduce respiratory stress. After arrival at the final destination, the horse should have its temperature monitored every 12 hours for the next 2 days to detect early signs of respiratory infection.

Another problem that occurs when shipping horses long distances is mild colic. Horses are reluctant to drink on the road and become dehydrated. It is best to stop and offer water every few hours to encourage drinking. Minimizing clothing on the horse during travel is better than allowing them to overheat with a blanket. This can help to reduce their chances of becoming dehydrated (Table 1.4).

Table 1.3. Farrier tools.

- Hoof testers
- Nail pullers
- Hoof knife (right or left handed)
- Shoe pullers
- Rasp
- Nippers

Table 1.4. Guidelines for long distance transport of horses.

- Take the temperature before and after transport to detect pyrexia.
- Offer water during the entire trip.
- Minimize clothing on the horse during travel.
- Plan for a recovery period after long transport. At least one overnight rest per 8 hours of road travel or one day of rest for every 2 hours of flying.

Shipping Sick or Injured Horses

- Horses that have severe colic should not be tied in the trailer during transport. If possible, they should be shipped in a box stall to have room to move around as needed.
- Sick neonatal foals should be separated from the mare with a divider if possible. If they are hypothermic, they should be placed in the cab of the vehicle or be covered in warm blankets.
- Neurologic horses do better if they are shipped in a confined space that supports them on all sides. However, if they are weak, they may not be able to remain upright during travel. It is important that they are shipped in a van that has removable paneling in case they fall during transportation. A ramp will help load and unload weak and ataxic horses. One person should be on the head and one person should take the tail to help stabilize the horse during loading.
- Horses with a distal limb fracture should be shipped similarly to neurologic horses. A snug fit may help them balance during the ride. The trailer should be equipped with removable panels that allow the horse to turn around in the trailer to exit.

Loading Ramps

If horses have not been well trained, loading them can be easy or challenging. Horses that are neurologic or have head injuries can be dangerous to load. Experienced horsemen should be in charge of this when possible. Often the veterinarian will be asked to sedate the horse to decrease the risk of the horse hurting itself.

Commercial vans will require the use of a loading ramp (Figure 1.8). Construction of a loading shoot should be considered for all hospitals to facilitate the safe loading of horses (Figure 1.9). The shoot keeps the horse from running backward and does not allow space for the horse to escape along the side of the trailer. The only option for the horse is to move forward onto the trailer. To minimize slipping and injury, it is best to load and unload horses in a dirt area, not a concrete area. The area where

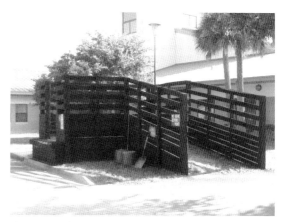

Figure 1.8. A loading ramp should have tall sides and good footing. Courtesy Dr. Dana Zimmel.

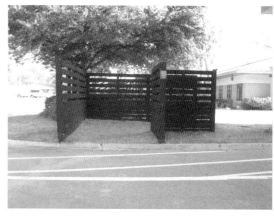

Figure 1.9. A loading shoot will help load difficult horses. Courtesy Dr. Dana Zimmel.

the horse is to be loaded should be completely fenced so if the horse becomes loose it does not get out on the road.

References and Further Reading

McCurnin, D., and J. Bassert. 2006. *Clinical Textbook for Veterinary Technicians.* 6th ed. St. Louis: Elsevier.

Marlin, D. J. 2004. Transport of horses. In *Equine Sports Medicine and Surgery,* ed. K. Hinchcliff, A. Kaneps, and R. Goer. St. Louis: Elsevier.

Equine Nutrition

Mary Beth Gordon, J. K. Young, K. E. Davison, and R. H. Raub

Introduction

Feeding horses to achieve optimal performance, whether that performance is work, growth, breeding, or simply living a healthy life, requires providing essential nutrients in optimal amounts and balance. Further, feeding management is a crucial factor in maintaining healthy horses. Horses are considered nonruminant herbivores, which means they are designed to eat plants (primarily grasses). In their natural state, horses spend most of their time grazing, moving freely over large distances, providing the digestive tract with a variety of forages in small amounts throughout the day. However, horses today are often kept in confinement with limited access to pasture and fed two or three meals per day. To maintain a healthy, contented horse under these conditions involves a complete understanding of the horse's distinctive digestive system, its nutrient requirements, and proper feeding management.

General Digestive Physiology and Architecture of the Gut

The digestive system of the horse is quite unique when compared to other livestock species. Horses are monogastric, which means that they have simple stomachs, unlike ruminants, which have several compartments to the stomach. However, there is a difference in the horse's digestive system when compared to other monogastric animals, such as humans and pigs, because the horse has a functional cecum. The cecum is a large sac located at the junction between the small and large intestines that is the site of a large amount of microbial digestion, similar to the rumen in cattle. Therefore, the horse is a nonruminant herbivore (an animal that eats plants but does not have a rumen).

The digestive tract of the horse includes the mouth, esophagus, stomach, small intestine, large intestine (cecum and colon), rectum, and anus. Obviously, the mouth is important for ingestion of feed. Efficient digestion starts when the food is taken in and chewed. If a horse does not receive proper dental care, the horse may not be able to chew properly, and digestion may be impaired. This could result in weight loss, a decrease in condition, and poor performance. Further, because chewing stimulates secretion of saliva, if a horse does not chew adequately, the ingesta passing through the tract may be too dry, possibly causing impactions.

The esophagus is a muscular tube extending from the mouth to the stomach. The saliva produced in the mouth lubricates the feed and helps prevent the feed from getting lodged. The muscles at the end of the esophagus are firm and strong, and the tube meets the stomach at a sharp angle, making it nearly impossible for the horse to belch or vomit. If a horse has colic, the stomach could rupture before the horse vomits. Also, because the horse cannot belch, the horse is unable to relieve gas pressure in some types of colic. From a management standpoint, it is quite important to understand that the horse does not appear to have a strongly functioning satiety center (i.e., alerts them when they have eaten enough and are full). Therefore, it is critical that a horse's intake be monitored closely and that the horse is offered small amounts of feed rather than be fed ad libitum.

The horse has a relatively small stomach when compared to the overall capacity of the gastrointestinal tract. The stomach holds only 7.5 to 15 L (2 to 4 gallons) of feedstuffs and is only about 8% of the total capacity of the digestive tract. The rate of passage of ingested feed through the stomach is rapid; usually less than 2 hours. Breakdown of several nutrients begins in the stomach, but there is little bacterial fermentation or nutrient absorption in the stomach.

The next segment of the gastrointestinal tract is the small intestine. The small intestine is about 21 m (70 ft) long and holds about 45 L (12 gallons). The rate of passage of ingested feed through the small intestine is fairly rapid, from 45 minutes to 8 hours. Many digestive enzymes are produced by the pancreas and released into the small intestine, and

more digestive enzymes are produced by the small intestine itself. In the small intestine, proteins are digested into amino acids, which are then absorbed into the bloodstream; fats are digested into fatty acids, and soluble carbohydrates are broken down into glucose and other simple sugars, which are absorbed into the bloodstream. There are no enzymes to break down fibrous carbohydrates, so those flow undigested into the hindgut. Digestion and absorption of some of the minerals and many of the vitamins takes place in the small intestine.

The large intestine includes the cecum and the colon. The large intestine comprises about 60% of the capacity of the digestive tract. The cecum alone can hold several liters (gallons) of digesta, and the rate of passage through the large intestine is slow, usually 50 to 60 hours.

The cecum is located at the junction of the small intestine and large intestine. Material not digested in the foregut passes into the cecum. The cecum is a large fermentation vat similar to the rumen in cattle and sheep. It houses billions of bacteria and protozoa, which digest fiber, cellulose, and the remainder of the soluble carbohydrates that were

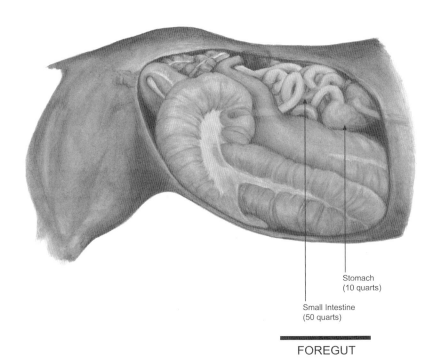

Stomach
(10 quarts)

Small Intestine
(50 quarts)

FOREGUT

Figure 2.1. Feedstuffs pass relatively rapidly through the stomach and small intestine of the horse, which is designed to handle small, frequent intake of feed.

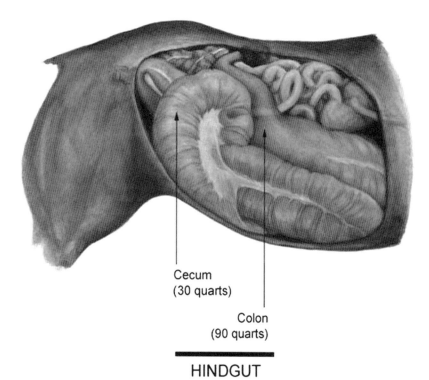

Cecum
(30 quarts)

Colon
(90 quarts)

HINDGUT

Figure 2.2. Fermentation of feedstuffs in the hindgut takes a longer period of time and is designed to digest and absorb fibrous portions of the equine diet.

not broken down and absorbed in the stomach and small intestine. Additionally, microbes in the cecum and colon synthesize B vitamins, which are then available to the horse to help meet requirements for those vitamins. Further, the microbes are able to metabolize nitrogen and produce protein, but little or no absorption of amino acids occurs in the large intestine. The digestive tract ends at the rectum and anus.

It is important to understand the horse's digestive system when feeding. The rate of passage of feedstuffs is fast through the foregut (stomach and small intestine) and slow through the hindgut (large intestine). This can be a problem because the majority of nutrient absorption occurs in the foregut. The horse's gastrointestinal tract was designed for, and is conducive to, grazing, where small amounts of forage pass through the gut almost continuously, and digestion is fairly efficient. However, because of convenience, most horse owners feed their horses in one or two meals per day. This means that large

amounts of food pass through the gastrointestinal tract at once. This can cause less efficient digestion and absorption and can predispose horses to colic.

Nutrient Requirements

Water

Water is necessary for almost every body process and is a major component of all fluids in the body. Water helps deliver nutrients to cells (as a component of blood), aids in digestion of feed and elimination of wastes, and plays a role in the regulation of body temperature via sweating.

Horses must have a source of fresh, clean drinking water at all times. Horses drink 37.85 to 45.42 L (10 to 12 gallons) of water per day during normal environmental conditions. During hot weather or when exercising intensely, horses may require up to twice that amount as a result of fluids lost through sweating and respiration. Pregnant mares require

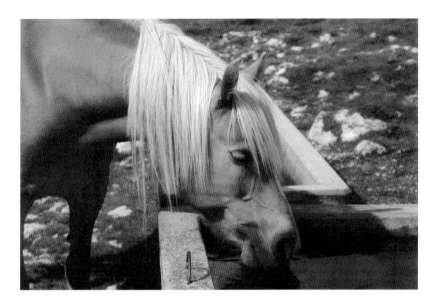

Figure 2.3. Horses need fresh, clean water at all times to help meet their intake requirements of 37 to 46 L per day.

more water (about 10%) than do nonpregnant mares, and lactating mares require 50% to 75% more water to replace that which is secreted in milk. Further, horses consuming dry feed drink more water.

Depriving a horse of water will decrease its feed intake. After 3 or 4 days, the horse will eat little if any feed. The reduction of feed intake is accompanied by rapid weight loss, primarily as a result of dehydration. This weight can be replaced in 3 to 4 days when water is again available to the horse. Horses should have free choice access to fresh, clean water at all times.

Energy

Energy is also an important nutrient requirement for a horse. Energy is the nutrient that allows the horse to maintain the most optimal body condition for performance, reproduction, or growth. Of the feed horses eat, 80% to 90% converts to energy. In the diet, digestible energy (DE) is measured in "megacalories" (Mcal) or "kilocalories" (Kcal).

The body condition scoring system is an effective way to monitor the horse's energy status. The level of condition that a horse possesses is determined by visual inspection and by the amount of palpable fat in the areas of the neck, along the withers, down the back, around the tail head, over the ribs, and behind the shoulder. Body condition scores range from 1 to 9, with 1 being extremely emaciated and 9 being extremely fat. The ideal body condition score is between 5 and 6.5, depending on the lifestyle of the horse. A description of the condition score system is given in Figure 2.4.

Dietary energy intake is the major nutrient that determines fatness in horses, as well as in other species. DE requirements are determined by the type of work or status of a horse. Energy balance is extremely important in the maintenance of a moderate level of body condition or a condition score of 5 (up to 6.5 in broodmares). Positive energy balance, when intake exceeds the DE requirements, results in deposition of fat in the previously mentioned areas on the horse. Zero energy balance, when intake equals DE requirements, results in maintenance of body weight and body condition. Negative energy balance, when requirements for DE exceed intake, results in mobilization of fat reserves in the body for use as a source of energy. Hence, the horse loses weight and becomes thinner because of the compromised DE intake.

Energy is possibly the most difficult requirement to meet in the performance horse. It is a challenge

Body Condition Scoring

Many physiological functions in horses are influenced by body condition, including horse's maintenance, reproductive and exercising requirements. A system called body condition scoring can be used to rate ideal body condition. This condition scoring system is based on visual appraisal and palpable fat cover on six areas of your horse's body.

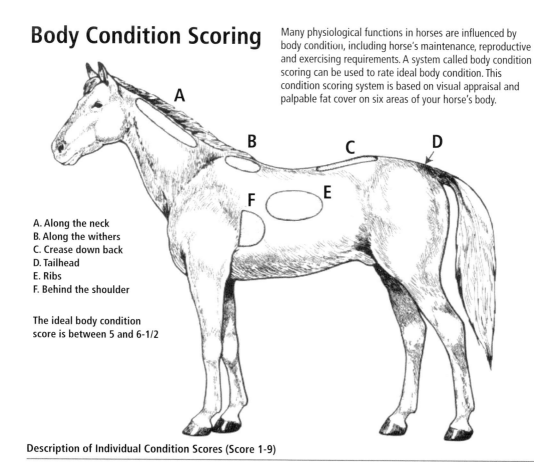

A. Along the neck
B. Along the withers
C. Crease down back
D. Tailhead
E. Ribs
F. Behind the shoulder

The ideal body condition
score is between 5 and 6-1/2

Description of Individual Condition Scores (Score 1-9)

1. Poor: Animal extremely emaciated; spinous processes, ribs, tailhead tuber coxae (hip joints), and ischia (lower pelvic bones) projecting prominently; bone structure of withers, shoulders and neck easily noticeable; no fatty tissue can be felt.

2.Very Thin: Animal emaciated; slight fat covering over base of spinous processes; transverse processes of lumbar vertebrae feel rounded; spinous processes, ribs, tailhead, tuber coxae (hip joints) and ischia (lower pelvic bones) prominent; withers, shoulders and neck structure faintly discernible.

3. Thin: Fat buildup about halfway on spinous processes; transverse processes cannot be felt; slight fat cover over ribs; spinous processes and ribs easily discernible; tailhead prominent, but individual vertebrae cannot be identified visually; tuber coxae (hip joints) appear rounded but easily discemible; tuber ischia (lower pelvic bones) not distinguishable; withers, shoulders and neck accentuated.

4. Moderately Thin: Slight ridge along back; faint outline of ribs discernible; tailhead prominence depends on conformation, fat can be felt around it; tuber coxae (hips joints) not discernible; withers, shoulders, and neck not obviously thin.

5 Moderate: Back is flat (no crease or ridge); ribs not visually distinguishable but easily felt; fat around tailhead beginning to feel spongy; wihters appear rounded over spinous processes; shoulders and neck blend smoothly into body.

6. Moderately Fleshy: May have slight crease down back; fat over ribs spongy; fat around tailhead soft; fat beginning to be deposited along the side of withers, behind shoulders, and along sides of neck.

7. Fleshy: May have crease down back; individual ribs can be felt, but noticeable filling between ribs with fat; fat around tailhead soft; fat deposited along withers, behind shoulders, and along neck.

8. Fat: Crease down back; difficult to feel ribs; fat around tailhead very soft; area along withers filled with fat; area behind shoulder filled with fat; noticeable thickening of neck; fat deposited along inner things.

9. Extremely Fat: Obvious crease down back; patchy fat appearing over ribs; bulging fat around tailhead, along withers, behind shoulders, and along neck; fat along inner things may rub together; flank filled with fat.

Figure 2.4. Body condition scoring.

for the horse owner to feed the proper amount of energy to acquire and maintain ideal body condition for the specific type of performance while providing enough fuel to support performance at the desired level of work. The diet must provide enough energy for the horse to maintain optimal body condition while performing at a light, medium, or heavy workload.

Energy may be supplied by carbohydrates, proteins, and fats. Carbohydrates include nonstructural carbohydrates (starches and sugars) from feed grain and structural carbohydrates (cellulose and hemicellulose) from forages and are readily used as a source of energy by horses. Protein is not an efficient source of energy for a horse. Therefore, adding protein to an already adequate diet will not benefit a performance horse. Fat is a dense source of calories for horses and is a useful way to increase energy in the diet without incurring many of the digestive disturbances that can occur with a diet that is high in nonstructural carbohydrates.

Carbohydrates and Starches

Many times, the terms *starch* and *carbohydrate* are used interchangeably. All starches are carbohydrates but not all carbohydrates are starches. Carbohydrates include sugars, starches, and fibers, all of which are found in plants, including grains, pasture, and hay. The term *carbohydrate* arises from the fact that most substances in this class have empirical formulas suggesting they are carbon "hydrates," with the ratio of carbon to hydrogen to oxygen being $1:2:1$. For example, the empirical formula of D-glucose, the precursor to all carbohydrates, is $C_6H_{12}O_6$. There are three major classes of carbohydrates: monosaccharides, or simple sugars; oligosaccharides, which are short chains of monosaccharides joined together by covalent bonds and are considered sugars as well; and polysaccharides, which consist of long chains having hundreds or thousands of monosaccharide units and are considered non-sugars. The most abundant polysaccharides, starch and cellulose, consist of recurring units of D-glucose, but differ in how the D-glucose units are linked together. In starch, the monosaccharides are linked together by α-linkages, which are subject to mammalian enzymatic digestion. Cellulose, on the other hand, contains monosaccharides linked together by β-linkages and can only be broken by cellulase, a microbial enzyme. Often, in the horse's diet, sugar and starch are referred to as soluble or hydrolysable carbohydrates and cellulose as insoluble or fermentable carbohydrate. This is in reference to whether the carbohydrate is hydrolyzed or digested in the small intestine, as with starch, or fermented in the hindgut, as with cellulose.

Dietary carbohydrates include those carbohydrates found as components of the cell walls of plants, or structural carbohydrates, and those found within the cell contents, or nonstructural carbohydrates (NSC). Sugars and starches (hydrolyzable carbohydrates) fall into the NSC category, whereas dietary fibers are considered structural carbohydrates.

Simple sugars are usually only a minimal presence in horse's diet, even when the horse is eating a sweet feed with molasses. In plants, simple sugars are used as fuel for growth or respiration; when excess sugars accumulate, they are stored as polysaccharides. In the horse, simple sugars are primarily digested and absorbed in the small intestine.

Starches are found primarily in grains and in the immature leafy portions of plants. During digestion, starches are broken down into the simple sugar building blocks (primarily glucose), which are then absorbed primarily in the small intestine. Glucose may then be used as fuel immediately, stored as glycogen by the horse, which is usually the major fuel source for aerobic and anaerobic activity, or stored as fat, which is also a fuel source for aerobic activity. Glucose is important for the horse to function properly because it is the only fuel that can be used by the brain; it is used to a large extent by the hooves; and it is the only substance that can be used for making glycogen. Studies have shown that horses that deplete their glycogen stores and are not provided dietary substrate to replenish the glycogen show reduced performance capabilities (Topliff, et al. 1983, 1985). So, glucose is vital to the health and well-being of the horse. Again, glucose comes primarily from NSC.

NSC that passes through the small intestine undigested will be fermented in the hindgut. If starch intake exceeds 0.2 to 0.4% of the horse's body weight per feeding, the amount of starch digestion in the horse's hindgut may increase considerably (Potter, et al. 1992; Radicke, et al. 1991). Starches that are fermented in the hindgut will not be broken down into glucose molecules but instead will result in volatile fatty acids (VFAs), which will then be absorbed. If a sudden increase in NSC to the hindgut occurs, it can result in a drop in cecal pH, causing a disruptive shift in microbial population. This situation may cause colic or laminitis in a horse.

Fibers are also formed by the linkages of simple sugars (again primarily glucose), but because the β-linkages can only be broken by microbial cellulase, fibers pass undigested through the upper gut and are subject to microbial fermentation in the horse's hindgut. Digestible fibers (including hemicellulose and cellulose) are fermented by the microbes into VFAs, which are then absorbed. These VFAs are also a source of energy for aerobic activity. Some fibers (lignin) are indigestible in the horse's digestive system and pass on through, providing bulk in the diet.

Concentrates and forages consumed by horses contain primarily starch and fiber (cellulose, hemicellulose, and lignin). Common feedstuffs eaten by horses contain only low levels of simple sugars. The best recognized source of dietary sugar for the horse is molasses. However, the most important source of dietary sugar for the horse is pasture grasses; and in comparison, molasses in feeds is a minor source.

Interestingly, legumes have lower soluble carbohydrate content than most pasture grasses. Drying the forage, as in making hay, especially conditioning or crimping the plant, reduces the soluble carbohydrate content as well (McDonald, et al. 1995). Fructans can be a large constituent of soluble carbohydrate in some grasses, depending on grass variety, time of year, and ambient temperature. There is no enzyme in the small intestine of the horse that is able to break down fructans to monosaccharides for absorption. Therefore, fructans from grasses will pass into the cecum where they are rapidly fermented, causing a drop in cecal pH similar to that from excess NSC in the hindgut.

Fats

Fats are included in the family of chemicals called *lipids*. Other lipids in the diet, which are not considered simple fats, include fat-soluble vitamins

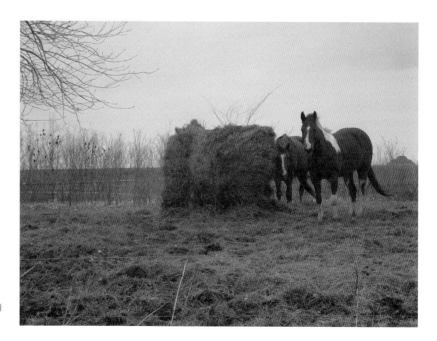

Figure 2.5. Adequate roughage (such as that found in hay) is essential to maintain the horses hindgut.

(A, D, E, and K), phospholipids, and cholesterol. Simple fats are usually present in the form of triglycerides, three fatty acids attached to a glycerol backbone, and are the major fuels for most organisms. Fatty acids vary in length, ranging from 4 to 24 carbons, usually containing an even number of carbons and are classified as saturated, containing no double bonds, or unsaturated, which contain double bonds. Fats are insoluble in water but soluble in organic solvents. In the small intestine, bile salts assist in breaking fat globules into smaller sizes and then pancreatic lipase hydrolyses the triglyceride molecules, successively splitting off one fatty acid at a time. Ultimately, this yields three free fatty acids and the glycerol backbone. These products are absorbed into the intestinal mucosa, where triglycerides are resynthesized. The resynthesized triglycerides, along with other lipids and some free fatty acids, are combined with protein to form chylomicrons. Chylomicrons leave the mucosal cells, enter the lymph system, and finally enter circulation. Chylomicrons are essentially cleared from circulation and taken up by the liver or adipose tissue within 2 to 3 hours following a meal.

The use of fats and oils in equine diets was delayed for a time because it was assumed that the horse would have limited ability to digest and use fats because of the absence of a gall bladder. However, the fact that mare's milk is around 15% fat on a dry matter basis was an indication that at least foals could digest and use fat. It has since been recognized that, instead of a gall bladder to store and release bile, the horse continuously secretes bile and is therefore capable of efficiently digesting fats in the small intestine. In the last 20 years, there has been much research investigating the palatability, digestibility, and use of dietary fats by the equine. Because fats and oils supply 2.25 times the energy as an equal amount of starch, the initial goal of this research was to use added dietary fats or oils to increase the energy density in rations for horses with high energy requirements. The idea was to be able to meet the energy demands with a smaller amount of grain required in the diet. Benefits in addition to the simple caloric value have since been shown.

Fat or oil can be added to a grain mix at up to 10% of the concentrate without impairing digestibility of the feed. Research has found that fat-supplemented diets increase fat percentage of mares' milk during early lactation and cause the fat content to remain higher as lactation advances (Davison, et al. 1991). Further, researchers have found that adding fat to the diets of racing or cutting horses may improve muscle glycogen storage and work performance (Webb, et al. 1987). Research has also shown that increased stamina and delayed onset of fatigue can result from adding fat to the rations (Oldham, et al. 1990).

When feeding fat-supplemented diets to horses, several factors must be considered. First, the horse needs at least 3 to 5 weeks to adapt to fat use (National Research Council [NRC] 2007). Second, a fat-supplemented diet provides more energy, so total daily feed intake must decrease if work level and body condition are to remain constant. Horse owners who plan to top-dress fat or oil on the feed should start with a small amount of added fat and gradually increase the amount, while keeping track of the horse's eating behavior and general well-being. Finally, supplementation of fats or oils requires reevaluation of the total dietary nutrient balance.

Essential fatty acid requirements have not yet been fully established for the horse, although the National Research Council (NRC; 2007) recommends a dietary minimum for linoleic acid of 0.5% of dry matter in the diet. It is thought that linoleic, linolenic, and arachidonic acids may be dietary essential fatty acids, although a fatty acid deficiency in the horse has not been reported in the literature. Further research is needed to determine the upper limit to fat digestion in the small intestine of the horse and to quantify the essential fatty acid needs of the horse.

Protein and Amino Acids

Protein is a necessary nutrient for growth and repair of body tissues. Proteins are composed of amino acids, and when dietary proteins are digested, they are broken down into their constituent amino acids. These amino acids are then recombined in various ways to provide specific proteins for muscle, blood, skin, and other tissues. Some amino acids can be synthesized by the horse, but some must be supplied in the diet and are considered essential amino acids. The dietary protein requirement of a horse is a function not only of the needs of that animal but also the quality of protein available (the amino acid profile) and the digestibility of that protein.

Evaluating rations for horses is commonly centered on percent protein, primarily in the concentrate portion of the diet. However, percent protein in the concentrate is a small piece of information in the total picture. First, horses do not have a protein requirement, but rather an amino acid requirement. Second, there is a need for an amount of protein and a quality of dietary protein source to supply the amino acid requirement. There has been much discussion regarding the relationship between energy and protein and some effort to fine-tune feeding programs for horses on a nutrient-to-calorie ratio (NRC 1989), but the current NRC (2007) bases crude protein recommendations on the actual protein required for a specific function and overall digestibility and efficiency of use.

Overfeeding of protein is a common practice in the performance horse industry. The NRC (2007) states that "not much evidence exists concerning the effect of excess protein consumption" (65). Excess protein will be metabolized, the nitrogen will be removed and excreted, and the remainder of the molecule will be used as fuel. However, although excess protein can be converted into fuel, it is an expensive way to provide energy to the horse. Therefore, it is not true that the most important consideration in a working horse's diet is a high level of protein. The balance of amino acids is important, but the total amount of protein necessary to maintain mature horses in optimal working condition is relatively low when compared to the protein needs of lactating mares and young, growing horses. Growing horses are more sensitive to quality of protein than mature horses at maintenance. For growing horses, the amino acid lysine is quite important. Research has shown that adding lysine to the diets of young growing horses allows the crude protein content of the total ration to be reduced (NRC 2007). Soybean meal and good-

quality alfalfa are good sources of protein with high lysine content.

A horse's protein, or amino acid, requirement may appear to be met from a ration analysis standpoint, yet other factors come into play influencing whether amino acid requirements are actually met. These factors include site of digestion, feedstuff variation and biological value, total amount and rate of protein consumption, and retention time in the digestive tract.

Amino acids are absorbed in the small intestine. No appreciable amount of amino acids from microbial digestion in the hindgut appears to be available for direct use by the horse (Reitnour and Salsbury 1976). Therefore, site of protein digestion is important in meeting amino acid requirements of the horse. Depending on the source of dietary protein, at least 60% to 70% of dietary protein may be digested and absorbed in the small intestine (Hintz 1975). In one study, horses were fed a 50:50 concentrate-to-hay diet, where two-thirds of the protein in the concentrates were supplied by either oats or sorghum grains, crimped or micronized. The remaining protein in the concentrate was supplied by a soybean meal-based supplement. On average, 67% of the nitrogen consumed was digested in the total tract. Approximately 70% of the digestible protein was digested in the small intestine (Klendshoj, et al. 1979). Compare this to work in which only 37% of the digestible protein was digested in the small intestine when ponies were fed an all hay diet (Gibbs, et al. 1988). In this study, ponies were fed 11.7% protein coastal Bermuda hay, 15% alfalfa hay, or 18% alfalfa hay. Dietary hay nitrogen was almost completely digested as the roughage passed through the entire tract. However, prececal digestibility was highest for the 18% alfalfa hay, next was the 11.7% coastal Bermuda hay, and lowest prececal digestibility was reported for the 15% alfalfa hay. The difference here is as a result of the quality of the hay within its type, not percent protein on an analysis. Coastal Bermuda hay that tests 11.7% protein is leafy and relatively immature, as is 18% alfalfa hay; however, 15% alfalfa hay is much more mature and stemmy and is therefore less available for enzymatic digestion in the small intestine. Lower quality alfalfa hay, although higher in protein than grass hay, will contribute little to the amino acid needs of the horse.

To evaluate common feeding practices for yearling horses, researchers fed one group of yearlings oats and alfalfa and another group were fed a balanced grain mix and alfalfa. Both groups were fed a 65:35 grain-to-hay ratio. The diet with oats provided more crude protein and lysine than NRC (2007) requirements. Upper tract digestible protein and lysine between the two treatments were 95% and 86%, respectively, for the oat diet and 124% and 140%, respectively, for the balanced grain mix. Yearlings in both groups showed similar gains in body weight, but those fed oats deposited nearly twice as much body fat and tended to gain less skeletal height than yearlings fed the balanced grain mix. Even though NRC (2007) requirements for protein were met when oats were fed, it was concluded that the higher protein-to-calorie and lysine-to-calorie ratios from the balanced grain mix appeared to support partitioning of available nutrients for skeletal growth as opposed to fat deposition (Gibbs, et al. 1989). Further work is needed on a wider variety of feedstuffs to more clearly define protein digestion in the small intestine and its impact on meeting the amino acid requirements of the horse.

Minerals

Minerals are involved in the formation of structural components in the body, muscular contraction, and energy transfer. Some minerals are also integral parts of amino acids, vitamins, and hormones. Levels of major minerals (macrominerals) are critical, especially for young, growing horses. Young horses may develop metabolic bone disease when mineral levels are inadequate.

Calcium and phosphorus are two macrominerals of great importance in the horse's diet. Horses require calcium and phosphorus in relatively large amounts for bone growth and maintenance. Growing horses, especially, need adequate amounts of calcium and phosphorus because they are still experiencing active skeletal growth and development. Deficiencies in calcium may lead to metabolic bone disease in young horses or weakening of the bones and lameness in mature horses. Phosphorus deficiencies also cause bone problems in young and adult horses.

Also of importance is the ratio of calcium to phosphorus in the horse's diet. Horses should receive diets that contain at least as much calcium as phosphorus. Diets containing inverted calcium-to-phosphorus ratios can contribute to weak bones and lameness in horses.

Other important macrominerals include sodium, chloride, potassium, magnesium, and sulfur. Hard-working horses may lose large amounts of sodium, potassium, and chloride in sweat. The increase in requirements for these electrolytes can normally be met with good-quality forage and top-quality commercially prepared horse feeds. Horses that are intensely exercised in hot, humid climates may lose large enough quantities of electrolytes in the sweat to require additional electrolyte supplementation in the feed. Magnesium and sulfur levels are usually adequate in typical diets fed to horses.

Trace minerals are those required in small amounts by the horse. Essential trace minerals include cobalt, copper, iodine, iron, manganese, selenium, and zinc. Deficiencies or imbalances of trace minerals may cause decreased growth rate, lowered resistance to disease, lack of stamina, and reduced reproductive rate. Osteochondrosis and osteodysgenesis have been associated with copper deficiency in young growing horses (NRC 2007). Selenium, along with vitamin E, functions as an antioxidant to protect body tissues. Depending on the region, forages may be either low or high in selenium content. Selenium deficiencies can cause vascular disorders, muscle degeneration, reproductive disorders, and neurological maladies (Lewis 1996). However, excess selenium is harmful, causing poisoning and possibly death as a result of pulmonary congestion and edema (Lewis 1996). The safest way to ensure that a horse is receiving adequate amounts of minerals in appropriate balance is to feed rations scientifically formulated by equine nutritionists.

Vitamins

Vitamins are required by the horse in small amounts to help use nutrients for growth, maintenance, reproduction, and performance. The horse is able to synthesize many of the needed vitamins from intestinal microorganisms, including vitamin K, and the B-complex vitamins, along with vitamin C that is synthesized in the liver.

Vitamins are divided into two general categories: fat-soluble vitamins (A, D, E, and K) and water-soluble vitamins (B-complex and C). High-quality pasture and forages are rich sources of vitamins; however, mature forage and forage that has been stored for an extended time lose much of this vitamin activity. Therefore, vitamin supplementation of these forages is often necessary.

Vitamin A requirements of horses can be met by carotene, which is found in all fresh green forages. However, the carotene content of forages decreases with time, so even if hay is stored properly, a significant amount of carotene will be broken down after as little as 6 months. Fortunately, the horse can store vitamin A in the liver, so horses feeding on green forage can store up to about 6 months' supply. Excessive vitamin A may eventually contribute to bone weakness, so horse owners must take care not to oversupplement vitamin A.

Vitamin D is not considered to be a dietary requirement because horses that receive normal exposure to sunlight will have sufficient vitamin D to meet their needs.

Vitamin E has received increased attention recently for its possible role in decreasing tissue damage. However, the influence of vitamin E on exercise and the muscle of the horse is currently under examination, and there are no concrete conclusions and therefore specific recommendations for additional supplementation of vitamin E at this time. Although vitamin E deficiency has been implicated as a causative agent in white muscle disease, current evidence indentifies selenium deficiency as the primary cause rather than vitamin E (NRC 2007).

The B-complex vitamins, except for vitamin B_{12}, are usually supplied in adequate amounts in high-quality forage. Vitamin B_{12} is not synthesized by plants typically grazed by horses, but it is synthe-sized by microbes in the hindgut of the horse. There is also abundant synthesis of other B vitamins by the intestinal microorganisms, and this source, along with the food supply, is usually adequate to meet the needs of most adult horses.

Some B vitamins play important roles in equine performance and may need to be supplemented in the exercising horse's diet. There is some evidence that exercising horses may need supplemental vitamin B_1 (thiamin) beyond what is normally required for maintenance. Another B vitamin, biotin, is often supplemented in the horse's diet for purposes of enhancing hoof growth or strength. There is limited evidence to support these claims, and more research is needed to determine exact recommendations for supplementing diets with biotin.

Vitamin C is synthesized in the liver of the horse and is therefore not generally considered a dietary essential nutrient.

Feeding Different Classes of Horses

Horses require differing amounts of nutrients in their daily rations depending on their nutritional class or lifestyle. What each horse does for a living determines the amount and balance of nutrients necessary for optimal performance, whether that performance is working, breeding, or growing. Dividing horses into classes relative to nutrient requirements is the first step in designing a workable feeding management program. This approach helps a horse owner meet each horse's nutrient requirements in the most manageable and economical fashion.

The NRC's Nutrient Requirements of Horses (2007) is the resource that most researchers, veterinarians, and nutritionists use in making feeding recommendations to horse owners. The NRC also provides a computer program that can be used to estimate nutrient requirements of specific horses more precisely than the tables in this chapter. The program may be accessed through the National Academies Press Web site (www.nap.edu). Table 2.1 provides the daily nutrient requirements for a

Table 2.1. Daily nutrient requirements of horses (500-kg mature body weight).

	DE (Mcal)	CP (g)	Lys (g)	Ca (g)	P (g)	Cu (mg)	Zn (mg)	Se (mg)	Vit A (kIU)	Vit E (IU)
Maintenance										
Minimum	15.2	540	23.2	20.0	14.0	100.0	400.0	1.00	15.0	500
Average	16.7	630	27.1	20.0	14.0	100.0	400.0	1.00	15.0	500
Elevated	18.2	720	31.0	20.0	14.0	100.0	400.0	1.00	15.0	500
Working										
Light	20.0	699	30.1	30.0	18.0	100.0	400.0	1.00	22.5	800
Moderate	23.3	768	33.0	35.0	21.0	112.5	450.0	1.13	22.5	900
Heavy	26.6	862	37.1	40.0	29.0	125.0	500.0	1.25	22.5	1000
Very heavy	34.5	1004	43.2	40.0	29.0	125.0	500.0	1.25	22.5	1000
Pregnant mares										
Early	16.7	630	27.1	20.0	14.0	100.0	400.0	1.00	30.0	800
5 months	17.1	685	29.5	20.0	14.0	100.0	400.0	1.00	30.0	800
7 months	17.9	729	31.3	28.0	20.0	100.0	400.0	1.00	30.0	800
9 months	19.2	797	34.3	36.0	26.3	125.0	400.0	1.00	30.0	800
11 months	21.4	893	38.4	36.0	26.3	125.0	400.0	1.00	30.0	800
Growing horses										
4 months	13.3	669	28.8	39.1	21.7	42.1	168.5	0.42	7.6	337
6 months	15.5	676	29.1	38.6	21.5	54.0	215.9	0.54	9.7	432
12 months	18.8	846	36.4	37.7	20.9	80.3	321.2	0.80	14.5	642
18 months	19.2	799	34.4	37.0	20.6	96.9	387.5	0.97	17.4	775

Ca, Calcium; CP, crude protein; Cu, copper; DE, digestible energy; g, gram; IU, international units; Lys, lysine; Mcal, megacalorie; mg, milligram; P, phosphorus; Se, selenium; Vit A, vitamin A; vit E, vitamin E; Zn, Zinc.
Source: National Research Council 2007.

500-kg horse at different lifestyle stages and workloads.

Maintenance

Maintenance horses are mature, idle horses that are neither pregnant nor lactating. The NRC (2007) suggests three categories of maintenance horses based on energy requirements—minimum, average, and elevated. An average maintenance energy requirement of 33.3 kcal/kg body weight is recommended for those horses with moderate voluntary activity and alert temperaments. For those horses that are more sedentary, possibly as a result of docile temperament or confinement, the daily energy requirement is 30.3 kcal/kg body weight. Horses with elevated maintenance energy requirements would be those with more nervous temperaments or

increased levels of voluntary activity. Suggested energy requirement for elevated maintenance horses are 36.3 kcal/kg body weight.

The NRC (2007) supplies formulas to calculate the crude protein requirements for the three classifications of maintenance horses:

Minimum: BW × 1.08g CP/kg BW/day
Average: BW × 1.26g CP/kg BW/day
Elevated: BW × 1.44g CP/kg BW/day

(CP = crude protein; BW = body weight)

There has been little research to determine the lysine requirement of maintenance horses. However, the following formula may be used to estimate the lysine requirement of horses at maintenance (NRC 2007):

Lysine (g/day) = CP requirement × 4.3%

Growth

The energy requirement of growing horses is the total energy required for maintenance plus the energy required for gain. The DE requirement for the growing horse is a function of the environmental conditions, horse's age, desired average daily gain (ADG), and the individual metabolic or health characteristics that may be unique to a particular individual. It is difficult to determine the energy requirement for growth because researchers have not yet defined optimal growth rates. If horses grow too fast in terms of increased body weight, soundness and longevity may be affected. However, insufficient energy intake will result in poor growth rates and unthrifty appearance of young horses. The NRC (2007) suggests a formula to calculate the daily DE requirement of growing horses:

$$DE \ (Mcal/day) = (56.5x^{-0.145}) \times BW + (1.99 + 1.21x - 0.021x^2) \times ADG$$

Where x is age in months, ADG is average daily gain in kilograms, and BW is body weight in kilograms.

Many horse owners, particularly of those growing horses to be shown at halter or for sale as yearlings, will feed to achieve ADG of 1.1 to 1.4 kg/day (2.5 to 3.0 lb/day) or more in some cases. The average energy concentration for total diets on an as-fed basis, fed to growing horses up to 1 year of age, can range from 2.5 Mcal/kg for diets containing 70% concentrate and 30% hay to approximately 0.72 Mcal/kg for some pasture feeding situations. Yearlings have been shown to derive enough energy from pasture to maintain adequate growth; however, forage type and quality, stocking rate, and level of training or exercise must be taken into consideration. In addition, protein level and quality, as well as vitamin and mineral intake provided by a given pasture may not be adequate to support a desired quality of growth. Restricting protein intake restricts growth rate in young horses. The equation to calculate crude protein requirements for young growing horses is:

$$CP \ requirement = (BW \times 1.44g \ CP/kg \ BW) + ((ADG \times 0.20)/E)/0.79$$

where E is efficiency of use of dietary protein, which is estimated to be 50% for horses 4 to 6 months of age, 45% for horses 7 to 8 months of age, 40% for horses 9 to 10 months of age, 35% for horses 11 months of age, and 30% for horses 12 months or older (NRC 2007).

In addition to quantity of protein fed, the quality of protein must be considered. Comparisons of sources of plant proteins showed soybean meal to result in the most favorable growth response in weanling foals. Information regarding specific amino acids and their effect on growth and development of the horse is quite limited. The addition of lysine to low-quality protein diets showed an improved growth response and is considered the first-limiting amino acid for growth in horses. Threonine has been suspected to be the second-limiting amino acid for growth when horses are fed a grass forage-based diet. Recent research has shown lysine/threonine supplemented low protein diets (9% crude protein [CP]) resulted in equal growth response when compared to higher protein diets (14% CP; Staniar, et al. 2001). This further emphasizes that protein quality (defined by amino acid composition) of protein sources can have significant effects on the growth of horses.

Breeding

Broodmare Nutrition

Broodmares have specific nutritional requirements that differ from other classes of horses. When feeding broodmares, the feeding program must meet the requirements of the growing foal, as well as the mare herself. As the mare progresses through the various stages of gestation, her nutritional needs change. There are differences both in the amount of feed mares need and the nutrient concentration needed in that feed. Throughout the year, the broodmare goes through three different phases, each with a different nutritional demand. She is either in early gestation, late gestation, or lactation. To keep this cycle going consistently requires that the mare receive the proper health care and nutrition.

Body condition may be the single largest factor affecting the reproductive performance of mares.

Research has shown that the body condition of a mare at the time of breeding can influence conception rate. Mares maintained in moderate to fleshy condition cycle earlier in the year, require fewer cycles per conception, have a higher pregnancy rate, and are more likely to maintain pregnancies than are thin mares (Henneke, et al. 1983). Using the body condition scoring system, research has determined that a condition score of less than 5 in lactating mares indicates that they may not have enough stored body fat to support efficient reproductive performance. Those mares are more likely to skip a breeding season than are mares with a condition score of 6 or more. This is especially prevalent in mares that are 15 years of age or greater (Gibbs and Davison 1991). Although no foaling difficulties have been shown in mares in obese condition (Kubiak, et al. 1988), there are no reproductive advantages to keeping mares in condition scores of 8 or 9, and there may be adverse metabolic consequences due to obesity. Therefore, scores of 5.5 to 7.0 represent the optimum (Henneke, et al. 1983).

Thin mares gaining weight at breeding time are twice as likely to conceive as thin mares maintaining weight. Mares in good-to-fat condition have high conception rates even when losing or maintaining body weight (Henneke, et al. 1984). Therefore, dietary energy requirements for reproduction depend on the body condition of the mare. Increasing energy intake 10% to 15% above the requirement should result in weight gain and a higher condition score. Protein requirements for brood mares are similar to those of maintenance horses.

Diets containing added fats or oils can be used to help mares in unsatisfactory condition gain the desired weight. The advantage of feeding these diets is that body condition can be improved without having to feed excessive amounts of concentrate, since the higher fat diets tend to have a higher digestible energy level.

Total daily feed intake by mares (hay plus concentrate) normally ranges from 1.5% to 3% of body weight, with 2% serving as an average. Actual daily feed intake depends on the type and quality of hay or grazing and on the crude fiber level and energy density of the concentrate. As the fiber level increases and energy density decreases, the amount of feed required to meet energy demands will go up. However, as forage quality decreases, voluntary intake often decreases as well. This can present a problem in providing enough energy to maintain the desired body condition. Furthermore, daily feed intake can vary. Feed intake may have to be increased for hard keepers or heavy milkers and decreased for other mares who are easier keepers.

A nonlactating, pregnant mare in the first 8 months of gestation has nutrient requirements quite similar to those of any mature, idle horse. The developing foal gains only 0.2 pounds/day during this time and does not present a significant nutritional demand on the mare. It is usually considered sufficient simply to meet the mare's nutrient requirements for maintenance.

As a mare enters the last 3 to 4 months of pregnancy, nutrient requirements increase because the unborn foal is growing more rapidly, averaging 0.45 kg (1 pound) per day. During this time, the intake of protein, energy, vitamins, and minerals needs to be increased. Even in situations where forage is sufficiently maintaining mares in acceptable condition, it is important that they receive quality concentrate supplementation. Although forage may be able to provide sufficient calories to maintain the body condition of the mare, other nutrients, particularly protein and minerals, will be inadequate. Therefore, simply having mares stay in good condition during late gestation does not guarantee proper foal development.

It is during the tenth month that the greatest amount of mineral retention occurs in the unborn foal. In addition to this, mares' milk is practically devoid of some trace minerals, such as copper, that are essential for proper bone development (NRC 2007). Therefore, adequate mineral nutrition of the mare is critical for normal fetal development and to provide sufficient minerals for the foal to be born with stores of these nutrients to draw on after birth. A supplemental feeding program that provides a good protein, vitamin, and mineral balance is necessary to properly support the growth and development of the foal.

At foaling, a mare's daily nutrient requirements increase significantly. The protein and energy requirements almost double from early gestation to lactation, as do requirements for calcium, phosphorus, and vitamin A. These nutrient needs must be met for the mare to recover from foaling stress, produce milk, and to rebreed, all without losing body condition. A lactating mare will usually consume between 2% and 3% of her body weight in total feed (hay plus concentrate) daily. Because of the significant difference in nutrient requirements from gestation to lactating, it is safer to gradually increase feed intake before foaling. This will prevent a drastic change at foaling time, which could increase the risk of digestive disorders. Also, providing the total daily feed in at least two equal feedings allows mares to more safely consume the amounts needed during lactation. Heavy milkers may require as much as 1.75% of body weight in concentrated feed each day, depending on the quality and nutrient density of that concentrate. This is a critical, nutritional period for the mare. Underfeeding of mares during early lactation can lower milk production and cause weight loss. This

may not pose a problem if the mare is in fleshy-to-fat condition. However, early lactation weight loss in mares that foal in thin condition will often affect the mare's ability to raise her new foal and become pregnant again.

Mares produce an average of 11 kg (i.e., 11 L, 24 lb, or 3 gallons) of milk daily during a 5-month lactation period. This represents 1,703 L or 1,587.6 kg (450 gallons or 1 3/4 tons) of milk over 150 days. High-producing mares produce as much as 14.51 kg (i.e., 14.5 L; 32 lb, or 4 gallons) of milk daily. The average production in the first 22 days of lactation is 12.02 kg (26.5 pounds) per day. Production appears to reach a peak at 30 days and slowly declines from there. Nutrient content of mares' milk follows a more drastic downward curve. In the fourth month of lactation, a mare's milk provides less than 30% of the total energy needed by her foal. Providing lactating mares with a concentrate that includes added fats or oils, and high-quality protein can help slow the downward curve of production and improve nutrient content of the milk. This will translate into an early growth advantage for the nursing foal.

In the fourth, fifth, and sixth months of lactation, daily requirements begin to decline. However, by

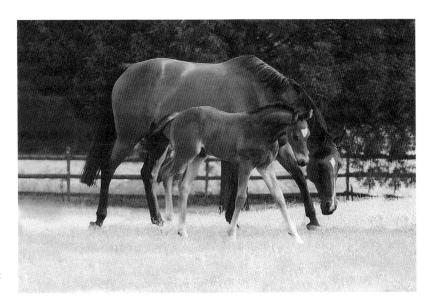

Figure 2.6. Energy requirements of the lactating mare may be double that of maintenance.

this time many owners will have had foals on a good creep feed to prepare them for weaning and will be weaning by the fourth or fifth month of age. There is no advantage for the foal to remain on the mare past this time. It is more nutritionally accurate for the foal and more economical for the owner to feed the foal a quality diet to meet needs directly than it is to feed the mare to produce milk. Once the foal is weaned, the dry, pregnant mare can be managed as an early gestating mare once again.

When possible, mares that are fed in groups should be sorted according to feed intake or body condition to ensure each mare receives the appropriate amount of concentrate to meet her needs. Providing individual feed troughs for each mare plus one extra trough for mares that get run off from their feed or providing plenty of space at group troughs will help insure that mares consume the feed they need.

Stallion Nutrition

Breeding stallions require more DE during the breeding season because they get more exercise. According to the NRC (2007), the DE requirement for breeding stallions in heavy use is approximately 20% higher than maintenance, and stallions are usually in the elevated maintenance category for energy requirements during nonbreeding season.

Protein requirements are slightly higher for breeding stallions than for horses at maintenance, but the increased feed intake as a result of increased energy demands should be adequate to meet the protein requirement.

Some stallions are young and may even still be growing so their nutritional needs will be different from a mature stallion. Those that are still showing through the breeding season will have different requirements from those that stay on the farm the whole season. Breeding season will place additional demands on each of them, but the base diet will be different. Basically, a stallion should be fed according to his current lifestyle, and then adjustments should be made based on how busy his breeding season may be and how hard he has to work.

It is important to monitor a stallion's body condition before and during the season. Results of one study showed that stallion body weight decreases during peak breeding activity when feed intake remains constant. So, feeding rates, and maybe even the product fed, may need to be adjusted for a heavy breeding season. Ideally, stallions should be kept in performance condition, where ribs are not visible but are easy to feel. A thin stallion is not receiving adequate calories in the diet and is possibly deficient in other important nutrients such as protein, vitamins, and minerals. This can affect libido and possibly fertility. On the other hand, overweight stallions may exhibit reduced libido, as well as, long-term negative effects on health as a result of excess weight on joints and other metabolic problems associated with obesity. Basically, a stallion should be treated as an athlete, which means that he should receive regular exercise and turn out. This is important for both physical and mental well-being.

For young stallions still growing or showing through the breeding season, good quality hay and a well-balanced feed that provides quality protein, vitamins, and minerals to support growth and performance will be important. Simply increasing the amount of feed to meet additional calorie needs will support the additional nutrient demands of breeding season. Older, more sedentary stallions can often maintain adequate condition in the off-season on hay or pasture alone and may not require the additional calories supplied in most feeds. However, hay or pasture will not provide all the nutrition needed for long-term health, and many of these stallions cannot eat the recommended levels of typical mixed feeds without getting overweight. If the feeding rates are reduced to prevent the weight gain, then they often become deficient in important nutrients. A general rule of thumb should be that if a horse does not eat at least 1.6 to 1.8 kg (3.5–4 lb) per day of a well-balanced, nutritionally fortified feed, then they are probably coming up short in some nutrients. In those cases, a product that is fortified to provide the needed protein, vitamins, and minerals in 0.45 to 0.9 kg (1–2 lb) per day would be a good choice.

For subfertile stallions, there have been studies looking at adding certain nutrients to the diet with the hopes of increasing fertility. Supplemental vitamins, including vitamin E, have been proposed to increase stallion fertility. However, controlled studies have failed to show any benefit, especially if these vitamins are added to an already well-fortified diet (Rich, et al. 1983). Several universities have reported improvement in motility of cooled or frozen semen from stallions fed a supplement containing docosahexaenoic acid (DHA), a marine-based omega-3 fatty acid. Similar benefit was not seen when supplementing with alpha-linolenic acid (ALA), an omega-3 fatty acid found in flax and other plant oils (Brinkso, et al. 2005; Harris, Anderson, et al. 2005; Harris, Baumgard, et al., 2005). This may be worth investigating for those stallions whose semen doesn't ship well. For most stallions, sticking to a well-balanced feed with good quality hay and providing regular exercise will meet all the requirements for a fertile and successful breeding season.

Performance

Feeding performance horses to provide essential nutrients to maintain condition, as well as supply the necessary energy and other nutrients to satisfy the requirements of intense exercise has received much research attention in the past several years.

To estimate the DE required by exercising horses, the amount of energy used during the exercise must be determined. The energy used depends on the duration and intensity of the exercise. Although the time of exercise is easy to measure, the intensity is not. Many factors that are somewhat difficult to quantitate can affect the intensity of work, including speed, terrain, incline, gait, and weight carried or pulled. To simplify the calculation of DE requirements for individual working horses, the NRC (2007) has divided work into four general categories: light, moderate, heavy, and very heavy.

According to the NRC (2007), light-working horses include recreational riding horses, horses at the beginning of training programs, and horses that

are occasionally shown. Such horses usually work 1 to 3 hours per week; 40% walking, 50% trotting, and 10% cantering. The mean heart rate is 80 beats per minute. The equation to calculate DE for light working horses is:

$$DE \ (Mcal/day) = (0.0333 \times BW) \times 1.20$$

Examples of moderate-working horses are school horses, horses that are frequently shown, polo horses, and ranch horses. The exercise consists of 3 to 5 hours per week; 30% walking, 55% trotting, 10% cantering, and 5% skilled work (e.g., jumping, cutting) The mean heart rate is 90 beats per minute. The equation to calculate DE for moderate working horses is:

$$DE \ (Mcal/day) = (0.03333 \times BW) \times 1.40$$

Heavy working horses include hard-working ranch, show and polo horses, low-to-medium-level event horses and horses in middle stages of race training. The work is 4 to 5 hours per week; 20% walking, 50% trotting, 15% cantering, and 15% galloping, jumping, or other skill work. The mean heart rate is 100 beats per minute. The equation to calculate DE is:

$$DE \ (Mcal/day) = (0.0333 \times BW) + 1.60$$

Very heavy-working horses are racing horses (Thoroughbred, quarter horse, standardbred, and endurance) and elite 3-day eventing horses. The work is varied, ranging from 1 hour per week of speed work to 6 to 12 hours per week of slow work. The mean heart rate is 110 to 150 beats per minute. DE is calculated as:

$$DE \ (Mcal/day) = (0.0363 \times BW) \times 1.9$$

These categories are arbitrary and may be helpful in classifying an individual horse, but many other factors influence the energy requirements of working horses, including level of fitness, skill and weight of the rider, environment, and breed. It is important to also monitor the body condition, weight, and performance of the individual animal to ensure that energy requirements are met.

Further, the type of work dictates the type of energy, or fuel, which will best fit the animal's needs. Some horses need quick bursts of energy,

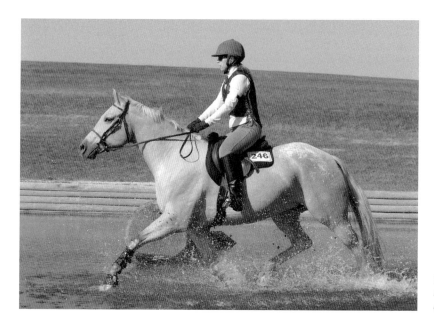

Figure 2.7. Lower level event horses are in the moderate-to-heavy working category depending on the individual.

whereas others require steady, sustained energy. Some horses need a combination of both, and all horses need energy that allows them to remain calm and focused and to maintain a "competitive condition" over the course of the athletic season. One factor to consider in meeting these requirements is the source of energy supplied in the horse's diet.

Dietary energy is supplied by nonstructural carbohydrates (NSC), fermentable fiber, fat, and protein contained in the daily ration. To accommodate the mixture of substrates used to fuel muscle activity during exercise, a mixture of dietary energy sources are needed in rations for performance horses. Muscle glycogen is a major source of stored energy used for exercise performance, so it is important that the diet contain adequate NSC to provide substrate for glycogen synthesis. As mentioned previously, protein is not a significant energy source, so dietary protein should not be considered for its energy content but more for its amino acid content.

All horses should be fed a minimum of 1% of body weight in hay or the equivalent in pasture to meet minimum fiber requirements for maintenance

of large bowel function. Energy supplied by forage is primarily from VFAs produced by microbial fermentation of fiber in the hindgut. VFAs provide the majority of the energy required for the horse at maintenance. However, only one VFA, propionic acid, can be used for gluconeogenesis (synthesis of glucose), and the amount of propionic acid produced is related to the level of starch in the diet. Therefore, fiber may be adequate for meeting maintenance energy requirements, but it has limited ability to supply glucose for work or quickly replenish depleted glycogen stores.

Fats are an excellent source of energy for working horses. Fats contain more than twice the calories per kilogram than either carbohydrates or proteins, so adding fat to the diet allows the horse to ingest more calories in a smaller quantity of feed, which helps prevent some digestive disturbances. Further, research has shown that adding fat to the diets of performance horses may improve performance, such as increased stamina and delayed onset of fatigue (Oldham, et al. 1990).

The protein requirements for exercising horses are increased over maintenance requirements as a result of additional muscle tissue gained during conditioning of the performance horse, repair of muscle tissue damaged during exercise, and nitrogen lost in the sweat. In the past, the increased protein requirement was usually met simply with increased feed to meet the higher energy requirement. However, with the fat-added energy-dense feeds available for performance horses, the amount of protein consumed by the working horse is important to consider.

A good recommended range in protein content for a performance horse feed is 10% to 14% crude protein. The actual amount of protein needed will depend on the age of the horse, amount of work and the type, and quality and quantity of forage provided. The amount of protein needed in the feed is also influenced by the energy content of the feed and how much has to be fed to keep the horse in good condition. For example, a horse eating oats, which are 11.5% protein, may require 4.5 kg (10 lb) of oats to maintain body condition. This horse would be eating 0.52 kg (1.15 lb) of protein per day. The same horse eating a more energy dense 14% protein feed may require 3.2 kg (7 lb) to stay in the same body condition. With this diet, the horse would be eating 0.44 kg (0.98 lb) of protein per day. So, in this case, the horse eating the higher percent protein feed is actually eating less total protein per day, and it may deliver a higher quality protein as well. It is important to consider the quantity of protein in the feed, the amount of feed needed to keep the horse in condition, and the quality of protein, or amino acid content, provided.

In addition to energy and protein, vitamin and mineral requirements also increase with increasing workloads. This is especially true for nutrients involved in energy metabolism such as B vitamins; electrolytes lost in sweat, including sodium, potassium, and chloride; and for antioxidants such as vitamin E. Although a well-balanced vitamin/mineral package is important in diets for performance horses, there is no evidence that feeding levels higher than requirements of any nutrient will result in enhanced performance. Often, oversupplementation becomes detrimental to performance as opposed to elevating the level of performance.

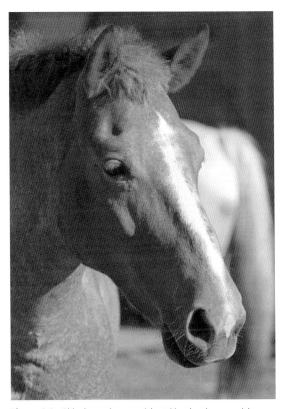

Figure 2.8. Older horses have special nutritional and managerial requirements that should be taken into consideration.

Aged Horse Nutrition

Before discussing diet requirements for the "older horse," it is necessary to determine when a horse is considered to become older. Although a horse in its teens is typically considered "aged," the reality is that the genetics of the individual plus how it was cared for during its life will dictate when its nutritional needs begin to shift from that of an adult mature horse to that of a geriatric horse. That point in life may be sooner for some horses than it is for others. It is also important to remember that aging is a gradual process and does not happen overnight.

The best manner in which to care for older horses is to address their special needs before any significant decline in condition or health. As always, the veterinarian plays a key role in helping to ensure the continuing good health and longevity of the older horse.

Many older horses have dental problems that can affect nutrition. Teeth that are worn or missing make chewing difficult for the horse. Poor dental care can also cause mouth ulcers resulting in pain. Poor teeth contribute to the horse not chewing its food long enough to produce the amount of saliva necessary for proper digestion and to help to lubricate the esophagus for ease of swallowing.

If the horse drops bits of feed or forage out of its mouth, it is probably time for a dental check. In addition to making sure that the horse's teeth are in good condition, feeds that are processed and are easy to chew will help the problem. Water can also be added to the feed to make gruel, which will be even more edible for the horse with poor dental condition.

One of the problems with aging is that the motility of the horse's digestive tract becomes compromised. One reason for this reduction in digestive motility may be because the horse itself has become less active. However, digestive concerns still can occur in those individuals that remain active even as an older horse. Gas production and impactions can lead to colic symptoms.

By feeding smaller meals more frequently, the horse can more easily digest and process its feed. Reducing starch or grain in the diet can be helpful in preventing excess gas and constipation. Increasing the amount of a high-quality, easily digestible fiber source may also assist in this regard. As always, offer plenty of clean, fresh water to keep food moving through the system. Consider adding 56.7 g (2 oz) of salt to the horse's diet to stimulate water consumption. Horses prefer tepid water from 7.2°C to 23.9°C (45°F to 75°F).

As part of the aging process, the older horse experiences a reduction in digestive efficiency, along with a decline in its ability to absorb nutrients. By feeding a processed feed, as opposed to whole grains, and by fortifying the nutrient levels in that feed, the horse is better able to absorb those nutrients that are made available in its diet. The diet that sufficed in the horse's earlier years simply will not provide adequate nutrition to the now older horse as the necessary nutrients are either not present or are no longer available to the changing geriatric digestive system.

Parasite infestation also hinders digestive capabilities, so a proper deworming and parasite control program must always remain paramount in proper maintenance and care of the horse at any age.

Feeding Management

Determining the nutrient requirements of a horse is only one part of the total feeding program. Following basic feeding management practices can contribute a great deal to the health and well-being of the animal, as well as, ensuring that the horse receives the most benefit from its feed.

It is important to determine how much feed a particular horse requires. To feed the correct amount to a horse, the owner must know the horse's body weight. To determine body weight, one can use a livestock scale, a weight tape (such as those available through local feed dealers), or a formula, such as:

BW (lb) = Heartgirth (in.) × Heartgirth (in.) × Body length (in.)/330.

(The heartgirth is measured as the circumference over the withers and around the barrel; the body length is measured from the point of the shoulder to the point of the buttocks.)

It is important to feed horses by weight, not volume. A scoop or coffee can of oats is not the same amount of feed as a scoop or coffee can of corn—the can of oats may hold 0.9 to 1.4 kg (2–3 lb) of grain, whereas the can of corn is actually 1.8 to 2.3 kg (4–5 lb) of corn. Further, because corn is more calorie rich than oats, the can of corn may contain 2 to 3 times the energy as the can of oats. Any time a horse owner changes feed, he or she must weigh the feed to make sure the horse gets fed the same amount of feed every meal.

Feed small amounts often. The horse has a small stomach in relation to its total size, and feeding too much grain in one meal can overload the stomach and cause problems such as colic or laminitis. A general rule of thumb is to feed no more than 0.5%

of the horse's body weight in grain per meal or no more than 2.5 kg (5.5 lb) of grain per meal for a 500-kg (1,100-lb) horse. To increase the feed, increase the number of meals rather than the amount per meal.

Horses need to consume at least 1% of their body weight per day as roughage (on a dry matter basis). Feeding adequate amounts of high-quality roughage can help prevent many digestive disturbances and behavior problems, as well as provide an important source of energy and other nutrients. It is important to note that the maturity at time of harvest is the major factor that determines the quality or nutrient content of hay. As a plant matures, it becomes higher in fiber and therefore less digestible in the upper gut and contributes less DE and protein. Further, many forages are deficient in several minerals, and hays are often low in some vitamin content. Even horses that maintain body weight on hay or pasture need appropriate vitamin, mineral, and possibly protein supplementation.

Changes in types of feed should be made gradually (4–7 days for small changes, up to 3 weeks for radical changes). Sudden changes in the diet may cause shifts in the microbial population in the hindgut, which may lead to digestive disturbances.

Horses that are fed on a consistent schedule are less likely to go off their feed or develop undesirable stall habits (vices). Further, horses that are fed on inconsistent schedules may get hungry and bolt their feed, possibly resulting in digestive disorders. It is a beneficial practice to feed horses at the same times every day.

Another good management practice is to avoid dust and mold and keep the feed manger clean. Proper feed storage reduces feed waste. Horses' digestive systems are not equipped to deal with dust, mold, and such, so poor quality hay or grain will not be digested efficiently and may cause health problems for the horse. It is imperative to provide the horse with top-quality feed.

Supplement with caution. Only supplement rations to correct specific deficiencies. When feeding a nutritionally balanced ration in adequate amounts, adding nutritional supplements may create imbalances or excesses with negative consequences.

Many horses are turned out in a herd. If horses must be fed as a group, use individual feeders spread far apart, put out extra feeders, and make provisions for timid horses (low in the pecking order).

Seasonal Nutrition Considerations

Cold Weather Feeding

Cold weather presents horses with some specific nutritional and management demands. It is a good idea to evaluate housing and feeding programs to ensure that horses get through the cold weather in good shape.

All warm-blooded animals have a critical temperature. This is the temperature below which the animal must produce additional heat to maintain normal body temperature. Mature horses in good flesh have a critical temperature around $-1.1°C$ (30°F) during early winter. After developing a winter coat and gaining 45.36 kg (100 lb), the critical temperature drops to $-9.4°C$ (15°F). It is estimated that young horses, horses in thinner condition, and those that have not developed a winter coat may have a critical temperature around 4.4°C (40°F). When wet, windy conditions are present, the critical temperatures will be higher as well. To produce extra body heat, an increase in feed energy is required. Horses will require an estimated 15% to 20% more calories for each $-12.2°C$ (10°F) the ambient temperature falls below critical temperature. However, thin horses or horses with short hair may need even greater increases in dietary intake to maintain normal body temperature (Cymbaluk 1990; Cymbaluk and Christison 1989, 1990; NRC 2007).

It is important that horses come into winter carrying adequate body condition. The additional body fat serves as insulation and energy reserves in times when the thermometer dips below the critical temperature. Once cold weather sets in, it is difficult to put weight on horses. Thin horses get colder and use so much energy trying to stay warm, there often aren't enough calories left for weight gain.

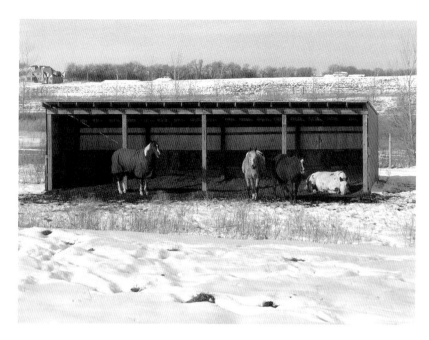

Figure 2.9. Horses can survive quite well during the winter months with adequate shelter and proper nutritional care.

Young horses and broodmares in late gestation may not be able to consume enough of a high fiber diet, such as hay, due to restrictions in digestive system capacity. These horses must have access to good-quality, highly digestible feeds to meet the additional energy requirements because of cold weather and higher production levels.

Historically, horsemen have often changed their rations from summer to winter to accommodate increased calorie needs. Typically, this is done by increasing the amount of hay and changing from oats to corn or a sweet feed. Feeding additional hay provides extra calories and also helps maintain body temperature due to the internal heat produced during digestion of fiber. The change from oats to corn or a sweet feed is based on the impression that corn or sweet feed is a "hotter" feed than oats. This concept of oats being a summer feed and corn a winter ration has some merit, but it also has some flaws.

One kilogram of corn has more energy and is lower in protein and fiber than 1 kg of oats. Not only does corn have more energy per kilogram than oats, corn also weighs more per unit of volume. One scoop full of corn has about 45% more calories than the same scoop full of whole oats. This has led to the idea that corn is a hotter feed than oats. Actually, because of the higher fiber level in oats, oats produce more internal heat during digestion than corn; it just takes more oats to provide enough calories.

Corn or oats alone can provide adequate calories but not adequate protein, vitamin, or minerals. The best option for the horse year-round is a nutritionally balanced diet of good-quality hay and a high-quality, well-fortified commercial feed. During the winter months, provide as much shelter as possible, especially from wind and wet weather, and increase feed intake to help maintain body condition. Then, as warmer weather arrives, continue to feed the nutritionally balanced diet, simply reduce the amount fed. When a well-balanced feed is used, the only adjustments necessary are to increase or decrease the amount fed, depending on body condition or energy demand.

Although grain does not provide as much of an internal warming effect as hay, it is often necessary to supplement a horse's winter ration with additional grain to boost calorie supplies. Cold temperatures increase the amount of calories a horse needs to maintain body weight, as well as, support activity or production. Because a horse may digest feed less efficiently as the temperature drops below the horse's comfort zone, additional feed may be required to maintain body weight and condition. It is important to maintain the horse in a body condition score of 5 to 6 (moderate to moderately fleshy) because a layer of fat under the skin provides insulation against the cold. Further, horses in moderately fleshy condition require less dietary energy for maintenance in cold weather than thin horses. In general, feeding an additional 1/4 kg (0.55 lb) of grain per 100 kg (220.5 lb) body weight to nonworking horses will provide adequate calories during cold, windy, and wet weather. Working horses may require up to an additional 1/2 kg (1.10 lb) per 100-kg (220.5-lb) body weight, depending on workload, to maintain body weight during cold weather.

Water should always be available to the horse. Monitoring water intake is another important consideration during winter weather. Snow is not a sufficient substitute for water because the horse cannot physically eat enough snow to meet its water requirement. Ideally, the temperature of the available water should be between 7°C and 18°C (45°F and 65°F). If the water is too cold, the horse may drink less, thereby decreasing water and lubrication in the gut and increasing the chance of impaction-induced colic. Mature horses in temperate climates will normally drink from 19 to 30 L (5–8 gallons) of water per day. Increasing the amount of hay in the diet will increase the water consumption, up to 34 or 39 L (9 or 10 gallons) of water with an all-hay diet. During cold weather, water intake can decline dramatically. Increased hay intake combined with decreased water intake contributes to the risk of impaction colic. This is especially a problem when horses are kept in stalls for several days because of inclement weather because confinement tends to slow intestinal motility. Further, if the horse drinks less water, it may also eat less feed, resulting in loss of body weight and condition. Finally, if a horse is forced to drink very cold water, its energy requirement will increase, because more calories are required to warm the water to body temperature inside the digestive tract. In cold weather, water should be kept fresh and free of ice to ensure adequate intake and horses exercised whenever possible. Also, adding 30 to 60 g (1 or 2 oz) of salt to the feed may stimulate water consumption.

Warm Weather Feeding

Heat and humidity put an added burden on horses during training, showing, and hauling. Horses are actually better equipped to work in cold weather than in the heat. They build up a tremendous amount of body heat because of the internal heat produced by fiber digestion and the large mass of working muscles, combined with insulation from their hair coat and body fat cover.

There are some nutritional concerns, however, during this season, and some management issues should be addressed to ensure the health and performance of horses.

First, as horses start working harder, the plane of nutrition must be increased to ensure that the horse's increased requirements are met. Energy is possibly the most important nutrient to consider in a working horse. As a horse works harder, its energy (calorie) requirement increases, and those additional calories must be supplied in a form that will not compromise the horse's digestive health. More calories can be added by increasing the amount of grain in the ration, but grain is high in starch, and too much starch (and other soluble carbohydrates) may lead to digestive disturbances such as colic or laminitis. Safer energy sources include fat and fermentable fibers. These performance feeds also contain the amino acids, vitamins, and minerals to support the increased demands of the performance horse. Keep in mind that all feeding changes must be made gradually, so it is important to gradually increase the amount of feed as the horse's workload increases.

If the horse will not be worked hard, however, or the horse is naturally an easy keeper, a concentrated feed may be the best way to meet the horse's nutritional needs without adding many calories. Next, because the forage portion of the horse's diet may be changing, some of these changes may be problematic for some horses. For some horses, the advent of spring means that the source of forage changes from hay to fresh grass. If this is the case, the horse owner should take care to minimize the risk of laminitis as horses are exposed to fresh pastures.

Why can fresh grass cause laminitis in horses? During the process of photosynthesis, plants manufacture sugars that are either used for metabolic processes such as growth or are stored as polysaccharides such as starch or fructans. The storage form of the sugars depends on the plant species. In certain situations, such as the warm sunny days and chilly nights that occur in the spring and the fall, the plants use fewer sugars for growth, and therefore store more as polysaccharides. This can cause problems for horses, especially when the sugars are stored as fructans because fructans are not digested in the horse's upper gut (where starch is digested and absorbed), but instead passes into the hindgut where it is fermented by the microbes. It is this fermentation of fructans that appears to be a trigger factor for colic or laminitis, similar to a grain overload. The fermentation of fiber carbohydrates in the hindgut is normal and does not cause digestive disorders. Other environmental conditions that can affect the amount of polysaccharide storage in plants include drought stress, duration, and intensity of sunlight, salinity (salt content) of soil, and overall health of the plant. Again, some species of grass, including cool season grasses, tend to store sugars as fructans, whereas others, the warm season grasses, tend to store sugars as starch and are less likely to cause problems.

How then should pastures be managed to minimize the risk of laminitis? Horses that are kept on pasture year-round usually adjust to the new grass as it grows. Nature does a fairly good job of making the pasture change gradually. The problems usually occur when horses have been confined and fed a hay and grain diet during the winter and are then abruptly turned out on the lush green pasture in the spring. Further, horses that have been kept up through the winter may overeat when turned out because of the palatability of the lush green foliage. This sudden change in the diet, especially when it includes a rapid

influx of the unfamiliar fructans into the hindgut, may trigger digestive upset.

There are several ways to prevent or minimize problems when introducing horses to spring pastures. Feeding hay immediately before turn-out may help keep horses from overeating because they are less likely to overeat on an already full stomach. Restricting grazing time will also help minimize risks. A suggested schedule is 30 minutes of grazing once or twice a day on the first day of grazing; then increase grazing time by 5 to 10 minutes per day until the horses are grazing 4 to 6 hours per day total. At this point, they have adapted to the green grass.

Horses working hard in hot, humid climates and sweating a great deal may need additional electrolyte supplementation. Electrolyte supplementation should be approached carefully. First, never give electrolyte supplementation to an already dehydrated horse. Second, the body has a set requirement for electrolytes but doesn't store any extra. If supplemental electrolytes are provided in excess amounts, the body will become efficient at eliminating them in the urine. This causes the horse to urinate more frequently, thus increasing water needs and making it more difficult to stay hydrated. Also, if the body is flushing excess electrolytes out of the system to keep the balance, on a day when additional electrolytes may be needed, they won't be available. Therefore, the best recommendation is to provide a well-balanced feed, good-quality hay and free choice salt and water on a daily basis. Provide additional electrolyte supplementation the day before, the day of, and the day after an event in which the horse works extremely hard and sweats excessively (Coenen and Meyer 1987; Hoyt, et al. 1995; Meyer 1987).

There are many commercial electrolyte supplements available. However, for the majority of working horses, the sodium and chloride requirements can be met with 30–60 g (1–3 oz) of supplemental salt per day and the potassium, calcium, and magnesium requirements will be met by a well-balanced quality feed and hay. Therefore, additional electrolyte supplementation is needed only at those times when a horse will be sweating large amounts for an extended time frame (Gibbs, et al. 2007).

Special Needs

The unique digestive anatomy of the horse requires somewhat thoughtful feeding conditions for optimal health. Overall, offering quality hay and a vitamin and mineral supplement to horses at maintenance can provide appropriate nutrients for the animal. If the horse has increased metabolic demands (e.g., from exercise, growth, or lactation), commercially prepared feeds provided at recommended rates in addition to quality hay will usually provide the additional calories and nutrients required in these cases. On the other hand, there are special situations when horses need more specific and specialized diets to meet their nutrient requirements, especially when horses are sick or suffering from certain medical conditions.

Sick horses require specialized nutritional management that varies depending on the illness or condition of the animal. More common ailments that veterinarians and technicians need to make dietary adjustments for include gastrointestinal disorders (mainly colic), laminitis, Cushing syndrome, insulin resistance, liver dysfunction, kidney dysfunction, respiratory disease, and starvation or emaciation among others. In some cases, parenteral or enteral nutrition are required, although these methods are not preferable to providing nutrients and calories through traditional oral feeding methods, if the horse will voluntarily eat. It is important to attempt to treat horses with different ailments on an individual basis, while both following currently recommended guidelines and remaining somewhat creative and flexible to help return the horse to health.

Gastrointestinal Disorders

Gastrointestinal disorders in horses can be categorized into disorders of the small intestine (i.e., enteropathies, malabsorption, small intestine resection, etc.) and large intestine (i.e., colitis, diarrhea, impaction, colon resection, etc.). For small intestinal disorders, enhancing hindgut fermentation and digestion should be emphasized. Feeding highly digestible fiber sources, such as beet pulp, certain fibrous by-products (soybean hulls, oat

hulls, wheat middlings), and quality alfalfa, will help to optimize this process. Horses with 50% small intestine resection have been successfully maintained on diets containing fermentable fibers and fat from oil and rice bran sources (Geor 2000). Horses with 70% distal small intestine resection have been successfully maintained on small feedings of complete (highly fibrous) pelleted feeds (Lewis 1995).

For large intestinal disorders, enhancing small intestine digestion should be emphasized. Unfortunately, many horses with large intestinal disorders suffer from complications with diarrhea and poor appetites, which require the horse to be maintained through enteral nutrition at first (Geor 2000). As soon as the horse is stabilized however, protein, carbohydrate, and fat should be provided through highly digestible grain sources. Fermentable fibers for proper hindgut health should also be fed as the horse's health improves. In cases of colon resection, vitamin production may be compromised, requiring supplementation of B-complex and K vitamins. Probiotic supplementation may be helpful in reestablishing hindgut microflora, although research in horses has not yet demonstrated efficacy.

With gastric ulcers affecting approximately 58% of show horses (McClure, et al. 1999) and an even larger percentage of racehorses (Murray, et al. 1989), horses suffering from gastric ulcers that also present with poor performance, appetite, poor hair coat, and such should be treated appropriately. In one study, inclusion of alfalfa hay in the diet appeared to have a protective buffering affect on nonglandular mucosa of the stomach (Nadeau, et al. 1999). Therefore, alfalfa hay given at 5- to 6-hour intervals has been recommended (Rich and Breuer 2002). Omeprazole treatment (GastroGard) has also been found to be effective and should be employed when necessary (Andrews, et al. 1999).

Laminitis

Laminitis can be caused by overconsumption of sugar and starches from concentrated meals or grasses; however it may also be a result of trauma, disease, or other factors. Feeding the horse with acute laminitis may be difficult if the horse's appetite is poor due to the painful condition. It is important not to starve laminitic horses but to provide nutrients through hays, vitamin and mineral supplements, and fat if necessary. Higher starch grain components of the diet should be eliminated. Obese horses are prone to laminitis, and slow weight loss should be a goal with these horses. There has been much consideration lately of the sugar, starch, and fructan concentrations of hays fed to laminitic horses. Some types of hays (grown under extreme conditions) may not be appropriate for laminitic horses due to their high starch and sugar content, and therefore, questionable hays may be tested for starch and sugar content before feeding them to horses with laminitis. Some preliminary research (Cottrell, et al. 2005) suggests that soaking hay may reduce starch and sugar content and may therefore be used to further decrease total carbohydrates in the diet.

Cushing disease caused by pituitary adenoma or dysfunction causes an increased risk of laminitis, and many horses with this condition also exhibit insulin resistance. Horses may also exhibit insulin resistance independent of Cushing disease, which is frequently correlated with obesity. The nutritional management of these horses is the same as with laminitic horses. Sugars and starches from grains and pasture grasses should be restricted in the diet. Quality hay and low-sugar and starch feedstuffs (e.g., non-molassed beet pulp, ration balancer pellets, low starch fat supplements) may be used to formulate the ration.

Liver Problems

Liver disease may compromise hepatic gluconeogenesis; therefore, diets should contain highly digestible starch sources to aid in the maintenance of glucose homeostasis (Lewis 1995). With acute hepatic failure, hepatoencephalopathy with neurologic signs may occur. Humans with this condition have benefited from diets higher in branched chain amino acids (i.e., leucine, isoleucine, and valine) and lower in aromatic amino acids. Horses, therefore, with this condition may also benefit from such a diet. Feeds such as ground corn cobs and

sorghum are appropriate, whereas legume hays, oats, and soybeans should be avoided (Lewis 1995). Grass hay may be fed as the fiber source (Geor 2000). Overall, horses with liver disease should have a low-to-moderate protein diet to help decrease problems with converting ammonia to urea that goes along with the condition (Geor 2000). Horses with hepatic failure may also benefit from daily oral B-complex vitamins and ascorbic acid because the liver is the site of niacin and vitamin C synthesis.

Kidney Problems

A reduction in kidney function as the result of disease can cause an increase in renal and bladder calculi, as well as a potentially lethal increase in blood calcium (Lewis 1995). Furthermore, phosphorus excretion may be impaired, and sodium deficits may develop as a result of poor renal conservation (Geor 2000). Therefore, feeds high in protein, calcium, and phosphorus (e.g., legumes, soybeans, wheat bran, and supplements containing calcium and phosphorus) should be avoided. On the other hand, hypoproteinemia can also develop in horses with renal failure in some cases, and protein supplementation may be necessary in this condition (Geor 2000). If an increase in energy density of the diet is required, calories can be provided by fat supplementation.

Respiratory Problems

Horses suffering from inflammatory airway disease or chronic obstructive pulmonary disease are sensitive to airborne allergens (i.e., mold, dust, fungi) and toxins (Geor 2000). Thoughtful management of these cases is critical to the health and comfort of the horse. Many horses do well living outside, removed from the dusty, poor ventilation of barns. Dust-free feeds and bedding should be used, as should countermeasures to reduce allergen and toxin exposure to these horses. For example, shredded paper or pellet bedding may be favorable, whereas sweeping and blowing barn aisles while affected horses are in the barn should be avoided. Some horses suffering from respiratory disease are intolerant to any type of hay and do well on a complete pelleted or beet pulp-based feed. Other horses may be able to tolerate hay or hay cubes that are soaked thoroughly before being offered to the horse.

Starvation and Neglect

In contrast to sick or postsurgical horses that may be in a hypermetabolic state, horses suffering from neglect in the form of emaciation or starvation are in a hypometabolic state. Undernutrition has detrimental effects on immune function, digestive tract health (especially enterocyte function and health), overall healing, and nutrient stores. Horses suffering from malnutrition may also suffer from hyperlipidemia, especially ponies and miniature horses. Increased plasma triglycerides, free fatty acids, and glycerol accompanied by cloudy serum or plasma and fatty infiltration of the liver and kidneys are hallmarks of the condition (Lewis 1995). Aggressive nutritional therapy is required in these cases and recovery is difficult.

If starved horses are willing and metabolically stable enough to eat on their own, Stull (2003) recommends the following program:

Days 1 to 3: Feed 0.45 kg (1 lb) of leafy alfalfa every 4 hours (2.72 kg/day or 6 lb/day) in six feedings.

Days 4 to 10: Slowly increase the amount of alfalfa and decrease the number of feedings so that by day 6 you are feeding just over 1.81 kg (4 lb) of hay every 8 hours (total of 5.896 kg or 13 lb/day in three feedings).

Day 10 to several months: Feed as much alfalfa as the horse will eat and decrease feeding to twice per day. Provide access to salt block. Do not feed grain or supplemental material until the horse returns to normal.

All changes should be made slowly and with extremely close monitoring of the sick horse. Sudden change from a poor-quality diet to a high-quality, digestible diet can cause death in starved horses within 3 to 5 days. Complications with mineral and electrolyte depletion and sequestering, along with laminitis and diarrhea are common problems when refeeding starved horses (Witham and Stull 1998).

Enteral and Parenteral Nutrition

For horses that are not healthy enough to voluntarily eat, enteral or parenteral nutrition may be employed. These methods are not preferred over encouraging the horse to eat via natural methods, but nevertheless are necessary in some situations. Enteral and parenteral nutrition, therefore, should be used for the least amount of time necessary to help the animal return to health.

Enteral nutrition via nasogastric tube has been used in hospital settings with varied success. Oral liquid diets formulated for human use have been used in horses, but these diets do not contain appropriate fiber and increase the risk of laminitis and colitis (Buechner-Maxwell, et al. 2003). Pellet slurries (alfalfa pellets) administered along with dextrose, amino acids, and oil helped to maintain horses' weight but also increase the risk of diarrhea and laminitis (Naylor, Freeman, and Kronfeld, 1984). The Naylor diet appears to be the most widely accepted for enteral nutrition and is composed of 454 g (1 lb) alfalfa meal, 204 g (0.5 lb) casein, 204 g (0.5 lb) dextrose, 52 g (0.11 lb) electrolyte mixture, and 5 L (1.321 gal) of water (Naylor 1977). The DE of this mixture is 2.77 Mcal, and therefore should be administered six times per day to meet the maintenance requirements of a 500-kg (1,100-lb) adult horse that requires approximately 16.4 Mcal/day DE. A pellet-vegetable oil slurry diet consisting of 454 g (1 lb) pelleted complete feed, 50 ml (1.69 oz) corn oil, and 2 to 3 L (0.528–0.793 gal) of water (1.76 Mcal DE per mixture) has also been used with some success (Geor 2000).

Unfortunately, enteral nutrition can often be problematic. Trauma resulting from the repeated passage of the tube and complications with indwelling tubes make this form of nutritional support challenging. Pellet slurries become lodged easily in the nasogastric tubes (even after initial blender grinding), and large amounts of water are needed to reduce the viscosity of the mixture (Geor 2000).

Parenteral nutrition is also an option and should be considered immediately if the horse suffers from ileus, shock, or peritonitis that prevents oral ingestion of feed (White n.d.). Horses with anterior enteritis or recovering from surgical correction of strangulation obstruction should also be initially provided nutrients via parenteral nutrition (Geor 2000). Glucose-containing fluids (i.e., 5% dextrose solution) are typically, used and are administered at a rate of 2 L (0.528 gallons) per hour and provide approximately 8 Mcal DE. Horses should be closely monitored for hyperglycemia and glucosuria, which requires a decrease in the rate of glucose administration (Geor 2000) and consideration of treatment with insulin (White, n.d.). It is recommended that intravenous glucose not be used as the sole source of nutrition for more than 2 to 3 days (Geor 2000). A mixture of glucose and amino acids may also be used, with inclusion of lipids in parenteral diets when insulin resistance is present (White, n.d.).

Appetite

Stimulating appetite in sick horses is a major goal postoperatively and during sickness to encourage voluntary oral ingestion of nutrients and to lessen the chances of reliance on enteral or parenteral nutritional support. It has been suggested that if an animal consumes at least 85% of optimal intake, no other nutritional support is required (Donahue 1992). Foremost, because pain or fever will certainly depress appetite, appropriate treatment with nonsteroidal anti-inflammatory drugs (e.g., phenylbutazone or flunixin meglumine) may help restore or improve feed intake (Geor 2000). Furthermore, "cafeteria style" feeding may be used to help stimulate appetite by offering novel and highly palatable feed stuffs (e.g., fresh grass, mashes, succulents, and molasses-based feeds), while keeping in mind individual horses' tolerability for certain types of feeds. Feeding a horse in the presence of other horses or feeding a horse with a decreased appetite shortly after feeding other horses in view (so the horse can see other horses excited and anticipating feed intake) may help to stimulate appetite and encourage additional intake.

Obesity

Obesity is a common problem in horses, with the United States Department of Agriculture (USDA) reporting as many as 4.5% of the equine population as overweight or obese (National Animal Health Monitoring System [NAHMS] 1998). Additionally, obesity can be related to complications of insulin resistance and devastating laminitis.

One study showed that horses with a body condition score of 7 or greater had a reduced insulin sensitivity to a higher sugar or starch feed (Hoffman, et al. 2003). Furthermore, obese ponies are less tolerant of a glucose load than normal weight ponies and standardbred horses (Jeffcott, et al. 1986). Hence, research suggests that overweight and obese horses (body condition score [BCS] >7) have a compromised ability to handle a glucose load. Research on a direct link between obesity and laminitis is not well documented, but widely accepted, especially because many horses that founder also tend to be overweight.

The main goal of managing the obese horse is to create a caloric deficit via exercise and carefully measured feed intake. Horses should be offered 1% to 1.5% body weight in moderate-quality grass hay and supplemental feed per day depending on size of horse or a specific weight control diet to balance the ration. Care should be taken not to feed rich, calorically dense hay because some horses can gain or maintain weight on small amounts of rich hay. Hay and grain should be measured to determine accurate allotments. Dry lot turnout or turnout with a grazing muzzle should be employed to limit pasture intake until appropriate weight loss is achieved. A dietary maintenance program should be followed once the horse loses weight to prevent pounds from being regained.

The horse should also undergo an incremental exercise program of significant vigor to burn calories, provided they are sound. An exercise plan of riding, longeing, or driving should be thoughtfully put together and strictly adhered to. Devices such as heart rate monitors and motorized "Equi-ciser" machines can be used to make sure horses are sufficiently "working," but they may not be available or used by many horse owners. Weight loss should

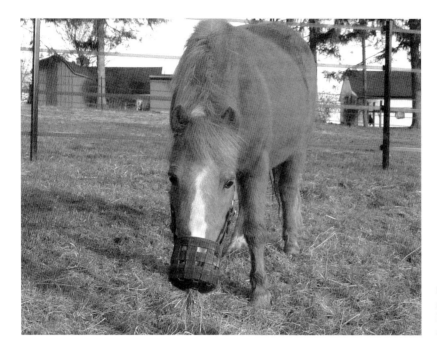

Figure 2.10. Turnout with a grazing muzzle can help restrict pasture and hay intake for horses and ponies that are prone to obesity.

be slow and steady to prevent problems with hyperlipemia (especially in ponies) (Jeffcott and Field 1985) and may take several months. Horses should be monitored with weight tapes and repeated body condition scoring weekly to adjust diet and exercise regimens appropriately.

Interestingly, keeping a horse physically fit and trim may be the best tool for staving off obesity and insulin resistance. In a study (Gordon, et al. 2007) comparing fit, standardbred racehorses, to their unfit, sedentary counterparts, the fit horses had hormone concentrations reflective of increased insulin sensitivity versus the unfit horses. This was evident despite the fit horses receiving large amounts of high NSC grain that some have suggested will lead to insulin resistance.

Metabolic Syndrome

Horse owners should work closely with their veterinarian if they suspect equine metabolic syndrome (EMS) because the condition is still being characterized. Horses that are diagnosed with EMS should be carefully managed. Because many EMS horses have a reduced glucose tolerance, a diet low in non-

structural carbohydrates may be of benefit. Presumably, a diet lower in NSC will blunt the glucose and insulin response to the diet, in hopes to not overload or exacerbate the ongoing problem with reduced glucose tolerance. Additionally, if the horse requires supplementation beyond hay and a small amount (0.454–0.908 kg or 1–2 lb) of supplemental pellets, the meals of concentrate should be broken up into many smaller meals throughout the day. Research is showing that rate of consumption and amount fed per meal are related to glucose and insulin responses to meals (Gordon, et al. 2008). The length of fasting time between meals may also impact responses (Gordon and McKeever, 2005) and should be kept to a minimum if possible. There have been arbitrary recommendations for total dietary NSC to be less than 12% to 15%; however, there are little data to back up a definitive number at this time. Some horses seem to be able to tolerate a 20% to 25% total NSC diet, whereas others fair better on less than 15%. Care should be taken when trying to get NSC very low (<10%). Horses in one research study on very low NSC diets (≤10% NSC) were found to be prone to colic, perhaps due to large amounts of undigestible fiber in the diet required to meet a 10% NSC requirement (Purina Mills research, Longview Animal Nutrition Center). Therefore, at this point, the goal is to provide feeds of lower NSC content than typical sweetfeeds, in ways that slow intake and provide more of a "grazing" scenario. For EMS horses requiring weight loss, they can be fed a diet as previously described for the obese horse. For horses requiring more calories, grass hay and a low NSC feed may be used. Pasture intake should be limited by time or availability via a dry lot or grazing muzzle. Under certain growing conditions, pasture can be very high in sugar content (Hoffman, et al. 2001) that is inappropriate for horses with metabolic conditions such as EMS.

There is some question regarding the NSC content of hays. The Dairy One Forage Laboratory reports an average NSC content of 13% for grass hay with a range of 8% to 18% (dry matter basis). Their database also reports an NSC content of 10% to 11% for legume hay/alfalfa cubes (with a range of 7% to 14%). Alfalfa hay is more calorically dense than grass hay and should be used judiciously as part of a ration so not to feed too many calories to the horse. A diet consisting mostly of hay is appropriate for the EMS horse because it is ingested slowly and results in a low glucose and insulin response to feeding.

Some hays (grown under extreme weather conditions) test higher in NSC and may not be suitable for the EMS horse. Soaking hay in water (approximately 30 minutes) can also reduce its sugar content (Cottrell, et al. 2005), as well as, decrease its palatability, resulting in a slower rate of intake. Caution should be taken when attempting to purchase very low NSC hay. Cool season hays with a quite low NSC content (<8%) were also poor quality, which could lead to an increased risk for digestive upset.

Supplements for Insulin-Related Issues

There have been anecdotal reports of horses doing well on diets containing supplementation of chromium, magnesium, or cinnamon. The recommendation of using these additives stems from human, as well as, some animal model research. An interesting review of chromium, magnesium, and

antioxidant supplementation for human diabetics deemed that there is insufficient clinical evidence at this time to warrant these supplements as a complement to treatment for diabetes (Guerroro-Romero and Rodriguez-Moran 2005). As for equine research, Ott and Kivipelto (1999) fed chromium to yearling horses and showed an increased glucose clearance in the supplemented group, yet no change in insulin sensitivity. Cartmill, et al. (2005) found that dietary chromium supplementation had no effect on glucose dynamics or insulin sensitivity in mature horses with high body condition scores and hyperinsulinemia. Although a small body of research suggests that cinnamon extracts may alter glucose metabolism in rats (Verspohl, et al. 2005), a recent study demonstrated no change in whole body insulin sensitivity or response to an oral glucose tolerance test in human subjects receiving cinnamon supplementation (Vanschoonbeek, et al. 2006).

Furthermore, at this time, cinnamon and chromium are not approved feed additives for horses, and therefore, cannot be legally included in formulated feeds. For magnesium, horses receiving balanced rations have little trouble meeting the NRC requirements for this mineral. Overall, this is not to say that certain supplements may not have a beneficial effect for some horses. However, at this time, there is not enough scientific evidence to completely support their use. Hopefully, research in this area will clarify if, how, and when these supplements may be of benefit. For now, focusing on feeding balanced rations and maintaining a healthy body condition score with a low NSC diet should be paramount.

Insulin Resistance

Although the conditions discussed thus far (e.g., obesity, EMS) may have the complication or symptom of reduced insulin sensitivity, the question arises if the conditions can be mutually exclusive. Is it possible for horses to be insulin resistant without also being obese or having other symptoms (e.g., regional adiposity, endocrine abnormalities, or laminitis)? It seems that some horses naturally become less insulin sensitive as they age, but that does not necessarily mean the horse has metabolic syndrome or is obese. Data on this topic in horses is scarce and research needs to be conducted to answer such questions. One of the foremost issues that should be addressed is a well-accepted definition and diagnostic test for insulin resistance. A broad definition of insulin resistance that can be found in the literature is that insulin resistance is the diminished ability of cells to respond to the action of insulin in transporting glucose from the blood stream into muscle and other tissues. This definition, unfortunately, is broad and does not help to decipher horses that respond to insulin in varying degrees. Work should be performed to further define extents of insulin resistance, so that horses can be categorized and risk factors for developing "true" insulin resistance can be created. Furthermore, there is debate over the appropriate and most beneficial diagnostic test for determining insulin resistance in horses. These testing protocols

are reviewed elsewhere (Hoffman, et al. 2003), and certain tests (e.g., minimal model testing, grain challenges) need to be selected depending on the variables of the research and the outcome being measured.

Whether the horse is insulin due to obesity, EMS, age, or some other condition, feeding management is similar to the previous recommendations. The goal of the feeding program is to blunt glucose and insulin response to meals in an effort not to exacerbate the insulin resistance state. Feeding a diet low in NSC by using long stem hay and low NSC feeds will help to achieve this goal. Concentrated meals should be split into as many feedings as possible to further mitigate hormonal and biochemical responses. Pasture grasses can be quite high in sugar (Hoffman, et al. 2001), so turnout on pasture should be limited with a grazing muzzle or eliminated from the insulin resistant horse's diet.

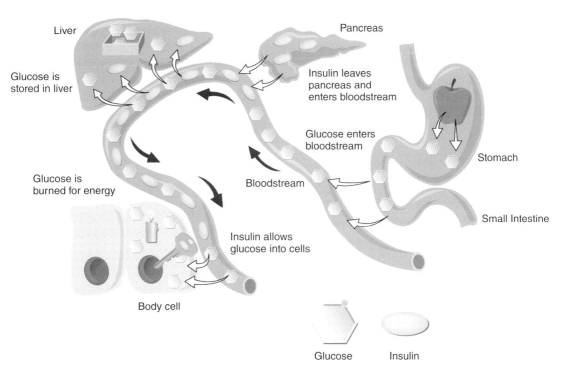

Figure 2.11. Simplified pictorial of glucose and insulin metabolism in the horse.

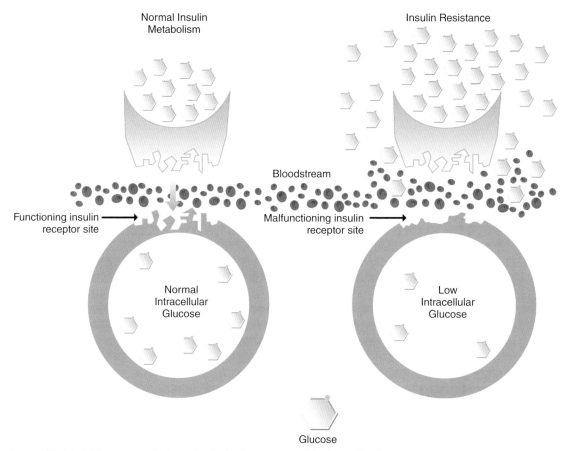

Normal Insulin
Metabolism

Insulin Resistance

Bloodstream

Functioning insulin
receptor site

Malfunctioning insulin
receptor site

Normal
Intracellular
Glucose

Low
Intracellular
Glucose

Glucose

Figure 2.12. Potential theory of causative factor related to insulin resistance, involving damaged insulin receptors.

Exercise is extremely important for managing horses with reduced insulin sensitivity. Exercise increases the transport of glucose into muscle cells by independently stimulating the transfer of glut-4 protein to the cell surface for glucose uptake (Lacombe, et al. 2003). Studies in horses have shown that exercise can improve insulin sensitivity, even with only three to five 30-minute sessions per week (Malinowski, et al. 2002; Powell, et al. 2002).

The parameters to measure include blood glucose, insulin, and triglycerides, as well as, body condition scoring. These tests can be conducted relatively easily in the field by clinicians. Research studies looking into the risk factors and mechanisms responsible for laminitis have increased in the past

few years. Hypotheses examined have centered on theories of inflammation, circulatory disruption, toxicity, and metabolic disturbances, among others (Bailey, et al. 2004; Field and Jeffcott 1989). With time, quality research should continue to elucidate mechanisms behind and appropriate treatments for this devastating illness.

Horses with acute laminitis are often in too much pain to eat. In this case, carefully administering oil via a syringe can provide some calories for a short period of time, although obviously not ideal. Extreme cases may require hospitalization where parenteral nutrition can be used if necessary. As the horse is recovering, one recommendation has been to feed only poor-quality hay and no grain whatsoever. Caution should be taken to not feed hay that is so poor quality that it leads to digestive upset or severe nutrient deficits. Laminitic horses should not be starved in an effort to stabilize the condition. A low NSC total diet, fed in small increments, as described previously is appropriate. Attention should be paid to nutrients that will help in the recovery process including protein to prevent muscle wasting and proper mineral fortification to support hoof regrowth. Some horses with a history of laminitis appear to fair better at lower body condition score of 4. A slow, progressive weight loss or weight gain program will help to accomplish this.

Pituitary Pars Intermedia Dysfunction (Cushing Disease)

Horses with pars intermedia pituitary adenomas have a resulting endocrine disorder of hyperadrenocorticism. This condition is also known as equine Cushing disease or pituitary pars intermedia dysfunction (PPID). Symptoms and biochemical alterations as a result of this disease include hirsutism, endocrine disruptions (e.g., insulin resistance, elevated endogenous cortisol, elevated hyperadrenocorticoid hormone, low thyroid hormone concentrations, among others), laminitis, polyuria/polydipsia, and weight loss (McCue 2002). Diagnosing the condition can sometimes be difficult, with several methods employed such as (a) measurement of resting plasma adrenocorticotropic (ACTH) concentrations, (b) an overnight dexamethasone suppression test, or (c) a combination dexamethasone suppression test, along with a thyrotropin-releasing hormone (TRH) stimulation test (Dybdal, et al. 1994; Eiler, et al. 1997). The suggested gold standard for diagnosis is histopathologic detection of a pituitary adenoma, but this method can only be used postmortem (Couetil, et al. 1996). Owners caring for horses with Cushing disease must work closely with their veterinarian to determine appropriate medical management of the horse. Many horses are stabilized with medication and proper management.

Feeding the horse with Cushing syndrome is similar to feeding horses with insulin resistance, EMS, or obesity as outlined previously. Horses pharmacologically treated for Cushing disease with a dopamine agonist (Pergolide) may suffer from inappetence. In these cases, it is important not to offer large amounts of high NSC feeds (i.e., sweetfeeds) that may entice the horse's appetite. Feeding smaller amounts of a low NSC feed or fresh grass, feeding in the presence of other horses, and keeping to a strictly timed feeding schedule may help in these cases. Maintenance of a healthy body condition score (ideal is 5) is very important and should be strived for.

Extensive mineral supplementation (i.e., magnesium, chromium, and specific chelated minerals) has been anecdotally recommended for horses with Cushing disease. There have been no published, peer reviewed bodies of research to support this recommendation at this time. Horse owners should beware of supplement companies making sensational claims to cure laminitis or Cushing disease with their products.

Conclusion

In summary, there are many factors to take into consideration when determining the proper way to feed horses. Keeping in mind the nature of the horse's digestive physiology, balancing forages with concentrate feeds properly formulated for specific stages of life and condition, and making special considerations for horses with medical needs will help to enhance the health and well-being of the horse. For further assistance, please refer to the References and Further Reading.

Acknowledgments

The authors would like to thank Jennifer Streltsova for her assistance with the preparation of this manuscript.

References and Further Reading

Andrews, F. M., R. L. Sifferman, W. Bernard, F. E. Hughes, J. E. Holste, C. P. Daurio, R. Alva, and J. L. Cox. 1999. Efficacy of omeprazole paste in the treatment and prevention of gastric ulcers in horses. *Equine Vet J Suppl* 29:81–86.

Bailey, S. R., C. M. Marr, and J. Elliott. 2004. Current research and theories on the pathogenesis of acute laminitis in the horse. *Vet J* 167:129–42.

Brinkso, S. P., D. D. Varner, C. L. Love, T. L. Blanchard, B. C. Day, and M. E. Wilson. 2005. Effect of feeding a DHA-enriched nutriceutical on the quality of fresh, cooled, and frozen stallion semen. *Theriogenology* 63:1519–27.

Buechner-Maxwell, V. A., C. D. Elvinger, M. J. Murray, N. A. White, and D. K. Rooney. 2003. Physiologic response of normal adult horses to a low-residue liquid diet. *J Equine Vet Sci* 23:310–17.

Cartmill, J. A., D. L. Thompson, Jr., W. A. Storer, N. K. Huff, and C. A. Waller. 2005. Effects of chromium supplementation on plasma insulin and leptin in horses with elevated concentrations of leptin. *Equine Science Society, Nineteenth Symposium Proceedings*, Tucson, Arizona, p. 352 (abstract).

Coenen, M., and H. Meyer. 1987. Water and electrolyte content of the equine gastrointestinal tract in dependence on ration type. *Proceedings of the Tenth Equine Nutrition and Physiology Society Symposium* pp. 531–36.

Cottrell, E., K. Watts, and S. Ralston. 2005. Soluble sugar content and glucose/insulin responses can be reduced by soaking chopped hay in water. *Equine Science Society, Nineteenth Symposium Proceedings*, Tucson, Arizona, p. 293 (abstract).

Couetil, L., Paradis, M. R., and Knoll, J. 1996. Plasma adrenocorticotropin concentration in healthy horses and in horses with clinical signs of hyperadrenocorticism. *J Vet Intern Med* 10:1–6.

Cymbaluk, N. F. 1990. Cold housing effects on growth and nutrient demand of young horses. *J Anim Sci* 68:3152–62.

Cymbaluk, N. F., and G. I. Christison. 1989. Effects of diet and climate on growing horses. *J Anim Sci* 67:48–59.

Cymbaluk, N. F., and G. I. Christison. 1990. Environmental effects on thermoregulation and nutrition of horses. *Vet Clin North Am Equine Pract* 6:355–72.

Davison, K. E., G. D. Potter, L. W. Greene, J. W. Evans, and W. C. MacMullan. 1991. Lactation and reproductive performance of mares fed added dietary fat during late gestation and early lactation. *J Equine Vet Sci* 11:111–15.

Donahue, S. 1992. Nutritional support of hospitalized animals. *J Am Vet Med Assoc* 200:612–15.

Dybdal, N. O., K. M. Hargreaves, J. E. Madigan, D. H. Gribble, P. C. Kennedy, and G. H. Stabenfeldt. 1994. Diagnostic testing for pituitary pars intermedia dysfunction in horses. *J Am Vet Med Assoc* 204:627–32.

Eiler, H., J. W. Oliver, F. M. Andrews, K. A. Fecteau, E. M. Green, and M. McCracken. 1997. Results of a combined dexamethasone suppression/thyrotropin-releasing hormone stimulation test in healthy horses and horses suspected to have a pars intermedia pituitary adenoma. *J Am Vet Med Assoc* 211:79–81.

Field, J. R., and L. B. Jeffcott. 1989. Equine laminitis—another hypothesis for pathogenesis. *Med Hypotheses* 30:203–10.

Geor, R. J. 2000. Nutritional support of the sick adult horse. *World Equine Vet Rev* 5(12):14–22.

Gibbs, P.G., and K.E. Davison. 1991. A field study on reproductive efficiency of mares maintained predominately on native pasture. *Proceedings of the Twelfth Equine Nutrition and Physiology Society Symposium*, Calgary, Alberta, pp. 71–76.

Gibbs, P. G., G. D. Potter, G. T. Schelling, J. L. Kreider, and C. L. Boyd. 1988. Digestion of hay protein in different segments of the equine digestive tract. *J Anim Sci* 66:400.

Gibbs, P. G., G. D. Potter, and B. D. Scott. (2007, November 12). Feeding the arena performance horse. Retrieved from Animal Computer Science Labs Web site: www.anslab.iastate.edu.

Gibbs, P. G., D. H. Sigler, and T. B. Goehring. 1989. Influence of diet on growth and development of yearling horses. *J Equine Vet Sci* 9(4):215.

Gordon, M.E., M. L. Jerina, S. L. King, K. E. Davison, J. K. Young, and R. H. Raub. 2008. The effects of nonstructural carbohydrate content and feeding rate on glucose and insulin response to meal feeding in Equine. *J Equine Vet Sci* 27:489–93.

Gordon, M. E., and K. H. McKeever. 2005. Diurnal variation of ghrelin, leptin, and adiponectin in Standardbred mares. *J Anim Sci* 83:2365–71.

Gordon, M. E., K. H. McKeever, C. L. Betros, and H. C. Manso Filho. 2007. Plasma leptin, ghrelin and adiponectin concentrations in young fit racehorses versus mature unfit standardbreds. *Vet J* 173:91–100.

Guerroro-Romero, F., and M. Rodriguez-Moran. 2005. Complementary therapies for diabetes: the case for chromium, magnesium and antioxidants. *Arch Med Res* 36:250–57.

Harris, M. A., C. R. Anderson, S. K. Webel, R. Godbee, S. R. Sanders, W. A. Schurg, L. H. Baumgard, and M. J. Arns. 2005. Effects of feeding an omega-3 rich supplement on the fatty acid composition and motion characteristics of stallion spermatozoa. *Equine Science Society, Nineteenth Symposium Proceedings*, Tucson, Arizona, p.239.

Harris, M. A., L. H. Baumgard, M. J. Arns, and S. K. Webel. 2005. Stallion spermatozoa membrane phospholipid dynamics following dietary n-3 supplementation. *Anim Reprod Sci* 89(1–4): 234–37.

Henneke, D. G., G.D. Potter, and J. L. Kreider. 1984. Body condition during pregnancy and lactation and reproductive efficiency in mares. *Theriogenology* 21: 897–909.

Henneke, D. G., G. D. Potter, J. L. Kreider, and B. Yates. 1983. Relationship between condition score, physical measurements and body fat percentage in mares. *Equine Vet J* 15:371–72.

Hintz, H. F. 1975. Digestive physiology of the horse. *J S Afr Vet Assoc* 46(1):13.

Hoffmann, R. M., R. C. Boston, D. Stefanowski, D. S. Kronfeld, and P. A. Harris. 2003. Obesity and diet affect glucose dynamics and insulin sensitivity in Thoroughbred geldings. *J Anim Sci* 81:2333–42.

Hoffman, R. M., J. A. Wilson, D. S. Kronfeld, W. L. Cooper, L. A. Lawrence, D. Sklan, and P. A. Harris. 2001. Hydrolyzable carbohydrates in pasture, hay, and horse feeds: direct assay and seasonal variation. *J Anim Sci* 79:500–6.

Hoyt, J. K., G. D. Potter, L. W. Greene, and J. G. Anderson. 1995. Mineral balance in resting and exercised miniature horses. *J Equine Vet Sci.* 15(7):310.

Jeffcott, L. B., and J. R. Field. 1985. Current concepts of hyperlipemia in horses and ponies. *Vet Rec* 116:461–66.

Jeffcott, L. B., J. R. Field, J. G. McLean, and K. O'Dea. 1986. Glucose tolerance and insulin sensitivity in ponies and Standardbred horses. *Equine Vet J* 18:97–101.

Klendshoj, C., G. D. Potter, R. E. Lichtnewalner, and D. D. Householder. 1979. Nitrogen digestion in the small intestine of horses fed crimped or micronized sorghum grain or oats. *Proceedings of the Sixth Equine Nutrition and Physiology Society Symposium*, p. 91.

Kubiak, J. R., J. W. Evans, G. D. Potter, P. G. Harms, and W. L. Jenkins. 1988. Parturition in the multiparous mare fed to obesity. *J Equine Vet Sci* 8:233–38.

Lacombe, V. A., K. W. Hinchcliff, and S. T. Devor. 2003. Effects of exercise and glucose administration on content of insulin-sensitive glucose transporter in equine skeletal muscle. *Am J Vet Res* 64:1500–6.

Lewis, L. D. 1995. *Sick Horse Feeding and Nutritional Support. Equine Clinical Nutrition.* Baltimore: Lea and Febiger.

Lewis, L. D. 1996. *Feeding and Care of the Horse.* 2nd ed. Philadelphia: Lippincott Williams & Wilkins.

Malinowski, K., C. L. Betros, L. Flora, C. F. Kearns, and K. H. McKeever. 2002. Effect of training on age-related changes in plasma insulin and glucose. *Equine Vet J Suppl* 34:147–53.

McClure, S. R., L. T. Glickman, and N. W. Glickman. 1999. Prevalence of gastric ulcers in show horses. *J Am Vet Med Assoc* 215:1130–33.

McCue, P. M. 2002. Equine Cushing's disease. *Vet Clin North Am Equine Pract.* 18:533–43.

McDonald, P., R. A. Edwards, J. F. D. Greenhalgh, and C. A. Morgan. 1995. *Animal Nutrition.* 5th ed. Singapore: Longman Singapore Publishers Ltd.

Meyer, H. Nutrition of the equine athlete. 1987. In *Equine Exercise Physiology*, ed. J. R. Gillespie and N. E. Robinson, 644–73. Davis, CA: International Conference on Equine Exercise Physiology.

Murray, M. J., C. Grodinsky, C. W. Anderson, P. F. Radue, and G. R. Schmidt. 1989. Gastric ulcers in horses: a comparison of endoscopic findings in horses with and without clinical signs. *Equine Vet J Suppl* 7:68–72.

Nadeau, J. A., F. M. Andrews, A. G. Matthew, R. A. Argenzio, and J. T. Blackford. 1999. Implications of diet in the cause of gastric ulcer disease in horses. *Proceedings of the Equine Nutrition and Physiology Society* pp. 258–59.

National Animal Health Monitoring System. 1998. *USDA Equine 98: National Animal Health Monitoring System Equine Mortality and Morbidity Info Sheet.* Retrieved from United States Department of Agriculture, Animal and Plant Health Inspection Service Web site: www.aphis.usda.gov.

Naylor, J. M. 1977. Nutrition of the sick horse. *J Equine Med Surg* 1:64–70.

Naylor, J. M., D. E. Freeman, and D. S. Kronfeld. 1984. Alimentation of hypophagic horses. Comp Cont Educ Pract Vet 6:S93–S99.

National Research Council. 1989. *Nutrient Requirements of Horses.* 4th rev. ed. Washington DC: National Academy of Sciences, National Research Council.

———. 2007. *Nutrient Requirements of Horses.* 5th rev ed. Washington, DC: National Academy of Sciences, National Research Council.

Oldham, S. L., G. D. Potter, J. W. Evans, S. B. Smith, T. S. Taylor, and W. S. Barnes. 1990. Storage and mobilization of muscle glycogen in exercising horses fed a fat-supplemented diet. *J Equine Vet Sci* 10:353–59.

Ott, E. A., and J. Kivipelto. 1999. Influence of chromium tripicolinate on growth and glucose metabolism in yearling horses. *J Anim Sci* 77:3022–30.

Potter, G., F. Arnold, D. Householder, D. Hansen, and K. Bowen. 1992. Digestion of starch in the small or large intestine of the equine. *Pferdeheilkunde (European Conference on Horse Nutrition)*: 109–11.

Powell, D. M., S. E. Reedy, D. R. Sessions, and B. P. Fitzgerald. 2002. Effect of short- term exercise training on insulin sensitivity in obese and lean mares. *Equine Vet J Suppl* 34:81–84.

Radicke, S., E. Kienzlel, and H. Meyer. 1991. Preileal apparent digestibility of oats and cornstarch and consequences for cecal metabolism. *Proceedings of the Twelfth Equine Nutrition and Physiology Society Symposium*, Calgary, Alberta, pp. 43–48.

Reitnour, C. M., and R. L. Salsbury. 1976. Utilization of proteins by the equine species. *Am J Vet Res* 37:1065.

Rich, G. A., and L. H. Breuer. 2002. Recent developments in equine nutrition with farm and clinic applications. *Current Concepts in Equine Nutrition, AAEP Proceedings* 48:24–40.

Rich, G. A., D. E. McGlothlin, L. D. Lewis, E. L. Squires, and B. W. Pickett. 1983. Effect of Vitamin E supplementation on stallion seminal characteristics and sexual behavior. *Proceedings of Eighth Equine Nutrition and Physiology Society Symposium,* Lexington, KY, pp. 85–89.

Staniar, W. B., Kronfeld, D. S., Wilson, J. A., Lawrence, L. A., Cooper, W. L., and Harris, P. A. 2001. Growth of Thoroughbreds fed a low-protein supplement fortified with lysine and threonine. *J Anim Sci* 79:2143–51.

Stull, C. 2003. Nutrition for rehabilitating the starved horse. *J Equine Vet Sci* 23:456–59.

Topliff, D. R., G. D. Potter, J. L. Kreider, T. R. Dutson, and G. T. Jessup. 1985. Diet manipulation, muscle glycogen metabolism and anaerobic work performance in the equine. *Proceedings Ninth Equine Nutrition and Physiology Society Symposium,* East Lansing, MI, pp. 224–29.

Topliff, D. R., G. D. Potter, J. L. Kreider, and G. T. Jessup. 1983. Diet manipulation and muscle glycogen in the equine. *Proceedings of Eighth Equine Nutrition and Physiology Society Symposium,* Lexington, KY, pp. 119–24.

Vanschoonbeek, K., B. J. Thomassen, J. M. Senden, W. K. Wodzig, and L. J. van Loon. 2006. Cinnamon supplementation does not improve glycemic control in postmenopausal type 2 diabetes patients. *J Nutr* 136:977–80.

Verspohl, E. J., K. Bauer, and E. Neddermann. 2005. Antidiabetic effect of Cinnamomum cassia and Cinnamomum zeylanicum in vivo and in vitro. *Phytother Res* 19:203–6.

Webb, S. P., G. D. Potter, and J. W. Evans. 1987. Physiologic and metabolic response of race and cutting horses to added dietary fat. *Proceedings Tenth Equine Nutrition and Physiology Society Symposium,* Fort Collins, CO, pp. 115–20.

White, N. A. (n.d.). *Update on perioperative nutrition.* Retrieved from American College of Veterinary Surgeons Web site: www.acvs.org.

Whitham, C. L., and C. L. Stull. 1998. Metabolic responses of chronically starved horses to refeeding with three isoenergetic diets. *J Am Vet Assoc* 212:691–96.

Applied Anatomy and Physiology

Amanda M. House, Kira Epstein, Laura Riggs, and Kelsey A. Hart

Hematology

The blood carries oxygen, nutrients, hormones, and other essential compounds to all of the cells throughout the body. It is classified as a fluid connective tissue. Blood is made up of plasma, erythrocytes (red blood cells), leukocytes (white blood cells), and thrombocytes (platelets). *Plasma* is the liquid matrix of the blood that consists of 90% water. Most of the substances transported by blood, such as nutrients, are dissolved in the plasma. When anticoagulated (unclotted) blood is spun down in a centrifuge, the red blood cells settle out at the bottom; the white blood cells make up the buffy coat in the middle; and the yellow, transparent fluid at the top is the plasma. If clotted blood is spun in a centrifuge, then the clear yellow fluid at the top is called *serum*.

Red blood cells are known as *erythrocyte*s and have a biconcave disc shape. Their primary function is to transport hemoglobin, a red pigment that contains iron. *Hemoglobin* is the essential molecule that carries oxygen from the lungs to the tissues. The formation of erythrocytes is called *erythropoiesis*. Red blood cells are formed in myeloid tissue in the bone marrow once animals are born. *Hematopoiesis* refers to the formation of all parts of the blood, which also occurs in the bone marrow. Erythrocytes are released into the circulation and survive approximately 120 days. At the end of their life span, they are removed from the circulation and broken down by the spleen and lymph nodes. *Erythropoietin* is the hormone secreted by the kidneys that stimulates erythropoiesis (red blood cell production) in response to low oxygen levels in the blood. *Anemia* is the term for a reduced number of erythrocytes in the blood. An interesting fact about equine erythrocytes is their tendency toward *rouleaux formation*, in which the cells stack one on top of another. Rouleaux formation results in rapid sedimentation in tubes of whole blood.

Leukocytes (white blood cells) are responsible for many of the immune functions of the blood and defend the body against foreign organisms. Leukocytes are classified as either granulocytes or agranulocytes, depending on the staining characteristic of their cytoplasm. *Granulocytes* contain stained granules in their cytoplasm when viewed on a blood smear. Neutrophils (light purple to neutral granules), eosinophils (red to dark pink granules), and basophils (dark blue granules) are the three types of granulocytes. *Neutrophils*, also known as polymorphonuclear cells (many-shaped nuclei), are the most numerous white blood cell in circulation. Their primary function is as a firstline of defense against foreign invaders by engulfing (phagocytizing) microorganisms and other debris in tissues. *Eosinophils* and *basophils* are present in the blood in much smaller numbers. Eosinophils are involved in inhibiting allergic reactions and are frequently increased with parasitic infections. The function of the basophil is not entirely understood, but basophilic granules contain histamine and heparin. Histamine acts to initiate inflammation and allergic reactions, and heparin acts as an anticoagulant.

Agranulocytes are white blood cells that have clear cytoplasm. Lymphocytes and monocytes are the two types of agranulocytes in the blood. *Monocytes* are the largest leukocyte and are responsible for cleaning up cellular debris. Monocytes migrate into the tissues at sites of inflammation or infection and are called tissue macrophages. Monocytes also process antigens (molecules that stimulate an immune response) and present them on their cell membrane so that lymphocytes can destroy them. *Lymphocytes* make up the majority of agranulocytes in the blood and are the only white blood cell with no phagocytic capabilities. Three types of lymphocytes are involved in the immune response: T lymphocytes (cell-mediated immunity), B lymphocytes (antibody production), and natural killer (NK) cells (defense against some cancers and viruses). The immune response will be covered in more detail in the next section.

Thrombocytes are commonly referred to as platelets and have an essential role in blood clotting. *Thrombocytosis* (increased platelets) can be seen in horses as a consequence of inflammation. *Thrombocytopenia* is a decrease in the number of platelets and can result in problems with blood clotting. Platelets are produced by megakaryocytes in the bone marrow.

Blood coagulation (clot formation) is a complex process that requires multiple clotting factors produced by the liver, plasma proteins (prothrombin and fibrinogen), calcium, vitamin K, and platelets. Blood vessel constriction is one mechanism that can help stop bleeding. Platelets stick to blood vessel walls and stimulate clot formation, while the coagulation cascade of clotting factors and enzymes results in fibrin formation. The fibrin matrix traps platelets and produces the clot. *Disseminated intravascular coagulation (DIC)* is a consumptive coagulopathy that results in increased coagulation of the blood and subsequent depletion of clotting factors and platelets. DIC can be a consequence of sepsis and ultimately results in fatal hemorrhage in late stages.

Immunology

The immune system functions to maintain health and protect the body from potential causes of disease. Any foreign molecule or organism not recognized as "self" is referred to as an *antigen*. Immunity can be divided into natural (nonspecific) and acquired (specific) immunity. *Natural immunity* involves the tissues, cells, and processes that protect the body from anything viewed as foreign. This includes the skin, mucous membranes, and blood leukocytes responsible for phagocytosis (such as neutrophils, monocytes, and macrophages). This type of immunity is generalized and does not initiate a response against a specific antigen.

Acquired immunity involves the immune system's ability to recognize and remember antigens for future encounters and generate a specific response. Acquired immunity is divided into cell-mediated immunity and humoral immunity. *Cell-mediated immunity* is a result of T lymphocytes, which attach to and destroy antigens on the surface of foreign cells. *Humoral immunity* is a result of B lymphocytes, which transform into plasma cells and produce antibodies against specific antigens. Five types of antibodies, also called *immunoglobulins*, have been identified: immunoglobulins G (IgG), M (IgM), A (IgA), E (IgE), and D (IgD).

The Lymphatic System

The lymphatic system is the series of ducts (lymph vessels or lymphatics) that returns excess tissue fluid, also called *lymph*, to the bloodstream. It includes lymph tissue that is found throughout the body in the lymph nodes, spleen, and thymus. The lymphatic system functions to remove excess fluid and waste material from tissues, filter foreign debris and bacteria from lymph, and transport large proteins and lipids to the blood from the tissues. Lymph fluid is excess tissue fluid that leaves blood capillaries and sits in the interstitial space (between cells). Although some returns back into the capillaries, most lymph is removed by the lymphatic duct system. The *thoracic duct*, which travels from the abdomen across the thorax, is the primary lymphatic duct that drains lymph into one of the large blood vessels entering the heart. Movement of lymph fluid through the lymphatics is a result of pressure on the ducts by muscles during activity and muscle contraction. The lymphatics contain valves to prevent backflow of lymph and keep it moving toward the heart. Lymph is filtered through lymph nodes before it enters into the blood.

Lymph Nodes

Lymph nodes are small kidney-shaped structures that are located along the lymphatic duct system (Figure 3.1). Lymph nodes filter foreign material and microorganisms from the lymph before emptying it in the blood. A connective tissue capsule surrounds the lymph node and sends branches (called *trabeculae*) into the center of the node. Multiple afferent lymph vessels will enter each node; however, only one efferent vessel exits each node with filtered lymph.

The lymph node is made up of three different areas: the cortex, the paracortex, and the medulla. The *outer cortex* contains primarily B lymphocytes within primary follicles (nodules of tissue). The

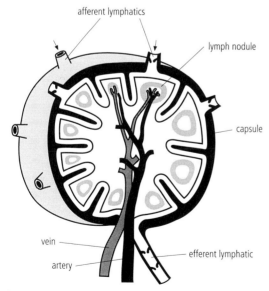

Figure 3.1. Lymph node anatomy.
Courtesy of Coumbe 2001.

paracortex is the middle layer made up of T cells and antigen-presenting cells. The *inner medulla* is the fibrous tissue "skeleton" of the lymph node, which makes up the center of the node and surrounds the follicles. It allows for lymph drainage out through the single efferent vessel.

Each region of the body has associated lymph nodes for drainage, but most are not easily palpable in the normal horse. The *submandibular lymph nodes* are palpable under the jaw within the intermandibular space and are the only readily palpable nodes in the horse. The parotid, superficial cervical, intra-abdominal (rectal palpation only), and superficial inguinal lymph nodes can only sometimes be palpated when they are enlarged. *Lymphadenopathy* is the name for enlarged or swollen lymph nodes. Lymphoid tissue (called *follicles*) is also found in the spleen and thymus. The thymus is located in the cranial mediastinum in the thoracic cavity. The thymus is involved in the differentiation of fetal T lymphocytes, but atrophies and is replaced by fat over the first year of life.

The Spleen

The spleen is a large hematopoietic organ that is located on the left side of caudal abdomen, behind the stomach and lateral to the kidney. The *nephrosplenic ligament* attaches the dorsal portion of the spleen to the left kidney. The large colon sometimes becomes trapped between the spleen and the kidney in the nephrosplenic space over this ligament, hence the term *nephrosplenic entrapment of the large colon* (also called a *left dorsal displacement*). The spleen is also attached to the stomach via the gastrosplenic ligament.

The spleen functions to store blood, remove foreign material from the blood, remove old or abnormal red blood cells, and produce lymphocytes. The spleen is made up of two types of tissue: the red pulp and the white pulp. The *red pulp* functions to store and remove red blood cells. The *white pulp* contains the localized areas of lymphoid tissue within the spleen and is responsible for the production of lymphocytes.

The Cardiovascular System

The Heart

The equine heart is a muscular organ that is located in the mediastinum primarily within the left thorax. It is responsible for pumping blood throughout the body within the circulatory system. The heart is made up of four chambers: the right atrium, the left atrium, the right ventricle, and the left ventricle. The right and left sides of the heart are separated by an interatrial and interventricular *septum*. The *atria*, which are more thin walled, receive and hold venous blood that is coming into the heart, whereas the *ventricles* act as the main pumps for blood away from the heart (Figure 3.2).

The heart is surrounded by the *pericardium*, which is a fibrous tissue covering that allows free movement of the heart within the thorax. The pericardium has two layers: the outer fibrous pericardium and the inner serous pericardium. A small volume of fluid is found between these two layers in the space called the pericardial sac. The fibrous pericar-

dium extends to the diaphragm and forms the sternopericardiac ligament. The pericardium also functions as a barrier to infection and prevents overexpansion of the ventricles during the cardiac cycle. The heart is made up of three layers:

1. The *epicardium* is the outer layer that is continuous with the serous pericardium.
2. The *myocardium* is the thick muscular layer of the heart, which produces cardiac contractions.
3. The *endocardium* is the thin membrane that lines the entire internal surface of the heart and forms the heart valves. The valves ensure unidirectional blood flow.

The *atrioventricular (AV) valves* separate the atria from the ventricles. The left and right AV valves are also called the *mitral* and *tricuspid* valves. The AV valves are attached to the heart by thin fibrous strands called *chordae tendineae*, which connect to the papillary muscles in the ventricles. These connections help prevent the valve leaflets (flaps) from everting into the atria. Blood flow out of the ventricles is controlled by the *semilunar valves*, also

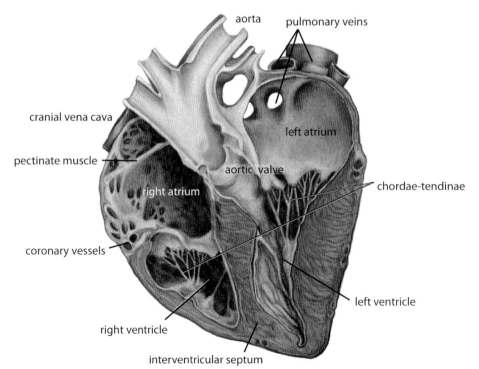

Figure 3.2. Longitudinal section anatomy of the equine heart. Courtesy of Dr. Robin Peterson.

known as the *aortic* (left-sided) and *pulmonic* (right-sided) valves. The aortic valve leads from the left ventricle into the aorta and the rest of the systemic circulation. The pulmonic valve leads from the right ventricle into the pulmonary artery and the lung circulation.

Cardiac Contraction and the Cardiac Cycle

The muscle cells of the heart are called *myocytes* and are connected to each other by *intercalated disks*. These close connections allow currents to transmit so quickly across the heart muscle that it can all contract essentially at the same time. For this reason, the heart is referred to as a functional *syncytium*. Cardiac contraction is coordinated by an internal conduction system within the heart. However, changes in heart rate are controlled by the autonomic nervous system. Parasympathetic nervous fibers in the vagus nerve slow the heart rate, and sympathetic nervous fibers increase the heart rate.

Electrical activity within the heart originates at the *sinoatrial node*, also known as the pacemaker of the heart, which is located within the wall of the right atrium. Nerve impulses spread across the right atrium and cause atrial contraction, as they move toward the *AV node* at the top of the interventricular septum. From the AV node, the nerve impulse is conducted to the *bundle of His*, which is located within the walls of the interventricular septum, and conducts the impulse to the *Purkinje system*. Purkinje fibers form a network of fast-conducting cells within the ventricular walls to enable the ventricular muscles to contract almost simultaneously.

The *cardiac cycle* represents the cyclical contraction and relaxation of the heart and has two phases. *Systole* is the phase of cardiac contraction, which generates the pressure that enables blood to be sent into the systemic and pulmonary circulation. *Diastole* is the phase of cardiac cycle when the heart is relaxed and fills with blood. The *stroke volume* is the volume of blood that is ejected by the ventricles in one beat. The *cardiac output* is the stroke volume multiplied by the heart rate, which calculates the volume of blood ejected by the heart in 1 minute. *Heart rate* is the number of times the heart beats in 1 minute, and ranges from 24 to 48 in the normal horse. *Blood pressure* is maintained through the cardiovascular system and is highest during systole (hence systolic blood pressure) and lowest during diastole (hence diastolic blood pressure).

Blood Vessels

Blood vessels enable blood flow around the body and back to the heart. Although blood vessels vary in size and thickness, essentially all vessels have three layers of tissue. The outer fibrous layer is the *tunica adventitia*. The middle layer is the *tunica media*, which consists primarily of smooth muscle and elastic tissue. The innermost layer of the blood vessel is the *tunica intima*, which is a single layer of epithelial cells known as the *endothelium*. The various blood vessels in the body are connected and allow for uninterrupted blood flow.

The *arteries* in the circulation are thick walled and elastic to allow blood flow at high pressures. Arteries carry oxygenated blood (except for the pulmonary artery, which is deoxygenated blood) away from the heart and branch into smaller arterioles. *Arterioles* connect the arteries to capillaries and affect peripheral resistance to blood flow, which can impact blood pressure. *Capillaries* are the smallest, thin-walled vessels that deliver oxygen and nutrients to the cells, as well as, collect cellular waste products. Capillary beds (networks of capillaries) are found within almost every tissue and are essential to the circulation. Diffusion of material in and out of capillaries is facilitated by their thin walls. The *capillary refill time* is an indicator of peripheral perfusion and is the amount of time it takes color to return to the mucous membranes after applying digital pressure. Normal capillary refill time is less than or equal to 2 seconds.

Capillaries combine to form *venules* on the outgoing side of the capillary bed. Venules collect deoxygenated blood and cellular waste products for return to the heart. Valves within the venules prevent backflow of blood, and these vessels are low pressure reservoirs for blood. Blood from the venules flows into larger veins and then back to the heart (Figure 3.3). The *veins* also carry deoxygenated blood, with the exception of the pulmonary vein, which carries oxygenated blood.

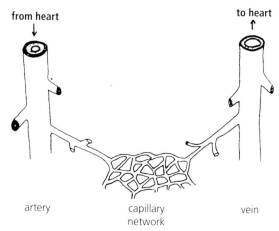

from heart   to heart

artery   capillary   vein
network

Figure 3.3. Anatomy of the peripheral circulation.
Courtesy of Coumbe 2001.

Blood Circulation

The circulatory system can be divided into the pulmonary circulation and the systemic circulation. Blood flow through the body is continuous and follows an organized circuit. Deoxygenated blood from the body enters the heart via the vena cava. The vena cava enters the right atrium, and the blood passes through the tricuspid valve into the right ventricle. Blood from the right ventricle is pumped through the pulmonary valve and into the pulmonary artery. The pulmonary artery enters the lungs for the blood to be oxygenated. The blood goes through arterioles, capillaries, venules, and finally comes back into the heart oxygenated via the pulmonary vein. This is known as the *pulmonary circulation*. The oxygenated blood travels into the left atrium, through the mitral valve, and into the left ventricle. The left ventricle pumps the blood through the aortic valve and into the aorta for delivery to the remainder of the body's tissues. The *systemic circulation* is where oxygenated blood is delivered to the tissues and deoxygenated blood is returned to the heart via the vena cava.

The Respiratory System

The function of the respiratory tract is to present air to the pulmonary circulation for gas exchange. This enables the uptake of oxygen into the circulation and the removal of carbon dioxide. Proper function of the intricate respiratory system is essential for oxygenation of all of the cells in the body.

Nostrils

The nostrils or *external nares* are large, paired openings into the respiratory tract, which, in the horse, are also quite flexible allowing increased airflow during exercise. The *alar cartilages*, present in the dorsal and lateral margins, provide support to the nares. Just inside the nostril, the skin meets the nasal mucosa at the *mucocutaneous junction*. The opening of the nasolacrimal duct is present at the ventral aspect of this junction and is a source of moisture within the nares. Beyond the opening, the nostril is divided into dorsal and ventral portions by the *alar fold*. The dorsal portion forms a 10-cm, hair-lined blind pouch known as the *false nostril* or *nasal diverticulum*.

Nasal Cavity

The nasal cavities extend from the nostrils to the nasopharynx. They are constricted spaces, when compared to the spacious nostrils, and are divided into two along the midline by the nasal septum. The lateral walls of the nasal cavity contain the dorsal and ventral turbinate bones, also called *conchae*, which are covered with a highly vascular mucosa. The conchae divide the nasal cavity into three parts: the dorsal, middle, and ventral meatuses. The widest of the three, the ventral meatus, is used for passage of nasogastric tubes and endoscopes. The dorsal concha forms the *ethmoturbinates* at the caudal aspect of the nasal cavity. The turbinates contain odor sensory cells, which transmit information to the brain via the olfactory nerve (cranial nerve [CN] I) producing the sense of smell (Figure 3.4).

Paranasal Sinuses

The paranasal sinuses are paired air-filled structures within the bones of the skull. There are seven paired sinuses: the *rostral* and *caudal maxillary*, the *frontal*, the *ventral* and *dorsal conchal*, the *sphenopalatine* and the *ethmoid* sinuses. The frontal, cranial maxillary, and caudal maxillary sinuses are the largest and

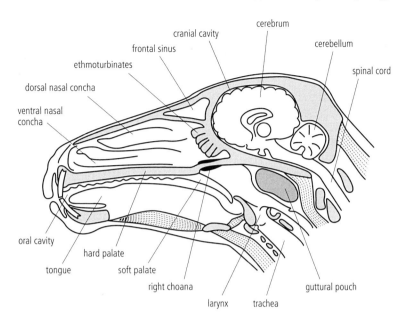

Figure 3.4. Median section of the equine head with nasal septum removed. The figure illustrates the passage of air from the nasal cavity, through the choana, and into the trachea.
Courtesy of Coumbe 2001.

those most often involved in clinical disease. The frontal sinus is triangular and is located rostral to the cranium and medial to the orbit (see Figure 3.4). The rostral maxillary sinus located dorsal to the fourth premolar and first molar and is separated from the caudal maxillary sinus by a bony septum. The caudal maxillary sinus is dorsal to the second and third molars (Figure 3.5). The roots of these cheek teeth extend into the maxillary sinuses.

The sinuses communicate both with each other and with the nasal cavity, allowing drainage into the nasal cavity. Both the frontal sinus and cranial maxillary sinus communicate with the caudal maxillary sinus. The caudal maxillary sinus communicates with the nasal cavity via the *nasomaxillary opening* in the caudal portion of the middle meatus. The nasomaxillary opening cannot be visualized directly with endoscopy but drainage from the sinus can be seen in the nasal cavity in cases of paranasal sinus disease.

Pharynx

The paired nasal passages combine caudally to form the *nasopharynx* and the *oropharynx*. The nasopharynx and oropharynx are separated by the soft palate but converge at their caudal extents to form

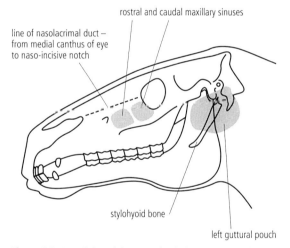

Figure 3.5. Lateral view of the equine head, showing position of the guttural pouch and maxillary sinuses.
Courtesy of Coumbe 2001.

the *pharynx*. In horses, the oropharynx is usually closed to the pharynx by the soft palate, except during swallowing when the soft palate moves dorsally. The position of the soft palate makes the horse an obligate nasal breather. The endoscopic examination of the pharynx allows visualization of the *dorsal pharyngeal recess* dorsally; openings of the *guttural pouches* laterally; and the soft palate, larynx, and *epiglottis* ventrally (Figure 3.6a). The nasopharynx is lined with pseudostratified columnar epithelium, whereas the oropharynx and caudal pharynx are line by stratified squamous epithelium. Additionally, the pharynx contains lymphoid tissue arranged into follicles. These follicles may become enlarged in young horses and is termed *follicular lymphoid hyperplasia*.

Guttural Pouches

The guttural pouches, unique to *equids*, are paired *diverticuli of the Eustachian tube*, which are separated by a thin membranous septum. Each pouch is air-filled and has a volume of 300 to 500 ml in the adult equine. The openings of the guttural pouches are evident as slits within the lateral walls of the pharynx (see Figure 3.6a). The pouches are bordered by the skull dorsally; the pharynx ventrally; and the caudal border of the mandible, parotid, and mandibular salivary glands laterally (see Figure 3.5). The pouches are divided into a large medial and a small lateral compartment by the *stylohyoid bone* and connect over the dorsal border of the structure (Figure 3.6b).

The function of the guttural pouch is unknown, but the walls contain an impressive list of neurovascular structures. The medial compartment wall contains the *glossopharyngeal nerve* (CN IX), *vagus nerve* (CN X), and *internal carotid artery*, and the wall of the lateral compartment contains the *external carotid artery*.

Larynx

The *larynx* consists of cartilage, muscles, and ligaments lined by epithelium. It is the junction between the upper and lower airways. The larynx is supported by the *hyoid apparatus*, a group of bones that attach the larynx and tongue to the base of the skull (Figure 3.7). The function of the larynx is to (a) protect the lower airway from aspiration of food during swallowing, (b) increase airflow into the lungs during exercise, and (c) phonation. The cartilaginous support of the larynx consists of the ring-shaped *cricoid cartilage*, the large *thyroid cartilage*, the paired *arytenoid cartilages*, and the triangular epiglottis (Figure 3.8).

(1) The epiglottis covers the *glottis* or opening into the trachea to prevent aspiration of feed material during swallowing.

(2) The paired arytenoid cartilages are positioned caudo-dorsal to the epiglottis. The paired *vocal*

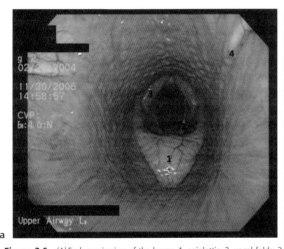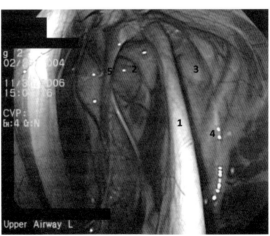

a   b

Figure 3.6. *(A)* Endoscopic view of the larynx. 1, epiglottis; 2, vocal folds; 3, arytenoid cartilages; 4, pharyngeal openings to the guttural pouches. *(B)* Endoscopic view of the left guttural pouch. 1, stylohyoid bone; 2, medial compartment; 3, lateral compartment; 4, external carotid artery; 5, internal carotid artery.
Courtesy of Dr. L. M. Riggs.

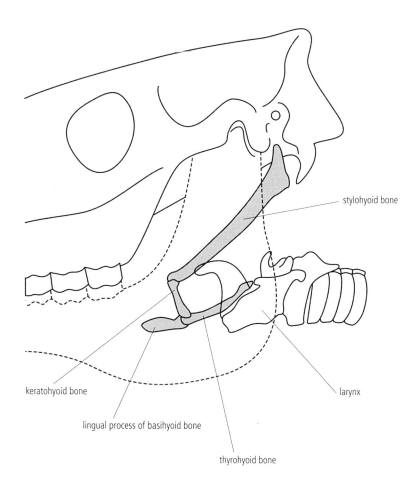

stylohyoid bone

keratohyoid bone

lingual process of basihyoid bone

thyrohyoid bone

larynx

Figure 3.7. The hyoid apparatus of the horse.
Courtesy of Coumbe 2001.

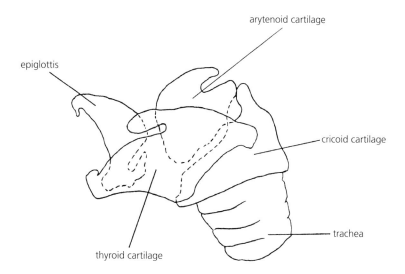

arytenoid cartilage

epiglottis

cricoid cartilage

thyroid cartilage

trachea

Figure 3.8. The cartilages of the equine larynx.
Courtesy of Coumbe 2001.

ligaments attach dorsally to the arytenoids and ventrally combine on midline at the caudal border of the thyroid cartilage. The *vocal folds* are formed by the membrane covered vocal ligaments. The arytenoids are abducted to increase or adducted to decrease the diameter of the laryngeal opening called the *rima glottidis*. This movement regulates airflow into the trachea. The failure of one or both of the arytenoids cartilages to abduct is termed *recurrent laryngeal neuropathy* and is a common cause of respiratory noise and exercise intolerance.

(3) The thyroid cartilage has attachments to each of the other laryngeal cartilages and the hyoid apparatus.

(4) The ring-shaped cricoid cartilage is the caudal most laryngeal cartilage and attaches to the first tracheal ring.

The Trachea

The trachea is the flexible connection between the larynx and the *bronchial bifurcation*. The trachea lies along midline through the neck and into the thorax. It is composed of C-shaped cartilaginous tracheal rings attached by elastic connective tissue. The dorsal trachea lacks cartilage and is composed of the *trachealis* muscle, a long band of smooth muscle. The trachea is lined with mucosa which contains many mucus secreting cells and *cilia*. Bacteria and foreign particles combine with the mucus, which is moved up the trachea by the cilia to protect the lower airway.

The Bronchi

The trachea divides into two main bronchi within the thorax. The bronchi further divide into *lobar bronchi* and again into smaller diameter airways called *bronchioles*. Both the bronchi and bronchioles contain smooth muscle, which allows dilation and constriction to regulate airflow. They are also lined with mucus producing cells and cilia to remove foreign material from the airway. The bronchioles can be differentiated from the larger bronchi because they lack cartilage. The bronchioles terminate into multiple alveolar ducts, which contain multiple alveoli. These terminal structures lack cilia. They have thin walls and comprise a large surface area for gas exchange with an extensive capillary network.

The Lungs

Once the bronchi bifurcate, they are almost completely surrounded by the right and left lungs. The lung tissue, or *parenchyma*, is elastic allowing the lungs to expand during respiration. The lungs of horses, unlike other domestic animals, are not divided into distinct lobes. Fibrous tissue within the lungs divides them into lobules but these lobules, like the lobes, are less distinct than in other species.

The Pleural Cavity

The thorax is lined by a thin layer of cells called the pleura. The pleura is a continuous sheet but is named according to the area of the thorax it covers. The *parietal pleura* covers the chest wall, diaphragm, and *mediastinum*. The mediastinum is a space surrounded by pleura, which contains the thoracic organs including the heart, the esophagus, and vasculature (Figure 3.9). The *visceral pleura* covers the

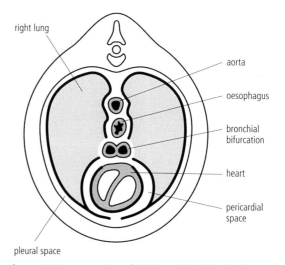

Figure 3.9. Transverse section of the thorax at the level of the heart. Courtesy of Coumbe 2001.

lungs. These pleural layers form two closed sacs within the thorax, which contain a small amount of *pleural fluid*. This fluid allows the layers to glide over one another during respiration.

Respiratory Physiology: Breathing

The lungs do not actively fill with air. Respiration is the result of muscle movement within the thorax. The diaphragm is the most important inspiratory muscle in the horse. The diaphragm contracts and flattens to increase the volume of the chest. This increased volume creates more negative pressure in the chest and forces the elastic lungs to expand. The expansion of the lungs causes the pressure within the alveoli to be lower than atmospheric pressure and air rushes into the lungs. The external intercostal muscles located between the ribs also participate in respiration, especially during intense exercise. These muscles expand to further increase the volume of the chest, and therefore, volume of air that enters the lungs.

Expiration occurs when the diaphragm and intercostal muscles relax, reducing the volume of the chest. This makes the pressure in the chest less negative. Subsequently, the lungs return to the non-stretched position, and the air is forced out.

Ventilation

Ventilation is the act of moving air into and out of the lungs. The *tidal volume* is the volume of air in liters inspired in a resting breath. The tidal volume of the average 500-kg horse is 4 to 5 L. The maximum amount of air that can be inspired above the tidal volume is the *inspiratory reserve volume*, whereas the maximum amount of air that can be exhaled below the tidal volume is the *expiratory reserve volume*. These volumes combined make up the *vital capacity*, which is important for ventilation during exercise when the tidal volume is inadequate. When the maximum volume of air has been exhaled the lungs still contain some air, termed the *residual volume*. The residual volume is important to allow alveoli to remain open and gas exchange to occur even during expiration (Figure 3.10).

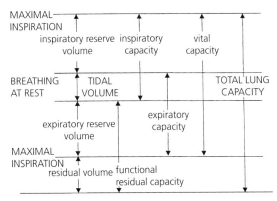

Figure 3.10. Respiratory terminology. Courtesy of Coumbe 2001.

Dead Space

Not all of the inhaled air is involved in gas exchange. The volume of air not participating in gas exchange is *dead space*. The areas which hold air but are not capable of gas exchange (nose, pharynx, and trachea) contain *anatomical dead space*. The alveoli do not all participate in gas exchange all the time. The volume of alveoli in which gas exchange does not occur is *alveolar dead space*. The two types combine to make up the *functional dead space*.

Gaseous Exchange

The alveoli and the pulmonary circulation participate in gas exchange, which is the intricate and essential purpose of the respiratory system. Inspired air contains a high concentration of oxygen when compared to oxygen-deficient venous blood. For this reason, oxygen moves from the alveoli and attaches to hemoglobin within the red blood cells. Oxygen is then transported by the blood to the tissues of the body, where it participates in the use of glucose for energy, termed *oxidative metabolism*. Without this process, cells are unable to produce energy efficiently and must rely on anaerobic respiration for energy. This can produce dangerous levels of lactic acid and result in cell death. At the same time oxygen is delivered to the tissues, carbon dioxide produced by the tissues is picked up and transported by the blood to the alveoli. The air in the alveoli has a lower concentration of carbon dioxide; thus, it moves from the blood into the alveolar air and is exhaled.

Respiratory Control

Respiration is, under most circumstances, involuntary. Control of respiration occurs both in the brainstem and in the lungs. The *respiratory center*, located in the *medulla* and *pons* areas of the brain, is most responsible for regulating respiration. Neurons from the respiratory center discharge rhythmically to send signals through the *phrenic nerve* to the diaphragm and *intercostal nerves* to the external intercostal muscles. The respiratory center monitors the levels of carbon dioxide and hydrogen ions in the blood. *Chemoreceptors* in the *carotid artery* and *aorta* monitor oxygen concentration and send this information to the respiratory center. The respiratory center is then able to immediately adjust the rate of alveolar ventilation to match the demands of the tissues. Increased hydrogen ion and carbon dioxide concentrations and decreased oxygen levels stimulate respiration.

The Gastrointestinal System

The gastrointestinal system is responsible for turning food into usable sources of energy and eliminating the waste products. As herbivores, horses' gastrointestinal tracts are specially adapted to be able to use components of plants that many other species cannot. The entire gastrointestinal tract is lined with *mucosa*, which is a specialized form of epithelium adapted to secretion and absorption. The mucosa has different characteristics depending on its location and related to the function of the region. Starting at the esophagus, the gastrointestinal tract is a modified tube. The tube has four layers: the *mucosa*, the *submucosa*, the *muscularis*, and the *serosa*. The organized contractions of the muscle layer are known as *peristalsis*.

Oral Cavity

The opening to the oral cavity is small in the horse. The lips of a horse are muscular and *prehensile* (adapted to grasping or holding food). The passage of food through the oral cavity is separated from the passage of air through the nasal passage by the palate. Rostrally, the palate is boney (*hard palate*) and caudally, the palate is muscular (*soft palate*).

Teeth

A tooth has two main portions: the *crown* and the *root*, which are separated by a *neck*. *Dentine* is the main mineralized tissue within a tooth. The crown can be identified by its characteristic *enamel* encasement making it hard, whereas the root is encased in *cement*. *Pulp* is the connective tissue within the hard encasement of a tooth. It is connected to the connective tissue in the tooth socket or *alveolus*. The initial teeth that erupt in young horses are temporary or deciduous. They are replaced over time with permanent teeth. Horses' permanent teeth are *hypsodont* (long crown). This means that their teeth are constantly, slowly erupting as they age to replace the crown that is worn off as they chew. This requires that young horses have a large reserve of crown that sits below the surface of the gum line that decreases as the horse ages. Wear of the *occlusal surface* (chewing surface) of the teeth is slowed by infolding of the hard enamel. The inner enamel of the fold is known as the *infundibulum*, and they are filled with cement. Additionally, to prevent exposure of the pulp, *secondary dentine* is formed as the tooth erupts.

Teeth at different locations in the mouth are adapted to the function they must perform. As herbivores, horses have two main functional groups of teeth: incisors (I) and cheek teeth. Incisors are used to cut food before it enters the mouth. A cross-section of a typical incisor can be seen in Figure 3.11. Cheek teeth are used to grind up the food in the mouth. Premolars (PM) and molars (M) are grouped as cheek teeth and serve the same function. The space not filled by teeth, between the incisors and the cheek teeth, is known as a diastema. Canine (C) teeth may or may not be formed and may or may not erupt (more commonly erupt in males). They do not participate in chewing. Incisors and canines have one root, whereas premolars and molars have multiple roots.

The dental formula is an expression of the types of teeth present on one side of the upper (maxilla) and lower (mandible) jaw. A generalized dental formula is:

$$\frac{\text{Upper I} - \text{Upper C} - \text{Upper PM} - \text{Upper M}}{\text{Lower I} - \text{Lower C} - \text{Lower PM} - \text{Lower M}}$$

The dental formula for the temporary teeth in horses is:

$$\frac{3 - 0 - 3 - 0}{3 - 0 - 3 - 0}$$

The dental formula for the permanent teeth in horses is:

$$\frac{3 - 1 - 3(4) - 3}{3 - 1 - 3 - 3}$$

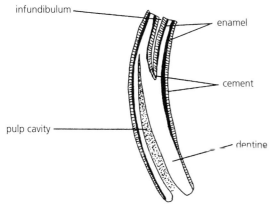

Figure 3.11. Cross-section typical incisor.
Courtesy of Coumbe 2001.

The first premolar is variably present on the maxilla and rarely on the mandible. It often referred to as the *"wolf"* tooth.

Individual teeth can be named by their location in the mouth (upper versus lower and right versus left), the type of tooth (I, C, PM, M), and the number of that type of tooth. The teeth are numbered rostral (front) to caudal (back). Thus, the right wolf tooth would be right upper PM1. To simplify the naming of teeth, the *modified Triadan system* can be used to give each tooth a number (Figure 3.12). All of the teeth in each quadrant of the mouth have the same first number. For permanent teeth, the upper right teeth are the 100s, the upper left are the 200s, the lower left are the 300s, and the lower right are the 400s. From rostral to caudal the teeth are numbered 1 (I1) to 11 (M3). In this system, the upper right PM1 would be 105. For temporary teeth, add 400 to the number of the coinciding permanent tooth. Thus, left lower I3 would be 703.

Estimation of a horse's age from their teeth is based on understanding the time of eruption of different teeth and the appearance of different teeth as a horse ages. Temporary incisors erupt at 6 days (I1), 6 weeks (I2), and 6 months (I3). Permanent incisors erupt at 2.5 years (I1), 3.5 years (I2), and 4.5 years (I3). Canines erupt at 4 years. Permanent premolars erupt at 2.5 years (PM2), 3 years (PM3), and 4 years (PM4). Molars erupt at 1 year (M1), 2 years (M2), and 3.5 years (M3). The shape of the infolding of enamel on the occlusal surface of the incisor leads to exposure of a *"cup"* of cement as the tooth is worn down. The shape of the cup can be used to

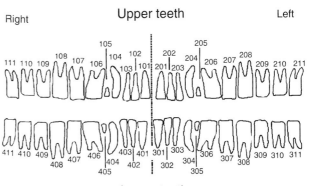

Figure 3.12. Modified Triadan System for naming teeth.
Courtesy of Auer and Stick 2006.

age a horse. The appearance and shape of the upper I3 also changes with age. Over time a dark line (*Galvayne's groove*) appears and disappears on the buccal surface (surface closest to the lip), and a "*hook*" appears and disappears on the caudal aspect distally. It is important to remember that these features can only estimate the age of a horse because they vary from horse to horse.

Salivary Glands

The horse has paired *parotid, mandibular, sublingual,* and *buccal* salivary glands. The saliva enters the mouth through salivary ducts (Figure 3.13). The saliva is important to moisten and begin the enzymatic digestion of food. The moisture lubricates the food to aid in chewing and swallowing. Salivation is stimulated by eating or thinking of eating.

Tongue

The tongue is responsible for moving food around in the oral cavity, combining it with saliva as it is chewed, and for creating a food bolus that can then be swallowed. Once the bolus is formed, the tongue brings the food back to the pharynx where a coordinated reflex allows it to be swallowed and enter the esophagus. *Taste buds* also reside on the tongue. The tongue is a made primarily of muscle and is shaped like the oral cavity. It is pointed at the rostral

aspect, or the *apex*. The tongue becomes thicker and wider as toward the caudal aspect, or *base*. The muscles of the tongue originate on the mandible and the hyoid apparatus.

Pharynx

The pharynx is an ill-defined anatomic region bordered rostrally by the nasal passage and oral cavity and caudally by the larynx and esophagus. The pharynx is divided into two compartments by the soft palate: nasopharynx dorsally and the oropharynx ventrally. Swallowing (*deglutination*) is controlled by a reflex initiated when food touches the pharyngeal mucosa. Proper deglutination requires coordination between the walls of the oropharynx and the soft palate to push the food caudally, the soft palate and the larynx to close off the nasal passages and the trachea, and the esophagus to accept the food bolus and move it toward the stomach.

Esophagus

The esophagus carries a food bolus from the oropharynx to the stomach. A sphincter is present at the oropharynx (upper esophageal sphincter) and at the stomach (lower esophageal sphincter, cardiac sphincter). The esophagus has a cervical, a thoracic, and an abdominal portion. The esophagus runs

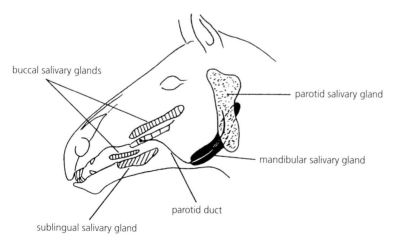

buccal salivary glands

parotid salivary gland

mandibular salivary gland

parotid duct

sublingual salivary gland

Figure 3.13. Major salivary glands of the horse.
Courtesy of Coumbe 2001.

along the dorsal aspect of the trachea in the cranial one-third of the cervical region, deviates to the left of the trachea in the middle one-third of the cervical region, and then back to the dorsal aspect of the trachea as it enters the thoracic inlet. In the cervical region, the serosal layer is replaced by a loose, fibrous connective tissue, the *adventitia*. The thoracic and abdominal portions are mainly covered by serosa. The muscular layer is composed of striated (skeletal) muscle from the oropharynx to the base of the heart (cranial two-thirds). The striated muscle then gradually blends into smooth (visceral) muscle in the caudal one-third.

Stomach

The stomach is a dilated portion of the intestinal tract between the esophagus and the small intestine where digestion begins (Figure 3.14). The stomach of the horse is relatively small (5–15 L volume) and is contained within the rib cage almost entirely on the left side of the body. The regions of the stomach are the *cardia* (adjacent to the opening of the esophagus), the *fundus* (a blind sac), the *body*, and the *pyloric* region. The horse's stomach has an acutely curved shape, which places the cardia and the pylorus close to one another. The longer side is known as the *greater curvature* and

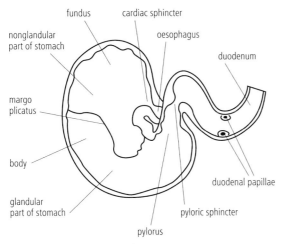

Figure 3.14. The equine stomach.
Courtesy of Coumbe 2001.

the shorter side is called the *lesser curvature*. The cardiac sphincter is quite strong in horses. This makes vomiting almost impossible, and thus rupture of the stomach is a potential consequence of gastric distension.

The muscular layer of the stomach is composed of three incomplete layers that work together to mix the food in the stomach and move it back into the small intestine. The mucosa of the stomach is adapted to create and survive in an acidic environment, as well as, secrete digestive enzymes and hormones. There are four mucosal regions within the stomach. The most oral region is the *nonglandular region*. It is covered with a stratified squamous epithelium that is protected from the acidic environment of the stomach by its impermeability to ions. It is not associated with any glands. The next mucosal region is the *cardiac epithelium*, which is a fairly thin band of mucosal tissue. The junction between the squamous epithelium and the cardiac epithelium is the *margo plicatus*. The function of the cardiac epithelium is not completely understood, but it does secrete bicarbonate (a base and acid buffer) in some species and a digestive hormone (*somatostatin*) that decreases acid secretion in horses. The next mucosal region is the *glandular* or *proper gastric mucosa*. In the glandular region, *parietal cells* are responsible for secreting hydrochloric acid, *zymogen cells* secrete *pepsinogen* (proenzyme for the digestive enzyme pepsin), and *enterochromaffin-like cells* that secrete a digestive hormone (called *histamine*) that increases acid secretion. The glandular mucosa protects itself from the acidic environment by secreting mucus and bicarbonate. The final mucosal region is the *pyloric mucosa*. In the pyloric region, *G-cells* secrete a digestive hormone (called *gastrin*) that increases acid secretion, and *D-cells* secrete a digestive hormone (called somatostatin) that decreases acid secretion.

Small Intestine

The small intestine spans from the pylorus of the stomach to the start of the large intestine at the cecum. On average, the small intestine of an adult horse is approximately 25 m (75 ft) in length. It is divided into three sections from oral to aboral: the duodenum, the jejunum, and the ileum. The small intestine secretes fluid and digestive enzymes that are mixed with the food and digestive products of the pancreas and liver to begin the process of digestion. As digestion progresses, the nutrients that are released and a portion of the secreted fluids are absorbed by the small intestine. Absorption and secretion by the small intestine also plays a role in electrolyte and mineral homeostasis. The majority of digestion and absorption occurs in the first half of the small intestine. Most of the reabsorption of fluid that occurs in the small intestine occurs in the distal one-third.

The mucosal surface of the small intestine is adapted to fulfill secretory, digestive, and absorptive functions. The surface of the mucosa is covered with innumerable fingerlike projections or villi. The villi dramatically increase the surface area of the mucosa. The cells responsible for digestion and absorption are enterocytes. Enterocytes are born at the base of the villi and mature as they migrate to the tip of the villi. The mature enterocytes are tightly adhered to each other and form microvilli or a brush border. Digestive enzymes are produced by the mature enterocytes and are referred to as brush border enzymes. The bases of the villi are surrounded by crypts of Lieberkühn. The crypts secrete large amounts of fluid into the lumen of the small intestine.

The muscular layer of the small intestine is divided into inner circular and outer longitudinal layers of smooth muscle. Ingesta is moved aborally by rhythmic contractions of different segments of the circular muscle and synchronized shortening of the longitudinal muscle.

The duodenum is short (approximately 1 m) and fairly immobile as a result of its tight attachment to the dorsal body wall by its mesentery. The duodenum can be separated into a cranial, descending, and ascending portion. The cranial portion is folded into an S-shaped or sigmoid flexure. Digestive enzymes from the pancreas (which breaks down carbohydrates, fats, and proteins) and bile salts from the liver (which emulsifies and aids in fat absorption) enter the small intestine at the major and minor duodenal papillae in the cranial flexure of the duodenum. The descending portion travels caudally along the right side of the abdomen adjacent to the liver until it reaches the level of the kidney and bends medial around the root of the mesentery and the cecum. The ascending portion of the duodenum runs cranially along the left mesentery until it reaches it's attachment to the transverse colon at the duodenocolic fold, where the duodeno-jejunal flexure occurs.

The jejunum comprises the majority of the small intestine. It has a long mesentery, which allows it to be fairly mobile within the abdomen. The ileum is the shortest section (0.7 m) of small intestine. It can be identified by an antimesenteric band of tissue that is continuous with the dorsal band of the cecum (ileocecal fold). It enters the cecum at the ileocecal orifice. Although no true sphincter is present at the ileocecal orifice, a third layer of muscle is present and the lumen size appears reduced.

Large Intestine

The large intestines can be identified by their external appearance (Figure 3.15). All portions of the large intestine have one to four longitudinal bands (taeniae) composed of a concentration of longitudinal muscle and elastic fibers. The bands are shorter than the surrounding tissue causing sacculations (haustra). In different portions of the large intestine, the haustra may be more or less apparent. The large intestine can be divided into the cecum and the colon. The colon can be divided into the large (ascending) colon, the transverse colon, and the small (descending) colon. The cecum and the large colon of horses is larger than in other species because they have been adapted to allow for the creation of an environment appropriate for microbial digestion of plant products (primarily cellulose), which are not able to be digested by mammalian enzymes. Microbial digestion produces volatile fatty acids (VFAs) that can be absorbed and used as nutrients.

The cecum is a blind sac between the ileum and the large colon. It is located primarily on the right side of the abdomen and has a capacity of approximately 30 L. It is made up of a base (attached dorsally), a body (travels cranioventrally), and an apex.

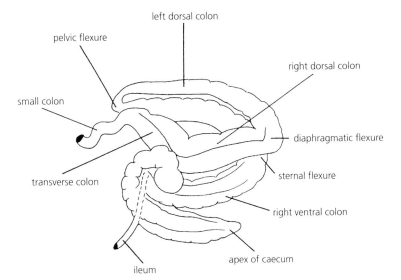

Figure 3.15. The large intestine.
Courtesy of Coumbe 2001.

The body has four bands: *medial*, *lateral*, *dorsal*, and *ventral*. As mentioned, the dorsal band is continuous with the ileocecal band. The lateral band is continuous with a band of tissue traveling to the large colon known as the *cecocolic band*. The primary functions of the cecum are the absorption of water and electrolytes and the creation of an environment for microbial digestion. Ingesta enters at the ileocecal orifice and exits at the *cecocolic orifice*. The cecocolic orifice is located in the cranial portion of the base of the cecum.

The large colon is approximately 4 m in length with a capacity of 50 to 60 L. The large colon is folded into dorsal and ventral halves that are attached by a short common mesentery. The colon begins on the right side of the abdomen at the cecocolic orifice as the *right ventral colon*. It travels cranially to the level of the sternum where it turns caudally (*sternal flexure*) and becomes the *left ventral colon*. When it reaches the caudal abdomen it turns dorsally (*pelvic flexure*) and becomes the *left dorsal colon*. The left dorsal colon runs cranially to the diaphragm where it turns caudally (*diaphragmatic flexure*) and becomes the *right dorsal colon*. The aboral portion of the right dorsal colon is adhered to the dorsal body wall. Thus, the large colon is only attached on the right side at its oral and aboral extents. The pelvic flexure is a common site for impactions of feed in the horse colon. The ventral colons have four bands and more pronounced sacculations. The function of the ventral colon is similar to that of the cecum. The pelvic flexure and left dorsal colon have one band, and the right dorsal colon has three bands. The dorsal colons have more muscular teniae and less pronounced sacculations. The muscular teniae are important to the regulation of transportation of ingesta into the transverse colon.

The transverse colon is the continuation of the right dorsal colon as it turns medially at the level of the seventeenth or eighteenth thoracic vertebra. It runs across the dorsal abdomen from right to left in front of the root of the mesentery. The lumen is much narrower than the right dorsal colon. It has a short mesentery and attached to the dorsal body wall.

The small colon is approximately 3 to 4 m long. It has a long mesentery that allows it to be fairly mobile within the abdomen. The small colon has two teniae; one is a wide antimesenteric band. The small colon is responsible for turning the ingesta from the transverse colon into fecal balls by completing the absorption of excess water and muscular contractions.

Rectum

The rectum of the horse is the continuation of the small colon through the pelvic canal. A variable portion of the rectum is present within the abdominal cavity (cranial to the peritoneal reflection). The remainder is retroperitoneal. The retroperitoneal portion is dilated to form the *rectal ampulla*. The rectal ampulla has thick longitudinal bundles of muscle. The rectum contracts to push feces out during defecation and is a location for storage of feces before defecation. The rectum and the gastrointestinal tract end at the *anus*. The anus is composed of internal and external sphincters that regulate the timing of defecation.

The Nervous System

The nervous system is the most complex system of the body and is responsible for sensing changes within the body and in the external environment and responding appropriately. The nervous system has sensory, integrative, and motor functions. The three divisions of the nervous system are the *central nervous system* (CNS), the *peripheral nervous system*, and the *autonomic nervous system* (ANS; which is a division of the peripheral nervous system).

The *neuron* is the functional unit of the nervous system and is responsible for transmitting information via impulses through the nervous system. Each neuron is made up of three parts: the soma (cell body), the axon, and the dendrites (Figure 3.16). The *soma* is the cell body that contains the nucleus and other cellular organelles. The *dendrite* is a short extension from the soma that receives impulses. Typically, each soma had multiple dendrites. Each dendrite has one of many possible specialized receptors at its tip to sense various types of nerve impulses or stimuli coming into the cell. The *axon* is the other type of extension from the soma, and each soma has only one axon. Axons carry nerve impulses away from the neuron to effector organs or other neurons. Axons are single, long extensions from the cell body and are covered by a white lipid

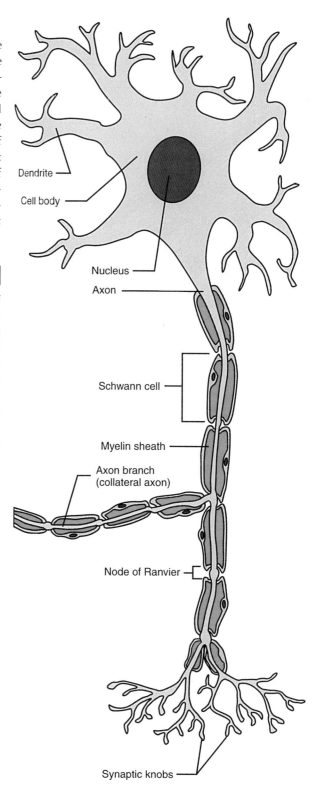

Figure 3.16. Anatomy of a neuron.
Courtesy of Colville and Bassert 2002.

(fatty) substance called *myelin*. Subsequently, nervous tissue containing primarily myelinated axons is called *white matter*, whereas nervous tissue not containing myelin is referred to as *grey matter*. The butterfly-shaped central core of the spinal cord is made up of grey matter.

Myelin acts as an insulator so that nerve impulses can move extremely fast. Specialized glial cells surround the myelin and make up the myelin sheath. *Glial cells* are the cells that support and protect the nervous system, but they do not transmit nerve impulses. In the brain and spinal cord, the specialized glial cells that surround the myelin sheath are called *oligodendrocytes*. Outside of the brain and spinal cord, the glial cells that make up the myelin sheath are called *Schwann cells*. Multiple glial cells are required to cover the entire length of an axon, and the small gaps that occur between the glial cells are called *nodes of Ranvier*. Nerve impulses move from one node of Ranvier to the next in a process called *saltatory conduction*, which allows rapid transmission of nerve impulses.

The *synapse* is the gap between the nerve axon and the target organ or nerve. *Neurotransmitters* are chemical substances that allow the release of impulses in one direction at the synapse. Nerve fibers can be classified as *sensory fibers*, which receive information, and *motor fibers*, which carry a nerve impulse and results in muscle movement. Sensory and motor fibers are classified as visceral if they innervate internal organs, smooth muscle, glands, or mucous membranes. All other structures are innervated by somatic fibers. A group of nerve cells where synapses occur, enabling the transmission of information, is called a *ganglion*.

Upper motor neurons are the neurons that originate in the cerebrum or brainstem and terminate in the spinal cord. Upper motor neurons are not responsible for directly stimulating a muscle to cause movement. Signs of upper motor neuron disease include spasticity, hypermetria (overreaching or high stepping gait), and exaggerated reflexes. *Lower motor neurons* are the neurons that bring nerve stimuli to the muscles. Lower motor neuron disease results in weakness, trembling, and neurogenic atrophy (decreased stimuli to the nerves at the level of the muscle).

The Central Nervous System

The CNS is made up of the brain and spinal cord. The brain is protected within the skull underneath the bony calvarium, whereas the vertebral column protects the spinal cord. The brain and spinal cord are surrounded by the *meninges*, composed of three layers of connective tissue:

- The *dura mater* is the outer fibrous protective tissue layer, which is connected to the periosteum in the inner surface of the cranium.
- The *arachnoid* is the middle tissue layer, which contains a network of collagen fibers. The *cerebrospinal fluid* (CSF) is contained within the subarachnoid space between the fibers.
- The *pia mater* is the inner layer of tissue covering the brain and spinal cord.

The meninges' blood supply provides nutrients and oxygen to the superficial tissues of the brain and spinal cord. Any inflammation of the meningeal membranes is called *meningitis*.

The CSF cushions the brain and spinal cord from the bones of the skull and vertebrae. It is produced from blood vessels within the ventricles of the brain and provides nutrient support to the nervous tissue. CSF circulates throughout the entire nervous system. Infection, inflammation, or cancer in the CNS can cause changes in the white blood cell count or protein concentration in the CSF. In the horse, CSF can be obtained by performing centesis at the lumbosacral (with standing sedation) or atlanto-occipital (with general anesthesia) spaces.

The Brain

The brain is divided into the *forebrain* (also called the *prosencephalon*), the *midbrain* (also called the *mesencephalon*), and the *hindbrain* (also called the *rhombencephalon*; Figure 3.17).

1. The forebrain (prosencephalon) is divided into the *telencephalon* (the cerebrum—two cerebral hemispheres) and the *diencephalon* (the thalamus, hypothalamus, optic tracts, pituitary, and pineal glands).
   - The *cerebral hemispheres* are made up of folds called gyri, deep fissures, and shallow grooves

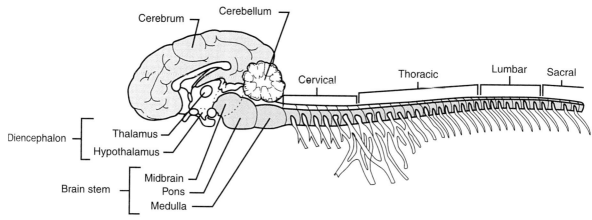

Figure 3.17. Anatomy of the central nervous system.
Courtesy of Colville and Bassert 2002.

called sulci. The longitudinal fissure is the prominent groove that divides the cerebrum into left and right hemispheres. The hemispheres are divided by their sulci into lobes, which each has a specialized function. The cerebrum is the largest portion of the brain and controls the highest mental activities (such as interpreting sensation and memory). The most rostral (forward) portion of the cerebrum is the olfactory bulbs, which are responsible for the sense of smell.

- The *thalamus* is deep within the forebrain and transmits impulses to and from the cerebral cortex (grey matter of the cerebrum).
- The *hypothalamus* receives and integrates nervous impulses and regulates the release of pituitary hormones. It acts as the interface between the endocrine and nervous systems, assists in controlling the autonomic nervous system, and helps maintain the body's homeostasis (constant internal environment).

2. The midbrain (mesencephalon) carries the nerve tracts between the forebrain and hindbrain. It is the most rostral portion of the brainstem and is made up of the *tectum* and *tegmentum*. It is associated with CNs III and IV.

3. The hindbrain (rhombencephalon) includes the *metencephalon* (cerebellum and pons) and the *myelencephalon* (medulla oblongata).

- The *cerebellum* coordinates movement through muscular activity and unconsciously controls balance.
- The *pons* and *medulla oblongata* form the brainstem. The medulla contains the respiratory center and nuclei of CNs VI to XII. The pons is associated with CN V.

The Spinal Cord

The spinal cord connects the brain with the peripheral nerves. It extends from the medulla oblongata at the foramen magnum of the skull to the second sacral vertebrae in the horse. At the end of the spinal cord, a group of spinal nerves forms the *cauda equina*, which supplies innervation to the tail, perineum, and rectum. The spinal cord is segmented corresponding to the surrounding vertebra and gives off a pair (left and right) of spinal nerves at each segment. The spinal nerves connect to the spinal cord by a dorsal and a ventral root. *Sensory nerves* enter at the *dorsal roots* of the spinal cord, whereas only *motor nerves* exit at the *ventral roots*. Sensory nerve cell bodies are contained within the dorsal root ganglion.

In cross-section, the spinal cord in composed of an outer area of white matter, a butterfly-shaped area of grey matter, and a central canal (Figure 3.18). The *white matter* consists of organized groups (called *tracts*) of nerves that run toward the brain (ascend-

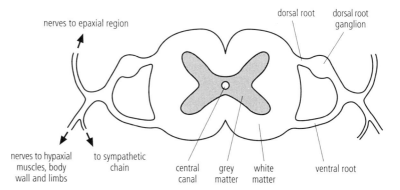

Figure 3.18. Cross-section of spinal cord. Courtesy of Coumbe 2001.

ing) or away from the brain toward other organs (descending). The *grey matter* contains *intercalated neurons* that link the incoming sensory nerves of the dorsal root with the motor nerves that exit through the ventral root. The central canal contains CSF and forms the ventricular system that extends into the brain. The *ventricular system* includes the fourth ventricle (where the central canal enters the hindbrain), the cerebral aqueduct, the third ventricle (within the forebrain), and the lateral ventricles (one in each cerebral hemisphere).

Reflexes are an involuntary fixed response for a particular stimulus and occur without involving the higher levels of the nervous system (brain). Reflex arcs may be simple (or monosynaptic), involving only two neurons at one synapse within the spinal cord or more complex (polysynaptic) with multiple neurons communicating. Reflexes can aid in the diagnosis of a region or nerve affected by neurologic disease. Reflexes may be overridden by the brain through conditioning.

The Reflex Arc
Reflexes occur instantaneously and demonstrate involuntary control over a group of muscles. A stimulus is received by receptors in nerve endings of the skin, joints, or muscles and sends an impulse to the spinal cord through the dorsal root. The impulse synapses with another nerve within the grey matter of the spinal cord and is sent out through the ventral root. The message sent out through the ventral motor root will effect a muscle (or other organ) response at the target site. An

example of a simple spinal reflex in the horse is the *panniculus reflex*. Pricking or pinching of the skin along the trunk sends sensory impulses to the spinal cord, which sends motor impulses to the cutaneous trunci muscle and results in muscle movement (twitching).

The Peripheral Nervous System

The peripheral nervous system is made up of all of the nerves given off by the brain and spinal cord. This includes the CNs, the *spinal nerves*, and the ANS. The ANS is made up of the spinal nerves which supply the smooth muscle, glandular tissue, and blood vessels associated with the body's viscera (internal organs). The ANS is further divided into the sympathetic and parasympathetic nervous systems.

Cranial Nerves
The cranial nerves originate from the brainstem and exit the skull at various foramina. They are numbered I to XII by Roman numerals from the front to the back of the brainstem. These nerves can contain sensory or motor fibers, or both. With the exception of the vagus nerve (CN X), all of the CNs innervate the structures of the head. The special sense nerves are olfactory (CN I) for smell, optic (CN II) for vision, and vestibulocochlear (CN VIII) for hearing. The twelve cranial nerves are:

• I, Olfactory: Sensory for smell.
• II, Optic: Sensory for vision.

- III, Oculomotor: Motor to the eye muscles and pupillary constriction.
- IV, Trochlear: Motor to the eye muscles, for position in orbit.
- V, Trigeminal: Sensory to the face and motor to the muscles of mastication.
- VI, Abducens: Motor to the eye muscles.
- VII, Facial: Motor to muscles of facial expression.
- VIII, Vestibulocochlear: Sensory for hearing and balance.
- IX, Glossopharyngeal: Sensory for taste and motor to the pharynx for swallowing.
- X, Vagus: Sensory and motor for the pharynx and larynx and motor to the heart, smooth muscle, and thoracic and abdominal viscera.
- XI, Accessory: Motor to the muscles of the neck and shoulder.
- XII, Hypoglossal: Motor to the tongue.

The Spinal Nerves

Each segment of the spinal cord has spinal nerves that exit the vertebral canal through the left and right intervertebral foramina. As previously discussed, the spinal nerves consist of a dorsal root carrying sensory fibers into the spinal cord and a ventral root carrying motor fibers away from the spinal cord. One or more *intercalated neurons* (interneurons) connect the sensory and motor nerves in the grey matter of the spinal cord.

The Autonomic Nervous System

The ANS is sometimes referred to as the *visceral nervous system*, and it directs many of the body's homeostatic functions. The ANS is made up of spinal nerves that innervate the internal organs and blood vessels. It is divided into the *sympathetic* and *parasympathetic* nervous systems. Most organs have both sympathetic and parasympathetic innervation, and normal function requires a balance between the two systems.

The *sympathetic nervous system* is responsible for the body's "fight-or-flight" response to emergencies. The chemical messenger (also called a *neurotransmitter* at the synapse) of the sympathetic system is *norepinephrine*. The sympathetic nervous system increases heart rate, opens airways, increases

blood supply to skeletal muscle, and dilates the pupils in response to potential life-threatening situations.

The *parasympathetic nervous system* controls the body during rest and digestive processes. The primary neurotransmitter is *acetylcholine*. This system functions opposite to the sympathetic system and slows the heart and respiratory rates, promotes increased secretion of glands, and increases gastrointestinal motility.

The Urinary System

The urinary system is made up of the kidneys, the ureters, the bladder, and the urethra. The urinary system is the primary mechanism for excretion of soluble waste products in the blood and excess water from the body. The urinary system maintains the body's balance of water and electrolytes and stimulates red blood cell formation through the production of erythropoietin.

The Kidneys

The kidneys are located in the middle of the abdomen on either side of midline in the retroperitoneal space. The left kidney is bean shaped and measures 15 to 20 cm long and 11 to 15 cm wide in the adult horse. The left kidney is medial to the spleen and connects to the spleen via the nephrosplenic ligament. The right kidney is wider (15–18 cm), sits more cranially than the left, and has a heart shape. The right kidney is located against the caudate lobe of the liver, forming the renal impression on the liver. The kidneys are covered by a connective tissue capsule and typically are surrounded by fat. On cut section of the kidney, the outer cortex, medulla, renal pelvis, and hilus can all be visualized (Figure 3.19). The outer *cortex* contains the glomeruli and convoluted tubules. The *medulla* is made up of the loops of Henle and collecting ducts, in addition to peritubular capillaries. The *renal pelvis* is the central area that collects urine for transport out through the ureters. The *hilus* is the location where blood flow enters and exits the kidney, and urine leaves the

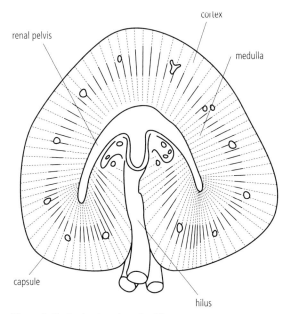

Figure 3.19. Section through equine kidney. Courtesy of Coumbe 2001.

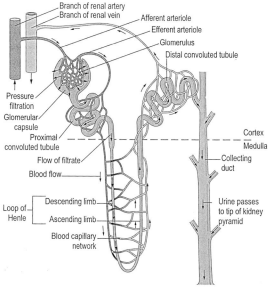

Figure 3.20. A renal nephron. Courtesy of Aspinall 2005.

kidney through the ureter. Oxygenated blood enters the kidney via the renal artery, and blood exits via the renal vein. The kidney has a tremendous blood supply that uses approximately 20% of the cardiac output.

The functional unit of the kidney is the *nephron*, and the equine kidneys contain approximately 2.5 million nephrons. Each nephron forms urine and is divided into different parts which are located in either the cortex or medulla of the kidney (Figure 3.20). The nephron is composed of:

- The *glomerulus* is located in the cortex and is made up of a network of blood capillaries surrounded by a capsule, also called *Bowman's capsule*. The glomerulus is responsible for filtration of fluid and small molecules through the kidney, ensures that the large proteins and blood cells do not get filtered into the urine, and produces the glomerular filtrate (also called *primitive urine*).
- The *proximal convoluted tubule* is connected to Bowman's capsule of the glomerulus in the cortex of the kidney. It functions to reabsorb sodium, glucose, and water from the glomerular filtrate. The convoluted tubule is also responsible for secretion of toxins and certain drugs, and concentration of nitrogenous wastes such as urea.
- The *loop of Henle* is the U-shaped tube that extends into the medulla of the kidney and is made up of a descending loop and an ascending loop. The loops function to concentrate or dilute the urine based on the body's homeostasis by controlling water and sodium levels.
- The *distal convoluted tubule* the ascending loop of Henle becomes the distal convoluted tubule in the renal cortex. The distal convoluted tubule is responsible for sodium reabsorption, potassium excretion, and hydrogen ion excretion. These functions are controlled by the hormone *aldosterone*.
- The *collecting ducts* of all of the individual nephrons travel through the medulla and empty into the renal pelvis, where urine is carried out through the ureter. The collecting ducts adjust the final urine concentration under the control of *antidiuretic hormone* (ADH).

In summary, the kidneys function to (a) excrete metabolic waste products through the production of urine, (b) help maintain the body's fluid, acid-base, and electrolyte balance, and (c) produce erythropoietin to stimulate red blood cell production. The kidneys also produce *renin* in response to low blood pressure. Renin converts the protein angiotensinogen to angiotensin. *Angiotensin* causes blood vessel constriction (to help raise blood pressure), stimulates thirst (to increase fluid volume), and stimulates the release of aldosterone from the adrenal cortex. Aldosterone acts on the kidneys to increase absorption of sodium, and excrete potassium.

The Ureters

A single ureter exits each kidney at the hilus and traverses the retroperitoneal space before entering the bladder within the abdominal cavity. The ureters enter on the left and right sides of the bladder neck at the *trigone*. The ureters are made up of three layers: an outer fibrous layer called the adventitia; a middle layer of smooth muscle; and an inner layer lined by transitional epithelium. Mucous glands contained within the mucosa of the ureter are responsible for the typical mucoid appearance of equine urine. Urine is transported through the ureter to the bladder by peristaltic contractions of the smooth muscle layer.

The Bladder

The bladder is the pear-shaped, saclike organ that functions to store urine between episodes of urination. The bladder wall is made up of three layers, similar to the ureter, and is also lined with transitional epithelium. The *transitional epithelium* allows the bladder to expand as it fills with urine. The ureters enter the bladder near the neck in the area known as the trigone. This is the caudal portion of the bladder near the pelvis. The ureters enter the bladder at an oblique angle to prevent backflow of urine. The bladder neck ends at the bladder sphincter, which opens into the urethra.

The Urethra

The urethra carries urine from the bladder to the external environment. The mare's urethra is relatively short and opens into the vestibule of the vagina. The stallion and gelding's urethra passes along the floor of the pelvis and into the penis. The urethra is accessible for catheterization through the vagina of the mare and penis of the gelding or stallion.

The Liver

The liver is the largest glandular organ in the body and has many functions vital for survival. The liver is located within the right cranial abdomen and is made up of four lobes: left, quadrate, right, and caudate. The liver is expandable and has a high blood flow; large quantities of blood can be stored within the vessels. Oxygenated blood enters the liver via the *hepatic artery* and leaves the liver via the *hepatic vein*. The portal vein also enters the liver and carries blood from the small intestine. The liver's *portal system* is responsible for filtering and detoxifying blood from the gastrointestinal tract. The liver also stores and metabolizes nutrients from the portal blood.

The primary cell within the liver is called the *hepatocyte*, and hepatocytes are arranged in hexagonal lobules within the liver tissue. Each lobule is associated with a branch of the hepatic artery and vein. The hepatocytes produce *bile*, which contains bile acids, cholesterol, and bilirubin. The bile flows continuously into bile canaliculi and into bile ducts. The bile ducts join together to form the *hepatic duct*, which empties into the cranial duodenum at the duodenal papilla. Unlike most other domestic species, it is important to remember that horses do not have a gall bladder.

Functions of the Liver

- Carbohydrate metabolism: the liver is responsible for glucose production, glycogen (stored form of glucose) storage, and the maintenance of normal blood glucose.

- Fat metabolism: the liver synthesizes fat from proteins and carbohydrates, oxidizes fatty acids (which can be used for energy), and forms cholesterol, phospholipids and lipoproteins.
- Protein metabolism: the liver produces the majority of the body's plasma proteins, including albumin, fibrinogen, and multiple clotting factors. The liver forms urea for removal of ammonia and can convert excess amino acids into useful substrates for glucose production.
- Storage: the liver stores vitamins A, D, E, and K and some of the water-soluble vitamins and minerals.
- Formation of bile: bile contains bilirubin from the breakdown of old red blood cells, which the liver performs. The liver also produces red blood cells in the fetus before birth.
- Detoxification and conjugation of substances for excretion in urine and bile.

Evaluation of the Equine Liver

Ultrasound examination can be helpful for evaluation of the size and echotexture (bright or dark appearance on ultrasound) of the equine liver. *Hepatomegaly* (an enlarged liver) can typically be identified if present, and ultrasound guided biopsies can be performed. Blood samples can be useful to determine whether hepatocellular (increased sorbitol dehydrogenase or SDH) or cholestatic (increased gamma-glutamyltransferase or GGT) disease is present. The best blood test to determine liver function is a *serum bile acids* concentration, which can be drawn at any time relative to a meal because horses do not have a gall bladder.

The Endocrine System

The endocrine system is comprised of a number of specialized glands that produce a variety of different "chemical messengers" called *hormones*. Endocrine glands secrete hormones into the systemic circulation, which allows the hormones to travel to distant sites and influence the activity of many different tissues and organs. The endocrine system helps maintain homeostasis, by regulating the fol-

lowing important functions: growth and development, metabolism and energy use, fluid and electrolyte balance, immune function, and sexual activity. The major components of the endocrine system include the pituitary gland, the adrenal glands, the thyroid gland, the parathyroid glands, and the pancreas. The *gonads* (ovaries and testes) also act as endocrine organs; these are discussed with the reproductive system.

The Pituitary Gland

The pituitary gland, also called the *hypophysis*, is arguably the most important endocrine gland because it produces a number of different hormones vital for regulation of the actions of many other endocrine glands. It is located in a small depression in the floor of the skull, the *pituitary fossa*, adjacent to the optic chiasm. It is attached to the ventral surface of the hypothalamus via the *hypophyseal stalk*, which contains blood vessels (*hypothalamic-pituitary portal* vessels) and nerve axons originating from hypothalamic neurons (Figure 3.21).

The pituitary gland consists of three distinct regions: (a) the anterior pituitary, or *adenohypophysis*; (b) the posterior pituitary, or *neurohypophysis*; and (c) the smaller *pars intermedia*, which is located between the anterior and posterior portions (see Figure 3.21). The pars intermedia is almost absent in humans, but is larger and has important functional significance in many veterinary species, especially the horse. These three distinct structural components of the pituitary gland each produce different hormones with many and varied effects.

The anterior pituitary gland produces a variety of *trophic hormones*, which stimulate the growth or activity of a number of different target organs. Anterior pituitary hormones include the following:

- *Growth hormone* (*GH* or *somatotropin*), which stimulates and regulates the growth of almost all the tissues in the body.
- *Adrenocorticotrophic hormone* (*ACTH* or *adrenocorticotropin*), which is released in response to a variety of environmental and physiologic stresses, and stimulates the adrenal glands to release cortisol, the body's primary stress hormone.

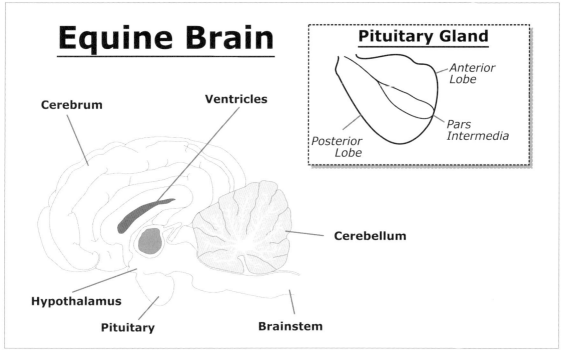

Figure 3.21. Saggital view of brain, cerebellum, brainstem, and pituitary gland, with inset of close-up of pituitary gland showing division into three components.
Courtesy of Dr. K. A. Hart.

- *Thyroid-stimulating hormone (TSH or thyrotropin)*, which acts on the thyroid gland to stimulate the synthesis and release of thyroid hormones.
- *Gonadotrophic hormones*, including both *follicle-stimulating hormone (FSH)* and *luteinizing hormone (LH)*. These hormones act on the reproductive organs and are required for normal testicular and ovarian function and sperm and ova development and maturation.
- *Prolactin (PRL)*, which acts on the mammary gland to stimulate milk production.

The posterior pituitary gland consists primarily of the terminal nerve endings of hypothalamic neurons. Thus, the posterior pituitary gland does not directly produce hormones itself, but it acts to store and release two different hormones produced in the cell bodies of these hypothalamic neurons. The two hormones released by the posterior pituitary are:

- *Oxytocin*, which acts on uterine smooth muscle to promote uterine contractions during parturition and on the myo-epithelial cells of the udder to stimulate milk release ("milk letdown").
- *Antidiuretic hormone (ADH* or *vasopressin)*, which is required for fluid resorption and urine concentration in the kidney.

The pars intermedia produces *melanocyte stimulating hormone* (MSH), which primarily acts to stimulate production of the skin pigment *melanin*. In horses, cells in the pars intermedia also produce beta-endorphin and ACTH. In *Equine Cushing disease*, dysfunction of the pars intermedia results in overproduction of all of these hormones, which ultimately stimulates excess cortisol release from the adrenal glands and produces the typical clinical signs.

In general, the release of pituitary hormones is regulated by the hypothalamus. The hypothalamus

Adrenal Glands in Situ

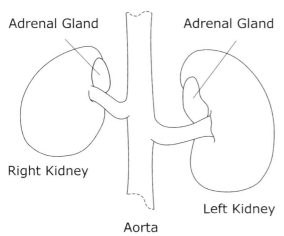

Figure 3.22. Adrenal glands in situ.
Courtesy of Dr. K. A. Hart.

Adrenal Gland

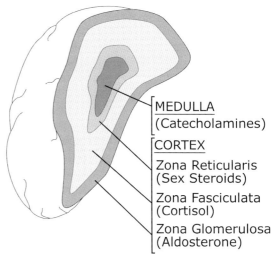

Figure 3.23. Cross-section of adrenal gland, showing three zones and corresponding hormones.
Courtesy of Dr. K. A. Hart.

receives and integrates input from the entire body and thus is able to regulate pituitary hormone secretion to levels adequate to meet the body's current needs. Release of anterior pituitary hormones is stimulated by specific hypothalamic "releasing hormones," which are secreted by the hypothalamus into the hypothalamic-hypophyseal portal vessels in the hypophyseal stalk. Release of posterior pituitary hormones, however, results from direct electrical activation of the hypothalamic neurons whose nerve endings terminate in the posterior pituitary gland. In the horse, release of hormones from the pars intermedia is controlled by both hypothalamic releasing hormones and hypothalamic neural input.

The Adrenal Glands

A small, irregularly shaped adrenal gland is located at the craniomedial aspect of each kidney (Figure 3.22). Despite their small size, the adrenal glands are vital for survival because they produce several different hormones needed to support the body's responses to various types of stress.

Each adrenal gland consists of two main functional parts (Figure 3.23): (a) the outer *cortex*, which produces several different types of *steroid hormones* that have a variety of systemic effects; and (b) the inner *medulla*, which produces the *catecholamine* hormones *epinephrine* and *norepinephrine* (see Figure 3.23). Catecholamines are necessary to support the fight-or-flight response in times of severe stress.

The adrenal cortex is divided into three layers, each of which produces a different type of steroid hormone (see Figure 3.23):

- The *zona glomerulosa* produces *mineralocorticoids*, which act on the renal tubules to regulate fluid and electrolyte balance by promoting sodium retention and potassium secretion. The most important endogenous mineralocorticoid is *aldosterone*.
- The *zona fasciculata* produces *glucocorticoids*, which act to support and modulate the body's response to physiologic and environmental stress. Glucocorticoids are necessary for appropriate regulation of the immune system, for

73

maintenance of blood pressure, and for ensuring available energy sources to tissues by promoting protein and fat breakdown and increasing blood glucose levels. *Cortisol* is the primary endogenous glucocorticoid in horses.

- The *zona reticularis* produces *sex steroids (adrenal androgens)*, which are important for fetal sexual development, and in conjunction with gonadal steroid hormones, support normal sexual activity in adult animals.

ACTH, released from the anterior pituitary gland, is the primary regulator of glucocorticoid secretion, and in concert with other hormones like PRL and estrogen, also stimulates adrenal androgen secretion. Mineralocorticoid secretion also requires the presence of ACTH, but it is predominantly regulated by *angiotensin II*, a hormone produced in the lungs in response to sudden drops in blood pressure. Other factors, such as increased blood potassium levels, also stimulate aldosterone secretion.

The *adrenal medulla* functions independently from the adrenal cortex. Activation of the sympathetic nervous system in times of stress results in direct release of epinephrine and norepinephrine from the adrenal medulla into the systemic circulation. These hormones then act on almost all the other organs and tissues in the body to perpetuate various aspects of the fight-or-flight response. Specific effects of adrenal medullary catecholamines include increased heart rate and cardiac contractility, increased blood flow to cardiac and skeletal muscle, bronchodilation, and increases in blood glucose levels.

The Thyroid Gland

The thyroid gland provides hormonal support for normal metabolism, growth, and development. In the horse, it is a bilobed gland located at the dorsolateral aspect of the proximal trachea. Each half of the equine thyroid gland is palpable as a smooth, slightly movable, oval structure—similar in size and shape to half of a plum—on either side of the trachea, a few centimeters caudal to the larynx. The thyroid gland is composed of numerous spherical *follicles* where the thyroid hormones are synthesized from dietary iodine by the *follicular cells*. Thyroid follicles contain a substance called *colloid*, which stores the two major thyroid hormones, *triiodothyronine (T3)* and *thyroxine (T4)*, until they are secreted into the systemic circulation.

Secretion of thyroid hormones is stimulated by release of TSH from the anterior pituitary gland as described previously. Once released into the systemic circulation, thyroid hormones exert a variety of diverse effects resulting in general stimulation of metabolic activity in almost every cell type in the body. Most importantly, thyroid hormones support skeletal and brain growth and development in early life, stimulate carbohydrate and fat metabolism, increase the basal metabolic rate, and support cardiovascular function.

In addition to the follicular cells that produce thyroid hormones, the thyroid gland also contains *parafollicular cells*. These cells produce a hormone called *calcitonin*, which helps regulate blood calcium levels. Calcitonin release is stimulated by elevated blood calcium levels and serves to decrease blood calcium levels by increasing renal calcium excretion and inhibiting bone resorption.

The Parathyroid Glands

There are four parathyroid glands, located adjacent to the thyroid gland. These glands are quite small and are often difficult to distinguish grossly from the thyroid gland and surrounding tissue. The parathyroid glands produce *parathyroid hormone (PTH)*, which works with calcitonin to regulate blood levels of calcium and phosphorous. PTH release is stimulated by low blood calcium levels and helps increase blood calcium levels by causing increased bone resorption, decreased renal excretion of calcium, and increased intestinal absorption of calcium.

The Pancreas

The pancreas is a small, irregularly shaped gland that lies, in association with mesenteric fat, adjacent to the proximal duodenum and stomach in the right cranial portion of the abdomen. In horses, it is smaller and more indistinct than in other species. It is a mixed *exocrine* and endocrine gland; exocrine

Pancreas Histopathology

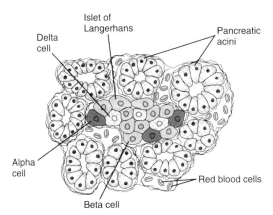

Figure 3.24. Pancreas histopathology.
Courtesy of Guyton and Hall 2005.

glands secrete their products, usually enzymes, into ducts rather than into the systemic circulation. Pancreatic endocrine tissue is composed of the *islets of Langerhans*, which are scattered among the *exocrine pancreatic acini* (Figure 3.24). Pancreatic acini join to form two main exocrine pancreatic ducts that empty into the duodenum; the *major pancreatic duct* joins the hepatic duct from the liver and forms the *major duodenal papilla*, and the smaller *accessory duct* opens into the opposite side of the duodenum on its own at the *minor duodenal papilla*.

The exocrine pancreas secretes the digestive enzymes *lipase* and *amylase* into the small intestine for digestion of fats and carbohydrates. The endocrine pancreas is composed of three distinct cell types—beta cells, alpha cells, and delta cells—which, like other endocrine organs, release hormones into the systemic circulation. The primary endocrine pancreatic hormones are *insulin* and *glucagon*, which work together to regulate blood glucose levels. Insulin is released from beta cells when blood glucose levels rise (such as after a meal); it promotes uptake of glucose into cells for energy use and also increases fat and protein synthesis and storage. Glucagon has essentially the opposite effects; it is released from alpha cells when blood glucose levels are low and acts

to increase blood glucose levels by stimulating glucose production and release by the liver. Glucagon also promotes breakdown of fat stores for energy use. Delta cells release somatostatin, which provides a more complex level of regulation by inhibiting the secretion of both insulin and glucagon.

The Skin

The skin is the largest organ in the body and is continuous with the mucous membranes at each orifice. The skin has three layers: the epidermis, the dermis, and the hypodermis (or subcutaneous layer).

1. The *epidermis* is the thin outer layer of keratinized stratified squamous epithelium. It can be divided into three layers of different cell types: the stratum corneum (top layer), stratum granulosum (middle layer), and stratum germinativum (bottom layer closest to the dermis).
2. The *dermis*, also called the *corium*, is the thick layer attaching the epidermis to the underlying tissues. This layer is composed of fibrous connective tissue, hair follicles, and cells. It contains blood and lymph vessels, nerves, and the erector pili muscles. The collagen and elastin fibers in this layer are responsible for the tensile strength and elasticity of the skin. The dermis is involved in maintenance, repair, and remodeling of the skin and provides support for the epidermis.
3. The *hypodermis* is the subcutaneous layer of the skin that blends with and is below the dermis. It contains areolar (loose connective tissue) and adipose tissues, which allows underlying bone and muscle to move easily without pulling on the overlying skin. The adipose tissue in this layer provides energy and insulation, and helps in maintaining the surface contours.

The Functions of the Skin

- *Protection*: The skin acts as a protective barrier from the external environment, bacteria, UV radiation, and trauma.

- *Thermoregulation*: The large surface area aids the skin in controlling body temperature via sweating, vasodilation, and movement of the hair shafts.
- *Sensation*: The skin enables monitoring of the external environment through nerve endings that are sensitive to touch, pain, and pressure.
- *Exocrine glands* within the skin allow for secretion and excretion of various products.
- Protects the body by *preventing loss of water* and electrolytes.
- *Vitamin D* is produced at the skin.
- *Immune function*: Lymphocytes and other cells form important components of the skin's immune system.

Hair

The hair functions as a protective barrier, a thermal insulator, a source for keratinocytes in wound healing, and facilitates distribution of apocrine gland secretions. Hairs are produced by simple follicles, which have roots that penetrate the dermis. The hair follicle shaft is the superficial portion of the hair follicle, which projects from the skin surface. All equine hair follicles are *primary*, meaning that they have large diameters and roots within the dermis. Most of the hair follicles have associated sweat and sebaceous glands, as well as, *erector pili muscles*. Hair growth in the horse is cyclical and happens biannually in the spring and fall.

Nutrition, overall health, genetics, and hormonal factors all influence the hair growth cycle. *Anagen* is the name of the growth phase, when hair is formed by differentiation of the matrix cells that divide, keratinize, and die. The hair becomes longer as new cells are added at the root. *Telogen* is the resting phase of the cycle, during which the primary follicle partially atrophies.

Sweat Glands

Apocrine sweat glands originate in the epidermis and are attached to the hair follicle by a long duct that empties near the skin surface. They are coiled and tubular. Of the domestic species, horses have the largest number of sweat glands. Although found almost everywhere in the skin, the sweat glands are less developed in the skin of the mane, middle of the back, limbs, and tail and are absent entirely in the lips close to the mucocutaneous junction and around the hoof and ergot.

The Eye

The eye is made up of the *globe* and the accessory structures around the eye, or *adnexa*. The eye and surrounding structures including the nerves, blood vessels, fat, tissues, and muscle are situated in the orbit. The *orbit* is the bony structure around the eye, which has a bony rim and acts to protect the eye from trauma. The equine eyes are positioned laterally on the skull, which results in excellent peripheral vision but reduced depth perception and binocular vision. The horse has about a 300-degree field of vision, with blind spots directly in front of and behind them. Movement of the head can easily compensate for any blind spots.

Three layers of tissue form the eyeball: the outer fibrous layer, the middle vascular layer, and the innermost nervous layer (the retina). The outer fibrous layer forms the *sclera*, which surrounds most of the globe. The anterior part of this outer layer is clear and forms the *cornea*. The junction between the cornea and sclera is the limbus. The middle vascular layer is also referred to as the *uvea*, and it forms the ciliary body, iris, and choroid (discussed later in the chapter). The innermost layer is the *retina*, of which the posterior portion contains the light sensitive nerve cells responsible for vision. The anatomy of the eye can be divided into the adnexa, the anterior (front) portion of the globe, and the posterior (back) portion of the globe (Figure 3.25).

The Adnexa of the Eye

The structures of the adnexa include the eyelids, the conjunctiva, the ocular muscles, and the lacrimal apparatus.

Ocular Muscles
The ocular muscles attach the globe to the orbit and facilitate movement of the eye. The four rectus

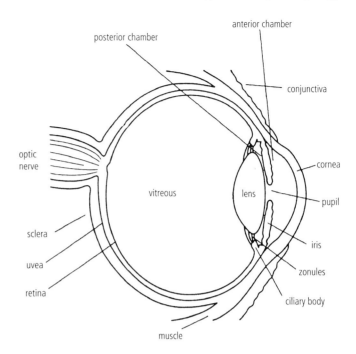

Figure 3.25. Anatomy of the eye.
Courtesy of Coumbe 2001.

muscles, two oblique muscles, and the retractor bulbi muscle all attach to the sclera and provide movement and rotation of the eye. The retractor bulbi muscle attaches at the posterior portion of the globe, surrounds the optic nerve, and is responsible for globe retraction in the orbit.

The Eyelids

The eyelids have several important functions, including protection of the cornea and anterior globe, tear production and distribution, and assistance in the control of light entry into the eye. The eyelids are divided into three basic layers: the skin, the musculofibrous layer, and the palpebral conjunctiva. The skin is the outermost layer, which is thin and generally haired. The *musculofibrous area* contains the orbicularis oculi muscle, the smooth tarsal muscle, the orbital septum, and the aponeurosis. This muscular layer assists with blinking of the eye. The deepest layer is the *palpebral conjunctiva*, which is an elastic tissue that touches the eye and facilitates movement of the lids. The upper and lower eyelid margins contain *meibomian glands*, which secrete the lipid component of the tear film

that lubricates the eye. Long eyelashes are on the upper lid only and help protect the eye from dust particles and sunlight.

The *third eyelid* is commonly referred to as the *nictitans* and is located between the lacrimal caruncle and the globe along the medial angle of the eye. The third eyelid is made up of cartilage, which is covered by conjunctiva on both surfaces. The *accessory lacrimal gland* is within the third eyelid and is responsible for tear production. Movement of the third eyelid occurs rapidly over the cornea and results in the distribution of tear film.

The Lacrimal Apparatus

The lacrimal apparatus is made up of the lacrimal gland, the accessory lacrimal gland, several small accessory glands, two lacrimal puncta, and the nasolacrimal duct. Lacrimal fluids (tears) are distributed over the eye during blinking to flush out foreign debris, lubricate the eye, and provide some nutritional components to the ocular tissues. Lacrimal fluid and secretions are drained at the medial angle of the eye through the *nasolacrimal duct* and into the nostril.

The Anterior Portion of the Eye

The anterior segment of the eye includes the cornea, anterior chamber, iris, iridocorneal angle, lens, and ciliary body. The *cornea* is the clear tissue that allows light into the eye. The cornea has four layers: the outer epithelium, the stroma (90% of corneal thickness), Descemet membrane, and the inner endothelium. The *anterior chamber* is a large space between the cornea and iris that is filled with aqueous humor. The *aqueous humor* is a clear fluid that supports corneal health. Aqueous humor drains from the eye and into the blood at the *iridocorneal angle*, which is the junction between the cornea, iris, and ciliary body. The *iris* is a circular structure that sits in front of the lens, with an opening in the center that forms the *pupil*. The iris is the front of the uveal tract and is quite vascular. The muscles in the iris allow the pupil to dilate (*mydriasis*) or contract (*myosis*) in response to light. The small black granules attached to the margin of the pupil are normal in horses and are called *corpora nigra*, or iridic granules. The *ciliary body* produces aqueous humor and is the middle portion of the uveal tract that is located behind the iris. The *lens* is the clear, round structure that sits behind the iris. The lens enables the horse to focus and is suspended from the ciliary body by zonular fibers.

The Posterior Portion of the Eye

The posterior segment of the eye is also called the *fundus*. It contains the vitreous chamber, the retina, and the optic disk. The *vitreous chamber* is the large space between the lens and the retina that contains a thick transparent fluid called the vitreous. The vitreous acts to transmit and refract light to the retina. The *retina* is the innermost layer of the eye and contains the nerve cells that enable vision. *Rod photoreceptors* are more numerous in the horse and are responsible for detecting light and dark differences. *Cone photoreceptors* are responsible for daytime and color vision, the latter of which is limited in the horse. The nerves originating from the rods and cones, as well as the nerve

endings from the retinal ganglion, form the optic nerve. The optic nerve head is also referred to as the *optic disk*, which contains ganglion nerve fibers and can be visualized with ophthalmoscopic examination.

The Ear

The ear is made up of three parts: the external ear, the middle ear, and the inner ear (Figure 3.26). The *external ear* includes the pinna and external auditory meatus. The ear pinna is made of cartilage and covered by skin. It is cone shaped and highly moveable, which allows the horse to focus on the source of sound. The cartilage of the pinna continues as the *external auditory meatus*, which travels vertically down the skull and then turns horizontally into the skull. The external auditory meatus is surrounded by cartilage rings and terminates at the tympanic membrane, or eardrum.

The *middle ear* is an air-filled cavity within the temporal bone that contains the *auditory ossicles* (the *malleus* or hammer, the *incus* or anvil, and *stapes* or stirrup) (Figure 3.27). The auditory ossicles transfer and amplify sound vibrations from the eardrum through the inner ear. The malleus, incus, and stapes form a chain of bones that are connected by synovial joints. The malleus is in contact with the eardrum and the stapes connects with the oval window of the inner ear. The *Eustachian tube*, which allows equilibration of pressure between the external and middle ear, opens into the middle ear and connects to the pharynx. The equine *guttural pouch* is a large diverticulum of the Eustachian tube.

The *inner ear* is made up of a *bony labyrinth* within the petrous temporal bone of the skull. It is connected to the middle ear via the round window and the oval window. The bony labyrinth is filled with perilymph fluid and surrounds the membranous labyrinth. The *membranous labyrinth* contains the endolymph and forms the organs of the inner ear: the vestibular apparatus and the cochlea. The *vestibular apparatus* contains two saclike structures, the *utricle* and *saccule*, and is responsible

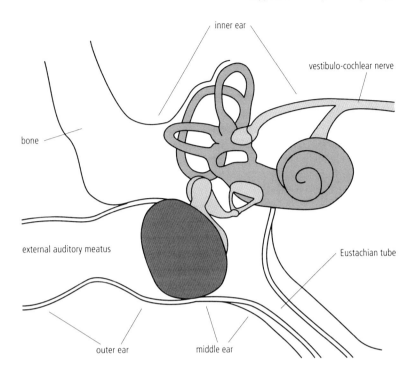

Figure 3.26. Overview of the ear.
Courtesy of Coumbe 2001.

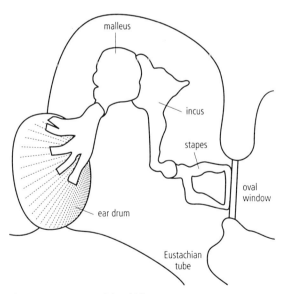

Figure 3.27. Anatomy of the middle ear.
Courtesy of Coumbe 2001.

for transmitting information about balance and acceleration to the brain. The utricle connects the three *semicircular canals* to the cochlea. The semicircular canals are perpendicular to each other and contain sensory receptor cells, which send signals to the brain based on endolymph movement. The *saccule* is the organ responsible for assessing balance and head position. The information from the vestibular apparatus is sent to the brain through the vestibular portion of CN VIII (the vestibulocochlear nerve). The *cochlea* is the blind-ended spiraling tube that looks like a snail's shell. The cochlea is filled with endolymph, which sends vibrations onto the sensory hairs. Within the cochlea, the area of sensory cells which have fine sensory hairs is the *organ of Corti*. A small nerve fiber from the base of each cell is part of the cochlear branch of CN VIII. The organ of Corti is stimulated by vibrations traveling through the ear canal, which are transmitted as nervous impulses to the brain and interpreted as sound.

79

The Musculoskeletal System

The musculoskeletal system is vital to the support, protection, and mobility of horses. It is composed of bone and muscle connected to one another by tendons and ligaments.

Skeleton

The skeleton is responsible for the rigid support and protection provided by the musculoskeletal system. It can be divided into an *axial* and *appendicular* portion.

The *axial skeleton* is composed of the bones of the head, vertebral column, ribs, sternum, and pelvis. It provides protection for the CNS, thoracic cavity, and portions of the abdominal cavity. The bones of the head include the *skull*, the *mandible*, the *hyoid apparatus*, and the *bones of the middle ear*

(Figure 3.28). The skull is made up of a large number of paired bones. The bones are firmly joined to one another to form the *cranium* (encases the brain and brainstem), *paranasal sinuses*, *nasal passage*, and *maxilla* (upper jaw). In the temporal region, the skull is connected to the lower jaw (*mandible*) at the *temporomandibular joint* and the *hyoid apparatus* (connected to the tongue and larynx and involved in swallowing) at the *temporohyoid joint*.

The vertebral column is separated into five regions from cranial to caudal: *cervical*, *thoracic*, *lumbar*, *sacral*, and *coccygeal*. The horse has 7 cervical, 18 thoracic, 6 lumbar, 5 sacral, and 15 to 20 coccygeal vertebrae. All vertebrae have similar basic architecture and are composed of a *body* and paired *arches* that converge dorsally (Figure 3.29). The body of the vertebrae is a round bone that is flattened dorsally and serves as the ventral floor of the spinal column, whereas the arch surrounds the

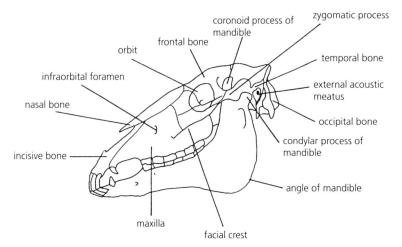

Figure 3.28. The equine skull. Courtesy of Coumbe 2001.

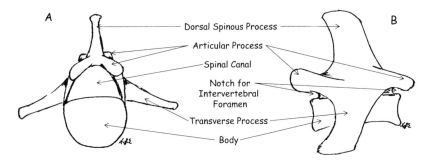

Figure 3.29. Generalized vertebra cranial view *(A)* and lateral view *(B)*. Courtesy of K. L. Epstein.

remainder of the spinal column. The arches have a *dorsal spinous process*, paired *transverse processes*, and paired *cranial* and *caudal articular processes*. There are also notches at the cranial and caudal edge of the arch that form *intervertebral foramen* for the passage of vessels and nerves. Modifications of the architecture occur to accommodate the function of different regions of the spine. For example, the first two cervical vertebrae, the *atlas* and the *axis*, are adapted to allow a specific range of motion for the head. In the thoracic region, the vertebrae articulate with ribs (18). The dorsal portion of the rib is boney, whereas the ventral portion is cartilaginous. The two portions join at the *costochondral junction*. The ventral aspect of the first eight ribs articulates with the sternum. The caudal 10 ribs are joined by overlapping the cartilaginous portions of the ribs with one another.

The *appendicular skeleton* serves as the structural support and lever arms for the front (thoracic) and hind (pelvic) limbs and is therefore primarily involved the mobility of the horse. Horses are have adapted to run with speed. The efficiency of their movement is increased because they have a decreased number of longer metacarpal and metatarsal (*cannon*) and phalangeal bones. Horses have retained the middle of five (third) phalangeal bones, the cannon bone. They have also retained the second and fourth metacarpal and metatarsal bones (*splint bones*) that bear a smaller amount of weight. The metacarpal and phalangeal bones are also oriented almost perpendicular to the ground. This leaves the horse to stand on the third phalangeal bone within the hoof capsule. The anatomy of the thoracic limb and pelvic limb are almost identical distal to the carpus (thoracic limb) and tarsus (pelvic limb). The bones of the appendicular skeleton can be seen in Figures 3.30 and 3.31.

The bones of the skeleton can be classified based on their shape into *long bones* (mostly in the appendicular skeleton and function as levers), *short bones* (bones of the carpus and tarsus are in this category and allow complex movement and reduce concussion), and *flat bones* (bones of the skull as well as the scapula and pelvis are in this category and are important in protection of underlying structures and for the attachment of muscles).

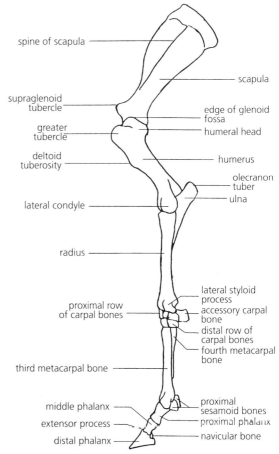

Figure 3.30. Skeleton of thoracic limb. Courtesy of Coumbe 2001.

The skeleton is a collection of individual bones related to one another by joints. Bone is a composite material comprised of an ordered deposition of *inorganic material* (mineral) onto an *organic matrix (osteoid)*. Calcium and phosphorus, primarily in the form of hydroxyapatite crystals, are the main inorganic components of bone. The organic matrix is composed mainly of type I collagen with a small percentage of proteoglycans and glycosaminoglycans. The structure of the collagen and its tight relationship with the hydroxyapatite crystals provides the mechanical strength of the bone. *Osteoblasts*, *osteocytes*, and *osteoclasts* are the predominant cell types in bone. Osteoblasts are responsible for depositing the osteoid onto bone surfaces. Osteoblasts

81

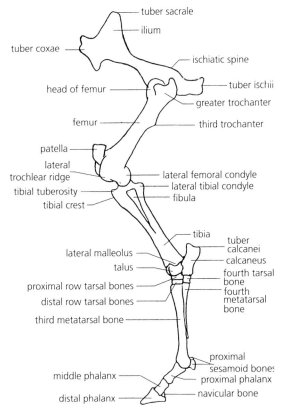

Figure 3.31. Skeleton of pelvic limb.
Courtesy of Coumbe 2001.

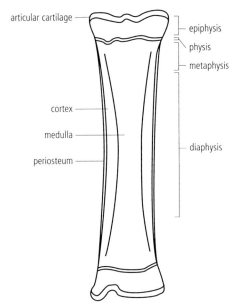

Figure 3.32. Immature equine tibia showing the different regions of a long bone.
Courtesy of Coumbe 2001.

that are incorporated into the osteoid become osteocytes. Osteocytes have numerous cytoplasmic processes to form a communication and transport network within bone. Osteoclasts are responsible for most bone resorption. Bone turnover by osteoblasts and osteoclasts is important in the homeostasis of healthy bone and the repair of damaged bone.

In general, bone can be divided into two main structural types: *cancellous (trabecular)* and *compact (cortical)*. Compact bone is dense and is the main component in the shaft of the long bones of the appendicular skeleton. Cancellous bone contains hematopoietic (makes blood cells) or fatty bone marrow divided by a network of fine boney partitions called *trabeculae*. Most of the bones of the axial skeleton and the end of the long bones of the appendicular skeleton contain cancellous bone. During

fetal development, bone can develop from either boney replacement of cartilage (*endochondral ossification*) or fibrous tissue (*membranous ossification*). In the fetus, long and short bones are initially made of cartilage whereas the flat bones of the skull, scapula, and portions of the pelvis are initially fibrous tissue. Ossification begins at a *center of ossification* and different portions of the skeleton are more or less ossified at birth. Long bones have at least three centers of ossification, one in the shaft (*diaphysis*) and one at each end (*epiphysis*; Figure 3.32). Short bones develop from one center of ossification. Following birth, longitudinal growth of long bones occurs via endochondral ossification at *physes*, or growth plates, whereas increase in diameter occurs from membranous ossification associated with the osteogenic layer of the *periosteum*.

Joints or *articulations* occur where one bone meets the next. Some joints provide a firm connection, whereas others allow motion is specific planes. Joints can be divided into three categories: *fibrous*, *cartilaginous*, and *synovial*. Examples of fibrous joints include the *sutures* of the skull in foals, which undergo membranous ossification with maturation; the *syndesmosis* (the sides of two bones connected by ligaments) between the cannon bone (third metacarpal or metatarsal bone) and the splint bones (second or fourth metacarpal or metatarsal bones); and *gomphosis* between a tooth and the underlying boney socket. Cartilaginous joints can be divided into *synchondroses* and *symphyses*. Temporary synchondroses occur in long bones between diaphysis and epiphysis before ossification. A permanent synchondrosis occurs between the hyoid bones and the base of the skull. A symphysis occurs when the bone ends are separated by tissue (generally fibrous in nature). Examples include the mandibular symphysis and intervertebral discs between adjacent vertebral bodies.

Most joints that allow for motion are *synovial joints*. Pain free, smooth, and efficient motion of each synovial joint depends on proper interaction and function of the components of the synovial joint "organ." Each joint is composed of specialized tissues designed to support the function of the joint including *subchondral bone, articular cartilage, synovial fluid* and *membrane, joint capsule*, and *periarticular ligaments* (Figure 3.33). The subchondral bone provides shape and stability for the overlying articular cartilage. Articular or hyaline cartilage is quite smooth to decrease friction during joint movement and designed to hold a large amount of water (70%–80% of wet weight), which allows the joint to function when loaded with the weight of the horse. In addition to water, articular cartilage is primarily composed of collagen (type II) and proteoglycans. Synovial fluid is vital to the lubrication of the joint. Components of joint fluid, such as hyaluronan and lubricin molecules, play a large role in decreasing friction during joint movement. The synovial membrane is responsible for the production and regulation of the composition of synovial fluid. The joint capsule and periarticular ligaments along with surrounding musculature are important to stabilize and allow a range of motion of the joint. Several synovial joints (temporomandibular and femorotibial) contain *menisci* composed of hyaline and fibro-cartilage and fibrous tissue within the joint capsule. The menisci are likely important for smoothing out incongruent joints and allowing different planes of motion within the same joint. Damage or dysfunction of any component of the synovial joint organ contributes to *degenerative joint disease* or *osteoarthritis*.

Muscles

Muscular contraction is responsible for almost all movement of and within a horse. Muscle can

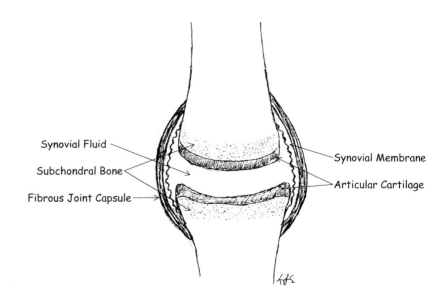

Figure 3.33. Cross-section of a synovial joint. Courtesy of K. L. Epstein.

Synovial Fluid
Subchondral Bone
Fibrous Joint Capsule
Synovial Membrane
Articular Cartilage

83

be classified as *smooth*, *cardiac*, or *skeletal*. Muscle within the internal organs and vascular system is primarily smooth muscle. Cardiac muscle is only present in the heart. The muscle in the musculoskeletal system is skeletal muscle. Thus, the description of muscle within this section applies to *skeletal muscle*.

An individual muscle is made up of many *muscle fibers*. Each muscle fiber is one giant, multinucleated muscle cell. Muscle fibers are made up of many parallel *myofibrils*. Myofibrils contain alternating thick and thin filaments. The thick filament is composed of *myosin* protein, whereas the thin filament is a combination of *actin*, *tropomyosin*, and *troponin* proteins. The interactions of these proteins in the presence of *adenosine triphosphate (ATP)* and *calcium* causes muscle contraction. Calcium binds to troponin, which allows a conformational change, such that actin can slide along myosin and shorten the muscle (Figure 3.34).

The myofibril can be divided lengthwise into contractile units known as *sarcomeres*. Myofibrils

are surrounded by the *sarcotubular system* composed of transverse tubules and sarcoplasmic reticulum. Each muscle fiber is innervated by a terminal motor nerve fiber. The *neuromuscular junction* is the region between the nerve and the muscle fiber. When an action potential is generated in the neuromuscular junction it travels via the transverse tubules to the sarcoplasmic reticulum and causes the release of calcium ions. All muscle fibers that are innervated by the same nerve fiber are called a *motor unit*.

Individual muscle fibers are covered by connective tissue known as *endomysium*. The fibers are grouped into bundles or *fasciculi* surrounded by connective tissue known as *perimysium*. The entire muscle belly is covered by a dense connective tissue known as *epimysium*. All of the connective tissue components of the muscle merge at the ends of the muscle belly to continue as the tendons which attach the muscle to the bones at either end (origin and insertion). When a muscle contracts, it causes the bone at either end of the tendon to move relative to one another leading to a change in the orientation of the joint between the two bones. Muscles can only contract, and to return to their original length, a muscle on the opposite side of the joint must contract. Thus, muscles must exist in antagonist pairs—some muscles increase joint angle (extensors), whereas other muscles decrease joint angle (flexors); some muscles move the leg toward the body (adductors), whereas others move the leg away from the body (abductors). Muscles of the body can be separated into different groups based on their location and function. Examples of muscles described by this system are given in Table 3.1.

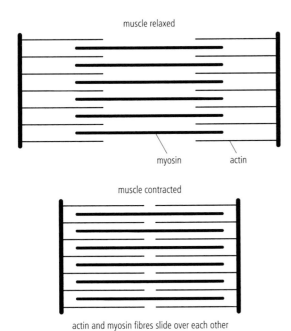

Figure 3.34. Muscle contraction.
Courtesy of Coumbe 2001.

Tendons and Ligaments

Tendons and ligaments are the connectors of the musculoskeletal system. As previously discussed, *tendons* connect muscle to the bones to allow the contraction of the muscle and result in a change in the angle of a joint. *Ligaments* attach bone to bone. They are often important to prevent excessive movement of joints in certain planes. The collateral

Table 3.1. Muscles grouped by location and function.

Location	Function	Selected individual muscles
Head	Facial expression	*levato labii superioris* (lift upper lip); *buccinator* (keeps food from accumulating in cheek); *orbicularis oris* (closes opening of mouth); *orbicularis oculi* (closes eyelids); and *levator anguli oculi* (opens upper eyelid)
	Mastication	*temporalis* (closes mouth); *digastricus* (opens mouth); *masseter* (cranial/caudal and side to side/grinding movement of jaw); and *pterygoideus* (grinding movement of jaw)
Neck	Turn neck to one side	*sternocephalicus* (unilateral contraction)
	Stabilize and retract hyoid	*sternothyroideus, sternohyoideus, omohyoideus,* and *thyrohyoideus*
	Join thoracic limb to body and move limb (girdle muscles)	*trapezius* (cervical portion, advance limb), *omotransversarius, brachiocephalicus, rhomboideus* (cervical portion, retract limb), and *serratus ventralis* (cervical portion, retract limb)
Vertebral column	Bending side to side	lateral column (*iliocostalis*)
	Extensors	middle column (*longissimus*) and medial column (*transversospinalis*)
	Flexors	hypaxial muscles (*longus colli, rectus capitis ventralis, longus capitis,* and *scalenus*), *sternocephalicus* (bilateral contraction)
Thorax	Respiration	*intercostal muscles*
	Join thoracic limb to body and move limb (girdle muscles)	*trapezius* (thoracic portion, advance limb), *latissimus dorsi* (retracts limb), *superficial pectoral muscles* (adduct limb), *rhomboideus* (thoracic portion, retract limb), *serratus ventralis* (thoracic portion, retract limb), and *pectoralis profundus* (retract limb)
Abdomen	Body wall	*external abdominal oblique, internal abdominal oblique, transversus abdominis,* and *rectus abdominis*
Thoracic limb	Girdle muscles	See neck and thorax
	Shoulder (scapulohumeral joint)	brace lateral aspect (*supraspinatus* [also extend], *infraspinatus* [also abduct]), brace medial aspect/adduct (*subscapularis, coracobrachialis*), flex (*deltoideus* [also abductor], *teres major, teres minor*), extend (no muscle has extension of shoulder as main function, but *brachiocephalicus, biceps brachii, supraspinatus,* and *pectoralis ascendens* may be involved)
	Elbow	flex (*biceps brachii* and *brachialis*), extend (*triceps brachii, tensor fasciae antibrachii,* and *anconeus*)
	Carpus	flex (*flexor carpi radialis, flexor carpi ulnaris, ulnaris lateralis* [flexes already flexed further]), extend (*extensor carpi radialis, extensor carpi ulnaris, ulnaris lateralis* [extends already extended], and *extensor carpi obliquus*)
	Carpus and digit	flex (*superficial digital flexor muscle, deep digital flexor muscle*), extend (*common digital extensor,* and *lateral digital extensor*)
Pelvic limb	Hip (coxofemoral joint)	flex (*sartorius, tensor fasciae latae, superficial gluteal*) adduct (*gracilis, pectineus, adductor, obturator externus*), abduct (*middle gluteal, accessory gluteal, deep gluteal*), extend joint/retract limb (*middle gluteal, accessory gluteal, biceps femoris, semitendinosus,* and *semimembranosus*)
	Stifle	flex (*tensor fasciae latae,* portions of the *biceps femoris, semitendinosus,* and *semimembranosus* that attach distal to stifle), extend (quadriceps femoris, portion of the *biceps femoris, semitendinosus,* and *semimembranosus* that attach proximal to stifle)
	Tarsus	flex (*tibialis cranialis, peroneus tertius*), extend (*gastrocnemius, biceps femoris,* and *semitendinosus*)
	Tarsus and digit	flex tarsus/extend digit (*long digital extensor, lateral digital extensor*), extend tarsus/flex digit (*superficial digital flexor muscle,* and *deep digital flexor muscle*)

Courtesy of K. L. Epstein.

ligaments of joints in the limb resist medial and lateral motion. The *suspensory apparatus* of the distal limb resists over extension of the fetlock joint. The suspensory apparatus spans from the cannon bone (third metacarpal or metatarsal bone) to the first and second phalanx. It is composed of the suspensory ligament, proximal sesamoid bones, and four pairs of distal sesamoidean ligaments.

Tendons and ligaments are composed primarily of type I collagen fibrils that are grouped into fibers that are parallel to one another. Cytoplasmic extensions of the tendon cells separated the individual fibers. The fibers are grouped into larger and larger subunits separated by loose connective tissue known as *endotenon*, which carries blood vessels and nerves. The endotenon is connected to the *epitenon*, which surrounds the entire tendon. *Paratenon* is a thicker layer of stretchy and resilient connective tissue that surrounds the epitenon in all regions not associated with a tendon sheath.

A *tendon sheath* encloses tendons as they change direction over high motion joints (i.e., carpus, tarsus, fetlock, interphalangeal; Figures 3.35 and 3.36). For example, the superficial and deep digital

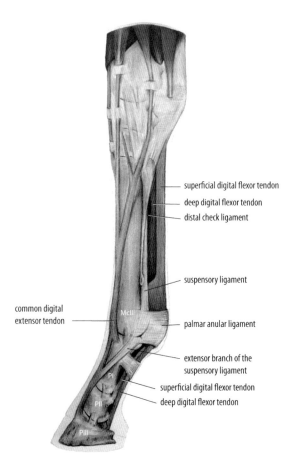

Figure 3.35. Tendons of the thoracic limb. Courtesy of Dr. Robin Peterson.

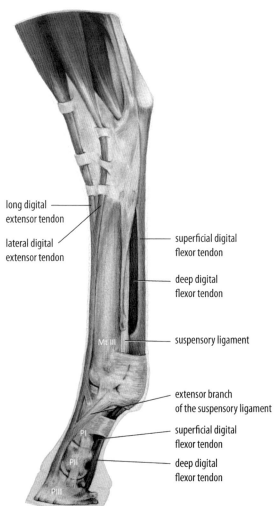

Figure 3.36. Tendons of the pelvic limb. Courtesy of Dr. Robin Peterson.

86

flexor tendons are protected by the carpal sheath in the region of the carpus, the tarsal sheath in the region of the tarsus, and the digital flexor sheath in the region of the fetlock and interphalangeal joints. Tendon sheaths are similar to a joint capsule with a synovial membrane to create synovial fluid to provide lubrication. They also generally contain a fibrocartilaginous pad that is smooth and covers boney prominences. Partitions composed of two layers of synovial tissue known as *mesotenons* often carry the blood supply to the tendon within the tendon sheath. A *bursa* is a synovial pouch between a tendon and a boney protuberance. Some examples include the *bicipital bursa* under the biceps tendon as it passes over the shoulder joint, the *cunean bursa* under the cunean tendon as it passes over the tarsus, and the *navicular bursa* under the deep digital flexor tendon as it runs over the navicular bone. The development of *sesamoid bones* (bones that develop within a tendon or ligament) also protects tendons and ligaments as they pass over areas of high motion and/or bony prominence.

The *passive stay apparatus* is an important adaptation of horses to allow them to rest and even sleep lightly in the standing position. The stay apparatus allows most of the weight of the horse to rest on tendons, ligaments, and deep fascia with minimal requirement of muscular energy. In the thoracic limb (Figure 3.37), the shoulder joint is prevented from flexion because of the internal biceps tendon from the scapula to the radius. This pull is transmitted to the lacertus and extensor carpi radialis to prevent the carpus from collapsing forward. The conformation of the carpal bones, the palmar carpal ligament, and digital flexor tendons and their accessory ligaments prevent overextension of the carpus. With the shoulder and carpus fixed, little force is required to keep the elbow in extension. Flexion is opposed by the tendinous components of the carpal and digital flexors, the collateral ligaments, and the triceps muscle. Overextension of the fetlock and pastern are prevented by the suspensory apparatus, digital flexor tendons, and their accessory ligaments. Flexion of the coffin joint as a result of the pull of the deep digital flexor tendon is pre-vented by the extensor branches of the suspensory ligament.

In the pelvic limb, the stifle must be locked in extension. This is accomplished by extending the stifle to bring the patella into a resting position and then rotating the patella medially to hook the parapatellar cartilage and medial patellar ligament over the medial trochlear ridge. Once the stifle is locked, the hock is locked because the *reciprocal apparatus* (Figure 3.38) that links the motion of the stifle to the hock. The reciprocal apparatus is composed of the tendonus cords of the peroneus tertius (cranially) and the superficial digital flexor (caudally). In the standing position, the superficial digital flexor is taught preventing flexion of the hock. The distal limb is stabilized similarly to the front limb.

The Hoof

The hoof protects the distal extremity of the limb, dissipates the concussive forces secondary to impacting the ground, and aids in venous return from the foot. The hoof is the result of a modified dermis and associated keratinized epidermis. The dorsal aspect of the hoof is referred to as the *toe*, the medial and lateral sides are referred to as the *quarters*, and the palmar or plantar aspects are referred to as the *heel*. The *coronary band* is region of tissue at the proximal edge of the hoof. It bulges because of a thickened region of subcutaneous tissue, the *coronary cushion*.

The portion of the hoof visible when a horse is standing is the *wall*. The wall is widest and thickest at the toe and decreases in height and thickness as it goes toward the heel. The wall forms a rounded heel and then continues forward as the *bars*, which are visible on either side of the frog from the bottom of the foot. The wall consists primarily of tubular horn growing toward the ground starting from the *coronary dermis* within the coronary band.

The external surface of the wall is covered by the *periople*. The periople is formed by the *perioplic dermis*, which is just proximal to the coronary dermis. It is widest proximal to the heels. The

87

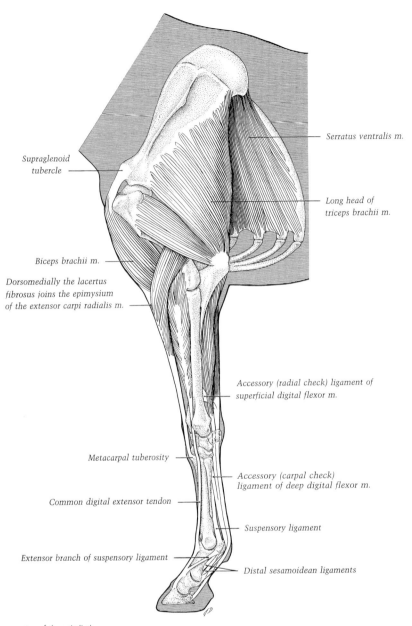

Supraglenoid
tubercle

Biceps brachii m.

Dorsomedially the lacertus
fibrosus joins the epimysium
of the extensor carpi radialis m.

Metacarpal tuberosity

Common digital extensor tendon

Extensor branch of suspensory ligament

Serratus ventralis m.

Long head of
triceps brachii m.

Accessory (radial check) ligament of
superficial digital flexor m.

Accessory (carpal check)
ligament of deep digital flexor m.

Suspensory ligament

Distal sesamoidean ligaments

Figure 3.37. Stay apparatus of thoracic limb.
Courtesy of Stashak 2001.

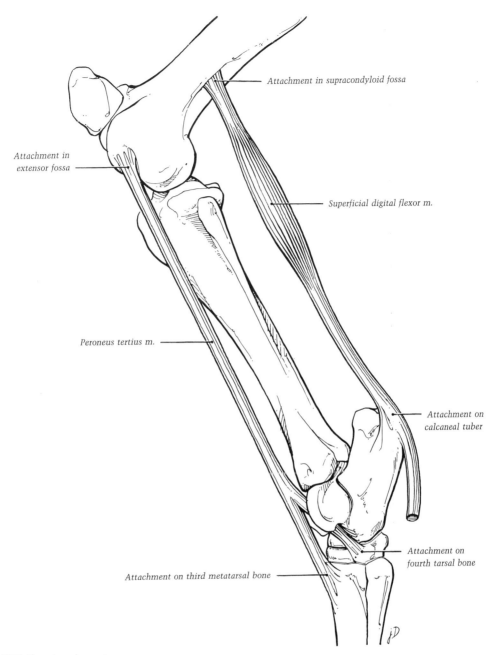

Attachment in supracondyloid fossa

Attachment in
extensor fossa

Superficial digital flexor m.

Peroneus tertius m.

Attachment on
calcaneal tuber

Attachment on
fourth tarsal bone

Attachment on third metatarsal bone

Figure 3.38. The reciprocal apparatus.
Courtesy of Stashak 2001.

periople has a rubbery consistency proximally and then becomes a thin glossy covering of the wall as it dries and moves distally.

Beneath the wall is the *laminar dermis*. The laminar dermis has many projections (laminae) that interdigitate with the laminae on the deep surface of the wall. Each laminae has many projections over its surface (secondary laminae) that make the connection even more secure. The connection holds the third phalanx (coffin bone) in place within the hoof capsule. The epithelium of the laminar dermis proliferates to allow the wall to slide past as it is being produced from the coronary dermis downward. Dysfunction of this connection is known as *laminitis* or *founder*.

The *frog* (cuneus ungulae) is a triangular shaped region of tubular, elastic horn on the underside of the foot. It grows from the aptly named *frog dermis*. The widest part is at the heel with the tip pointing dorsally. It has a central sulcus or groove and a medial and lateral collateral sulcus that separates it from the bars of the hoof. The subcutaneous tissue under the frog is known as the *digital cushion* and contains and internal spine (frog stay) under the central sulcus.

The *sole* fills the remaining space between the wall and the frog on the underside of the hoof. The region between the bar and the quarter is the *angle* of the sole. The sole is slightly concave to allow the majority of weight bearing to occur through the wall and the frog. It is softer than the wall horn. It grows from the aptly named *sole dermis*, which is firmly attached to the distal aspect of the third phalanx. Figure 3.39 illustrates the portions of the hoof when viewed from the ground surface and Figure 3.40 is a cross-section of the hoof.

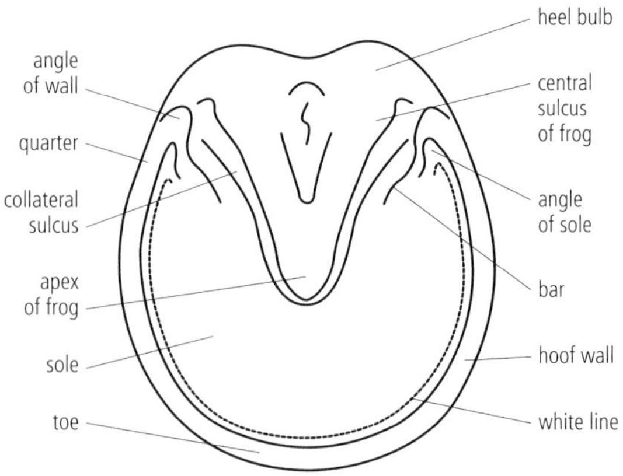

Figure 3.39. Solar view of the hoof.
Courtesy of Coumbe 2001.

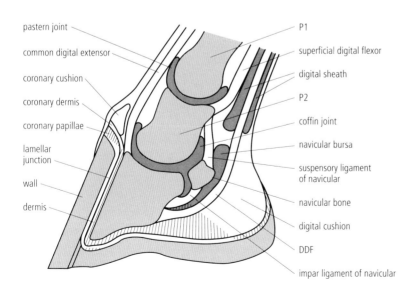

Figure 3.40. Sagittal section of the equine digit.
Courtesy of Coumbe 2001.

References and Further Reading

Aspinall, V. 2005. *Essentials of Veterinary Anatomy and Physiology*. London: Elsevier Ltd.

Auer, J. A., and J. A. Stick. 2006. *Equine Surgery*. 3rd ed. St. Louis: W.B. Saunders Company.

Colville, T., and J. M. Bassert. 2002. *Clinical Anatomy & Physiology for Veterinary Technicians*. St. Louis: Mosby, Inc.

Considine, R. V. 2003. The Adrenal Gland. In *Medical Physiology*, 2nd ed., R. A. Rhoades and G. A. Tanner, 607–22. Baltimore: Lippincott Williams & Wilkins.

Coumbe, K. M. 2001. *The Equine Veterinary Nursing Manual*. Oxford: Blackwell Science, Ltd.

Dybdal, N. O. 2002. Endocrine and Metabolic Diseases. In *Large Animal Internal Medicine*, 3rd ed., B. P. Smith, 1233–65. St. Louis: Mosby, Inc.

Guyton, A. C., and J. E. Hall. 2005. *Textbook of Medical Physiology*. 11th ed. Philadelphia: W.B. Saunders Company.

Riegel, R. J., and S. E. Hakola. 1999. *Illustrated Atlas of Clinical Equine Anatomy and Common Disorders of the Horse*. Volumes 1 and 2. Marysville: Equistar Publications, Limited.

Schott, H. C. 2002. Pituitary pars intermedia dysfunction: equine Cushing's disease. *Vet Clin North Am, Equine Pract* 18: 237–70.

Stashak, T. S. 2001. *Adams' Lameness in Horses*. 5th ed. Baltimore: Lippincott Williams & Wilkins.

Equine Reproduction

Michelle LeBlanc and Audrey Kelleman

Reproductive Anatomy of the Mare

The mare's reproductive organs are situated within the pelvic and abdominal cavities. The *perineum* is the area that includes the anus, vulva, and adjacent skin under the tail. The normal conformation of the perineum prevents the ingress of air and bacteria into the genital tract. This area is important because conformational defects due to genetics, trauma, or repeated foaling results in aspiration of contaminates into the vagina that will eventually result in uterine infections. Three anatomical seals protect the genital tract from contaminants entering the reproductive tract:

- The vulvar seal.
- The vestibulovaginal seal.
- The cervix.

The *vulva* forms the external opening of the reproductive tract. It is directly ventral to the anus. The two vulvar lips should be full and firm and meet evenly in the midline (Figure 4.1). The normal anatomic arrangement of the anus and vulva are that the vulva should be vertical (less than 10% off vertical; angle of declination) and that more than 80% of its length should lie below the level of the pelvic bone. Variations in either of these parameters results in a tendency for the vulva to be drawn forward into the perineum below the anus, especially during late pregnancy (Figure 4.2). Mares with an inadequate vulvar seal, abnormalities in the relative length of the vulva below the pelvic bone, or an increase in the angle of declination may aspirate air, feces, or bacteria into the vestibule, vagina, or uterus resulting in uterine infections.

The *clitoris* is contained within a depression (the clitoral fossa) at the bottom of the vulva. Many types of bacteria reside in this space, some of which cause potentially serious venereal infections. Infected mares show no outward signs. Disease is detected by swabbing the clitoral area and submitting the sample for culture. Mares in estrus (heat) will stand for the stallion, urinate, and expose their clitoris repeatedly. This is termed *winking*. It is common for there to be an accumulation of moist smegma in this area.

The *vestibule* is the tubular portion of the tract between the lips of the vulva and the vestibulovaginal seal (hymen). Sometimes, the hymen has not broken before a maiden mare is presented for breeding and needs to be manually broken to allow breeding. The vestibulovaginal seal may be stretched or torn from either natural breeding or during foaling. If damaged, air and contaminants can enter into the anterior vagina and through the cervix.

The *vagina* is the portion of the reproductive tract between the vestibulovaginal seal and the cervix. The cervix projects into the vagina at its anterior aspect. The majority of the vagina is retroperitoneal (i.e., lies outside the peritoneal cavity) so penetrating injuries usually do not enter the peritoneal space. However, in some maiden mares bred by

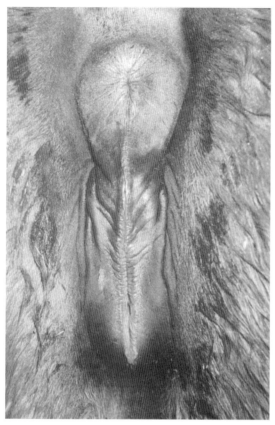

Figure 4.1. Normal perineal conformation.
Courtesy Dr. LeBlanc.

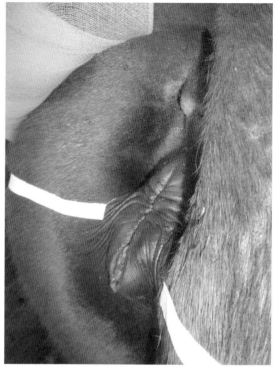

Figure 4.2. Poor perineal conformation. Note the cranial ventral tilt to the vulvar lips.
Courtesy Dr. LeBlanc.

natural cover, an aggressive, vigorous stallion may rupture the anterior wall of the vagina near the cervix. This injury may result in death of the mare to peritonitis. Therefore, mares that have blood on their vulva after natural cover should have a vaginal examination performed to evaluate the integrity of the anterior vaginal wall. The vagina must be able to dilate sufficiently to allow delivery of the foal, so scarring from a previous foaling or breeding must be noted because it will hamper delivery. Accumulation of air, urine, or feces in the vagina can result from an abnormality of the anatomical arrangement of the caudal structures and is a common cause of infertility. A vaginal examination is commonly performed during estrus with a cardboard or glass speculum and bright light to determine if there is any abnormal discharge or inflammation of the vaginal walls and to determine if the cervix appears normal for stage of cycle. If abnormalities are noted additional diagnostics are performed.

The *cervix* is a muscular tubular structure that is between 5 to 8 cm long and 2 to 5 cm in diameter. It is the third protective physical barrier and last line of defense between the uterine lumen and the external environment. The cervix changes size and shape depending stage of the estrous cycle. It is short and open during estrus and long, and tightly closed during diestrus and pregnancy. Any damage to the cervix incurred at breeding or during foaling will adversely affect the mare's ability to carry a foal until term. Some maiden mares, especially those greater than 10 years of age, do not properly open their cervix during estrus. This problem results in either not enough semen entering the uterus if the mare is bred by natural cover or if bred by either natural cover or artificial insemination, the closed cervix inhibits clearance of uterine inflammatory debris associated with breeding.

The *uterus* is a T-shaped structure that consists of a large body and two horns. It is suspended in the pelvic cavity by two ligaments and can freely move within the confines of the ligaments similar to a hammock suspended between two trees. Distension and movement of the intestines and bladder, as well as, pregnancy influence the position of the reproductive tract. The uterus consists of a secretory epithelial lining, a glandular endometrium, and a muscular portion that also contains blood vessels and lymphatics. Blood flow to the endometrium changes during the estrus cycle resulting in changes in uterine tone and appearance on ultrasonography. It is extremely important to be able to determine stage of estrous cycle, especially if there is no stallion to tease the mares for estrus detection.

The *oviduct* is a muscular long tube that extends from the uterine horns to the ovaries. The oviduct is divided into an infundibulum, ampulla, and isthmus. At ovulation, the ova drop into the funnel-shaped infundibulum. It quickly travels to the midportion of the oviduct (ampulla) where it is fertilized. The fertilized ovum remains there for 5.5 days before traveling through the narrow isthmus and entering the uterine horn at the uterotubal junction. Unfertilized ova rarely enter the uterus.

The *ovaries* are kidney shaped with a prominent depression (the ovulation fossa) on the free border.

They are suspended in the broad ligaments and are located below the third and fourth lumbar vertebrae. The ovaries of the mare are larger than other domestic species and vary considerably in size during the year. In the spring and summer, the ovary has several follicles ranging in size from 10 to 50 mm in diameter. Mares will ovulate the largest follicle usually on the third to fifth day of estrus. Some breeds such as Thoroughbreds ovulate two large follicles about 25% of the cycles. In winter, the ovaries are small, firm, and contain few if any follicles greater than 15 mm in diameter. The corpus luteum forms in the crater that was previously filled with follicular fluid. Unlike other species, it does not project from the greater surface of the ovary and is therefore not palpable during rectal examination.

The reproductive tract is suspended in the abdomen by two large *broad ligaments* that extend along the lateral walls of the sublumbar region of the abdomen and the lateral walls of the pelvis. The broad ligaments serve as attachments to the body wall and support blood vessels, lymphatic vessels, and nerves. There are three main vessels that supply blood to the uterus and ovaries that lie within the broad ligament. Occasionally, in late gestation, at foaling or in the first few days after foaling, one of the vessels ruptures resulting in severe hemorrhage and in some cases death of the mare (Figures 4.3 and 4.4).

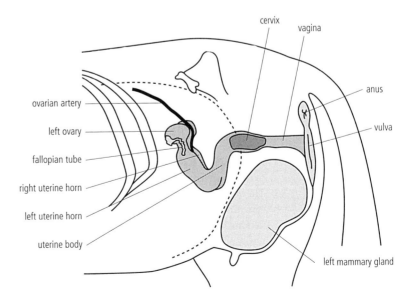

Figure 4.3. Equine reproductive tract.

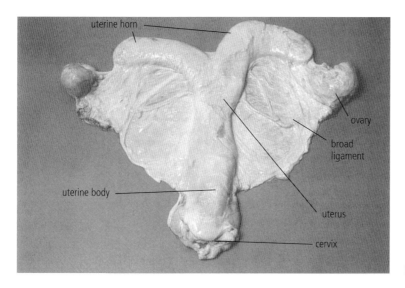

Figure 4.4. Equine reproductive tract.

Puberty

Puberty is the onset of reproductive activity. The onset of puberty occurs from a combination of endocrinological events within the hypothalamus, the pituitary gland, and the gonads. The onset of puberty occurs at around 12 to 24 months of age but can be affected by several factors including: age, photoperiod, nutritional status, and contact with other horses of breeding age.

Reproductive Endocrinology in the Mare

Seasonality

Mares are long day, seasonally polyestrous breeders, meaning that they exhibit a distinct breeding season characteristically during the spring, summer, and early autumn months. During this period, normal nonpregnant mares show repeated estrous cycles lasting about 21 days. Nondomesticated, feral mares and breeds of northern European descent do not normally undergo cyclical ovarian activity during the winter and early spring months. However, some domesticated breeds, such as Arabians, may cycle regularly throughout the year. This seasonality means that foals are born in the spring and early summer, which is the time when the environmental conditions should be optimal for foal survival. Therefore, the natural breeding season of the horse is from May until August. This is the time when highest pregnancy rates are likely to occur.

The mare does not suddenly start to cycle regularly in the spring but enters what is known as a "transitional phase." This period lasts from 30 to 90 days and is primarily determined by the length of daylight. Long day length (15 to 16 hours), such as occurs during the summer, stimulates ovarian activity. The effects of day length are mediated negatively by melatonin secretion from the pineal gland within the brain. Prolonged periods of high melatonin secretion during the short winter days suppress gonadotropin-releasing hormone (GnRH) from the hypothalamus in the brain. Increasing day length in spring causes shorter periods of high melatonin production, allowing an increase in the frequency and amplitude of pulsatile GnRH release. Other factors such as body condition, ambient temperature, and stress also affect the timing of the first ovulation of the year. Thin mares, mares that are housed outdoors when temperatures are below freezing, and maiden mares that are stressed in their new environment tend to cycle later in the year. During the transitional phase, a mare makes three to four waves of follicles, but only a follicle in the fourth wave is capable of ovulating. Mares in transition may show constant estrous behavior, erratic estrous behavior, be passive, or hateful to the stallion.

During the winter, most mares pass through a period of anestrus or sexual inactivity, when neither follicles nor corpora lutea are present. The period of sexual quiescence centers on the shortest day of the year, December 21. Physical characteristics and behavioral signs include: Small, firm ovaries, an atonic, thin walled uterus, and pale, dry vaginal walls and cervix. The cervix appears closed on vaginal speculum examination; however, it may gape open because there is no progesterone to keep it tightly closed. The behavior patterns of seasonal anestrus are not predictable. Most mares are passive to mildly resistant in the presence of a stallion. It is not unusual, however, for a mare in deep anestrus to be sexually receptive to the point where she accepts the stallion at any time.

The Estrous Cycle

The ovulatory season is from late April or the beginning of May to the end of September in the northern hemisphere. The middle of the mare's natural breeding season is around the 21st of June. As autumn approaches, cyclical activity normally wanes. As mares age, the ovulatory season shortens and may only last 3 months.

The estrous cycle consists of two phases:

- The *follicular phase* (also known as estrus) is when the mare will allow the stallion to mate her. Estrus may last from 3 to 7 days during the ovulatory season. Mares will ovulate a follicle that ranges in size from 35 to 50 mm in diameter about 12 to 48 hours before the end of standing estrus. Some breeds, such as Thoroughbreds, have a high incidence of double ovulations (25%) and will consistently ovulate two follicles. This

trait appears to be passed down from mother to daughter. After ovulation, the cavity occupied by the previously mature follicle becomes filled with a blood clot to form the corpus luteum, which produces progesterone.

- The *luteal phase* (also known as diestrus) is when the mare is not receptive to the stallion and a corpus luteum is present on the ovary. Diestrus lasts 14 to 16 days on average and is more consistent in duration than the estrous phase.

The estrous cycle is defined as the interval from one ovulation to the subsequent ovulation when ovulation is accompanied by behavioral estrus or plasma progesterone concentrations below 1 ng/ml. Cycle length ranges from 21 to 24 days. However, it can be variable between a group of mares, and it tends to be longer in the spring and shortest from June through September.

The Hormones of the Hypothalamic-Pituitary-Gonadal Axis Control the Estrous Cycle

These hormones can be divided into:

- The *brain hormones*—melatonin and GnRH produce signals that directly stimulate the pituitary gland.
- The *pituitary hormones*—follicle stimulating hormone (FSH), luteinizing hormone (LH), prolactin, and oxytocin exert a direct trophic action on the ovaries, uterus, and other parts of the genital tract.
- The *genital* or *sex hormones*—estrogen, progesterone, inhibin, and prostaglandin $F_{2\alpha}$ are secreted in response to stimulation by pituitary hormones and control functional changes in the genital tract and behavioral changes in the mare.

Hypothalamus

GnRH is secreted by cells in the hypothalamus and is released in brief pulses. After GnRH reaches the pituitary gland via a portal venous system, it stimulates the secretion of FSH and LH. The frequency of the GnRH pulses is mediated by melatonin release. A low frequency occurs during anestrus when melatonin release is high because of the shortened day length. The frequency of GnRH release is also reduced during diestrus as a result of negative feedback effects exerted by progesterone. The frequency of the GnRH pulses controls which gonadotropin (FSH or LH) is released from the anterior pituitary. High frequency pulses stimulate LH, whereas low-frequency pulses stimulate FSH release.

Pituitary Function
FSH stimulates the growth and development of follicles in the ovary. During the estrous cycle, there are two peaks of FSH. The first peak of FSH occurs near the end of estrus, while the second peak occurs in midestrus about 10 to 11 days later. The rise in FSH stimulates a group of follicles to develop. This phenomenon is referred to as follicular waves. The follicles initially grow in synchrony, and then one follicle eventually becomes dominant and produces inhibin that inhibits further development of the other follicles within the group.

LH is involved in the final maturation of the follicles, maturation of the oocytes within the follicles, and ovulation. Plasma LH levels begin to rise steadily at the end of diestrus with levels peaking 1 to 2 days after ovulation. Progesterone produced by the corpus luteum suppresses LH after ovulation.

Oxytocin is released from the posterior pituitary by the estrous mare in response to sexual arousal. It is frequently administered as a postbreeding treatment to stimulate uterine contractions and speed up emptying of the uterus. It is also used to induce parturition in the mare.

Ovarian Hormonal Production
Follicles produce estrogen, which causes the mare to be receptive to the stallion and induces major changes in the reproductive tract including:

- Softening and relaxation of the cervix.
- Increased uterine and vaginal secretions.

- Uterine edema.
- Growth of the primary follicle.

Estrogen concentrations are low during most of the estrous cycle but rise in early estrus to peak 12 to 36 hours before ovulation and the LH surge.

Progesterone is produced by the corpus luteum during days 1 to 17 after ovulation. It is associated with:

- Contraction of the cervix.
- Increased viscosity of vaginal secretions.
- Loss of the uterine edema.
- Prepares the uterus for entry of the embryo.
- Increases activity of the secretory endometrial glands.
- Acts on the brain to induce rejection-type behavior.

Progesterone is routinely measured in some veterinary practices to confirm ovulation and to determine plasma concentrations during diestrus and pregnancy. Normal values between 5 and 15 days of the estrous cycle and during early pregnancy range from 8 to 20 ng/ml.

Mature follicles secrete inhibin during their maturation. This hormone exerts a direct, negative feedback effect on FSH release and blocks the further development of other follicles within the follicular wave.

The Uterus
The uterus produces two reproductive hormones

- *Prostaglandin $F_{2\alpha}$* is released by the endometrium around day 16 to 17 of the estrous cycle if the mare is not pregnant. Prostaglandin lyses the corpus luteum causing the mare to return to estrus. It is also released where there is inflammation or infection within the uterus.
- *Equine chorionic gonadotrophin* (ECG; see Pregnancy)
- The endocrine, behavioral and physical changes that occur during the estrus cycle are presented in Table 4.1. When these changes do not occur in synchrony, infertility can result.

Table 4.1. Basic endocrine, physical, and behavioral changes during the estrous cycle.

	Endocrine changes		Physical changes		
Stage of cycle	Pituitary	Ovary	Ovary	Tubular tract	Behavioral changes
Early estrus	FSH rise	Estrogen rise	Follicle develops; ovaries large	Uterine edema, cervical relaxation	Beginning receptivity
Late estrus	LH surge	Estrogen peak	Follicle matures	Maximum uterine edema and cervical relaxation; vulva relaxed and long; cervix pink and moist	Strong receptivity; raised tail, urinating, everting clitoris (i.e., "winking")
Ovulation	LH near peak	Estrogen fall begins, progesterone rise begins	Follicle collapses, fresh "crater" palpable	Loss of uterine edema, vulva shortens, cervix still relaxed, pink and moist	Variable, usually still receptive
Early diestrus	LH fading	FSH rise	CH palpable	Firm uterine tone, cervix closed, pale and dry	Rejects stallion
Midcycle	FSH rise	Progesterone peaks	May detect follicular activity, CL may be palpable	Maximum uterine tone, cervix firm, pale and dry	Rejects stallion
Late diestrus		Luteolysis; rapid demise of CL causes progesterone fall	No palpable changes	Early softening of uterus	Rejects stallion

CH, corpus hemorrhagicum; CL, corpus luteum; FSH, follicle-stimulating hormone; LH, luteinizing hormone.
Adapted from LeBlanc, M. M., Lopate, C., Knottenbelt, D., and Pascoe, R. 2003. The Mare. In *Equine Stud Farm Medicine* and *Surgery,* ed. D. C. Knottenbelt, M. M. LeBlanc, C. Lopate, and R. R. Pascoe. United Kingdom: Saunders.

Controlling the Estrous Cycle

Artificial Lighting

Artificial light, applied 60 days before the intended breeding season, is the best method of shifting the vernal (spring) transition forward from April to February (northern hemisphere). Light needs to be added at the end of the day to provide a minimum of 14.5 hours of light daily. Mares exposed to lights from December 1 usually cycle within 60 to 75 days or by February 15. Older mares (>18 yr of age) and mares in poor body condition (body condition score less than 4.5) will take longer to being cycling. Cold winter weather will adversely affect the timing of the first ovulation of the year because mares will expend calories to keep warm. Young mares off the racetrack may not respond to lights because of stress, low body weight, and the possible use of anabolic steroids. They also may not be able to handle the group dynamics (placed in pasture with older mares), and if so affected, should be maintained in a small paddock with a buddy and fed a high fat diet to maintain or increase body weight during the transitional phase.

Many lighting schemes have been advocated. The standard approach for mares that need to be bred in February is to place mares in a 12′ × 12′ box stall (3.6 × 3.6 m box stall) at around 4:30 to 5 pm and leave the lights on until 10 pm. Each stall is fitted with a 100-lux white light. This size light will provide approximately 12 to 15 foot candles of light. The minimum intensity of light required to stimulate cycling appears to be about 2 foot candles. Mares that don't need to be bred until March or April should be placed under lights around the winter solstice. Putting mares under lights in January will not move the natural breeding season forward from late April to March. Breeders who wish to expose mares to artificial photoperiod in a paddock situation must consider the shape and size of the paddock to determine the number, type, and strength of the lights and the height and angle at which they must be placed.

Hormonal Methods for Inducing Cyclicity

Although photoperiod is the most efficient nonhormonal method for manipulating the first ovulation of the year, hormonal treatment schemes added to the end of the lighting regime can advance the first ovulation or can also be used to synchronize the first ovulation in a group of mares. The efficacy of these drug regimes in advancing the first ovulation depends on the stage of the transition period and follicular status at the onset of treatment. The likelihood of mares ovulating successfully after therapy is low if the treatment is started early in the transitional period or when mares are in anestrus. Before treatment with any of the drugs is instigated in late transition, several 25- to 35-mm follicles should be present on the ovaries. If progestins (either altrenogest or progesterone) or progesterone and estradiol are to be given, mares need to be under 14.5 hours of light for at least 60 days if the lighting regime was started on the first of December or for at least 45 days if a lighting regime was begun on December 23. Mares administered either progesterone in oil intramuscularly or altrenogest orally for 10 to 12 days usually exhibit the onset of estrous behavior within 1 to 5 days of the last treatment. Mares given progesterone and estradiol injections daily for 10 to 12 days need to given prostaglandin on the last day of treatment. Mares will begin to show heat around the fifth or sixth day after the last injection and will ovulate around the ninth or tenth day after the last injection. Not all mares will respond favorably to progesterone (P) and estradiol (E) therapy, and they will not exhibit good estrous behavior, even though they have a follicle present that ovulates. Recently, a long acting P and E product has been introduced to the market. One injection is given in late transition. Mares will begin to show heat about 15 to 17 days after the injection. Estrous behavior is better with the long acting P and E than after treatment with daily P and E injections. Ovulation will occur between 18 to 25 days after the injection.

FSH may be given to mares in late transition if they have follicles that are at least 18 mm in diameter. The drug is given twice daily until a 30-mm follicle is present on the ovaries. Treatment typically lasts for 5 to 6 days. The mare is then given human chorionic gonadotropin (HCG) when there is a 35-mm follicle to induce ovulation.

Dopamine antagonists block dopamine. Dopamine is a neurotransmitter that inhibits the release of GnRH and prolactin so there are minimal signals from the brain to the pituitary to release FSH and to upregulate the LH receptors on the ovaries. Dopamine antagonists are most successful in inducing follicular development in February or March if mares are placed under lights for at least 16 hours for 14 days before treatment is begun. Daily injections of sulpiride or oral administration of domperidone are given until the mare begins to develop a follicle greater than 30 mm and shows signs of estrus. If the mare does not develop a follicle in 16 days, treatment is stopped (Table 4.2).

Induction of Ovulation

Ovulatory drugs are used in mares to ensure that the mare will ovulate within a predictable time. This is exceedingly important if a mare has only one opportunity to be bred by natural mating or is to be bred once with cooled or frozen semen. The ovulatory agent is given so that the mare will ovulate within 24 hours when mated naturally, within 18 hours if bred with cooled semen, and within 8 hours if bred with frozen semen. Two types of hormones are used to induce ovulation, GnRH agonists and LH (HCG). Mares need to be in estrus when the drug is given. The first group of drugs (GnRH agonists) causes the release of LH which hastens follicular development and ovulation. Deslorelin is the GnRH agonist that is currently used in equine practice. It comes either as a liquid that is injected into the neck of the mare or as an implant that is placed in the vulvar lip. It is given when the mare has a follicle of at least 30 mm in diameter. If the implant is used, it must be removed after ovulation is detected as it may adversely affect future follicular development and delay the next estrous cycle if the mare does not get pregnant. HCG has LH activity and is given when the mare has a 35 mm or greater follicle on her ovary. Ovulation can occur between 12 to 48 hours when HCG is given. Failure

Table 4.2. Hormonal methods for hastening the first ovulation of the year, inducing ovulation or lysing the corpus luteum.

Drug	Dose	Frequency	Indications
Hormones			
Progestins			
Altrenogest	0.044 mg/kg PO	Once daily for 10–14 days	Estrus suppression
Progesterone	150–300 mg IM	Once daily for 10–14 days	Estrus suppression
Long-acting progesterone P and E	1,500 mg IM	Once every 7 days	Estrus suppression
Long-acting P and E	150 mg/10 mg IM	Once daily for 10 to 12 days	Estrus synchronization
Prostaglandins			
Cloprostenol (Estrumate)	62.5–250 μg IM	Once; give 4 or more days after ovulation	Lyse corpus luteum
Dinoprost (Prostin)	5–7.5 mg IM	Once; give 4 or more days after ovulation	Lyse corpus luteum
Ovulatory agents			
Deslorelin (compounded)	1.5 mg IM	Give when follicle greater than 30 mm	Induces ovulation in 42 to 50 hours
Deslorelin (Ovuplant®)	2.1 mg/implant; place in vulvar lip	Give when follicle greater than 30 mm	Induces ovulation in 42 to 50 hours
HCG	1,500–3,000 IU IV	Give when follicle greater than or equal to 35 mm	Induces ovulation in 24 to 48 hours
FSH	6.5 mg IM	Give twice daily when follicle is longer than 18–20 mm; stop treatment when follicle reaches 30 mm	Induces follicular development (anestrus); induce ovulation with HCG
Dopamine antagonists			
Sulpiride	200–400 mg IM	Once daily for 10–16 days	2 weeks of 14.5 hours of light in January then start treatment; induces follicular growth and hastens ovulation during transition
Domperidone	440 mg IM or orally (paste formulation)	Once daily for 10–16 days	

E, estradiol; FSH, follicle-stimulating hormone; HCG, human chorionic gonadotropin; IM, intramuscularly; IU, intrauterine unit; IV, intravenously; P, progesterone; PO, by mouth.

of HCG to induce ovulation increases with increasing age of the mare. Approximately 15% of mares greater than 16 years of age will not respond to HCG.

Lysis of the Corpus Luteum
Prostaglandins (prostaglandin $F_{2\alpha}$ or an analogue) can be used to shorten the normal luteal phase (diestrus). Estrus will occur between 2 and 10 days of drug administration. The time from drug administration to estrus is determined by the size of the largest follicle on the ovary at the time the drug is given. Mares routinely have follicles that range from 5 to 35 mm on their ovaries during the diestrus phase. The larger the follicle on the ovary when prostaglandin is given, the quicker the mare will return to estrus and the quicker she will ovulate. Mares with follicles of 35 mm or greater may come into estrus and ovulate within 48 hours of drug administration, making it difficult to time

insemination. Therefore, the reproductive tract should be palpated per rectum before prostaglandin is administered to determine when to order semen or when to book the mare to a stallion. It is advisable not to give mares with follicles that are 35 mm or greater prostaglandin to shorten the diestrus phase because they may ovulate before they can be inseminated or bred and the cervix may not be properly dilated at breeding.

Prostaglandins need to be given when the corpus luteum is sufficiently mature or 4 to 5 days after ovulation. Prostaglandin can have unpleasant side effects such as sweating, transient colic, diarrhea, and respiratory distress within minutes of its administration. These signs usually last about 20 to 30 minutes. To avoid these side effects, a small dose of cloprostenol (Estrumate; 60 µg) may be given instead of dinoprost (Prostin).

Pregnancy

Fertilization

Pregnancy occurs as a result of fertilization of an oocyte with a spermatozoa and subsequent maturation of the ensuring embryo with its passage into the uterus. Fertilization of the oocyte occurs in the ampulla of the oviduct. Fertilized oocytes remain in the oviduct for 6 days after which time it enters the uterus through the utero-tubal junction. Unfertilized eggs do not pass from the oviduct into the uterus.

Embryonic and Fetal Development

Once the embryo enters the uterus, it migrates throughout the uterine body and both horns until day 16 to 17 day after ovulation. The migration signals to the dam that she is pregnant (maternal recognition of pregnancy). During migration, the embryo contacts the entire endometrial surface repeatedly as a result of uterine contractility, and movement through the uterus continues until it becomes too large to pass through the horn, around 16 to 17 days. The cessation of movement of the embryo is called *fixation*. Embryos typically are found at the base of one of the two horns when

migration ceases. The embryo produces factors that prevent the release of prostaglandin from the uterus at day 15 of the cycle, thereby allowing maintenance of the corpus luteum. The embryo produces estrogens at about day 12 of pregnancy. The production of estrogen from the embryo and the follicles on the ovaries in combination with progesterone production from the corpus luteum results in a marked increase in tone in the uterus. Increased tone in the uterus is one of the cardinal diagnostic signs of early pregnancy.

The term *embryo* is used up to day 40, and the term *fetus* is used, thereafter. Between 60 days and about 7 months of gestation, the fetus grows slowly because this period is focused on fetal organ development. At the eighth month, the fetus begins to increases dramatically in size and will gain about 60% of its weight in the last 3 months. Proper placental function is extremely important for adequate fetal development. If the placenta is not functioning efficiently or there is infection in the last 3 months, the fetus will be compromised at birth, will be born prematurely, or will be aborted.

Placentation

The placenta consists of fetal and maternal tissues that are apposed for gas and nutrient exchange and for removal of toxic wastes produced by the fetus. Attachment of the placenta to the endometrium occurs relatively late in the mare and begins around day 40 of gestation and is not complete until about 120 days. Endometrial cups are a unique feature of the equine placenta. They begin to form around day 25 of pregnancy, are fetal in origin, and originate from a girdle of cells that are present around the outer shell of the embryo (trophoblast). These cells invade the dam's endometrium starting at about 35 to 38 days of pregnancy. Once in the endometrium, they enlarge and become clumped together to form a horseshoe-like ring of white cups of tissue in the pregnant horn (look like horse teeth). They produce ECG (formerly known as pregnant mare serum gonadotrophin), which stimulates the primary corpus luteum to produce progesterone and causes follicles to ovulate or luteinize. Because progesterone production remains high, mares do not show signs of estrus at the time of these secondary ovulations. The cups continue to increase in size until day 70 of pregnancy at which time they begin to degenerate. They continue to produce ECG until days 120 to 150 when degeneration is complete. Mares that lose their pregnancy after 40 days will not come back into heat until day 120 to 150 even after repeated injections of prostaglandin because endometrial cups block the effect of prostaglandin (lysis of the corpus luteum). Endometrial cups also appear to have an immunological function that may interfere with the mare coming back into heat. Therefore, loss of a pregnancy after 40 days usually results in the mare remaining barren for the year. A decision on whether to abort a mare with twins needs to be made before 38 days of gestation to avoid the complication of the mare not returning to estrus until after 120 days.

The placenta of the mare is epitheliochorial and noninvasive. These terms are used to describe the fact that the maternal endometrial epithelium and the fetal chorion are intact and there is no loss of maternal tissue at parturition. The placental attachment is diffuse in that the membranes are attached to all portions of the uterus with the exception of the cervix when there is no attachment. The membranes that are passed with the fetus are commonly called the *placenta;* however, the correct terminology is *fetal membranes* because the placenta consists of both the maternal and fetal portions of gas exchange. The fetal membranes of the mare include:

- The chorioallantoic: the thick, large outer fetal membrane. The chorionic side, that is, the side that attaches to the dam, is red and velvety in color, whereas the allantoic side, the fetal side, has a bluish gray tinge. The placenta is usually passed inside out so that the bluish side is what is observed once it is passed. The placenta should always be inspected for completeness and then turned inside out to evaluate the maternal side. If there is placental inflammation (placentitis) or infection (discharge, thickening, and discoloration of the membrane) the abnormalities will be present on the maternal or red, velvety side, usually near the cervical star region.

- The amnion is the thin, white membrane the covers the fetus. A foal that is normal at birth will break this bag during the delivery process. If the foal is weak or there is inflammation of the sac, the foal may be born within the sac and die from suffocation.
- The umbilical cord is usually 45 to 65 cm in length and will contain many twists. It consists of two portions, the amnionic and allantoic portions. Umbilical cord torsions can occur and will result in abortion. Usually the torsion is due to an excessively long or very short cord. If a torsion is suspected its length should always be measured.
- Hippomane is a soft putty-like brown to yellowish brown disc-shaped structure. It is usually about the size of a small shoe. It contains urinary calculi that form throughout pregnancy. It will have a layered appearance when cut.
- Yolk sac remnant is sometimes identified within the allantoic part of the umbilical cord. It is hard in consistency and can be mistaken for a deformed remnant of a twin pregnancy.

Endocrinology of Pregnancy

The hormonal profile during the first 2 weeks of pregnancy is similar to that of the nonpregnant mare. Differences start at 14 days, when prostaglandin would normally increase with a subsequent decrease in progesterone. Maternal recognition of pregnancy accounts for the continued production of progesterone by the primary corpus luteum, which is the sole source of progesterone until day 35. The endometrial cups contribute to the production of progesterone through the actions of ECG. In addition to its effects on progesterone production, ECG blocks the estrous cycle for the duration of the life of the endometrial cups or around day 120 to 150 of pregnancy.

For the first half of gestation, progesterone from luteal tissue supports the pregnancy. Luteal progesterone levels peak at about day 100 and subside to baseline by about day 180 to 200. After day 200, levels of progesterone are negligible in the dam's serum. The fetus and placental unit begin to contribute to the endocrine patterns of pregnant mares around day 60 of gestation. The unit is responsible for the production of progestins, estrogens, and relaxin. Measurement of these hormones in the dam's circulation after day 150 of gestation reflects hormonal production by the feto-placental unit and not the mare's ovaries. Progestins produced by the feto-placental unit begin to rise around day 90 of pregnancy and level off at about 180 days of gestation. Concentrations remain constant in maternal serum until days 305 to 310 of gestation, when they begin a dramatic rise, peaking about 5 days before parturition. The rise in progestins in the last 3 weeks of gestation is thought to be associated with maturation of the fetal adrenal glands. If the fetus is stressed the progestin concentration in the dam's serum will rise prematurely. If the fetus is dying due to an in utero crisis such as acute placental infection or hypoxemia (lack of oxygen) during a colic surgery, the progestins will fall. Because of the changes in the progestin pattern during disease or fetal stress, they are measured in mares at risk of abortion or premature foaling if the condition affects the mare before 305 days of gestation. Three blood samples can be drawn at 48- to 72-hour intervals. If the progestin concentration changes by more than 50% from sample to sample, an in utero crisis is occurring. Progestins can be measured using an assay that measures progesterone because progestins are metabolites of progesterone, and they cross-react with both radioimmunoassays and enzyme-linked immunosorbent assay (ELISA) designed for measuring progesterone. Progestin concentrations range between 3 and 12 ng/ml between day 180 and 305 of gestation in mares carrying normal fetuses.

Estrogen remains relatively low in pregnant mares until day 35, when it suddenly increases. The source of estrogen production in early pregnancy is ovarian luteal tissue. Estrogen production by ovarian tissue may be stimulated by ECG because it rises and falls in concert with the rise and fall in ECG. A second rise in maternal estrogens begins around day 60 of pregnancy when estrogens synthesized by the feto-placental unit appear in the dam's circulation. A massive rise in estrogens continues from day 70 to 100 of gestation with levels peaking around day 210 to 240 and gradually decreasing as gestation continues to term. The fetal gonads are the source of the estrogen precursors, which are then synthesized by the feto-placental unit into eight types of estrogens. The elevated levels of total estrogens can be used as a pregnancy test in the horse by immunoassay of blood, urine, or milk from day 45 to term.

The equine fetus only matures in the last 5 to 7 days of gestation. Therefore, inducing parturition must be carefully considered in each mare because it performed too early it will result in a premature foal that will likely die in the first few weeks of life (see Induction of Parturition).

Diagnosis of Pregnancy

Pregnancy diagnosis is determined by a veterinarian via rectal palpation and ultrasonography. The first examination is usually conducted around day 14 or 15 after ovulation with the day of ovulation considered as day 0. The 14-day conceptus is 13 to 16 mm in size and lies most commonly in the uterine body but can also be found in the uterine horns. The uterus must be evaluated carefully to determine if the mare has twins. Frequently a second examination is performed on day 16 or 17 to ensure that only one vesicle is present in mares with a history of twinning or in a mare that ovulated two follicles. If a twin is present, one of the two vesicles is then crushed manually by the veterinarian. The next examination is conducted on day 28 after ovulation. The embryo is highly echogenic and clearly visible ultrasonographically. The heart of a normal embryo should be beating at a rapid consistent rate. Highest pregnancy loss occurs between the 14 and 28 day examination so the examination must be thorough. The size and shape of the vesicle should be measured and recorded. There are tables depicting normal growth and development. Any pregnancy that is not conforming to appropriate measurements should be reevaluated. Twins are sometimes missed and not identified until the day 28 examination. Mares are not allowed to carry twins because most mares will abort them between 7 to 8 months and serious complications to the mare's health can occur. Twins identified at 28 days can be successfully managed if there is space between the two vesicles. If the twins are side by side or on top of each other, success at reducing the pregnancy to one viable vesicle is poor. However, the mare can be brought back into heat with prostaglandin before the formation of the endometrial cups. Any decision to abort a pregnancy needs to be made before day 35 of gestation to avoid the effects of ECG.

Pregnancy can be reconfirmed at 35 to 42 days. If the pregnancy is to be insured an ultrasonographic examination must be conducted between 42 and 45 days of gestation. Additional pregnancy examinations may be conducted during the autumn and early spring. Large breeding operations routinely perform ultrasonographic examinations on mares at days 14, 17, 28, and 45 and reconfirm pregnancies by rectal palpation on days 60, 120, and then in the winter or late autumn.

Fetal Assessment

Problems may occur during mid- to late gestation that adversely affect the fetus. These include placentitis, umbilical cord torsion, and secondary complications due to a medical or surgical crisis, such as colic or a viral infection. A pregnancy may be evaluated in late gestation by rectal palpation, transrectal and transabdominal ultrasonography, vaginal examination, and by measuring total estrogens or progestins. Rectal examination is the simplest method for fetal monitoring; however, it does not provide much information on fetal well-being other than the fetus is moving or not moving. Foals that are compromised continue to move so movement alone is a poor index of viability. In addition, the fetus will go through periods of sleep in utero so one can not assume that a fetus that is not moving is a dead fetus.

Transrectal ultrasonography is used most commonly to measure utero-placental thickness, to determine if there is placental separation, and to evaluate fetal fluid clarity. Increased placental thickness in the last 3 months of gestation is associated with placental abnormality including placentitis. Transabdominal ultrasonography is most commonly performed to measure fetal heart rate, monitor fetal movement, and to determine if there is twins or placental separation within the uterine horns or uterine body. Mares that develop a vaginal discharge during pregnancy may have ascending placentitis. A vaginal examination will determine where the discharge is from, if there is vaginitis, and if the cervix has opened prematurely. Any discharges arising from the vagina should be culture, and the swabs submitted for bacterial or yeast isolation.

Measurement of total estrogens or plasma progestins will provide data on fetal well-being. The fetal gonads produce the precursors for a number of estrogens, and these precursors are metabolized by the placenta into estrogens. Measuring total estrogens between 5 and 9.5 months of gestation can provide information on fetal well-being. Progestins remain at baseline levels in a normal pregnancy (2–12 ng/ml) until 3 weeks before foaling when they begin to rise dramatically in the maternal circulation. The rise in maternal progestins is thought to be due to maturation of the fetal adrenals as research has shown progesterone output by the fetal adrenal glands in the last 3 weeks of pregnancy. Progesterone is the precursor to cortisol and the fetal adrenals lack the necessary enzymes to convert the progesterone to cortisol until the last 5 days of pregnancy. Therefore, the progesterone produced by the fetal adrenals is metabolized by the placenta into many progestin compounds. During the last 5 days of pregnancy, the enzyme needed to convert fetal adrenal progesterone to cortisol becomes available and fetal adrenal progesterone is converted to cortisol. Because of this unusual endocrine finding, final maturation of the equine fetus only occurs in the last week. If the foal is born before this final maturation it has a poor chance at survival even if it is in a neonatal unit. Changes in the progestin pattern before day 305 of gestation can be used to determine a premature stimulation of the fetal adrenals. A premature rise indicates fetal stress, whereas a fall is most commonly associated with fetal demise. A minimum of three blood samples taken at 48- to 72-hour intervals are needed to identify changes in the progestin pattern.

Mammary Secretion Electrolyte Concentrations

Mammary secretion concentrations of sodium, potassium, and calcium change in the last week of pregnancy. Measurement of these electrolytes can be used to determine when a mare will foal. About 5 days before the normal foaling day, sodium begins a rapid drop, while potassium rises such that the concentrations flip flop with potassium being higher than sodium. In the 72 hours preceding parturition, calcium begins a rapid rise, peaking after she delivers the foal. Mares can be safely induced to foal if the following criteria are met:

- No maternal illness, no premature dripping of milk from the udder.
- Colostrum in the udder.
- Mare is at least 330 days of gestation.
- Characteristic mammary secretion electrolyte changes have occurred.
  - Sodium level is less than potassium level.
  - Calcium level is greater than 12 mmol/l or 60 mg/dl or 300 parts calcium/million in the Foal Watch test.

There are two types of test kits that can be used to monitor mammary secretion electrolyte concentrations, the strip test or the fluid test. The former is associated with false-positive determinations (i.e., that the mare will foal and she does not). This finding is due to the strip measuring both calcium and magnesium. Magnesium rises before the calcium, and if high enough, gives a false-positive result. The fluid test is a modification of the water hardness test used in the water purification industry. It only tests for calcium and it also gives the level of calcium within the colostrum. Mares that have a calcium concentration of 250 parts/million have a 95% likelihood of foaling within the next 72 hours.

Induction of Parturition

Inducing parturition is a procedure that should not be taken lightly because many complications can occur. If the procedure is elected the criteria mentioned previously must be absolutely followed. Mares are induced with small doses (5 to 10 IU) of oxytocin intravenously. A catheter should be placed in the mare's jugular vein before the procedure and one must have all equipment available to handle a possible dystocia (see Dystocia). Drugs for sedation and anesthesia must be available so if difficulties arise the mare can be rapidly anesthetized. The time from administration of the first injection of oxytocin until the foal is delivered is usually 30 to 45 minutes. The procedure is most commonly performed in mares that have had repeatedly delivered stillborns, mares that have had foals that developed neonatal isoerythrolysis, mares that have experienced rectovaginal tears, and mares over 410 days of gestation.

Abortion

Abortion is not common in mares. It will occur, however, more frequently in mares greater than 14 years of age than in young mares. Mares carrying twins will abort about 90% of the time but abortion due to twins in not commonly seen anymore because most twins are detected early in pregnancy by ultrasonography and one of the vesicles is manually removed. Twins used to be the number one cause of abortion in mares. Abortion in mid- to late gestation may occur in a single mare or may occur in many mares. The latter is referred to as an "abortion storm." Because viral or bacterial infections can spread rapidly through a group of mares, any mare that has aborted must be separated immediately from the herd until the cause is identified. The fetus and placenta should be placed on ice and examined by a veterinarian within 12 hours or sent off immediately to a diagnostic laboratory. The mare that aborted should be examined for retention of a twin, for placental retention and for bruising, tearing, or infection of the reproductive tract. Blood may be needed to measure titers. The Table 4.3 below presents information on the most common causes of abortion in mares.

Table 4.3. Causes of abortion in the mare.

Cause	Contagious or non-contagious	Clinical signs	Time of abortion	Gross placental changes	Method of identification	Control methods
Equine herpes virus-1	Contagious	Usually none; clear nasal discharge weeks before abortion	6+ months	none	Changes to fetal liver and lung	Vaccination Isolation post-abortion
Equine viral arteritis	Contagious Venereal disease	Fever, limb edema, conjunctivitis, nasal discharge	6+ months	None	Virus isolation in fetus; high titers in maternal blood	Vaccination Isolation post-abortion
Leptospirosis	Contagious	Fever, depression, icterus	5+ months	Thickened placenta Exudate	Fetal liver swollen; titers in maternal blood	No vaccine approved Isolation
Mare reproductive Loss syndrome	Not contagious	None	45–120 days; 10+ months	Thickened placenta	Fetal and placental changes	Remove Eastern Tent caterpillars
Ascending placentitis	Not contagious	Vaginal discharge; premature udder development	5+ months	Thickened cervical star region; exudate	Culture fetal stomach contents;	Caslick; breed young mares
Nocardioform placentitis	Not contagious	Premature udder development	9+ months	Exudate over uterine body	Classic exudate on placenta; white patch on placenta	None
Umbilical cord torsion	Not contagious	None	Anytime	Swollen, twisted cord greater than 65 cm	Swollen cord	None
Twins	Not contagious	Premature udder development	5+ months	Large white area on placenta	Two fetuses	Ultrasound early in pregnancy
Stress	Not contagious	None	Anytime	None	None	Decrease stress
Endotoxemia	Not contagious	Sick	Anytime	None	None	Determine cause and avoid

Parturition

Preparation for Foaling

Gestation is extremely variable in the mare with normal gestation length ranging from 325 to 360 days. The primary signs that a mare is nearing foaling are development of an udder, wax on the teats, and elongation of the vulva. The vulva will also become soft and flabby to the touch. The tail-head will appear to rise as the ligaments around the tail head soften.

The mare should be moved approximately 2 weeks before the anticipated due date, the mare should be moved to her foaling location. If she has had a Caslick operation, the vulva should be opened after local anesthesia has been infiltrated along the previous incision line. A daily and nightly routine should be established and followed so that she become accustomed to the routine and will not be disturbed by normal occurrences when she is ready to foal. The mare is remarkable capable of postponing active labor when she does not feel safe or secure. Most mares foal between 10 pm and 6 am, when there is minimal activity. A common saying is that the foal picks the day to be born and the mare picks the time. The foaling attendant should quietly observe the mare and look in on her about every hour when the mare has developed wax on her udder or shows other signs of imminent foaling. Monitoring systems may be used. These include video cameras, birth alarm systems that are either strapped over the mare's girth like a surcingle or are sown into the vulvar lip. The latter are activated when either abdominal contractions begin or when the amnion parts the vulvar lips.

Some mares in late gestation will exhibit abdominal discomfort. It is difficult to differentiate these signs from colic in some mares. Discomfort in late gestation due to fetal movement will frequently resolve by walking the mare or administering a nonsteroidal anti-inflammatory drug. As parturition approaches the mare will usually decrease feed intake. She may also separate herself from the group if she is with other mares.

Mares should foal in a clean, dry environment. Small grassy paddocks are ideal. If foaling in a stall, the stall should be at least 12' × 12'. The mare should be monitored closely to ensure that she does not get cast in a corner.

Parturition in the mare is divided into three stages. Stage 1 is the preparatory stage where the fetus is rotating from lying on its back to lying on its abdomen. Average duration is about 1 hour. If the mare is disturbed, she can postpone stage 2 for hours or a few days. During stage 1, the mare may be found rolling, pawing, kicking at her abdomen, and looking back at her flanks. Sweat will appear on her flanks and neck. She will frequently urine and defecate, get up and down, and exhibit the flehmen response (curling the upper lip). Once one recognizes that the mare is in stage one, the tail should be wrapped and the vulva washed with soap and dried. The mare should then be left alone and watched from a distance.

Stage 2 is defined as delivery of the foal. Stage 2 usually lasts about 5 to 20 minutes, though it may be as long as 60 minutes. The mare actively contracts during this stage and is usually lying down. There usually are several contractions in succession and then a period of rest lasting 2 to 3 minutes before the next set of contractions. The mare may reposition herself, getting up and down many times. Shortly after the waters break, the amnion, a bluish-white sac that looks like a balloon, is presented. A healthy, normal foal will break the amnion before it is delivered, whereas a weak, ill, or compromised foal may be born in the sac. If the head has passed through the vulva and the sac remains closed over its head, it should be opened and pulled back over the foal's head. If necessary the mare can be assisted by gently pulling on the foal's front legs. Amnionic fluids are honey colored. A brown to deep yellow amnionic fluid is indicative of meconium staining. This is a serious complication especially if the foal is stained as it is indicative of stress in utero. Inhalation of meconium is extremely irritating to the lungs and can cause pneumonia.

Emergencies at Foaling

The presence of a red velvety or a brown granular membrane at the lips of the vulva is an emergency. The membrane is the chorioallantois that has separated from the dam's endometrium prematurely. The membrane must be cut immediately and the foal assisted in the delivery as the foal has lost its oxygen supply. This is referred to as a "red bag" delivery (Figure 4.5). It is common in mares with placentitis, with mares that have been induced to foal, and in mares that appear not to be contracting properly. A source of oxygen should be available for the foal. Many of these foals may appear to be normal for the first 12 to 18 hours of life only to become a "dummy" after that time (see Chapter 6).

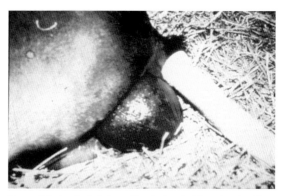

Figure 4.5. A red velvety bag will protrude out of the vulva when the chorioallantois separates prematurely from the endometrium during labor. It must be cut and the foal delivered immediately. Courtesy Dr. LeBlanc.

When to Assist

If any of these situations occur, the veterinarian should be contacted immediately. If the mare can be stood up, she should be walked (Table 4.4). If the mare is to be transported to a hospital, advise the client on sedation protocols. The technician should have the room ready for the arrival of the mare and all equipment needed to assist the veterinary. Equipment that should be included is detailed in Table 4.5.

Most mares transported to a hospital are anesthetized if the foal is alive and hung from a hoist to relieve pressure on the caudal abdomen thereby assisting delivery. The technicians should assist the veterinarian as requested and be ready to care for the foal. See Chapter 6 on neonatology.

The foal has a relatively long umbilical cord, which remains intact through the delivery process. It is left intact for a few minutes as blood continues to leave the placenta into the foal. The mare should not be disturbed at this stage to avoid her from rising and rupturing the cord. The cord usually ruptures at a predetermined place due to movements of the mare or foal. Once the umbilical cord has ruptured the stump should be examined for hemorrhage and the end of the cord dipped in (1:4) solution of chlorhexidine. The stump should be disinfected several times during the first few days of life.

Stage the of parturition involves the passage of the fetal membranes, often termed *delivery of the afterbirth*. It usually occurs within 2 hours of foaling, and if the fetal membranes are not passed by 5 hours, the mare should be examined. Retention of fetal membranes can result in metritis, septicemia, and laminitis. When the mare stands, a knot should be placed in the fetal membranes so that it hangs just above the hocks so that the mare does not step on it before it is completely passed.

Evaluation of Fetal Membranes (Placenta)

Fetal membranes need to be examined and preferably weighed after every foaling to ensure that all have passed from the dam and to note any abnormalities. Mares that retain a piece of placenta may become severely ill within hours or days of foaling and develop metritis, septicemia, and laminitis. In addition, abnormalities in fetal membrane color or texture or areas containing brown thick or purulent discharge reflect placental infection or premature separation from the endometrium. These abnormalities will compromise oxygen exchange to the fetus or result in the foal being born with an infection. Fetal membranes should be weighed within a few hours of foaling. Normal weight ranges between 12 and 16 lb or 10 to 12% of the foal's body weight. Fetal membranes that are infected will usually be edematous and weigh more than 18 lb. Mares may abort their fetus because of excessive twisting of the umbilical cord (umbilical cord torsion), and in some cases this occurs because it is longer or shorten than normal (normal 40–65 cm). It is, therefore, advisable to measure the length of the umbilical cord after an abortion.

Table 4.4. When to assist in delivery.

- No progression in the delivery process 5 minutes after rupture of the chorioallantoic (water breaking).
- No straining for lengthy period once the amnion has appeared.
- The mare continually gets up and down and rolls from side to side.
- One foot and the head, two feet and no head, or only the head.
- If the foal is coming through the rectum.
- "Red bag" delivery-cut membrane and delivery immediately.
- The foal is stuck at the hips once the head, legs and chest are out.

Table 4.5. Equipment needed for a dystocia.

- A bucket of warm water.
- Soap.
- Obstetrical lubricant.
- Roll cotton.
- Chains or straps for the foal's legs.
- Towels.
- Fetotomy equipment.
- Resuscitation equipment for foal.
- Clippers to clip abdomen if a cesarean section must be performed.
- Anesthetic equipment.

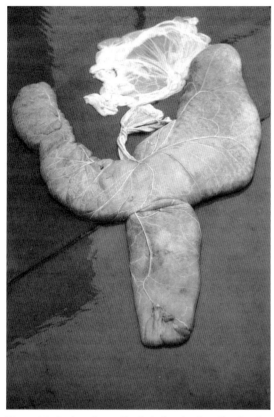

Figure 4.6. Fetal membranes. The chorioallantois, a large blue-tinged sac, is attached to the endometrium. Fetal side is shown in picture. The smaller white tissue is the amnion. It surrounds the fetus during pregnancy.
Courtesy Dr. LeBlanc.

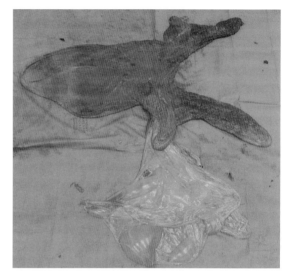

Figure 4.7. Fetal membranes from a mare with ascending placentitis. Note the brown, granular appearance of the maternal side of the chorioallantois in the area of the cervical star.
Courtesy Dr. LeBlanc.

Placental membranes are made up of the chorioallantois (the sac attached to the dam's endometrium), the amnion (whitish blue sac surrounding the foal), and the umbilical cord. All these tissues are of fetal origin and must be passed from the uterus within 5 hours of birth to avoid the dam becoming ill. Placental membranes are normally passed inside out so that the membrane closest to the foal (allantoic portion of the chorioallantoic membrane that has a bluish-gray color) is visible. Because almost all lesions are on the maternal side of the placenta (chorionic portion of the chorioallantoic membrane), the placenta must always be turned inside out to view the red,

velvety side. When examining the placental membranes, they should be laid out in an F formation so that the membranes can be evaluated completely (Figure 4.6). The tip of the fetal membranes that is attached to the end of the uterine horn closest to the ovary is most commonly retained so if there is a tear in the membranes in these areas one should assume that a portion is retained in the mare. The veterinarian should be notified immediately so that the mare can be thoroughly examined. Because most infections arise from bacteria ascending through the vagina and cervix, the placental area that is closest to the cervical star is most commonly affected (Figure 4.7). It may be thickened, brown, and granular in appearance. White areas within the chorioallantois indicate that the placenta was not attached to the endometrium. If the area is large, one must suspect that the mare was carrying twins. Any abnormality should always be reported to the veterinarian so that the mare and foal can be properly attended to.

Reproductive Management of Mares

Maiden Mares

As a group, maiden mares should have the highest degree of potential fertility as long as they are less than 10 years of age. Assuming normal reproductive development, they have the best resistance to bacterial contamination and tolerate marginal breaches of management better than barren mares.

Specific Problems with Maiden Mares Mainly Relate to

Estrus Detection

Psychological factors—fear or stress may prevent maiden mares that are cycling normally from exhibiting estrous behavior. These mares need to be patiently worked with, presented to the stallion slowly, and rewarded if they stand quietly. Handlers need to be careful when working with these mares as they may leap forward, rear, or kick back suddenly. In some cases when the mare needs to be bred naturally, sedation may be needed.

Breeding

Young mares are often nervous and don't tolerate manipulation of their vulva and vagina. If the mare does not tolerate these procedures when twitched, placed in a stock, or when a lip chain is placed over her gum, sedation is recommended. Mares that need to be bred by natural mating can be given partial, small doses of tranquilizers for calming. In some cases, diazepam is given. A full dose of tranquilizer should not be give because the mare may fall when mounted by the stallion.

Adjustment to Life as a Broodmare

Fillies with extensive athletic careers or show-circuit backgrounds may be difficult to convert to broodmares. They may require a separate paddock or a small paddock with a buddy. After long periods of confinement, rigidly scheduled training, or other established routines, many maiden mares deteriorate in condition on retire-

Table 4.6. Complete reproductive examination.

- Attention should be directed to the size and function of the ovaries and uterus during rectal palpation.
- The vaginal examination should, in addition to the routine inspection, evaluate remnants of the hymen that might cause problems in breeding.
  - A persistent hymen is simply treated by stretching or incision.
  - An imperforate hymen traps mucus and uterine secretions in the cranial vagina causing irritation.
- Uterine cultures of maiden mares may be required before breeding on some farms.
- The chance of endometritis occurring in a maiden mare is remote.
- In the absence of clinical signs of inflammation, a positive culture should be viewed skeptically.
- Occasionally, young mares have pneumovagina and concurrent vaginitis, cervicitis, and even a vulvar discharge.
- Such cases respond quickly to a Caslick operation.

ment to the breeding farm. Special handling, feeding, and close observation may alleviate this problem. Turning a nervous filly out into a large pasture with mature barren mares almost guarantees the filly will receive physical punishment, be located at the bottom of the pecking order, and receive inadequate nourishment.

A complete reproductive examination of all maiden mares before breeding is advisable (Table 4.6). Breeding maiden mares by natural service presents a challenge even to experienced handlers. The unpredictability of the mare poses a potential for injury to the stallion, mare, and attendants. After suitable restraint is applied, before breeding the mare with a valuable stallion it is wise to allow a teaser stallion to mount the mare a few times. A breeding roll, which limits intromission, is advisable when breeding maiden mares.

Foaling Mares

Following prolonged suppression of pituitary and ovarian function by gestation, mares respond with a dramatic, fertile, cycle within 8 to 14 days after foaling. This estrus is called foal heat. Mares can conceive on this heat as long as they have foaled normally, at term, had not retained their placenta and have no fluid in their uterus

10 days after foaling. Mares bred by artificial insemination during foal heat will have pregnancy rates that are similar to those at the 30-day estrus as long as they foaled normally, did not retain their placenta, and had no intrauterine fluid on day 10 after foaling. In the Thoroughbred industry, mares are rarely bred on foal heat because pregnancy rates are lower, and early embryonic death rates are higher in mares bred by natural cover on foal heat. Thoroughbred mares are most commonly bred at the next estrus that occurs around 28 to 30 days after foaling (lay term: 30-day heat) or they are given prostaglandin 5 to 6 days after they ovulate their foal heat follicle.

Before a foaling mare is bred a thorough reproductive examination should be conducted. Mares can aspirate feces, air, and other contaminants into their uterus during foaling, especially if they foal in a small stall. They can experience severe bruising or tearing of the walls of the vagina or cervix or they may hemorrhage before, during, or after foaling from their uterus, blood vessels in the broad ligaments, or from the vagina or cervix. The examination should include evaluation of the perineal area for cuts, bruises, and swelling; a rectal and ultrasonographic examination of the reproductive tract; a vaginal speculum examination; and evaluation of the cervix for tears, bruising, or adhesions. If there is any indication during the examination that there may be an infection, a uterine cytology and culture is warranted.

Estrus detection in mares that are nursing foals presents potential problems. The protective nature of some mares is such that they do not exhibit estrus behavior when approached by a teaser stallion. This is a particular problem of mares with their first foal. Restraint in various forms may be of value. The presence or absence of the foal and its location during teasing are variables to consider.

Barren Mares

Management of mares with a history of endometritis should be directed so that as few matings as possible are used. Semen induces an inflammatory response, and most mares that are infertile because of endometritis are unable to quickly clear the uterus of the by-products of insemination. It is the prolongation of the normal physiological inflammatory response that renders these mares subfertile. If the inflammation persists 5 days after ovulation when the embryo enters the uterus, the inflammatory by-products will damage the embryo, resulting in pregnancy loss.

It is extremely important that the stallion to which barren mares are to be bred is fertile. If the mare is to be bred with shipped, cooled semen, semen quality must be excellent; otherwise the mare will need to be bred on repeated cycles. It is not advisable to breed mares with a history of endometritis with frozen semen because pregnancy rates are poor, especially if she is more than 12 years of age.

The cause of the infertility should be diagnosed before the breeding season. A complete reproductive examination should be performed during the summer or early autumn of the previous year. Because treatments vary depending on the type of endometritis, it is extremely important to discover the cause of the infertility before instilling antibiotics into the uterus. Antibiotic treatment is not benign and can cause secondary infections with yeast or fungi if used indiscriminately. Not all infertility is due to the mare. Data on the stallion must be obtained especially if the mare was bred the previous season with either shipped cooled semen or frozen semen.

Artificial Insemination

The vast majority of mares in the United States and Canada are bred by artificial insemination, with the exception of racing Thoroughbreds, in which natural mating is required. Mares may be bred with fresh semen, cooled, or frozen semen. Most breeding programs that use artificial insemination incorporate the administration of an ovulatory agent and repeated ultrasonographic examinations of the reproductive tract to time ovulation. If the stallion resides on the farm, it is not uncommon to breed the mare every other day beginning on the second or third day of estrus until they stop showing estrous behavior. Caution should be used with this method if the mare is an old, barren mare that had foaled many times previously and has a history of uterine fluid accumulation. The technique for artificial insemination is similar with fresh, cooled, or frozen semen. Most commonly, mares are bred with an artificial insemination pipette attached to a syringe when fresh or cooled semen is used. An artificial insemination gun or a flexible long catheter for deep horn inseminations may be used with frozen semen. The syringe used for delivering the semen should be one without a rubber stopper because the rubber contains compounds that are toxic to semen. All equipment should be maintained at 37° C (Table 4.7 and Figure 4.8).

Breeding with Cooled Semen

To breed mares successfully with cooled semen all parties involved, mare owner, stallion manager, and veterinarians need to cooperate when coordinating the semen shipments with the timing of the mare's ovulation. A technician can be extremely helpful to the veterinarian in organizing information about the mare, stallion, breed specifics, and making the appropriate phone calls to the stallion owner and working out the logistics with pick up or drop off of semen. This section details what must be known before breed-

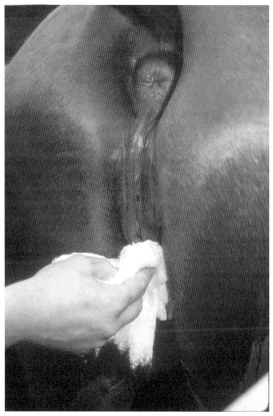

Figure 4.8. The vulva of the mare needs to be washed three to four times and then dried before one passes a hand into the vagina. Courtesy Dr. LeBlanc.

Table 4.7. Artificial insemination technique.

- The mare should be prepared for insemination before the semen is drawn into the syringe or before the semen is thawed. It is preferable to have the mare in stocks when breeding.
- The mare's tail is wrapped and pulled to the side so that the perineum can be thoroughly washed and not contaminated with particulate matter from the mare's tail.
- The vulva and anus are washed three to four times with soap and water and then dried thoroughly. The vulvar lips should be parted to determine if there are feces within the vestibule, and if feces or debris are present, the vestibule should be rinsed with water. Cooled semen does not need to be warmed before breeding unless it has been extended in a cream gel extender.
- The operator applies sterile obstetrical lubricant to a gloved hand. The tip of the insemination pipette is covered by the hand, which is inserted into the vagina.
- The cervix is located with the fingers and the tip of the insemination pipette is inserted into the cervix and advanced into the uterus.
- Semen is slowly injected into the uterus. If there is pressure on the syringe during infusion, the pipette should be gently pulled back 1 to 2 cm because the tip may be lodged against endometrium.
- The bandage on the tail is removed after the veterinarian removes the gloved hand.

ing is conducted. Before shipping semen, the owner should clarify several points with the stallion manager.

- The cost of stallion collection.
- The cost of preparing the semen for shipment, the number of collections provided gratis (if any), the cost of shipping semen tanks by air, and when and how the semen tanks must be returned.
- The days of the week the stallion is collected.
- Times during the breeding season when the stallion will not be available.
- The number of days notice that the stallion manager needs before the semen shipment.
- The latest time one can call to obtain semen (for example-one must call by 9 am to receive semen by the next day)
- The longevity of the semen—does it live in the tank for 12, 24, or 36 hours
- First-cycle conception rate of the stallion.
- The method of air transport used (same-day air or overnight shipment).
- Number of times the mare can be bred if she does not conceive (is the contract limited to 1, 2, or 3 years).
- The breed registry requirements, and the number and timing of postinsemination clinical (pregnancy) examinations must be established.

Management of mares for breeding has changed in the last 15 years because more mares are bred on farms where there are no means for teasing the mare to determine where she is in her estrous cycle. Stabling the mare at a veterinary clinic or at a breeding operation that is visited daily by a veterinarian saves money on veterinary travel fees. Many of these facilities have a stallion to tease the mare to determine when she is in heat, thereby limiting the number of examinations. Once the mare is in heat, she will need to be examined at least every other day and bred within 24 hours of ovulation.

Pregnancy rates are highest when mares are bred within the 24 hours that precede ovulation using semen of high fertility. The quality of the semen is of paramount importance: Stallions with low fertil-ity usually have much lower first cycle pregnancy rates than those with high inherent fertility. In addition, the handling of the semen is critical; failure to prepare it correctly, as well as, poor subsequent handling at the mare end can make the process quite disappointing. Timing of the breeding with the ovulation can be difficult especially if the stallion is collected only three times a week. Ovulation should be induced with drugs such as HCG or Deslorelin. Mares may ovulate as quickly as 12 hours, as late as 48 hours, or they may not respond at all after administration of HCG. The window from injection of Deslorelin to ovulation is tighter than that of HCG with most mares ovulating between 42 and 48 hours; however, it costs about 2 times more than HCG.

There are standards that semen needs to meet to be considered of adequate quality. A dose of semen should contain a minimum of 500 million progressively motile sperm with at least 30% of the sperm being progressively motile. Semen should always be examined under a microscope after a mare is bred and the progressive motility should be recorded. If semen is of poor quality, the stallion manager or veterinarian for the stallion should be notified.

After insemination, the reproductive tract of the mare should be examined daily until she ovulates. If she does not ovulate within 24 hours, she should be bred a second time. Some mares are problem breeders. The most common cause of low pregnancy rates in mares is decreased clearance of uterine fluid and the by-products of breeding. When semen is deposited in the uterus, the mare responds with an inflammatory response because the semen is recognized as a foreign substance. Reproductively normal mares clear the fluids that are associated with the inflammation within 12 to 18 hours of mating; those that do not, accumulate fluid. The inflammatory products in the fluid are harmful to the uterine lining as they have a low pH (acid). Old mares (>14 years of age) that have had many foals may have a pendulous uterus that does not drain well, so the mare accumulates fluids in her uterus after breeding. Some maiden mares do not open their cervix properly when they are in heat, which also results in fluid accumulation in the uterus. Both of these conditions will lead to low pregnancy rates. If a mare does not become pregnant after two breeding attempts she should be considered a problem mare and reevaluated. Treatment after breeding with oxytocin, uterine lavage, or steroids may be needed to increase a mare's chances at becoming pregnant. Keep in mind that the stallion may contribute to the low pregnancy rates so one should always record the number of progressively motile sperm that is in an insemination dose.

Breeding Mares with Frozen Semen

Breeding a mare with frozen or thawed semen often results in a lower first-cycle pregnancy rate than if the mare was bred with either fresh or cooled semen. Pregnancy rates of 0% to 70% per estrous cycle have been reported with an average pregnancy rate per cycle of 35% to 40%. Pregnancy rates are highest when a full dose of frozen semen from a stallion of known fertility is placed in a young mare of known fertility. Mares that are more than 14 years of age when they are bred with frozen semen have a pregnancy rate of about 20%. It is more costly to breed mares with frozen semen because the mare needs to be inseminated within 8 hours of ovulation. Therefore, many of these mares need to be examined more often than if they are bred with cooled or fresh semen.

Points that must be clarified before buying frozen semen:

- What is the first cycle conception rate of the stallion when breeding with frozen semen?
- What is the cost of semen?
- What constitutes a dose—number of straws?
- Is semen sold by the dose or by the straw?
- Will there be directions with the semen on how to thaw the straws?
- Are nitrogen tanks available to store the semen?
- What is the rental fee for the dry shipper?
- What paperwork is required by the breed organization?

One needs to understand the difference between a dose of frozen semen and a straw of frozen semen.

Semen is packaged in either 0.5- or 5-ml straws. If the smaller straw is used, more than one straw will be needed because the 0.5-ml straw does not always hold enough motile semen. The number of straws needed for breeding varies between stallions, but 250 progressively motile sperm is commonly recommended as the minimum number of sperm needed for an insemination. Stallions with highly concentrated semen with high sperm motility require less straws for a dose than stallions that are not as fertile. Four to eight 0.5-ml straws are usually required for a dose. Some clients wish to use only a half of a dose or a quarter of a dose of frozen semen as semen is frequently sold by the straw and not by the dose. If a mare is bred with only a quarter or a half of dose of semen, the semen should be inseminated deep within the horn on the side where the dominant follicle is located using a flexible pipette made specifically for these types of inseminations.

A number of methods for managing mares with frozen semen have been reported. If only one dose of semen is available, mares need to be bred after ovulation. They are usually examined every 8 hours after they have been given an ovulatory agent. Either HCG or Deslorelin is given when the dominant follicle is 35 mm in diameter and soft to the touch. As soon as ovulation is detected the mare is bred. If more than one dose is available, a timed breeding protocol can be followed. This method will incur lower veterinary fees and less stress on the mare because she will need fewer examinations. If HCG is used to induce ovulation, the mare is first bred 24 hours after she was given HCG and then a second time at 36 hours after HCG, if she has ovulated by 36 hours. If she has not ovulated at 36 hours, the veterinarian may elect to breed after ovulation has been confirmed. In the latter instance the mare should be examined every 8 hours from hour 36 (time 0 = time when HCG was given) to ovulation. If Deslorelin is used as the ovulatory agent, the mare is first bred at 36 hours and then again at 48 hours.

Pregnancy rates of 50% to 70% per cycle can be obtained routinely with frozen semen *if* the mares are carefully chosen for fertility and *if* the stallion's fertility (with frozen semen) is high. If either requirement is not met, then breeders often are frustrated because costs are high and the mare does not get pregnant.

Equine Embryo Transfer: Technique, Expectations, and Results

Embryo transfer has become a relatively commonplace procedure in the equine industry, especially with the establishment of large recipient herds throughout the country. In addition, breed associations have amended their rules governing the number of foals derived from embryo transfer that may be registered each year. Most associations now allow for more than one foal to be registered.

Success rates vary and depend on the fertility of the stallion and mare and on the synchronization and quality of the recipient mare. Pregnancy rate per cycle when a grade 1 or 2 embryo is transferred is 50% to 65% with rates of up to 80% reported. The embryo recovery rate of a reproductively normal mare should equal the per cycle conception rate of the stallion. If the rate of recovery is 15% or lower than the per cycle conception rate, one needs to reevaluate the technique. Embryo recovery rates do drop though when the mare has fertility problems or semen quality is poor. Pregnancy rates associated with nonsurgical transfer depend on the ability of the veterinarian and proper synchronization and reproductive soundness of the recipients. Highest rates are achieved when a grade 1 or 2 embryo is transferred into a recipient that ovulates 1 to 2 days after the donor mare and the recipient mare has a tightly closed cervix and a toned uterus. Some individuals consider the management and quality of recipient mares to be the most important factor in obtaining high pregnancy rates.

The average costs associated with producing a foal by embryo transfer if the stallion and mare are fertile and the recipient is reproductively normal and synchronized properly, ranges from $5,500 to $7,500. These costs include veterinary fees associated with breeding the mare on two cycles (pregnancy rates are approximately 50%), collection of an embryo, transfer of the embryo into a recipient, and the cost of the recipient from a commercial herd. If the owner elects to use their own recipients, pregnancy rates are highest when the donor's estrous cycle is synchronized with that of three recipients. Because most owners do not include the cost of maintaining their own recipients, their costs will appear to be lower. It is important to communicate this information to clients because their perception of what success rates should be may be unrealistically high.

Donor Mare Management

A complete reproductive examination should be conducted on donor mares before breeding. This examination should be conducted during estrus and should include evaluation of external perineal conformation to determine if the mare needs a Caslick, a vaginal examination, and ultrasonographic evaluation of the reproductive tract. If abnormalities are noted, such as poor uterine tone, a long, narrow cervix during estrus, excessive uterine edema or intrauterine fluid, a uterine cytology and culture should be performed. Cervical competency can be evaluated when the culture instrument is passed manually. Mares with "manageable" reproductive problems need to be bred to highly fertile stallions and in some cases, the use of frozen semen should be avoided. Mares with clinical signs or histories of endometritis need to be aggressively managed after breeding and may require treatment before breeding. Treatments include uterine lavage, judicious use of ecbolics such as oxytocin or cloprostenol and intrauterine antibiotics.

Breeding management of embryo transfer donors is more intensive than in mares that are left to carry their pregnancies. Many of these mares will have repeated uterine flushes in order to obtain three to five embryos in a season. Extra efforts to avoid contamination of the vagina and uterus are needed to avoid bacterial infections that may occur from repeated entry into the uterus during diestrus. During each estrus that the mare is to be bred, the reproductive tract should be examined by rectal palpation and ultrasonography every other day until insemination, after which time the mares should be examined daily until 24 hours after ovulation. Ovulation should be induced with either HCG or Deslorelin. Ovulation should be timed such that the mare ovulates within 24 hours of insemination. Repeated use of HCG has been associated with a lack of response (ovulation within 48 hours) when it was administered for three or more estrous cycles in one season. Therefore, most veterinarians that use HCG will administer it for the first two cycles of the year and then give Deslorelin in subsequent cycles to induce ovulation.

Semen quality needs to be evaluated at breeding and if found not to be adequate, a second dose of semen should be inseminated. Recommended minimum dose is 500 million progressively motile sperm. Time of ovulation and the number of follicles that ovulate need to be recorded. An embryo flush is conducted on either the seventh or eighth day after ovulation. Young mares are routinely flushed on day 7, whereas mares that are older than 15 years of age and those bred with frozen semen are flushed on day 8. If a mare ovulates two follicles, flushing the uterus 7 days after the second ovulation is preferred. In situations where no embryo was recovered and the mare was inseminated with high-quality semen, ovulated within 36 hours of breeding, and had good uterine tone on the day of uterine flush, it recommended that the uterus be flushed the next day.

Embryo Flush Procedure

Before the embryo flush attempt, the reproductive tract of the donor mare needs to be evaluated by rectal palpation and ultrasonography. This is especially important if the mare was managed for breeding by another individual. The cervix should be evaluated for length and tone, the uterus for tone, presence of endometrial edema or intrauterine fluid, and the ovaries for a corpus luteum. If the examination identifies an open cervix, endometrial edema, and only follicles, then the flush attempt may be cancelled. Preparation of the mare for an embryo flush attempt includes:

- Mare should be placed in stocks.
- The tail bandaged and pulled to the side (the tail can be wrapped with long gauze, pulled laterally and toward the mare's head, and then tied around the horse's neck).

- It is preferable to sedate the mare with a small dose of detomidine and butorphanol (0.25 ml of each drug) because it facilitates rectal manipulation of the uterus during the flushing procedure. Detomidine is used because it is associated with waves of uterine contractions in a pattern that is similar to that produced by oxytocin.
- The perineal area is thoroughly washed and dried. The vulvar lips are parted and the vestibule is washed with wet cotton.
- Complete flushing media and transport media are available from a number of commercial sources. The uterus is routinely flushed three to four times using a total of 3 L of embryo flushing media. The liter of flushing media should be hung on the stocks and the tubing attached. One line of the tubing is attached to a uterine catheter and the second line to a specialized filter that will catch the embryo.
- The tubing and the catheter are then filled with flushing media before the catheter is placed in the uterus so that no air is infused into the uterus.
- The veterinarian passes the catheter through the vagina and into the uterus. The cuff on the uterine catheter is then filled with between 35 and 60 ml of air and water. The amount is determined by the size of the uterus. The cuff is not filled to capacity so as not to interfere with movement of the catheter tip during the procedure.
- The uterus is filled with flush media three times. The volume of media needed is determined by uterine size. After the uterus is filled, it is palpated per rectum to ensure that both horns have filled. The uterus is also balloted as the embryo is sticky and may adhere to the endometrial surface.
- The efflux passes through the catheter and is collected in a graduated cylinder. The amount of flush media recovered is recorded. On the second and third flushes, the catheter tip is inserted into each horn while the fluids are being drained. The horn is massaged during the recovery phase.
- After the uterus is flushed, the catheter is removed and the tubing flushed by running unused flush media directly from the holding bag through the filter (Figure 4.9).

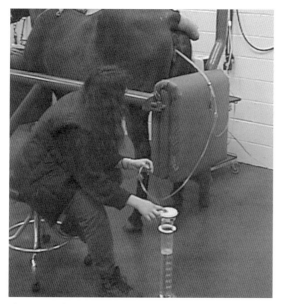

Figure 4.9. The uterus is filled with flush media for collecting an embryo. The volume retrieved is recorded.
Courtesy Dr. LeBlanc.

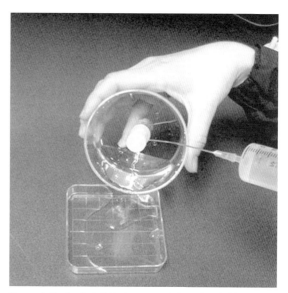

Figure 4.10. The flush fluids that remain in the embryo holding cup are poured into a dish and examined under a dissecting microscope for an embryo.
Courtesy Dr. LeBlanc.

Embryo Evaluation

The contents of the filter are emptied into a dish with gridlines. The type of search dish used is at the practitioner's discretion. The filter is flushed with 30 to 50 ml of flush media that has been previously set aside and this fluid is placed in a second dish. A stereomicroscope for searching for and grading embryos is recommended. Once an embryo is identified, it is aged and graded for quality and stage of development. It is then removed from the wash fluids, placed in a dish containing transfer media and washed a number of times. If the embryo flush media is cloudy, it is cultured for the presence of bacteria or yeast. The donor is given prostaglandin unless a second attempt is to be performed the next day (Figure 4.10).

Transfer Procedure

Almost all embryos are transferred nonsurgically through the cervix. The technique requires strict cleanliness as the operator can iatrogenically inoculate the mare's uterus or cervix during the procedure. Following embryo recovery, the reproductive tract of the recipient is palpated per rectum and fecal material removed. The recipient has been chosen previously from her ultrasonographic findings. The recipient mare is prepared as previously described for the donor mare. The perineum is thoroughly washed and the vestibule wiped with clean moist cotton. The mare is lightly sedated to facilitate the procedure.

The embryo is transferred through a transfer gun specifically made for horses. Day 6 and early day 7 embryos fit readily into a 1/4-ml straw that is slid through the barrel of the transfer gun. Larger embryos, day 7.5 or day 8, may need a 1/2-ml straw or even an artificial insemination (AI) pipette for placing in the uterus of the recipient mare. The embryo should not occupy more than 60% to 70% of the diameter of the straw or pipette. To place the embryo into the uterine horn, a technician parts the dried and cleaned vulvar lips as the veterinarian carefully places his or her hand into the vestibule. The cervix is located and gently manipulated to find the opening in the external os, and the embryo transfer (ET) gun is placed into the cervical canal. The veterinarian then removes his or her arm from the vagina and locates the ET gun via rectal palpation. The ET gun is slowly and gently guided up a uterine horn and the embryo released. After the procedure the straw is flushed with media into a dish and the dish searched to ensure that the embryo was discharged into the uterus. The recipient mare may be placed on a non-steroidal anti-inflammatory drug and given an antibiotic and supplemental progesterone based on the discretion of the veterinarian. The decision of when to discontinue medication is made after pregnancy examination.

Some embryos are collected by veterinarians and then shipped by air to an embryo recipient herd. If an embryo is to be shipped to a recipient unit, airline connections need to be identified in advance. If one chooses to ship by commercial airline and not by an overnight express company, the veterinarian needs to have their facility approved by the airline. Some recipient facilities will forward an airline bill to the veterinarian for embryo shipment. The embryo is packaged by placing it in a 5-ml tube containing embryo holding media (also referred to as transfer media). The cap of the tube is sealed with parafilm wax paper and is then placed in a 50-ml conical tube that contains either embryo flushing or holding media. The screw top of the 50-ml conical tube is also wrapped in parafilm wax paper. The 50-ml tube is then placed in an equitainer that has properly cooled cans. Paperwork identifying mare, owner, day of collection, and grade of the embryo needs to be furnished.

Recipients

The veterinarian has the option of using recipients provided by the client, using recipients owned by the hospital, or shipping the embryo to a recipient facility. Criteria for recipients that receive embryos need the following: On the day of transfer, there should be a large corpus luteum on the recipient's ovary as visualized by ultrasonography. The uterus

should have good tone and not be edematous, doughy, or thick walled. There should be no evidence of uterine edema, that is, intrauterine fluid or air. The cervix should be long and narrow. It is preferred that the recipient ovulate 1 to 2 days after the donor. Mares that ovulate before the donor or more than 72 hours after the donor are less desirable. Recipients should be sound of limb and a body condition score of 4.5 to 6.5. They need to have satisfactory perineal conformation and an udder that palpates normally. If possible, they should be quiet and easy to work around. Many clients feel that the mare's disposition influences the foal's disposition.

There are many, large, well-managed recipient herds through the country. The mare owner needs to discuss options with their veterinarian and then contact the recipient facility that they wish to work with in the future. A contract will be sent detailing the specific costs, what will be covered including number of attempts allowed, when the pregnant recipient must be picked up, if the recipient can be returned, and the price that will be paid to the mare owner for returning the recipient. Some facilities include three embryo flush attempts in their fee after which time the mare owner pays for each attempt. Once a contract is signed a holding fee, usually $1,500, needs to be paid. The remainder of the fee ($2,500–$3,500) is paid when the mare is declared pregnant.

If a mare owner prefers to use their own recipient mares, it is best to have three mares synchronized for every transfer attempt. Three mares are preferred because there is wide variation in the length of estrus, in the rate of follicular development, and in the timing of ovulation after administration of HCG or Deslorelin. Mares should be reproductively sound and less than 15 years of age. If maiden mares are to be used, they should be less than 10 years of age and have normal cervical function. Pluriparous mares need to be examined to ensure that there are no anatomical defects that may have occurred from a previous foaling or uterine degeneration. Highest pregnancy rates are obtained when the recipient ovulates 12 to 48 hours after the donor.

Attention to detail, cleanliness, and dedication are needed to obtain pregnancies by using embryo transfer techniques. The donor will require intensive management to optimize the change of pregnancy. Semen quality must be known before used for insemination and the number of progressively motile sperm recorded at time of insemination. Cleanliness during all procedures is of paramount importance because any mishandling of the embryos can result in degeneration or death.

Infertility

A number of factors have contributed to low reproductive efficiency in the horse, despite the high level of stud farm management and veterinary attention that they receive.

- Man has superimposed a January 1 birth date on foals in the northern hemisphere, creating a disparity between the physiological breeding season of mares and the breeding season arbitrarily impose by racing and performance industries. For some breeds, notably Thoroughbreds and quarter horses, an operational breeding season exists, which is February 15 until the first week of July. This "artificial man-made" breeding season means that mares are in the transitional period between winter anestrus and the regular cycles of summer when they are bred.
- Horses are not selected for fertility but for performance. In doing so, breeding stock with heritable defects that reduce fertility is retained in the breeding pool.
- Geriatric mares and stallions are bred.
- Prohibition of artificial insemination in Thoroughbred horses.

Few mares are permanently infertile, but subfertility of varying degrees is a major problem. There are many causes of subfertility, which can either act along or in combination with each other. For convenience and ease of diagnosis, fertility problems are divided by "client complaint." The three most common complaints are:

- Mares that don't cycle: This indicates that the signal from the brain is not reaching the reproductive tract. Endocrine dysfunction is the cause. Common conditions include: winter anestrus, transition into the breeding season, granulosa cell tumors (ovarian tumor), poor body condition, lactational anestrus, anovulatory follicles, and pituitary abnormality.
- Mare gets pregnant and then loses her pregnancy: the signals from the brain to the reproductive tract are functioning properly. There is a defect within the reproductive tract itself. This problem can be due to anatomical or functional problems. Common causes include: uterine degeneration, endometritis, delay in uterine clearance after breeding, cervical defects, lymphatic drainage problems, poor blood flow, infectious causes of abortion, early embryonic death, "old egg" disease in mare older than 16 years.
- Mare does not get pregnant after frequent breedings: the most common causes are inflammation or infection or poor quality semen. Other causes include: delay in uterine clearance after breeding, conformational defects (e.g., vulva, vaginal, or cervical), resulting in aspiration of air, urine, or contaminants (e.g., bacteria, yeast, or feces) into the uterus.

To determine the cause of the infertility a breeding soundness examination must be performed. The basic examination consists of taking a complete history, evaluation of the physical condition of the mare, evaluation of the perineum (e.g., vulva, perineal musculature in relationship to the anus), rectal and ultrasonographic examination of the reproductive tract, a vaginal speculum examination, and a cervical examination. Laboratory diagnostics that may be needed include: hormonal analysis, uterine culture, uterine cytology, biopsy, or endoscopic evaluation of the uterus. The latter diagnostics are used on a case-by-case basis. The findings of the examination are then compiled to make a diagnosis and to then make recommendations on mare management.

Veterinary technicians can be extremely helpful during and after the examination by setting up the room for the examination, completing the necessary paperwork, recording findings of the procedures for the veterinarian, preparing and evaluating the cytological specimens, and sending off samples. In addition, they can collect reports after samples have been analyzed, call clients, and review recommendations.

Breeding Soundness Examination

The general physical condition of the mare should be appraised. Systemic problems, poor body condition, laminitis, or pain may adversely affect fertility. Lame or painful mares may accumulate intrauterine fluid because they have limited mobility. Abnormal estrous cycle length or no estrous cycles during the mare's natural cyclic season may be associated with uterine infection, pain, ovarian tumors, or systemic endocrine abnormality such as Cushing disease or insulin resistance. Farm management should be assessed because group dynamics may adversely affect body condition of young or old mares, especially if mares are fed in pens. Mares housed in cold climates require more energy in the cold months (December–March) because they expend more calories. Mares that lose weight in the winter or early spring tend not to cycle properly even when placed under 14.5 or more hours of artificial light in December.

Because most uterine infections are due to bacteria or yeast ascending through the vagina, the anatomy of the pelvic region and perineum must be evaluated critically. Mares that pool fluid after breeding (especially Thoroughbred mares) often are long and weak in their loin, flat over their croup with a high tail setting that is level with the sacral iliac joint, and have a sunken anus. The perineum is best evaluated during estrus, when relaxation and elongation of the vulvar lips are greatest. After the external examination is performed the mare's tail should be wrapped and pulled laterally out of the field of work. The basic order of the examination is:

- External evaluation.
- Rectal/ultrasonographic examination.
- Vaginal examination.
- Cervical examination.

- Uterine culture and cytology (samples collected by swab culture or by small volume flush).
- Uterine biopsy (not always performed).
- Endoscopic procedure (this may be performed directly after the rectal examination because mares may be presented only for the endoscopic procedure).

The rectal examination provides information as to when a mare may ovulate; where she is in her cycle; if she is pregnant; if there is cervical, uterine, or ovarian pathology; and if there is an inconsistency between cervical findings, uterine tone, and follicular development. Uterine tone—thick, doughy, edematous, flaccid—is associated with changes in the estrous cycle, seasonality, and pathological processes. Size, shape, and turgidity of follicles on the ovary are used to predict ovulation and identify abnormal structures such as suspected anovulatory follicles or tumors. Repeated ultrasonographic evaluations of the reproductive tract during the estrus cycle may be needed to identify the cause of infertility because the reproductive tract changes dynamically during the estrous cycle, and subtle abnormalities may be noted only during a specific portion of the cycle. The findings should always be recorded as should stage of estrous cycle.

After the rectal or ultrasonographic examination, the perineum of the mare should be thoroughly washed and dried so that a vaginal and cervical examination can be performed. The perineum can be washed a minimum of three times with wet roll cotton or thick paper towels and a mild soap. The area should be dried thoroughly with clean, dry paper towels. Vaginal examinations are usually performed with disposable cardboard speculums or glass speculums. A small amount of lubricant should be placed on the end of the speculum that is placed in the vagina. A vaginal speculum examination should always be performed in infertile mares because the integrity of the vestibulo-vaginal sphincter, the presence of fluid such as pus or urine in the vaginal vault, or discrepancies between cervical relaxation and stage of estrous cycle and the color and moisture of the vaginal mucosa are identified visually. The external os of the cervix may be adhered to the vaginal fornix or the cervix may be inflamed, closed, and located off the vaginal floor during estrus in a mare with endometritis.

If the veterinarian suspects a cervical lesion, a manual cervical examination should be performed. The veterinarian will require a sterile sleeve and in some cases will ask for a sterile glove to be placed over the sleeve. A small amount of sterile lubricant should be placed on the back of the hand to facilitate entry into the vagina.

Laboratory Diagnostics

Diagnostics most commonly used to determine the cause of infertility in mares are uterine cytology and culture. In some cases, endometrial biopsy or uterine endoscopy are also performed. Uterine culture samples are usually obtained by a guarded culture swab, whereas cytological specimens are obtained by passing a second swab into the uterus, collecting cells on the cap of a guarded swab, or by using a cytology brush. The swab collected for uterine culture should be immediately placed in a transport media, labeled, and placed in a cooler until it can be taken to the laboratory. After the culture swab is prepared, the swab or the cap of the swab guard that is to be used for cytology smear is rolled (swab) or tapped (cap) onto a glass slide (Figures 4.11 and 4.12). The glass slide can be fixed with a cytological spray or it can be air-dried and placed into a slide case for transport to the laboratory. Slides for cytological evaluation are stained with a Diff Quick Stain, air-dried, and then looked at under a microscope using high power (40×) and oil (100×). The number of inflammatory cells and epithelial cells identify bacteria or yeast and estimate the degree of debris. Cytological smears are twice as sensitive as culture swabs in identifying mares with inflammation.

Culture swabs have been found to only identify about 60% of bacterial infections. Reasons for this low accuracy are that a swab only comes into contact with a small area of the endometrium directly in front of the cervix, thereby missing focal infections or those infections centered in the uterine horns. Some bacteria adhere tightly to the endometrium and do not produce fluid

so a dry swab placed into the uterus may not adequately collect the required specimen. Because of these deficiencies, a small volume uterine flush technique has become the method of choice for collecting culture specimens from infertile mares. In this technique, a uterine catheter is placed into the uterus and 60 to 150 ml of sterile saline are infused into the uterus. The veterinarian then rectally massages the uterus for 1 minute and then drains the fluid into a sterile bag or sterile 50-ml conical tube. The clarity of the fluid is recorded.

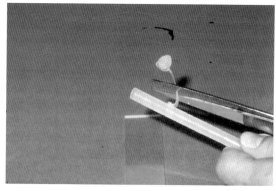

Figure 4.11. Tapping cap of guarded uterine culture instrument onto glass slide for cytology is one method for collecting secretions to make a smear for cytological evaluation.
Courtesy Dr. LeBlanc.

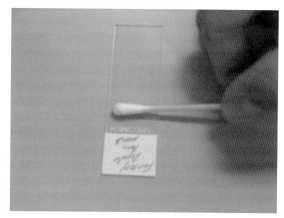

Figure 4.12. Cytology smears can be made by rolling a swab with uterine secretions unto a glass slide.
Courtesy Dr. LeBlanc.

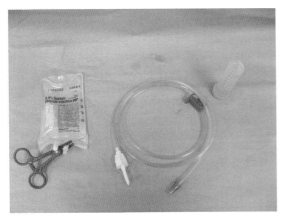

Figure 4.13. Equipment needed to perform a small volume flush of the uterus for uterine culture.
Courtesy Dr. LeBlanc.

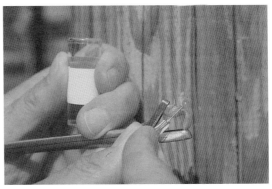

Figure 4.14. Endometrial tissue sample collected for histological evaluation needs to be lifted gently out of the basket and then placed in Bouin's solution.
Courtesy Dr. LeBlanc.

Cloudy efflux or efflux with mucus strands is highly correlated with bacterial or yeast infections. The efflux is centrifuged and the pellet cultured. A sample of the pellet can be placed on a swab and the swab rolled on a glass slide to make a cytological specimen (Figure 4.13).

Endometrial biopsies provide valuable information on whether a treatment reduced inflammation, if there is uterine degeneration that adversely affects uterine clearance or blood flow and if additional therapy is required. Biopsies can be taken during estrus or diestrus. They are usually reserved for mares that have been barren for at least one season and not obtained in the cycle that the mare is bred. They also may be taken as part of a prepurchase examination or to determine if the mare will be an adequate recipient mare for embryo transfer or if the mare should be embryo donor candidate. Endometrial biopsies are taken with a specially designed biopsy forceps. The forceps has a basket that is approximately 3.5 cm in length and 2 cm in depth. For a tissue specimen to be considered of adequate size, the sample needs to be at least 2 cm in length. The tissue is gently lifted out of the basket with a 25-gauge sterile needle and placed in Bouin's solution (pitric acid). The specimen is transferred into alcohol (70% or greater) and shipped to a pathology laboratory for cutting the tissue appropriately and

placing on a slide. The biopsy specimens are read either by a board certified pathologist or theriogenologist (Figure 4.14).

Uterine endoscopy is usually limited to mares with possible focal infections, uterine adhesions, or foreign bodies. The procedure can be performed during diestrus or in early estrus. The uterine lumen may be filled with either air or saline. Visibility is best with air insufflation, however, air can be irritating to the endometrium. On completion of the examination, the infused air should be removed through a catheter or pump, the uterus lavaged with saline, and in some cases, antibiotics infused if the mare has a history of endometritis. These diagnostics should provide the information needed to make a diagnosis. The question that arises is how to best treat the mare.

Uterine Therapies

Many therapies have been advocated for infertile mares. Some have a scientific basis; others have been used out of frustration. As more is learned about uterine function, how systemic disease or pain adversely affects uterine function, and how uterine degeneration interferes with normal function, treatment protocols have improved. Uterine therapies for inflammation, infection, or fluid retention include:

- Uterine lavage with 2 to 3 L of saline or lactated Ringer's.
- Oxytocin or prostaglandin administration to induce uterine contractions.
- Intrauterine or systemic antibiotics for uterine infection (also used in Thoroughbreds as a postbreeding treatment).
- Dexamethasone or prednisolone treatment around breeding for chronic inflammation or fluid accumulation within the uterus.
- Uterine lavage with disinfectants such as 25 ml of provodone iodine (2%) in 1 L saline; dimethyl sulfoxide (DMSO; 100 ml) in 1 L saline.
- Mucolytics (acetylcysteine—20 ml in 250 ml of saline).
- Calcium chelators such as TRIS-EDTA for *Pseudomonas*, *Klebsiella*, or *Escherichia coli* infections (120 ml IU).

Mares that have had bacteria or yeast isolated from their uterus should be treated for a minimum of 4 to 5 days. Treatment typically consists of uterine lavage followed by infusion of the appropriate antibiotics. In some cases, the uterus is lavaged and the mare treated with systemic antibiotics. It is recommended that the mare not be bred during the estrus that bacteria or yeast have been recovered.

Technicians that work in equine reproduction should become familiar with the common uterine therapies, how to properly dilute antibiotics, and what antibiotics can and cannot be placed in the uterus. New antibiotics will be brought to the market and some are not suitable for intrauterine use (Table 4.8a and 4.8b).

Caslick Operation

The most important procedure in the treatment of pneumovagina and infertility caused by infection of the genital tract is the suturing of the upper lips of the vulva (Caslick operation). With numerous foals, loss of condition and aging, the shape of the perineal area of the mare changes. There is usually an insidious loss of fertility, but continuous contamination of the reproductive tract with air and fecal material lowers the mare's ability to get pregnant. A Caslick operation should be performed when the dorsal vulvar commissure is located more

Table 4.8a. Antibiotics that can be infused into the uterus.

- Ampicillin.
- Amikacin.
- Ceftiofur.
- Gentamicin.
- Potassium penicillin.
- Ticarcillin.
- Timentin (ticarcillin + clavimox).

Table 4.8b. Antibiotics that have been given systemically.

- Ampicillin.
- Amikacin.
- Chloramphenicol.
- Ceftiofur.
- Enrofloxacin.
- Gentamicin.
- Procaine or potassium penicillin.
- Trimethoprim sulfa and other sulfonamides.

than 4 cm (1.5 in.) dorsal to the pelvic floor. The vulva lips should be sutured such that the new dorsal vulvar commissure is preferable at the level of the pelvis and not further than 1 cm ventral to the pelvis. Mares sutured below this point may reflux urine. A mare must remain sutured for the remainder of her reproductive career. Incision and resuturing for breeding and foaling are needed; a delay in resuturing for as little as a few days may allow reinfection.

The technique consists of restraining the mare, preferably in stocks, twitched or tranquilized. The tail is wrapped and held to one side. The vulva and perineum are carefully cleaned with soap and water or a dilute surgical scrub. The labial margins are infiltrated with local anesthetic. An 8- to 10-mm strip of mucosa and skin is removed from the labial margin. The raw edges of the right and left labia are sutured together, starting at the dorsal vulvar commissure. Various suture patterns have been used.

The sutured labia must be reopened before foaling to avoid the mare tearing her vulva. The Caslick is usually reopened about 10 days to 2 weeks before the mare's foaling date. The labia is infiltrated with anesthetic and opened with a pair of sharp scissors. The vulva should be resutured 5 to 7 days after foaling.

The Stallion

Anatomy

The reproductive organs of the stallion include both the internal and external genitalia. The external genitalia consist of the prepuce, penis, and the scrotum (Figures 4.15 and 4.16). The internal genitalia consist of the accessory sex glands, the deferent ducts (ductus deferens), and the inguinal canals.

The prepuce consists of the skin folds that cover and contain the retracted penis. The penis consists of three main portions and is of the musculocavernous type. What this means is that the penis contains both cavernous spaces, which fill with blood during erection, and also muscle tissue. The glans penis is the distal free end (tip) of the penis. The shaft (body) is the main portion of the penis. The base of the penis is the portion that attaches the penis to the body. The cavernous tissues of the penis are the large corpus cavernosum and the smaller portion surrounding the urethra and extending into

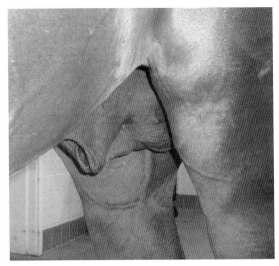

Figure 4.16 The external genitalia of the stallion. Courtesy of Dr. Kelleman.

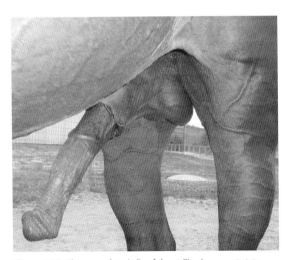

Figure 4.15. The external genitalia of the stallion in an erect state. Courtesy of Dr. Kelleman.

the glans, the corpus spongiosum. The urethra is contained within the penis. It is the tube by which both urine and also semen are excreted. Just dorsal to the urethral opening on the tip of the penis is a space called the urethral fossa and a slightly deeper area of this fossa called the urethral sinus. This sinus is a site of smegma accumulation. Smegma often accumulates in a small pellet of debris called the "bean," which can be removed by gentle washing of the penile fossa and sinus. The sinus of the urethral fossa is a site often sampled for culture for bacterial venereal pathogens.

The scrotum contains the two testes (testicles), as well as the epididymides and the spermatic cords. The testes are the site of spermatozoa production. The two testes should be symmetric oval-shaped organs with the bilaterally similar slightly turgid texture. The length, width, and height of each testis should be measured in breeding stallions at least annually. Using these measurements, the volume of each testis then can be calculated using the geometric formula for the volume of an ellipsoid. Testicular volume can then predict how many spermatozoa can be produced on a daily basis. Regular measurements of testicular size can help identify conditions in which testicular size is decreasing. A decrease in testicular size is often associated with a decrease in sperm production and semen quality.

Dorsal and lateral to each testes is the epididymis. The epididymis is a long thin convoluted tube in which the spermatozoa pass through on the way from the testes to the deferent duct. The epididymis can be used as a landmark for determining the orientation of the testes within the scrotum. The tail of the epididymis is the largest and most easily palpable section of the epididymis and thus is used most commonly for this purpose. The tail of the epididymis is normally found on the caudal end of the testis (the tail of the epididymis toward the stallion's tail).

In some stallions, the testis may be found with the tail of the epididymis pointing cranially. This finding indicates that the spermatic cord is rotated 180 degrees relative to its normal position. If this finding is not causing vascular compromise, then the testis should not be inflamed and should be nonpainful. When spermatic cord rotations are not associated with clinical signs, they should be noted in the stallion's medical record but are considered variations of normal. However, some reports suggest they may be associated with slight decreases in sperm production in some cases. Less often, spermatic cord rotations may cause the cord to torsion to the point that it impairs blood flow to the testis. When this occurs, the scrotum is usually edematous, enlarged, and painful. In these cases, treatment, usually in the form of unilateral castration, is indicated.

The spermatic cords are cordlike structures from which the testes are suspended and contain several structures including arterial and venous blood vessels, nerves, the cremaster muscle, lymphatics, and the deferent duct. For normal spermatogenesis to occur, the testes need to be maintained at a temperature that is a few degrees cooler than body temperature. The blood vessels and cremaster muscle are important in maintaining this thermoregulation. The pampiniform plexus is a web of veins that surrounds the testicular artery and acts via counter current exchange to cool the warm arterial blood flowing to the testes. In addition, the cremaster muscle will raise and lower the testes to modulate their temperature; the testes are held closer to the body in cold weather and dropped more during hot weather.

The internal genitalia consist of the accessory sex glands, the deferent ducts (ductus deferens), and the inguinal canals. The stallion has a full complement of accessory sex glands that contribute fluids (seminal plasma) to the ejaculate (semen). The bulbourethral glands produce watery fluids that often are expressed in part during sexual stimulation before ejaculation. These fluids may act to cleanse the urethra. The prostate contributes fluids to the sperm rich portion of the ejaculate. The seminal vesicles add the thick gel to the later, sperm poor fraction of the ejaculate. The deferent duct is the tube for sperm transport that connects each of the epididymides to the urethra. The ampullae are glandular thickenings of the deferent ducts that are found just before the ducts connect to the urethra. The ampullae are primarily sites of spermatozoa storage. Inspissated sperm may form a mechanical blockage that causes the ampullae to become occluded in some stallions. When this occurs, sperm are unable to pass through the ductus deferens in this area and cannot reach the ejaculate. Affected animals present for infertility in association with few or no sperm in the ejaculate. Frequent ejaculations can help to clear these blockages.

The inguinal canals are slits in the abdominal wall musculature, which allowed for the spermatic cord and fetal testes to descend out of the abdomen and into the scrotum. The testes normally descend into the scrotum before birth or by several weeks after birth. If one or both testes do not descend properly then the horse is called a cryptorchid.

Physiology

The testes produce several important hormones including testosterone and estrogens. Although estrogens are typically thought of as female hormones, they also are produced by the testes in males. The role of estrogens in the male is not well understood. One confirmed role of estrogens in males is the regulation of the secretion of other hormones. The Leydig cells of the testes produce testosterone primarily under the influence of LH from the pituitary gland. The Sertoli cells are the primary producers of estrogen, primarily under the influence of FSH from the pituitary." Testosterone is necessary for the production of spermatozoa via the process called spermatogenesis. Testosterone and other androgens also are responsible for development of the male genitalia, male body type, and male behavior.

Spermatozoa develop from spermatogonia in the testes. The testicular Sertoli cells are considered "nurse cells" and also provide support factors for the developing spermatozoa. Spermatozoa need approximately 57 days to form and mature in the testes and then take about a week to travel through the epididymides where further maturation occurs. Spermatogenesis is dependent on proper testicular hormonal environment and temperature. In addition, the size of the testes determines the number of sperm that can be produced, in that testes of larger size produce more sperm than smaller testes.

Semen Collection

Semen can be collected from stallions and then used to artificially inseminate one or multiple mares. The most common way to collect an ejaculate from a stallion is by means of an artificial vagina (AV). The stallion is teased to a mare in estrus to sexually arouse the stallion and achieve penile erection. The penis is then washed with warm water and blotted dry. The goal of washing the penis is not to sterilize it but simply to remove gross debris. In addition, washing the penis before each semen collection allows for regular examination of the penis for any abnormalities.

After washing, the stallion is then allowed to either mount a dummy mount (phantom) or an estrous mount mare. An AV is placed on the erect penis of the stallion, the stallion thrusts multiple times in the AV, and accompanied by urethral pulsations and tail flagging, an ejaculate is obtained. Note that proper handling of the stallion in the breeding situation is necessary for the safety of personnel, as well as of the stallion and mare. A good stallion handler has the stallion calmly in control at all times, while still allowing the animal to exhibit normal sexual behaviors such as calling to the mare, prancing, and arching of the neck.

Semen Evaluation and Extension (Dilution)

The semen that is collected is then evaluated. It is filtered to remove the viscous gel that was produced by the seminal vesicles. The appearance of normal semen can vary from creamy to milky to watery white, depending on the concentration of spermatozoa. It should be free of obvious blood or urine contamination. The volume in milliliters is measured, as is the concentration of sperm per milliliter. Volume is quite variable and depends on many factors, including the degree of sexual arousal of the stallion. Several automated devices are available, which will determine the concentration of sperm in the ejaculate. In addition, diluted semen can be placed in a hemacytometer (a special microscope slide used for blood cell counting), and a manual sperm count performed. The total number of spermatozoa contained in the ejaculate is found by multiplying the volume by the concentration.

Spermatozoal motility is also determined. The total percentage of spermatozoa that are moving are determined, as well as, the percentage of sperm that are moving progressively, in a relatively straight line. Higher motility is better than lower motility.

The morphology or shape of the spermatozoa is also evaluated under the microscope at 1,000× magnification. Spermatozoa consist of a head and a tail (also called the *flagellum*). The tail is divided into three parts: the midpiece, the principal piece, and the end piece (Figure 4.17). The head contains the nuclear DNA. The midpiece is the proximal portion of the tail and contains mitochondria necessary for energy. The tail undulates and allows the sperm to move. The shape of each of these portions is examined

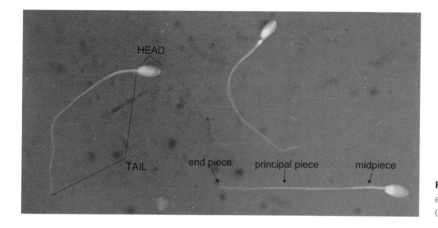

Figure 4.17. Spermatozoa fixed with eosin-nigrosin stain (1,000×). Courtesy of Dr. Kelleman.

for normalcy. Generally, at least 100 spermatozoa are examined and classified as normal or abnormal and the specific defect is recorded.

Depending on the time interval to insemination of the mare, the semen may be diluted (extended) various ways to preserve and extend the life span of the spermatozoa. Semen extender is often a milk based liquid, which contains various sugars, electrolytes, and antibiotics. If the ejaculate is to be used for artificial insemination within a couple hours, then the fresh semen may be extended with semen extender in the proportion of one part extender to one part semen. If the ejaculate is to be stored for any period of time, it is extended to an appropriate concentration of approximately 25 to 50 million spermatozoa per milliliter and then cooled slowly to approximately 4°C. The extended semen may be packaged in various shipping containers, which both cool and maintain the semen at a chilled temperature. This chilled semen may then be transported by various means, such as overnight express services (i.e., UPS or FedEx) or even same day counter to counter airline shipment.

An ejaculate, depending on total number of spermatozoa contained, motility, and morphology, may be used to artificially inseminate one or multiple mares. In general, at least 500 million progressively motile spermatozoa are required in a standard intrauterine insemination dose to achieve good pregnancy rates in mares. When morphology is also taken into account, at least 250 million progressively motile morphologically normal spermatozoa are desired. Note that not all stallions will have spermatozoa that will survive cooling and transporting of the semen. Ability to withstand the cooling process and maintain adequate motility should be determined before commercial shipping of a given stallion's extended ejaculates. When properly extended and cooled, semen from most fertile stallions will maintain good motility for 24 to 48 hours after ejaculation.

Semen may also be frozen for long-term storage. When properly extended and processed, frozen semen can be stored indefinitely. Before freezing, the ejaculate is evaluated and the semen extended with cryopreservation (freezing) extenders, which may be either milk- or egg-yolk-based. The semen is then packaged in plastic straws of various sizes, cooled, and then frozen in liquid nitrogen. Note that the semen in the straw is frozen solid and is no longer in the liquid state as for chilled extended semen. After freezing, a straw is thawed and evaluated to assess whether the spermatozoa have survived the freezing and thawing processes. Not all stallions' semen will adequately survive these processes. Per cycle pregnancy rates with frozen-thawed semen typically are lower than pregnancy rates with fresh or cooled semen. Additionally, the timing of insemination of the mare must be more precise and closer to ovulation when using frozen-thawed semen.

Stallion Diagnostics

In addition to semen analysis and physical examination of the genitalia, various tests may be performed on the normal stallion or as a part of a workup for subfertility (lower than normal fertility) or infertility. These can include culture of specimens obtained from the semen and external genitalia for bacterial or viral venereal diseases, ultrasonographic examination of the internal and external genitalia, and blood work to assess circulating hormones. Ultrasonographic examination of the scrotal contents is often performed in addition to manual palpation of the scrotal contents to determine the size of the testes and to examine the scrotal contents for normalcy. Palpation and ultrasonographic examination of the internal genitalia of the stallion may also be performed by the veterinarian.

Veterinary Technician's Role

The veterinary technician may be asked to assist the veterinarian with such procedures as semen collection; washing of the penis; specimen collection for culture; AV preparation and subsequent cleaning; semen evaluation; and semen extension, packaging, and preparation for shipment or for freezing.

References and Further Reading

Knottenbelt, D. C., M. M. LeBlanc, C. Lopate, and R. R. Pascoe. 2003. *Equine Stud Farm Medicine and Surgery*. United Kingdom: Saunders-Elsevier Science Limited.

Pycock, J. F. 1997. *Self Assessment Colour Review of Equine Reproduction and Stud Medicine*. London: Manson Publishing.

Samper, J. 2000. *Equine Breeding Management and Artificial Insemination*. Philadelphia: W.B. Saunders.

Schatten, H. and G. M. Constantinescu. 2007. *Comparative Reproductive Biology*. Ames, IA: Blackwell Publishers.

Younquist, R.S., and W. R. Threlfall. 2007. *Large Animal Theriogenology*. 2nd ed. St. Louis: Saunder Elsevier.

CHAPTER 5

Equine Wellness Program

Dana Zimmel

The components of an equine wellness program that require veterinary intervention include immunizations, internal parasite control, annual Coggins testing, and dental care. An annual physical examination should be part of every wellness program. This is an opportunity for the veterinarian to evaluate the horse for any changes in condition that can affect health or performance.

Vaccination Guidelines

Routine vaccination is a fundamental component of disease prevention in the horse. Vaccines can prevent fatal diseases, or they can help minimize or eliminate contagious diseases that can affect athletic performance. A "standard" vaccination program does not exist. The risks of contracting an infectious disease should be evaluated against the risk, efficacy, and cost of vaccination.

The type of vaccine will dictate the frequency of vaccination and duration of immunity. Vaccines fall into one of two categories, live vaccines or killed vaccines. *Live vaccines* are altered versions of the infecting agent that stimulate the immune system and require fewer doses. Examples of live vaccines are modified live vaccines (MLV) or recombinant vector vaccines. In contrast, *killed vaccines* are unable to replicate within the horse, and these vaccines must be given multiple times to induce protection. The best current source to review equine vaccine technology and vaccination recommendations can be obtained at the American Association of Equine Practitioners (AAEP) Web site at www.aaep.org.

Vaccines should be administered with aseptic technique using a new needle and syringe for each horse. Vaccines should be stored at 35° F to 45° F. A thermometer should be placed in the refrigerator with the vaccines and the temperature recorded daily. Vaccines should not be frozen. A vaccine inventory log should include the name of the vaccine, the manufacturer, serial lot, and the expiration date. This information should be recorded in the patient's chart plus the location (e.g., neck, semimembranous, or left or right side) in which the vaccine was injected.

Intramuscular (IM) vaccines can be given in the neck, pectoral, semimembranous, or semitendinous muscles. The gluteal muscles are often avoided due to the difficulty in draining a postinjection abscess in that location. The neck is often preferred by veterinarians in horses that kick. A disadvantage of giving a vaccine in the neck is muscle soreness that results in the horse refusing to lower their head to graze. Other adverse reactions include swelling at the site of injection, transient fever, anorexia, or lethargy. Anaphylactic reactions are rare. Clinical signs of an anaphylactic reaction range from hives and limb edema to severe colic and laminitis. Adverse reactions should be reported to the U.S. Department of Agriculture Center for Veterinary Biologics at 1-800-752-6255.

Frequency of vaccination varies with the age and use of the horse. All broodmares should be vaccinated 4 to 6 weeks before foaling. This will maximize the concentration of antibodies in the colostrum that the foal will suckle. Passive transfer of immunity to the foal through the colostrum will provide protection against disease for the first few months of life. As a general rule, foals will require a series of three vaccinations for each disease to acquire adequate protection. If the mare was not vaccinated 4 to 6 weeks before foaling or the foal did not receive colostrum, the foal should start the vaccination series at 3 to 4 months of age. If the foal did receive colostrum from a properly vaccinated mare, the vaccination series should begin at 5 to 6 months of age. Research on foal and pregnant mare immunity is active changing vaccination recommendations frequently.

When planning the vaccination schedule for the year, any events such as horse show or sale should be listed on the calendar. For vaccinations to be protective they must be administered at least 2 weeks before the possible exposure to the pathogen. Thus, advance planning of special events and knowledge of the mosquito season are important in the timing of vaccination programs.

Vaccination for Prevention of Fatal Diseases

The most important vaccines to administer are those that prevent a fatal disease, such as tetanus, encephalomyelitis (i.e., eastern equine encephalomyelitis [EEE], western equine encephalomyelitis [WEE], and West Nile virus [WNV]), and rabies.

Tetanus is caused by a potent neurotoxin derived from anaerobic, spore-forming bacterium (*Clostridium tetani*) that lives in the soil. Horses are at risk of contracting tetanus if they receive a puncture wound to the foot, laceration, or any surgical procedure such as a castration. The neurotoxin causes muscle rigidity and spasticity also called "lock jaw." If a horse becomes injured and has not received a tetanus shot in the last 6 months, a booster shot is recommended at the time of injury. If a horse becomes injured and has never received a vaccination for tetanus, it should be treated with tetanus antitoxin. Tetanus antitoxin induces immediate passive protection that lasts about 3 weeks. Tetanus antitoxin is associated with Theiler disease (fatal hepatic failure) and should be used only under certain circumstances such as an unvaccinated

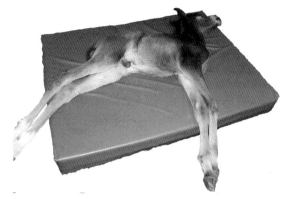

Figure 5.1. Foal with tetanus. Courtesy Dr. Dana Zimmel.

horse with an injury or a foal born to an unvaccinated mare (Figure 5.1).

Adult horses should be vaccinated with tetanus toxoid once a year. Pregnant mares should be vaccinated with tetanus toxoid 30 days before foaling. Foals born to vaccinated mares that received adequate passive transfer of colostral antibodies should be vaccinated three times starting at 6 months of age. The first two doses should be 4 weeks apart and the last dose 12 to 16 weeks later. For example a foal would be vaccinated with tetanus toxoid at 6 months, 7 months, and 10 to 11 months of age.

Encephalomyelitis is a viral disease that affects the central nervous system, which results in clinical signs such as lethargy, behavior changes, ataxia, blindness, and seizures. EEE and WEE are also known as "sleeping sickness" because the initial signs of the disease can be as simple as lethargy, depression, inappetence, and fever. The disease is transmitted by mosquitoes, and the reservoir is wild birds. It can also be fatal. The mortality rate for EEE can approach 75% to 95%. The mortality rate for WEE is significantly less, around 50%. EEE occurs east of the Mississippi river and WEE occurs west of the Mississippi river. Venezuelan equine encephalomyelitis (VEE) occurs in South and Central America. Texas and Florida encountered outbreaks of VEE in the 1970s. Because it has been over 30 years since VEE has invaded the United States, it is not considered a necessary vaccine.

Adult horses should be vaccinated for EEE or WEE in the spring of each year. In areas of the country in which the mosquito population is constant, such as in Florida, horses should be vaccinated every 4 to 6 months. Pregnant mares should be vaccinated 30 days before foaling to induce colostral antibodies. Foals born to mares that were appropriately vaccinated should begin their vaccination series for EEE or WEE at 5 to 6 months of age. They should receive three vaccines with 3 to 4 weeks between the first two doses and the last booster should follow 8 to 12 weeks later. For example, a foal would be vaccinated for EEE or WWE at 6 months, 7 months, and 9 to 10 months of age. The next dose would be in the spring of the year before mosquito season.

WNV emerged in the United States in 1999 and is now endemic in the United States. WNV is not as lethal as EEE, but infected horses may require several days of intensive care to survive. The mortality rate for horses that contract WNV is approximately 32% to 35%. Horses infected with WNV may have a fever, show muscle fasciculations, ataxia, and behavioral changes (Figure 5.2).

Vaccination frequency for WNV depends on the vaccine administered. There are three vaccinations currently approved for WNV; a killed vaccine, recombinant vaccine, and modified live chimera vaccine. Adult horses should receive annual vaccination before the beginning of each mosquito season. Foals born to mares that were vaccinated 30 days before foaling should begin their vaccination series at 4 to 6 months of age. The number of boosters and the age they should be administered varies with the vaccine used.

Humans can contract both EEE and WNV from infected mosquitoes. Horses do not acquire the level of viremia necessary to serve as a reservoir of infection. Humans cannot get EEE or WNV from horses. If a horse is infected, that indicates that the infected level of mosquitoes in that area is increased, which makes human infection more likely.

Rabies is an infrequent but fatal neurological disease for humans and animals. In 2006, the American Veterinary Medical Association (AVMA) reported 6,940 rabies cases detected in animals in

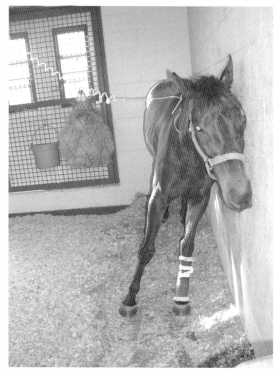

Figure 5.2. Horse infected with West Nile virus. Notice the loss of balance as the horse is leaning against the wall. Courtesy Dr. Genevieve Fontaine-Rodgerson.

the United States. Raccoons composed 38%, bats 24%, skunks 21%, foxes 6.2%, cats 4.6%, cattle 1.2%, and dogs 1.1%. Horses can be bitten by a rabid animal and develop rabies; it is transmitted through the saliva of the infected animal. Although the incidence of rabies is low in horses, it is a serious public health concern. Vaccination of horses is prudent not only for the health of the horse but also the safety of all the people working with the horse. Horses should be vaccinated annually for rabies. None of the rabies vaccines are licensed for use in pregnant mares; however, they are routinely administered by veterinarians without complications. Foals born to mares that have been vaccinated should receive the first vaccine at 6 months of age and the second dose 1 month later. The third dose should be administered between 10 and 12 months of age.

Vaccinations to Minimize Illness

There are several vaccines available to prevent
infection of respiratory diseases, such as influenza,
equine herpesvirus (rhinopneumonitis), and Strangles *(Streptococcus equi equi)*. These diseases can
cause severe illness that may require veterinary care
and definitely will result in lost days of productivity. For example, a horse that contracts influenza
may be sick for 3 to 7 days and may take 2 to 3
weeks to recover before returning to work.

Influenza is a common contagious respiratory
disease that is transmitted by aerosolization and
inhalation. The most susceptible population is
young horses (<3 years) and in stressful conditions
(i.e., shows, crowding, or shipment). The common
clinical signs include serous nasal discharge, coughing, anorexia, and fever (103°F–106°F). It can
take 21 days for the respiratory epithelium to regen-
erate after contracting influenza. Vaccination for
influenza is important for horses that travel frequently or are exposed to many horses. Influenza
can be self-limiting, often requiring only supportive
nursing care such as anti-inflammatory medication,
oral or intravenous fluids, and potentially antibiotics to prevent secondary bacterial infection. If the
horse contracts influenza and is forced to continue
to work or travel long distances, severe life-
threatening pneumonia can develop.

There are three vaccinations available for influenza: killed, MLV, and canary pox-vectored vaccine.
The frequency of administration depends on the
vaccine. The adult horse that is exposed to other
horses should be vaccinated twice a year. Broodmares should be vaccinated 30 days before foaling
with the killed or canary pox-vectored vaccine to
induce colostral immunity. The modified live intranasal vaccine does not produce high-circulating
serum titers, thus, it does not produce colostral protection for the foal. Foals born to mares that were
appropriately vaccinated should begin influenza
vaccination at 6 months of age. The number of
doses required to achieve protective immunity is
dependent on the type of vaccine used. The inactivated vaccine requires three doses at approximately
6 months, 7 months, and 10 and 12 months of age.
The MLV only requires two doses starting at 6 to 7

months and the second dose between 11 and 12
months of age.

Equine herpesvirus/rhinopneumonitis has three
clinical forms that include respiratory disease, abortion, and neurological disease. Equine herpesvirus
type 1 (EHV-1) results in respiratory disease, abortions, and neurological disease. Equine herpesvirus
type 4 (EHV-4) can cause respiratory disease and
infrequent abortions.

Respiratory disease caused by EHV-1 and EHV-4
occur in young horses, usually weanlings and yearlings. Widespread outbreaks can occur in high-
density and stressful environments. Older horses
are important in the outbreak because they may
become subclinically infected but shed virus. Clinical signs of respiratory disease include mild fever,
coughing, and nasal discharge. The discharge is
clear but progression to a yellow thick exudate is
common. The incubation period may be as short as
2 days and as long as 10 days. The outcome is dictated by minimization of stress and rest.

Abortion caused by EHV-1 occurs without
warning signs as early as 90 days of gestation with
most abortions occurring be between 7 and 9
months of gestation. Red-bag abortions are common
in horses infected by EHV.

The neurological form of the disease caused by
EHV-1 can be fatal and is the greatest cause for
concern at boarding facilities, racetracks, and horse
shows. Most horses experience respiratory signs for
1 to 2 weeks before development of neurologic
signs. Stress (e.g., shipping or surgery) may trigger
the onset of neurologic signs. The virus will attack
the spinal cord and brainstem. Neurological signs
include rear limb weakness, incoordination, toe-
dragging, dog-sitting, and urinary/fecal incontinence (Figure 5.3).

Transmission is via the respiratory route with
infective droplets obtained from coughing and
snorting horses. Shedding of the virus in nasal secretions can occur for 14 days. The virus can be spread
by contaminated hands and equipment and from
aborted tissues, fluids, and tissues. Even mares that
abort transmit infection by the respiratory route.
Without disinfection, the virus can actually survive
several weeks. All horses can be carriers of the virus
whether or not they demonstrated clinical signs.

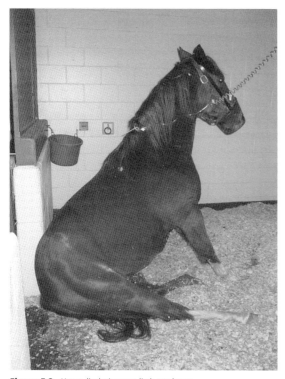

Figure 5.3. Horse displaying rear limb weakness.
Courtesy Dr. Rob Mackay.

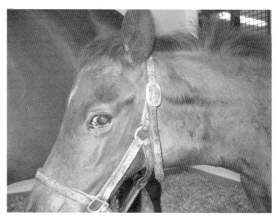

Figure 5.4. Weanling with enlarged lymph nodes infected with strangles.
Courtesy Dr. Dana Zimmel.

Vaccination for the respiratory form of EHV may not prevent the disease, but it will decrease the frequency and severity of clinical signs and more importantly decrease shedding of the virus to other horses. Adult horses less than 4 years of age or performance horses that travel frequently should be vaccinated every 6 months with EHV-1 and EHV-4. Broodmares should be vaccinated with EHV-1 at the beginning of the fifth, seventh, and ninth month of pregnancy to prevent abortion. Foals should begin vaccination at 6 months of age. The second dose should be given at 7 months of age and the third dose at 10 to 12 months of age. There is no vaccination currently available that is labeled to protect against the neurological form of EHV.

Strangles is a common contagious bacterial infection that usually affects young horses. The term *strangles* refers to the clinical signs of severe cases in horses that suffocate from enlargement of

the retropharyngeal lymph nodes. The first clinical sign of strangles is fever, which persists as the lymph nodes become infected and form abscesses (Figure 5.4). The lymph nodes become painful and enlarged about 1 week after infection. The most common lymph nodes affected are the mandibular lymph nodes (located under the jaw) and the retropharyngeal lymph nodes (located deep to the throat latch). Identification of enlarged retropharyngeal lymph nodes is difficult by palpation of the throat area. Some horses may be painful on palpation of the throat. The best methods to visualize enlargement of these lymph nodes is to radiograph the head or perform endoscopy of the guttural pouch. Often enlarged retropharyngeal lymph nodes will rupture into the guttural pouch and drainage is seen in the nostrils. Nasal discharge from the infected horse is the largest source of contamination (Figure 5.5). Sources of infection can be nose to nose contact with an infected horse, sharing contaminated water buckets, feed tubs, twitches, tack, and clothing, and equipment of handlers who work with infected horses. Horses can be infected by subclinical shedders that harbor the organism in their guttural pouch.

Once the horse comes into contact with a potential source of infection it may take 3 to 14 days after exposure before the horse will show the first clinical

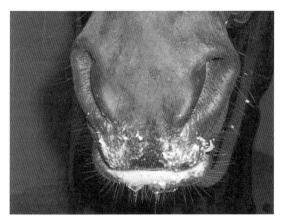

Figure 5.5. Adult horse with nasal discharge from a strangles infection. Courtesy Dr. Dana Zimmel.

sign of strangles (fever). Based on this information, a minimum isolation period for introduction of new horses to the farm should be 14 days. The rectal temperature for all new horses should be monitored twice a day. If an elevation in rectal temperature is detected that horse should be immediately isolated from the rest of the herd. An infected horse will start shedding the bacteria 1 to 2 days after the onset of fever. Isolation of that horse can stop the spread of the disease to other horses. This is one measure to minimize the spread of the disease on a farm.

Approximately 75% of horses that contract the disease develop solid immunity after they recover for 5 years or longer. There are two vaccine types currently available: M-protein-based inactivated vaccine for IM use and a modified attenuated live bacterial intranasal vaccine. The inactivated vaccines and the modified attenuated live vaccine require two to three initial vaccinations depending on the specific vaccine. Adult horses should be vaccinated one to two times a year depending on the vaccine used. All of the vaccines decrease the severity of the disease in experimental challenges, with a more significant reduction in clinical scores observed with the intranasal product. Pregnant mares should be vaccinated 30 days before foaling with the inactivated IM vaccine to induce colostral antibody production. Foals should begin their vaccination series between 4 and 6 months of age when

using the inactivated IM vaccine. They will require three doses 4 to 6 weeks apart. Foals vaccinated with the modified attenuated live vaccine should start the series at 6 to 9 months of age and require two doses 3 weeks apart. For example, a foal vaccinated with an MLV for strangles should receive vaccines between 6 and 9 months of age, 3 to 4 weeks later for the second dose, and at 11 to 12 months of age for the third dose.

There are additional risks in vaccinating horses for strangles. Both the intranasal vaccination and the IM vaccination can cause purpura hemorrhagica. This is an immune-mediated vasculitis resulting in severe swelling of the limbs. The limb edema is painful, and the horse may lose large areas of skin on the extremities. This condition can occur after a natural infection of strangles or secondary to the use of vaccination.

Additional risks with the intranasal vaccine include mild clinical disease or abscess formation at the site of concurrent injections. The vaccine strain is presumably able to overcome natural pharyngeal barriers and create a temporary bacteremia, which leads to the colonization at inflamed muscle sites. To avoid this potential complication, administration of intranasal vaccines should not occur at the same time of any other vaccinations. Horses that have signs of strangles should *not* be vaccinated. The American College of Veterinary Internal Medicine (ACVIM) consensus statement recommends vaccination of horses during an outbreak only if they have no clinical signs and if the horses have no contact with infected or exposed horses. If the horse has had strangles within the last year it should *not* be vaccinated.

During an outbreak of strangles, all personnel should use protective clothing when working with infected horses. The infected horses should be treated last if the same personnel have to care for the entire farm. Dedicated equipment should be used for infected horses (e.g., pitch forks, rakes, and tack) and thoroughly disinfect equipment between horses. To disinfect stables and vans, remove all manure and debris first. Soak all surfaces with liquid disinfectant or steam treat the area and allow the area to dry. All water troughs should be disinfected daily that are used by infected horses. Pastures used to house infected horses should be rested for 4 weeks under ideal circumstances.

Vaccines Occasionally Used in Equine Practice

Botulism *(C. botulinum)* is an endemic disease in Kentucky and along the mid-Atlantic seaboard states. Botulism toxin acts by blocking transmission of nerve impulses at motor end plates, resulting in weakness that progresses to paralysis, inability to swallow, and death. Horses can become infected if the toxin contaminates a wound or if the toxin is ingested. "Forage poisoning" results from ingestion of the toxin produced by decaying plant or animal material in feed. "Shaker foal syndrome" occurs when a foal consumes vegetative spores that produce the toxin are ingested. *C. botulinum* type B and C are related to most outbreaks in horses. Vaccination is recommended in pregnant mares in endemic areas (type B toxoid) such as in Kentucky. Mares that have been previously vaccinated need one dose 30 to 45 days before foaling. If the mare has never been vaccinated, then she should receive three doses at 8, 9, and 10 months of gestation. Foals born to vaccinated mares in endemic areas should receive three doses, 4 weeks apart starting around 3 months of age.

Potomac horse fever (PHF; *Neorickettsia risticii*) causes mild to severe diarrhea, laminitis, and fever. It can cause abortion between 90 and 120 days of gestation. PHF was first described in 1979 in horses living by the Potomac River, and it is now endemic in the eastern United States and California. It has been documented by serologic surveys (IFA) in forty-three states. Affected horses have exposure to rivers or creeks where they can consume caddis flies that hover near the water or end up in the grass near the stream or river. The vaccination is safe but has questionable efficacy. The vaccine has not been tested in horses that have been challenged with infected aquatic insects. Also, one study described horses that have been vaccinated with the killed *N. risticii* vaccine and subsequently developed the clinical disease after natural exposure. Adult horses in endemic areas should be vaccinated every 6 to 12 months depending on the risk of infection. The vaccine has not proven to protect mares from abortion induced from *N. risticii*. Foals should be vaccinated after 5 months of age and again 4 weeks later.

Equine viral arteritis (EVA) is a contagious viral infection of horses throughout the world that can result in abortion or respiratory illness. EVA can infect all breeds of horses, but standardbreds have been found to have the highest infection rate. The disease has the potential to cause significant economic losses in breeding herds, resulting in abortion outbreaks, and a significant number of stallions may become carriers that transmit the virus quite efficiently. In addition, horses that test positive for EVA antibodies may be prohibited from entering foreign countries, despite appearing clinically normal.

The clinical signs of EVA include fever, depression, edema (swelling) of the limbs or mammary gland, abortion, nasal discharge, urticaria (hives), and conjunctivitis. The respiratory signs can mimic influenza. Many horses infected with EVA may not show any clinical symptoms. The disease can be transmitted by respiratory secretions, or stallions can shed the virus in their semen, which means it can be transmitted via cooled or frozen semen. Most horses at racetracks, sales, and horse shows contract the virus through the respiratory route. On breeding farms, the most common form of viral transmission is through breeding.

The United States is the only major horse breeding country that does not have an EVA import restriction and control policy. Although this virus occurs infrequently, it can affect the future of breeding operations. The virus gained notoriety in a 1984 epidemic in Kentucky affecting forty-one Thoroughbred breeding farms. In 2006, a large outbreak of EVA occurred in ten states. The occurrence was significant and the first time the quarter horse population was involved.

The common method of diagnosis is blood analysis for the presence of antibodies against EVA. The detection of antibodies against EVA does not indicate an active infection but exposure to the virus only. A single blood test with a high antibody titer may be diagnostic, or a paired blood sample 4 to 8 days after infection reflecting a significant rise in the antibody titer can indicate active infection. The best diagnostic test is isolation of the virus from nasal secretions, semen, placenta, or fetal tissue. Sample handling is crucial for recovery of the virus, which makes this method of diagnosis difficult to perform. There is no specific treatment for EVA other than supportive care for respiratory signs. Adult horses should recover fully from the infection.

There is one MLV vaccine available in the United States that has been proven safe for use in stallions and nonpregnant mares. The vaccine has been effective at controlling disease outbreaks if administered 7 to 10 days after exposure. The AAEP emphasizes the vaccination of all colts intended to be breeding stallions between 6 to 12 months of age. Breeding stallions and teasers should be vaccinated at least 1 month before the start of the breeding season each year. The purpose of vaccination is to prevent the establishment of the carrier state.

If an adult stallion has never been vaccinated, a blood sample should be drawn before the first vaccination to prove he has not been exposed to the virus. This is important with regard to exportation rules and regulations. If a stallion is positive on a blood test for the antibodies to EVA and has never been vaccinated, a semen sample must be tested for the virus to determine if he is a carrier. Open mares should only be vaccinated if they are to be bred to a carrier stallion. They should then be isolated for 21 days after breeding to a carrier stallion. The vaccine is not approved for use in pregnant mares. The new policy created by U.S. Department of Agriculture Animal and Plant Health Inspection Service (APHIS) is to serve as a standard for handling EVA in breeding situations. The new publication contains minimum standards for detection, control, and prevention of EVA and can be found at www. aphis.usda.gov/vs/nahss/equine/eva/index.htm.

Rotavirus is a contagious disease that causes severe diarrhea in the neonatal foal. It is rarely fatal but can require supportive care, including fluids and electrolyte replacement. The virus is transmitted by the fecal-oral route. To control outbreaks on breeding farms pregnant mares should be vaccinated at 8, 9, and 10 months of gestation. The foal must get adequate levels of colostral antibodies to acquire protection.

Equine Internal Parasites

A heavy burden of parasites can cause weight loss, a rough hair coat, poor performance, diarrhea, and colic. Deworming plans should be implemented to minimize costs, prevent the development of resistant parasite, and maintain a healthy horse. The internal parasites that are most devastating to the horse are small strongyles (cyanthostomes), large strongyles (bloodworms), ascarids (roundworms), and tapeworms. Less important are bots, pinworms, stomach worms, lungworms, and threadworms.

Small and large strongyles are the most debilitating parasites in the adult horse. They are divided into two groups based on their size. Large strongyles are 2 in. in length and small strongyles are the size of small hairs (Figure 5.6). They share the same life cycle outside of the horse, but it varies dramatically once the larvae enter the horse. The life cycle begins with the strongyle eggs deposited in manure. Strongyle eggs on the pasture are not capable of infecting horses. The egg must go through three distinct larval stages before it can infect the horse. The larvae feed on bacteria in the manure for 5 to 14 days and then emerge onto a blade of grass where they are consumed by the horse in the third larval stage (L3). Removing manure in the pasture quickly can minimize the infestation on the grass. As the larvae emerge onto the grass, they are swallowed by the horse when

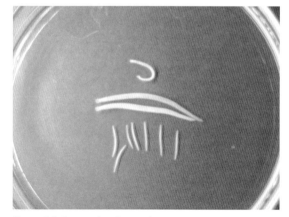

Figure 5.6. Large and small strongyles.
Courtesy Dr. Dana Zimmel.

eating. In the southeastern United States larvae survive poorly on grass during the summer months due to the extreme heat. Horses develop infection by ingesting larvae on the pasture from September to March in hot regions. In colder climates, the freezing temperatures will not kill strongyle eggs and the larvae can persist over the winter.

Small strongyles are the most common and abundant parasite of horses with infections exceeding 100,000 worms per horse. Once swallowed the small strongyle larvae migrate through the wall of the gastrointestinal tract for 4 to 6 weeks before emerging as an adult in the large colon and cecum where they lay eggs. When the parasite is migrating through the gastrointestinal wall of the large colon and cecum, it can become encysted. When the larvae become encysted, they are protected from the horse's immune response and the effects of many anthelmintics. The larvae may remain encysted for a long period of time and when they erupt can cause a severe inflammatory reaction in the wall of the gastrointestinal tract. Small strongyles can cause colic, diarrhea, and ill thrift. The encysted larval stage of the parasite can only be eliminated by the use of moxidectin at 0.4 mg/kg or fenbendazole at 10 mg/kg orally once a day for five treatments.

Large strongyles (*Strongylus vulgaris, S. edentatus,* and *S. equinus*) are referred to as bloodworms. Large strongyle larvae are swallowed and exit the intestine soon after infection. They migrate in various tissues for 6 to 11 months before returning to the intestine. The paths they take depend on the species of parasite. For example, *S. vulgaris* larvae migrate into the lining of the arteries of the intestine; *S. edentatus* larvae migrate through the liver and peritoneum; and the *S. equinus* migrates through the liver and pancreas. The migrating stage of this parasite can cause severe colic. Treatment at 6-month intervals with ivermectin, moxidectin, or fenbendazole will control large strongyle infections.

Ascarids *(Parascaris equorum)* can be deadly to young horses less than 1 year of age; adult horses develop immunity to this parasite. Transmission occurs by shedding large numbers of eggs in the manure. The eggs can live for several years in the environment. Ascarids migrate from the gastroin-

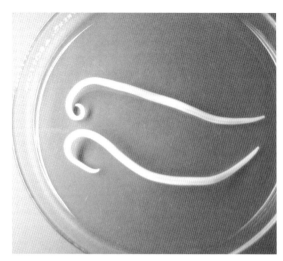

Figure 5.7. Adult ascarid (roundworm). Courtesy Dr. Dana Zimmel.

testinal tract through the liver to the lungs, and then they are coughed up and swallowed. The adult ascarid lives in the small intestine and ranges from 1 to 14 in. in length (Figure 5.7). A weanling infected with ascarids can have a poor hair coat, pot belly, and poor weight gain. During the migration of the larvae in the lungs weanlings may present with coughing, fever, or a nasal discharge. Weanlings with a large burden of ascarids are at risk for an impaction of adult parasites in the small intestine. It takes 60 to 75 days for the life cycle to be complete at which time eggs can be detected in a fecal floatation. Thus, early infections are not detectable.

Ascarid eggs can live in the soil and the stall floor. The eggs are difficult to kill with disinfectants. The best control method is to pick up manure frequently in paddocks and feed hay and grain off the ground. Foals should be dewormed for the first time between 30 and 60 days of age. Then they should be dewormed every 60 days until they are 15 months old. The adult and juvenile worms are sensitive to pyrantel, ivermectin, moxidectin, and benzimidazoles (10 mg/kg). The migrating larvae are only sensitive to ivermectin and moxidectin. Moxidectin products are not labeled for use in horses younger than 6 months of age.

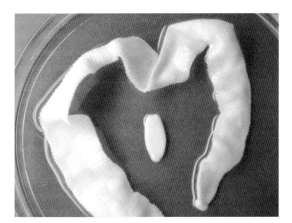

Figure 5.8. Tapeworms: *Anoplocephala perfoliota* (small) and *Anoplocephala magna* (large). Courtesy Dr. Dana Zimmel.

Tapeworms (*Anoplocephala perfoliota* an *A. magna*) can cause colic in horses by affecting the motility of the gastrointestinal tract in the area of the ileo-cecal valve (Figure 5.8). Specific conditions include spasmodic colic, ileal impactions, and intussusception (telescoping of one section of intestine into another). In the United States, the exposure rate for tapeworms is 54%. Young horses (<5 years) and older horses appear to have the highest infection rates. The life cycle of the tapeworm includes the orbatid mite as an intermediate host. Infection is acquired when the horse swallows the mite that contains tapeworm eggs. Worms mature within the horse in 6 to 10 weeks. It is difficult to detect tapeworm eggs in the feces. Special fecal tests (centrifugation/flotation) or an enzyme-linked immunosorbent assay (ELISA) test performed on the blood are the best diagnostic tests to identify the parasite. The parasite can be eliminated by deworming twice a year with praziquantel at 1 mg/kg or greater.

Bots (*Gastrophilus intestinalis* and *G. nasalis*) are flying insects that lay their eggs on the leg hairs of horses. The horse will scratch its legs with its muzzle, and the eggs gain access to the mouth. The first- and second-stage larvae will spend a month in the oral cavity before migrating into the stomach. The larvae will attach around the margo plicatus of the stomach. These parasites do not cause significant damage to the stomach but can cause gastric ulcers in some horses. The only anthelmintics that kill these larvae are ivermectin or moxidectin. Bots are observed in horses during the middle of summer. Removal of the bot eggs from the horse's legs can reduce infection. A pumice stone or a bot knife is the most common methods to remove the eggs from the hair. Hand washing is important after the removal of bot eggs because the hatched bot larvae can infect the eyes of humans.

Stomach worms (*Habronema muscae, H. microstoma*, and *Draschia megastoma*) live in the glandular portion of the stomach along the margo plicatus. Transmission of stomach worms occurs by stable or house flies. When the fly lands on the horse's muzzle, eyes, sheath, or an open wound the larvae are transferred into the horse. These parasites do not cause significant internal damage, but they do cause skin conditions known as cutaneous habronemiasis or summer sores. This condition is caused by the larvae forming granulomas in moist areas of the skin, such as around the eyes. These parasites can be eliminated by administration of oral ivermectin to the horse.

Pinworms (*Oxyuris equi*) generally cause tail rubbing and a rat-tailed appearance. The female worm will discharge about 60,000 eggs in a thick yellow fluid around the rectum. As this fluid dries and cracks, it will cause the horse to itch the area. Severe infections with third- and fourth-stage larvae can cause inflammation of the cecum and colon resulting in mild colic symptoms. The life cycle will take 5 months to complete. These parasites can easily be killed by most anthelmintics.

Threadworms (*Strongyloides westeri*) can cause diarrhea in young foals up to 5 months of age. The foals can become infected by passage of the parasite thorough the dam's milk. These parasites can be eliminated by deworming the mare before foaling with ivermectin or oxibendazole. Horses develop immunity to *S. westeri* after 6 months of age.

Lungworms (*Dictyocaulus arnfieldi*) is a problem for horses that share a pasture with donkeys. Horses infected with lungworms can have a cough or decreased performance. Donkeys can harbor the infection without any clinical signs. Lungworm infections in the horse can be eliminated by treatment with ivermectin or moxidectin.

A Guide to Anthelmintics

A major concern among scientists is the excessive use of anthelmintics leading to drug-resistant parasites. Anthelmintic use in the United States changed in the 1960s and 1970s when benzimidazole (i.e., fenbendazole and oxibendazole) anthelmintics were introduced. The products were available over the counter, and for the first time, parasite control was available to horse owners without interaction with a veterinarian. Deworming horses every 8 weeks became standard in the equine industry. Research studies in the last few years have a confirmed a single dose of fenbendazole has demonstrated greater than 90% resistance to cyathostomes. In addition, scientists report that some farms have pyrantel-resistant cyathostomes. To avoid the development of resistant parasites, a new approach is needed. Investigation of fecal eggs counts on large farms has proven that there are only a few individual horses that carry all the parasites and the rest of the herd has a minimal parasite burden. Parasitologists recommend that all horses should not be treated the same and dewormed at arbitrary intervals. Instead horses should be dewormed based on the individual parasite load.

The best diagnostic test to evaluate parasite burden is the McMaster fecal egg count (FEC). A routine fecal egg float only identifies the presence or absence of parasite eggs but not the quantity present in the feces. A McMaster FEC counts how many eggs per gram (EPG) of feces. This test is easy to perform and requires a compound microscope, a McMaster's egg counter slide (Chalex Corporation, available at www.vetslides.com), sodium nitrate solution, balance, graduated beaker, and plastic pipettes. The feces should be collected from the horse and refrigerated until the examination can be performed. The test will provide a quantitative measurement of the nematode egg burden, which can be used to identify the horse that truly need deworming, as well as, the response to specific anthelmintics. In this way a farm can monitor for the development of resistant parasites. Most parasitologists agree that a horse does not need to be dewormed until the FEC is at least 200 to 500 EPG. This specifically applies to deworming for strongyles.

The interval between deworming depends on the anthelmintic used because each drug has a different egg reappearance period (ERP). This is the time period from deworming to the time in which the parasite can reproduce and the eggs can be detected in the feces. The ERP of oxibendazole, fenbendazole, and pyrantel is about 4 weeks. The ERP of ivermectin is 8 weeks and 12 to 16 weeks for moxidectin.

The mechanism of action for killing parasites varies with each drug group. Horse owners are often confused about the difference between the drug class, generic name, and the brand name of anthelmintics. There are dozens of products on the market but only four major drug classes of anthelmintics currently used (Table 5.1).

1. Macrocyclic lactones: Avermectins are macrocyclic lactones. The mode of action is to modulate the chloride ion channel activity in the nervous

Table 5.1. Common anthelmentics.

Drug	Brand name product	Comments
Ivermectin	Eqvalan, Zimectrin, Equimectrin, Rotation 1, and Ivercare	
Moxidectin	Quest	Must be older than 6 months
Oxibendazole	Anthelcide EQ	
Fenbendazole	Panacur and Safe-Guard	
Oxfendazole	Benzelmin	
Pyrantel pamoate	Strongid P, Strongid T, and Rotation	
Pyrantel tartrate	Strongid C, Strongid C2X, and Continuex	
Ivermectin/praziquantel	Equimax and Zimecterin Gold	Must be older than 5 months
Moxidectin/praziquantel	Quest Plus and ComboCare	Must be older than 6 months

system of nematodes and bind to receptors that increase chloride ion permeability, inhibiting electrical activity of nerve cells causing paralysis and death. The parasite will die because it can no longer take in nutrients. In mammals the receptors are only in the central nervous system, usually avermectins do not cross the blood-brain barrier, making them safe to use in horses. The mechanism to induce death takes 3 to 4 days before the adult worms are killed and fecal eggs counts are lowered.

2. Tetrahydropyrimidines: Tetrahydropyrimidines include pyrantel tartrate or pyrantel pamoate. This drug is a depolarizing neuromuscular blocking agent in nematodes. Pyrantel will induce muscle contraction within the parasite that is not reversible. The worm will quickly die as it is unable to eat.

3. Benzimidazoles: The mode of action is to bind to nematode dimeric tubulin to prevent polymerization of tubulin during microtubule assembly. Microtubules are essential in mitosis and energy metabolism, thus benzimidazoles are most effective against actively dividing cells that are present in nematode ova and larvae. The parasites will die by interfering with its ability to metabolize energy. This class of anthelmintics has developed a wide range of resistance.

4. Isoquinoline-pyrozines: Praziquantel is the only drug used in horses in this category. It has a narrow spectrum of activity and only is effective at eliminating tapeworms. It disrupts the worm's ability to maintain equilibrium of its body fluids. This affect on motility impairs their ability to attach to the intestinal wall.

How to Determine Drug Resistance on a Farm

The best way to determine anthelmintic resistance on a farm is to perform a fecal egg count reduction test (FECRT). A McMaster FEC is performed before deworming. Ten to 14 days following deworming, another McMaster FEC is preformed. For benzimidazoles and pyrantel, anything less than 80% is considered resistant. For ivermectin, anything less than 98% is considered resistant.

$$FECRT\% = \frac{pre\,FEC - post\,FEC}{pre\,FEC} \times 100$$

For example:

pre-FEC $= 200\,eggs/g$

post-FEC $= 125\,eggs/g$

$$\%\,FECRT = \frac{(200-125)}{200} \times 100 = 37.5\%$$

Summary of Parasite Control Measures

- Perform a McMaster FEC on each horse to determine the parasite load for each individual and to monitor for resistance to strongyles.
- Remove manure from small paddocks twice a week.
- Dragging or harrowing pastures to break up manure can spread parasite larvae. Make sure to remove horses from a harrowed pasture for 2 to 4 weeks.
- Do not spread fresh manure on pastures.
- New horses added to the farm should be dewormed with moxidectin or ivermectin if they are staying less than 6 weeks.
- New or visiting foals should be treated with 10 mg/kg of fenbendazole for 5 days in a row to kill both the adult and migrating ascarid larvae.
- Deworm foals every 60 days until they are 15 months old.
- Deworm for bots once a year in autumn with ivermectin or moxidectin.
- Deworm for tapeworms in late autumn and early spring using praziquantel.
- Use an accurate body weight; underdosing is an ideal way to develop resistant parasites.
- If the horse will not swallow the paste dewormer, have the veterinarian administer the medication via nasogastric tube.

Annual Components of an Equine Wellness Program

Equine Infectious Anemia

Equine infectious anemia (EIA) is an infectious viral disease. Horses that contract the infection can be subclinical carriers or they can die from the disease. The clinical signs are anemia, weight loss, petechia, depression, fever, icteric mucous membranes, and limb edema. No vaccine is currently available. Transmission occurs by biting insects such as horse-flies or deerflies. Humans can spread the virus by sharing blood contaminated instruments or needles between horses. In 1970, Dr. Leroy Coggins developed a serologic test to detect antibodies to the virus. This test is an agar-gel immunodiffusion assay now called the Coggins test. A negative Coggins test is required for crossing state lines, health certificates, horse shows, sales, and events. A Coggins test should be performed annually. The Agar gel immunodiffusion assay (AGID) test takes 24 hours to perform. There is an ELISA test available that can be completed in 2 to 4 hours. Some states offer an electronic copy of the Coggins test, which is similar to a driver's license containing pictures of the horse. This card can be carried by the owner and contains the negative status of the horse for EIA and the date the sample was collected. Any test that is positive is immediately reported to the state veterinarian. The horse and the property will be quarantined by the state veterinarian.

Health Certificates

Health certificates are legal documents signed by a licensed veterinarian in the state in which the certificate is generated. Health certificates are required for interstate travel, sales, and horse events. The information on the health certificate generally includes the name and address of the owner and the name and address of the destination the horse will be traveling to. The certificate requires a physical examination by a veterinarian, which verifies the horse was healthy at the time of the examination. The certificate will require proof a negative Coggins test, vaccination record, and the horse's vital signs. There are variations in the data requested from state to state. International health certificates are different and are dependant on the destination country.

Routine Dental Care

Horses' dentition has evolved to suit a lifestyle of grazing. They have hypsodont teeth that continue to erupt from the jaw over many years. This type of tooth is well designed to handle the increased wear from consuming abrasive grass and small amounts of sand and grit. The tooth will erupt 3 to 4 mm a year to compensate for daily wear and tear of eating. Most horses' teeth will last until they are 25 to 30 years old.

A dental examination should be performed on all newborn foals to examine the bite and look for evidence of congenital defects. Identification of an abnormal bite at an early age will provide time to correct the defect before it will affect the foal's entire life. It is recommended for horses to undergo a dental examination twice a year for the first 5 years of their life. They many not require significant dental work, but during this time, the horse will lose 24 deciduous teeth and 36 to 44 permanent teeth will erupt. This is an important time for training young horses. Abnormalities of their teeth may cause them to misbehave from the discomfort in their mouth with the use of a bit. Between the ages of 5 and 15 years of age a dental examination performed once a year is adequate for a horse with a normal mouth. After 15 years the probability of developing dental problems will rise because the teeth begin to wear out. Most veterinarians recommend twice a year evaluation of these older horses to keep on top on new problems.

To perform a good dental examination, a speculum, dental mirror, and quality light source are a must (Figure 5.9). Most horses will require sedation to safely apply the speculum and facilitate the

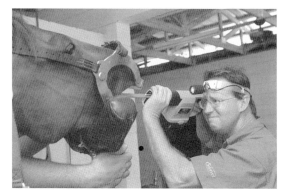

Figure 5.9. Equine dentist using a speculum and headlamp. Courtesy Dr. Toots Banner.

EQUINE DENTAL CHART

NOTES: _____
_____
_____
_____
_____
_____
_____

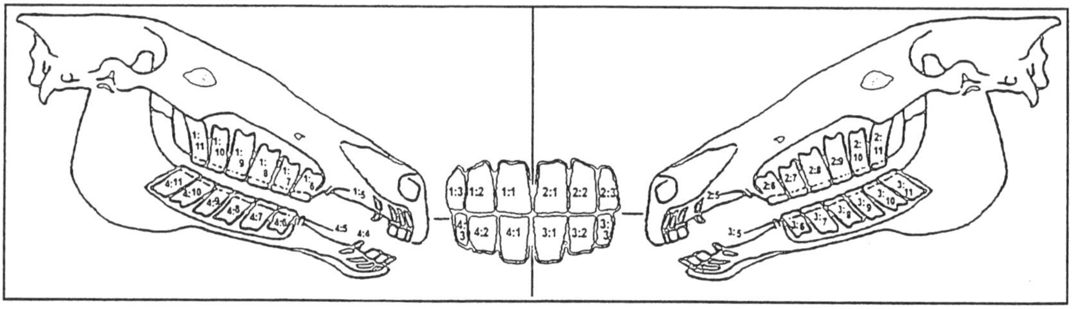

HISTORY

- ☐ WEIGHT LOSS
- ☐ RESISTING
- ☐ COLIC
- ☐ DROPPING FEED
- ☐ QUIDDING
- ☐ ABNORMAL CHEWING
- ☐ HEAD TILT
- ☐ HEAD TOSSING
- ☐ LARGE STEM IN FECES
- ☐ OTHER _____

EXAM OBSERVATIONS

☐ SHARP POINTS ☐ VERY SHARP POINTS ☐ LACKS LATERAL EXCURSION ☐ TMJ SENSITIVITY ☐ HOOKS ☐ RAMPS ☐ STEP ☐ WAVE ☐ CUPPED

☐ EXCESSIVE TRANSVERSE RIDGES ☐ RETAINED DECIDUOUS ☐ FRAGMENT ☐ UNERUPTED ☐ MISSING ☐ EXCESSIVE WEAR ☐ OVERLONG INCISORS

_____
_____
_____
_____
_____

INCISORS				CANINES		WOLF TEETH	
☐ Reduction ____		**EXTRACTION:**		☐ Reduction ____		☐ Extraction ____	
☐ Realign ____		☐ Deciduous ____		☐ Tartar ____		☐ Erupted ____	
☐ Balance ____		☐ Fragment ____		☐ Elevate ____		☐ Unerupted ____	
☐ _____		☐ Decayed ____		☐ Extract ____		☐ Fragment ____	
		☐ _____ ____		☐ Gingivitis ____		☐ _____ ____	
				☐ _____ ____			

MOLARS

					RECOMMEND	MAINTAIN	
☐ Float ____	☐ Ridges ____	**EXTRACTION:**				☐ YEARLY	
☐ Bit Seat ____	☐ Cupped ____	☐ Deciduous ____				☐ EVERY 6 MONTHS	
☐ Hooks ____	☐ Gingivitis ____	☐ Fragment ____				☐ EVERY 3 MONTHS	
☐ Ramps ____	☐ Decayed ____	☐ Decayed ____					
☐ Waves ____	☐ Balance ____	☐ _____ ____				NEXT APPOINTMENT:	
☐ Step ____						____ / ____ / ____	

Original - Record   Pink - Service   Yellow - Doctor   White - Client

Figure 5.10. Dental examination chart.
Courtesy Dr. Dana Zimmel.

144

examination. The mouth is rinsed with water to remove all debris between the teeth and tongue. The mouth is evaluated for any evidence of ulceration or laceration of the tongue, cheeks, and lips. The horses' bite is evaluated for proper chewing motion. Each tooth and the surrounding gum are examined and palpated to determine if they are loose or cracked. The gums can be closely evaluated with the aid of the dental mirror to rule out periodontal disease.

Dental charting is widely accepted using the Triadan system of dental nomenclature (Figure 5.10). This system uses three digits to identify each tooth. The first digit represents the quadrant, with 1 for the upper right, 2 for the upper left, 3 for the lower left, and 4 for the lower right. The deciduous (permanent) teeth are similarly identified using the prefix 5 to 8 for the four quadrants.

Many veterinarians specialize in equine dentistry. The demand for good work and knowledgeable veterinarians and their technicians is quite prevalent. Dental equipment has advanced beyond hand floats, and now routine work is performed with several types of motorized equipment which can deliver a faster and safe job when appropriately applied.

Preventative Health Care for the Neonatal Foal

Careful assessment of the neonatal foal can identify problems before they become life threatening. A physical examination, immunoglobulin G (IgG) measurement, administration of an enema, and dipping the umbilicus at birth are the key features to a wellness plan for a newborn foal. Understanding normal foal behavior will help to recognize when the foal may be in trouble.

A normal foal should be able to sit on its sternum in 2 to 3 minutes after birth and stand within 60 minutes. If the foal is not standing by 2 hours, someone should intervene. Most foals will have a suckle reflex by 30 minutes of age. They should be standing and suckling within 2 hours of age. If a foal does not nurse in 3 to 4 hours after birth, they can become hypoglycemic and are too weak to stand. Then a vicious cycle can begin resulting in a recumbent, hypoglycemic, and a dehydrated foal. Most foals will sleep within 1.5 to 4 hours after birth. Foals lay down about 33% of the time compared to 5% to 10% of the adults. Normal foals are able to gallop by 6 to 7 hours of age. During the first week of life foals spend 85% of their time within 1 m of the dam. If a foal is seen off by itself, this would be considered abnormal. Lack of affinity for the mare is one of the first signs of hypoxic ischemic encephalopathy (HIE), which can be a life-threatening problem in neonates.

All neonates should receive a physical examination by a veterinarian within the first 8 to 24 hours of age. The examination should evaluate general health status of the foal and to look for congenital or developmental defects such as a cleft palate and umbilical or scrotal hernia. It is quite common to administer an enema in the first few hours of life to help the foal pass meconium. Over-the-counter enemas are acceptable for this purpose. They are simple to use and require proper restraint of the foal while inserting the soft applicator into the rectum.

All newborn foals will need to have the umbilical stump dipped at birth. The use of straight (tincture) iodine on the umbilical stalk is contraindicated because it can cause severe scalding of the skin. Dilute iodine (the color of ice tea) or a 1:4 solution of chlorhexidine can be used. Fill a 6- or 12-ml syringe case with the solution and hold it over the umbilical stalk for 30 seconds. Dipping the umbilicus one to two times a day for the first 2 days is adequate. Inspection of the umbilicus for purulent debris, sudden enlargement, bleeding, or urine should be part of daily monitoring.

All foals should have the IgG (antibody or immunoglobulin) level checked between 8 and 24 hours of age. This test reflects the level of antibody absorbed by the foal through the process of pinocytosis in the small intestine. The absorption of these antibodies is crucial for the prevention of disease. The foal will rely on these antibodies for protection against disease during the first 3 to 4 months of life. The quality and quantity of colostrum directly influence the IgG level. Commercial test kits are readily available and can be easily performed stall side in less than 20 minutes. Failure of passive transfer is diagnosed when the IgG is less than

800 mg/dl. If the foal is older than 24 hours of age, the only method to provide adequate immunity is administration of plasma because of gut closure. After 24 hours of age, the foal can no longer absorb the immunoglobulins into the bloodstream because the gut is "closed" and the immunoglobulins are digested. Failure to acquire adequate immunity puts the foal at high risk for development of serious consequences, such as septicemia, pneumonia, and infectious arthritis/physitis.

References and Further Reading

Baker, G., and J. Easley. 2005. *Equine Dentistry.* 2nd ed. Philadelphia: Elsevier Limited.

Kania, S. A., and C. R. Reinemeyer. 2005. Anoplocephala perfoliata coproantigen detection: a preliminary study. *Vet Parasitol* 127(2):115–19.

Kaplan, R. M., T. R. Klei, E. T. Lyons, G. Lester, C. H. Courtney, D. D. French, S. C. Tolliver, A. N. Vidyashankar, and Y. Zhao. 2004. Prevalence of anthelmintic resistant cyanthostomes on horse farms. *J Am Vet Med Assoc* 225(6):903–10.

Kaplan, R. M. 2002. Anthelmintic resistance in nematodes of horses. *Vet Res* 33(5):491–507.

Scollay, M.C., W. Bernard, G. W. Brumbaugh, B. S. Carroll, N. Cohen, T. Cordes, R. M. Dwyer, et al. 2008. Guidelines for the vaccination of horses. Retrieved from the American Association of Equine Practitioners Web site: www.aaep.org.

Smith, B. P. 2001. *Large Animal Internal Medicine.* 3rd ed. St. Louis: Mosby.

Sweeney, C. R., J. F. Timoney, J. R. Newton, and M. T. Hines. 2005. *Streptococcus equi* infections in horses: guidelines for treatment, control, and prevention of strangles. *J Vet Intern Med* 19:123–34.

Wilson, J. H. 2005. Vaccine efficacy and controversies. *AAEP Proceedings* 51:409–20.

CHAPTER 6

Foal Care

Bonnie S. Barr, DeeAnn Wilfong, Laura Javsicas, Tanya M. Balaam-Morgan, and Dana Zimmel

Basic Foal Care

Normal Foal Behavior

Careful assessment of the neonatal foal can identify problems before they become life threatening. An important aspect of good husbandry is to understand normal behavior and recognize subtle changes in the foal's condition that may indicate a problem. A normal foal should be able to sit on its sternum in 2 to 3 minutes after birth and stand within 60 minutes. Most foals will have a suckle reflex by 30 minutes of age. They should be standing and suckling within 2 hours of age (Figure 6.1). If a foal does not nurse within 3 to 4 hours after birth, they can become hypoglycemic and unable to stand. A vicious cycle can begin resulting in a recumbent, hypoglycemic, and a dehydrated foal. Most foals will sleep within 1.5 to 4 hours after birth. Foals lay down about 33% of the time compared to 5% to 10% in adults. Normal foals are able to gallop by 6 to 7 hours of age. During the first week of life, foals spend 85% of their time within 1 m of the dam. If a foal is seen off by itself, this would be considered abnormal. Lack of affinity for the mare is one of the first signs of hypoxic ischemic encephalopathy (HIE).

Neonatal Physical Examination

All neonates should receive a physical examination within the first 8 to 24 hours of age (Table 6.1). Be sure to look for congenital or developmental defects such as a cleft palate and umbilical or scrotal hernia.

Colostrum: A Critical Component for a Healthy Foal

The fetus is unable to receive immunoglobulins via transfer from the placenta due to the epitheliochorial type of equine placentation. The foal relies on the ingestion of colostrum for absorption of and initiation of humoral immunity. Immunoglobulins and other large molecules are selectively absorbed by specialized epithelial cells in the newborn small intestine. After intestinal absorption, (primarily immunoglobulin G [IgG]) will enter the circulation via lymphatic vessels. These cells are replaced approximately 12 to 24 hours postpartum, which results in loss of ability to absorb immunoglobulins. The maximal absorptive capacity occurs within the first 8 hours postpartum and results in maximal blood levels approximately 18 hours postpartum. In the mare's mammary gland, colostrum is replaced by milk, which contains little to no immunoglobulins, within 24 hours postpartum. Considering the preceding time line, it is important to make sure newborn foals nurse an adequate quantity of colostrum within the first 24 hours of life and preferably by 8 to 12 hours postpartum to maximize IgG absorption for initial immunity. *All foals should have their IgG measured between 8 and 24 hours of age. To achieve adequate immunity the foal should have an IgG*

147

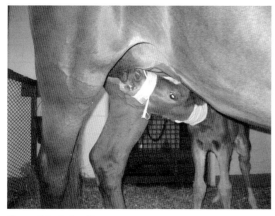

Figure 6.1. Foal suckling.
Courtesy Dr. Dana Zimmel.

greater than 800 mg/dl. The risk of life-threatening bacterial infection is substantially increased when the foal has failure of passive transfer (IgG <200 mg/dl).

The quantity of IgG absorbed depends on the quality of colostrum, the volume of colostrum available, the volume of colostrum ingested, the timing of ingestion, and the health status of the foal.

The quality of colostrum should be measured when the foal is born. The specific gravity can be measured with a colostrometer. Good-quality colostrum should have a specific gravity greater than 1.060 and contain at least 50 g/L of IgG. The volume of colostrum produced by the mare will vary with regard to the number of previous foals, health of

Table 6.1. Foal physical examination.

Physical examination	Normal	Abnormal
Attitude, behavior	Bright, alert, responsive	Depressed, sleepy, hyperexcitable, and seizures
Body posture	Erect head and neck	Hypotonia with sepsis, extensor rigidity with asphyxia or meningitis
Temperature	99.0° F–102.0° F	Hypothermia—sepsis, prematurity, and asphyxia; fever—indicates infection
Heart rate	70–110 beats per minute, normal rhythm	Tachycardia—dehydration, sepsis, asphyxia, pain, shock, and fever; bradycardia—septic shock, hypothermia, and hypoglycemia
Capillary refill time	<2 seconds	Prolonged CRT—dehydration and shock
Mucous membranes	Pink, moist	Red/injected—sepsis and endotoxemia; Pale pink—anemia; Brown/orange—hemolysis, liver disease, and sepsis; White/grey—shock
Pulse quality—distal extremities	Strong, warm extremities	Poor quality, cool limbs—hypotension and hypovolemia
Respiratory rate	30–40 breaths per minute	Tachypnea—stress, pain, pneumonia, shock, fever, and acidosis; slow or irregular-asphyxia, shock, hypothermia, and prematurity
Auscultation of lungs	Easily heard over the entire thorax	Crackles, wheezes, absent lung sounds—pneumonia and atelectasis
Gastrointestinal motility	Borborygmi present bilaterally	Absent or increased borborygmi/abdominal distension—enteritis, ileus, hypoxic damage to gastrointestinal tract, meconium impaction, and uro-abdomen
Feces, quantity, color, and consistency	Pasty yellow or tan in color, 2–4 times a day	Constipation-meconium impactions; diarrhea—viral, bacterial, and parasite induced; bloody diarrhea—*Clostridium* or *Salmonella* enterocolitis
Suckle reflex	30 minutes after birth	Absent or weak—sepsis, asphyxia, and immaturity
Urine	Clear, urinates frequently, USG <1.008	Decreased volume with dehydration, renal failure, and uro-abdomen
Umbilicus	Dry and small	Swelling or purulent discharge—umbilical infection; wet (urine)—patent urachus
Eyes, eyelids	Clear cornea	Tearing, miosis, blepharospasm can indicate corneal ulceration that can occur with recumbency or entropion
Joints	No evidence of lameness or distension	Pain, heat, joint swelling or lameness can be caused by septic arthritis/physitis
Limbs	Straight	Angular limb deformity, contracted tendons, and joint/tendon laxity (common with premature foals)
Palpation of ribs	smooth, nonpainful	If broken there may be increased RR rate, edema or crepitus over thorax

CRT, capillary refill time; RR, respiratory rate; USG, urine specific gravity.

the mare, and previous damage or disease of the mammary gland. Primiparous mares will produce less colostrum than multiparous mares, and mares with illness or stress will produce less colostrum. Mares that prematurely leak colostrum before parturition will have less available colostrum for the foal. Foals that are compromised will have a reduced appetite, which translated into a delay in ingestion of colostrum.

The volume of colostrum required for each foal depends on the quality of the colostrum and on the size of the foal. An average 50-kg foal will need between 2 and 3 L of high-quality colostrum. In general the amount of colostrum required to be ingested by neonatal foals is defined as "as much as possible."

A normal foal will nurse up to five to eight times per hour per day and ingest approximately 80 ml per feeding. Total colostrum and milk consumption in the first 24 hours postpartum is approximately 150 ml/kg body weight. For an average 50-kg foal this is calculated to be approximately 8 L with 2.5 to 3.5 L being colostrum. If foals are unable to naturally ingest an adequate quantity of colostrum, it is up to the owners and veterinary staff to make sure an adequate quantity of immunoglobulins gets absorbed. This can be accomplished through bottle feeding, bucket or pan feeding, or nasogastric tube feeding.

As long as the foal is stable and can systemically handle the administration of colostrum, the volume administered should mimic that of natural nursing. Within the first 24 hours the foal should be fed every 2 hours with a volume of approximately 400 to 500 ml (12–16 oz) at each feeding for a total rate of at least 5 L/day. If colostrum is unavailable from the dam or it is of poor quality, colostrum from a frozen bank or a donor mare is advisable. Fresh colostrum is better than frozen colostrum due to the denaturing of complement in the freezing process. If frozen colostrum is available, it should be thawed in a warm water bath not a microwave. The quality of the colostrum should be evaluated after it is room temperature to determine if the specific gravity is greater than 1.060.

If the foal has an adequate suckle response, a bottle can be used for administration of colostrum.

Most foals will readily accept the bottle as a newborn. Lamb nipples work quite well because they are of similar shape to the mare teat. Care must be taken to ensure that the foal has a strong suckle response to avoid potential aspiration of colostrum or milk. In addition, make sure the opening in the nipple is not too large so that the rate of colostrum or milk running out of the nipple doesn't exceed the rate of swallowing the foal. If milk is observed in the foal's mouth immediately after swallowing or if the foal coughs while suckling, the nipple should be examined.

Bucket or pan feeding is best when the foal is too weak to hold its head in a position to nurse the teat. Bucket or pan feeding is beneficial for foals with pneumonia that are unable to interrupt respiration for prolonged periods while nursing the teat. Feeding from a pan or bucket requires less energy for the foal due to the position of the head and neck, which also can decrease the likelihood of milk going down the trachea via gravity flow. As an added benefit, bucket and pan feeding is less labor intensive when raising an orphan foal.

Foal Umbilical Care

The umbilical cord is composed of the umbilical vein, two umbilical arteries, and the urachus. The umbilical vein extends from the umbilical remnant to the liver. Over time the umbilical vein becomes the falciform ligament. The umbilical arteries travel from the umbilical remnant around the bladder to the aorta. Later they will form the round ligaments of the bladder. The urachus is positioned between the two umbilical arteries and runs from the umbilical remnant to the bladder. In utero, the urachus connects the urinary bladder to the allantois of the placenta. During fetal life the umbilical cord supplies nutrition and oxygen to the growing fetus and functions to relieve the waste products from the fetus.

Birth of the newborn will rupture the umbilical cord at a predetermined level when the mare stands. Little hemorrhage results due to contraction of the muscle in the vessel wall. It is best to allow the cord to rupture naturally versus cutting the cord and suturing the bleeding cord.

The remaining portion of the umbilical stump is a potential portal of entry for bacteria into the bloodstream. Neonatal foals are born with a naïve immune system, making them vulnerable for many infectious insults. Until they have ingested adequate colostrum foals are at risk for infection. It is important to treat the umbilical remnant with an antibacterial solution to keep bacteria from colonizing the area.

Supplies that are needed for effective umbilical care include a small spray bottle or a small container, such as a specimen cup or a large syringe case, sterile water, 2% chlorhexidine solution, and examination gloves. The greatest reduction in bacterial colonization has been shown with a 0.5% solution of chlorhexidine. Strong solutions of iodine or tincture of iodine can result in rapid desiccation of the umbilical stump with burning and necrosis of the surrounding skin. This can predispose to local infection, as well as, patent urachus. It is recommended to use a 0.5% solution of chlorhexidine as a navel dip for newborn foals.

To make a 0.5% solution of chlorhexidine, dilute one part 2% chlorhexidine solution with three parts sterile water. To make a large volume of solution for multiple dosing, an empty clean chlorhexidine gallon container can be used. For ease of an accurate concentration of chlorhexidine solution draw a line with a permanent marker for the level of 2% chlorhexidine solution needed to make the desired 0.5% solution. The remainder of the container will be filled with sterile water. To avoid misuse of the chlorhexidine solution be sure to adequately label the container with the concentration of chlorhexidine and "foal navel treatment/dip." From the bulk supply of 0.5% chlorhexidine solution pour the solution into a smaller container, such as a specimen container or large syringe case.

The procedure for treatment of the umbilical stump should first involve adequate restraint of the foal. This is easiest if performed with two people but can be accomplished by a single individual. Dip the entire length of the umbilical stump into the solution for 20 to 30 second (Figure 6.2). Alternatively, the navel dip solution can be sprayed onto to stump using a spray bottle. This may be a desirable method if performing the procedure alone.

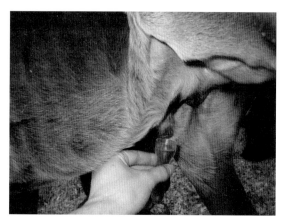

Figure 6.2. Dipping the umbilicus with chlorhexidine. Courtesy of Dr. Steeve Giguère.

Ideally, treatment should be initiated as soon as the umbilical cord has ruptured and the mare and foal have had a chance to become acquainted. Treatment should be repeated every 6 to 8 hours for at least the first 24 hours. If the foal appears normal and healthy, the veterinary examination is normal and the IgG level is adequate (>800 mg/dl) umbilical treatment is usually not necessary after 48 to 72 hours. Treatment should continue until the stump is dry.

Although treating the umbilical stump, it is important to examine the structure each time for the detection of any abnormalities such as redness, heat, pain, swelling, excess moisture before treatment, or urination. If any of the aforementioned abnormalities are noted, it is important to notify the veterinarian for further examination and diagnostics. Further diagnostics should include complete blood count with fibrinogen, chemistry profile, and ultrasound examination of the umbilical structures. Omphalophlebitis, or inflammation of the umbilical remnants, is a common infection of newborn foals. This condition requires immediate treatment and diagnostics.

Treatment with 0.5% chlorhexidine solution does leave the umbilical stump moist for a greater period of time compared with the iodine preparations. This can result in a longer period of time for the stump to desiccate. Careful daily examination of the umbilical stump is necessary until the stump has completely desiccated.

Administration of Enemas

Many farms administer enemas to newborn foals prophylactically in an effort to prevent the discomfort and straining that often accompany passage of meconium. In the hospital setting, enemas are commonly administered to a neonatal foal that is displaying signs of abdominal discomfort, straining to defecate, or that has a meconium impaction.

Types of Enemas
There are several different types of enemas that can be administered. The most commonly used commercial enema is the Fleet enema. These enemas are composed of electrolytes or mineral oil. Administration of one or two of this type of enema is safe. Enemas commonly used in a hospital setting consist of warm water and a gentle nonirritating soap such as Ivory. Excessively harsh detergents should not be used because the rectal mucosa is easily irritated and may become edematous. A retention enema with acetylcysteine may be administered if routine enemas are unsuccessful in resolving the impaction. Barium enemas are administered to provide contrast for radiography if there is a suspicion of obstruction of the rectum or small colon or a congenital defect.

Commercial enemas are packaged in a container with an applicator. Lubrication should be used on the application tip to prevent rectal perforation. Materials needed for homemade enemas include 5 ml mild detergent (Ivory), a soft stallion catheter or Foley catheter, warm water, an enema bag or enema bucket, and lubricant.

How to Perform an Enema
The enema should be administered with the foal in lateral recumbency or standing. A Foley catheter or some other type of soft flexible tubing is generously lubricated and gently inserted into the rectum until resistance is met, which is usually 3 to 7 in. Care should be taken to not use excessive force. A volume of 200 to 400 ml for a 50-kg foal may be administered by gravity flow. It is normal for

some fluid to be pushed out around the sides of the tubing. After administration the foal may benefit from standing or walking.

The administration of a retention enema may require the foal to be sedated and placed in lateral recumbency. A lubricated 30 French Foley catheter is inserted 2 to 3 cm into the rectum and the cuff is inflated to prevent backflow. Approximately 100 to 200 ml of a 4% concentration of acetylcysteine is administered by gravity. To make the 4% solution, mix 160 ml of warm water with 40 ml of commercial 20% acetylcysteine (Mucomyst). To adjust the pH, 20 g of baking soda is added to the mixture. The Foley catheter should be left in place for 10 to 15 minutes if possible. The cuff should be deflated prior to removing the catheter.

The administration of a barium enema is similar to the instructions for a homemade enema except 180 ml of barium is administered by gravity slowly while holding the anus closed around the tube. A lateral radiographs is taken immediately after all of the barium is administered.

A routine enema may be repeated several times if it is unsuccessful in resolving the impaction. It should be noted that repeated enemas may cause rectal irritation and should be administered only if clinically warranted.

Complications
Possible complications include irritation to the rectal mucosa. This can happen with repeated enemas or if excessively harsh detergents are used. Repeated administration of the commercially prepared over-the-counter enemas can result in electrolyte disturbances, specifically hyperphosphatemia. Rectal perforation may occur if the tubing used is too rigid or if the tubing is aggressively forced into the rectum.

Foal Nutrition

Neonatal foals are born with minimal nutritional and energy stores compared to adult horses. A readily available nutritional source is required to fuel organ systems, red blood cells, and to support thermoregulation and growth. This is true whether the foal is born normal and healthy, born compromised, or becomes affected by illness in the neonatal period. Energy is stored in the form of glycogen and is predominately stored in the liver and muscle tissue. In the newborn foal these energy stores are adequate to maintain body temperature for approximately 1 hour or less postpartum. After this time frame, energy is derived from endogenous fat which is also limited in the newborn. Fat-derived energy is adequate to maintain body temperature for approximately 24 hours or less.

Energy Requirements for Healthy Foals

Foals grow rapidly and require a great deal of energy to support this growth. During the first 30 days of life normal healthy foals gain approximately 1.3 to 1.5 kg/day and within the first 6 months Thoroughbred foals reach 83% or their adult height and 46% or their adult weight. Healthy foals suckle approximately five to eight times per hour and will consume 20% to 28% of their body weight in mare's milk per day. They usually ingest approximately 80 ml per feeding. As an example, a 50-kg foal may consume 12.5 L of milk per day. During the first few days postpartum, most foals will consume approximately 5 L of milk, which is 10% to 15% of its body weight. Daily energy requirements for foals are measured in kilocalories (kcal). Estimated caloric requirement based on age of a 50-kg foal is as follows: 7,500 kcal from birth to 7 days (150 kcal/kg/day); 9,800 kcal from 8 to 14 days; 11,000 kcal from 15 to 28 days (about 120 kcal/kg/day); 12,500 kcal for 1 to 2 months (80–100 kcal/kg/day). These values demonstrate that the energy requirements per kg of body weight decrease as the foal's body weight increases. Normal foals nursing mares with good quality milk can easily achieve the daily energy requirements for maintenance of basal metabolic needs and ongoing growth.

Energy Requirements for Sick Foals

The energy requirement of a sick neonatal foal is significantly lower compared to healthy foals. This is based on the fact that sick neonates are often recumbent with decreased activity, and there is a temporary reduction in growth rate. In these foals the energy expenditure exceeds the gross energy intake, and as a result, energy is unavailable for growth. In a diseased or compromised state foals quickly develop a negative energy balance resulting in protein catabolism. One study reported that the resting energy requirement of clinically ill foals was 45 kcal/kg/day (roughly one-third of a healthy foal). When managing a critically ill neonatal foal it is often preferable to achieve a hypocaloric diet to prevent a catabolic state and accept that all nutritional needs may not be met. There has been little evidence in human patients that providing a hypocaloric diet for several days will negatively impact the outcome of the patient.

Advanced Nursing Care for Neonates

Neonatal nursing care can range from administration of colostrum to management of a critical foal in the intensive care unit. Fluid therapy and critical care monitoring are discussed in Chapter 11.

Enteral Nutrition

Administering nutrition to a foal using a nasogastric tube may be required if the foal has not consumed colostrum in a reasonable time frame or is unable to nurse milk from the mare due to systemic illness or injury. The feeding tube permits access to the gastrointestinal tract of foals that can tolerate enteral nutrition but have a poor suckle reflex. For single or short-term use a 14 or 16 French stallion catheter can be placed in the foal's esophagus. The rigid nature of these tubes can cause significant laryngeal inflammation and trauma if left in place for more than a few days. The larger diameter of these tubes necessitates placement in the esophagus rather than the stomach to prevent gastric reflux between feedings. Feeding tubes that are made of polyurethane are less traumatic and can be left in place for several weeks. A common feeding tube used in veterinary practice is the 14 French × 50-inch nasogastric feeding tube. Another feeding tube used frequently is the Rhyles tube. These feeding tubes are generally smaller in diameter and can be placed in the stomach. Another benefit of using a small diameter tube is the availability for the foal to suckle the mare while the tube is in place. The

Table 6.2. Supplies needed to place a nasogastric tube.

- Nasogastric tube.
- 2-in. Elastikon tape.
- 1-in. white tape.
- Suture material (2-0 to 0 size).
- Permanent marker.
- Stethoscope.
- Radiographic equipment.

supplies needed to insert a nasogastric tube are listed in Table 6.2.

How to Place a Nasogastric Tube

The foal should be restrained in a standing position or in sternal recumbency. The feeding tube is passed into the nose and through the ventral meatus. Because of the small diameter of the tube, it is often difficult to palpate the tube in the esophagus. Suction can be applied to the end of the tube. If air is difficult to aspirate, the tube is likely in the esophagus, where as if air is easily aspirated, the tube is likely in the trachea. To confirm proper placement of the tube into the esophagus or stomach, air can be introduced into the end of the tube while a stethoscope is placed on the abdomen over the stomach area. If air is easily auscultated in the stomach, the tube has been properly placed. Another way to assess proper placement of the tube is to take a radiograph of the foal's thorax and abdomen; the end of the feeding tube is generally easy to visualize in the esophagus or stomach.

Once the tube has been confirmed in the esophagus or stomach, it will need to be secured to the foal's head. This can be accomplished by various methods. One method is to place a piece of white tape around the tube distal to the marked line in a butterfly fashion. The tape can then be suture to the lateral aspect of the external nares. Alternatively, 2-0 suture is used to form a loop over the lateral aspect of the nares, and a Chinese finger snare suture pattern is used to hold the nasogastric tube in place (Figure 6.3). After securing the tube, it is beneficial to place a mark on the tube with a permanent marker at the level of the external nares to designate and monitor proper placement of the tube.

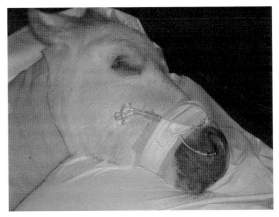

Figure 6.3. Nasogastric tube secured with a Chinese finger snare. Courtesy Dr. Dana Zimmel.

How to Feed Through a Nasogastric Tube

Normal foals can consume up to 27% of their body weight in milk on a daily basis by 1 week of age, whereas sick foals generally are unable to tolerate this volume during the acute phase of illness. For sick full-term foals, the goal is to provide 10% to 15% of the foal's weight in multiple small feedings. Initial feedings should be every hour and then decreased to every 2 hours, with double the volume, once the condition of the foal has stabilized. A suggested or recommended initial rate for the first 24 hours is 2 to 3 ml/kg body weight/hour, which is approximately 100 to 150 ml/hour for a 50-kg foal. The feeding rate can be gradually increased over the next 2 to 3 days such that on day 2 the rate may be 4 to 5 ml/kg per hour and on day 3 the rate may be 6 to 8 ml/kg per hour (about 10%–15% of body weight). This rate and feeding level will typically meet the resting energy requirements of hospitalized clinically ill foals.

Nutrition for enteral feeding should ideally be mare's milk. If mare's milk is unavailable commercial milk replacers, goat's milk, or cow's milk can alternatively be used. Commercial foal milk replacers are preferable as a second choice to mare's milk as the composition is formulated to closely match that of mare's milk with regards to energy, protein, mineral, and vitamin content. Goat's and cow's milk are less dilute and contain nearly twice as much as fat compared to mare's milk. Goat's and cow's milk also contain less lactose and carbohydrates. Cow's milk may cause diarrhea so either 2% milk or diluted whole milk should be used with the addition of 20 g of dextrose per liter to each (40 ml of 50% dextrose per liter of milk).

These feeding rates and types of nutritional supplementation can also be applied to feeding foals with a bottle or a bucket or pan. If you are feeding a healthy orphan foal, the rates will likely be able to be increased to a greater degree and more rapidly than previously mentioned for feeding the clinically ill foal.

Careful clinical monitoring is important and should include frequent assessments of the gastrointestinal function of the foal. This should include gastric reflux, intestinal sounds, abdominal distension, and quantity and quality of feces. Before each feeding the presence of gastric reflux should be checked. If reflux is present the scheduled feeding should be skipped and the volume of feedings should be decreased until the foal can handle the larger volumes. Feeding through the nasogastric tube should be accomplished using gravity flow or gentle pressure via a dosing syringe (Figure 6.4).

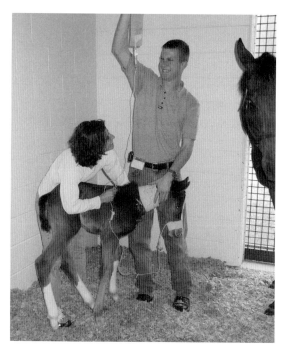

Figure 6.4. Gravity feeding of milk through a nasogastric tube. Courtesy Dr. Dana Zimmel.

Complications

The most common complications associated with enteral feeding include mismanagement of the feeding tube and overfeeding. Tubes with a large diameter can allow gastric reflux to enter the esophagus if placed in the stomach. These larger tubes should be placed in the esophagus or smaller diameter tubes should be used for placement in the stomach. Active foals can dislodge the placement of the tube between feedings. Careful examination of the tube before each feeding is essential to make sure the tube remains in the esophagus. Monitoring the position of the previously marked line on the tube will help with this process. It is important to monitor for abdominal bloating, which could indicate overfeeding. Careful monitoring can be accomplished by marking an area on the foal's abdomen and measuring the diameter using string or tape before each feeding.

Oxygen Therapy

The addition of oxygen therapy to the treatment plan of a compromised foal is common in intensive care units. Adequate oxygen content, oxygen tension (PaO_2), and oxygen saturation (SaO_2) are important for maintaining normal pulmonary, tissue, and organ perfusion. Maintaining pulmonary perfusion allows for adequate ventilation-perfusion matching that is necessary for effective gas transport in the lungs.

Indications for Oxygen Therapy

Oxygen therapy may be indicated in any foal that suffers from hypoxemia or hypoxia. Hypoxemia is defined as subnormal blood oxygen tension levels. Hypoxia is defined as lack of oxygen content at the tissue level and may occur with or without concurrent hypoxemia. Hypoxia may result from hypoxemia, hypoperfusion, or below normal oxygen-carrying capacity of blood such as occurs with anemia or abnormal hemoglobin. Hypoxemia may result from low inspired oxygen tension, hypoventilation or abnormal ventilation, ventilation-perfusion mismatch, diffusion impairment, and right-to-left shunting of blood. Conditions that create hypoxemia or hypoxia include septicemia, perinatal asphyxia syndrome (PAS), prematurity, pneumonia, neonatal isoerythrolysis, and cardiac abnormalities.

When presented with a foal that requires oxygen therapy it is important to obtain an arterial blood sample to asses the respiratory and metabolic status. Arteries that are most commonly used for blood sampling are the dorsal metatarsal artery in the lateral aspect of the hind limb and the brachial artery in the front limb. See Chapter 11 for a detailed description of evaluating patients with hypoxemia and hypoxia.

Oxygen therapy can be delivered through an intranasal cannula or via an endotracheal tube with full respiratory support and mechanical ventilation. This section will cover delivery using intranasal oxygen insufflation.

How to Administer Intranasal Oxygen

Supplies needed to set up for intranasal oxygen insufflation include nasal oxygen tubes, 2-inch Elastikon, tongue depressor wrapped in tape, 1-inch white tape, suture, oxygen supply, humidifier, and a permanent marker. Small-bore flexible rubber feeding tubes with a diameter of less than 1 cm are useful for the intranasal oxygen cannula. The oxygen supply can be from in house supply lines or from portable oxygen tanks. If short-term delivery of oxygen if required, anesthesia face masks can be used for the delivery of oxygen.

Before passing the intranasal cannula, it is helpful to mark the proper distance for placement with a permanent marker. The cannula should be inserted to the level of the medial canthus of the eye. Measure the distance from the external nares to the medial canthus and mark a line on the tubing at the external nares to designate the correct length. The cannula is inserted in the foal's nostril and passed through the ventral meatus to the predetermined distance.

Once the cannula is in place it can be secured to the foal's head using one of two methods. One method involves attaching the tube to a tongue depressor that has been wrapped in tape. The cannula tubing is taped to one side of the tongue depressor and then looped around to run parallel with the previously taped tubing. The cannula tubing and tongue depressor are then taped to the foal's nose using Elastikon that wraps circumferentially around the nose caudal to the nostrils (Figure 6.5). Care must be taken not to wrap the Elastikon too tight inhibiting the foal from opening its mouth. The other method involves suturing the cannula tubing to the external nares. Place a piece of white tape around the tube distal to the marked line in a butterfly fashion. The tape can then be sutured to the lateral aspect of the external nares

If oxygen therapy will be administered longer than 1 hour, the oxygen gas should be humidified before delivery to the foal. A humidifier functions to bubble the oxygen gas through water to increase the absolute humidity of the gas. The smaller the bubbles are the greater the contact surface is and the more efficient the humidification of the gas. An increase in the oxygen flow rate results in less contact time and less efficient humidification process.

The flow rate should be titrated according to the response of the patient and results of blood gas analysis. If the PaO_2 is greater than 120 mm Hg, the flow rate should be decreased. Foals that are unable to stand should remain in sternal recumbency. Foals in lateral recumbency will develop atelectasis and ventilation-perfusion mismatching. The PaO_2 on foals in lateral recumbency can be 10 to 20 mm Hg lower than foals that are in sternal recumbency or standing. If the foal is unable to stay in sternal

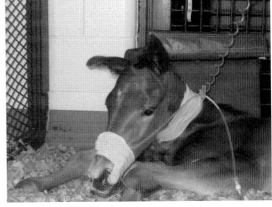

Figure 6.5. Oxygen cannula placed in the left nostril. Courtesy Dr. Dana Zimmel.

recumbency it should be turned every 2 to 3 hours. The use of V-shaped pads can help maintain a foal in sternal recumbency (Figure 6.6).

Complications

Complications associated with intranasal oxygen insufflation include nasal irritation and rhinitis and airway drying. Airway drying results in excess tracheal and nasal discharge. This is caused by inadequately humidified oxygen gases. The most common complication is nasal irritation and rhinitis. Foals will typically grind their teeth, have increased upper airway moisture, and develop nasal discharge that can be quite profuse. The irritation and inflammation is caused by the physical presence of the intranasal cannula and the drying effect of the oxygen flow. The airway drying and nasal irritation often go together and can occur in the presence of a humidifier due to larger bubbles and a high flow rate. To try and avoid this irritation and inflammation the flow rate should be adjusted to the lowest rate needed to maintain a normal PaO_2. The nasal cannula should be cleaned every 4 to 6 hours to remove nasal discharge that can block the fenestrations in the tubing preventing oxygen flow.

Eye Care

The neonatal foal has decreased corneal sensitivity compared to an adult. Foals with eye injuries may not display the common clinical signs of blepharo-

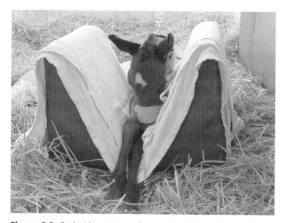

Figure 6.6. Foal with respiratory disease placed in sternal recumbency. Courtesy of Dr. Steeve Giguère.

spasm and epiphora. Problems can develop especially if the foal is recumbent. Prevention through careful nursing care is the key to eliminate or minimize eye problems. In many intensive care units, part of the daily examination is fluorescein staining of the eye to rule out corneal trauma. See Chapter 11 for details on performing a complete evaluation of the eye.

A recumbent foal's head should be maintained on a soft, surface to avoid injury to the down eye. If the foal is thrashing, "donuts" can be made out of 6-in. stockinet, cotton, and tape to prevent trauma to the eyes. The donut encircles the entire eye socket, leaving an open hole for the foal to see through. The eyes of these patients should be examined closely several times a day because they are prone to traumatic injuries, corneal ulcers, and entropion.

The technician should wash their hands when applying medication to the eye. The foal should be effectively restrained when treating the eye to avoid further injury. Do not share tubes of ointment or bottles of solution among foals. The ointment or solution may be transferred to a tuberculin syringe (1 ml) to apply to individual patients. If a needle is on the end of the syringe remove it before applying the medication. With one hand, open the foal's eye. Hold the medication in the other hand, placing the back of the hand near the lateral canthus for stability, and deposit the medication on the cornea, the sclera, or on the inside of the lower lid. Do not rub the cornea with the tip of the ointment tube or syringe.

Management of Entropion

Entropion or inversion of one or both eyelids is occasionally seen in the foals (Figure 6.7). The lower lid is much more commonly affected. Entropion can occur as a congenital or as an acquired defect. Most often entropion is acquired secondary to dehydration or eyelid trauma in the compromised foal. The rolled-in skin may cause irritation of the cornea and conjunctiva with subsequent corneal ulceration, lacrimation, and conjunctivitis. Clinical signs include increased lacrimation and blepharospasm. It is important to stain the cornea because secondary corneal ulceration is often present. In mild cases

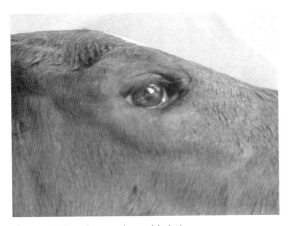

Figure 6.7. Entropion secondary to dehydration. Courtesy Dr. Dana Zimmel.

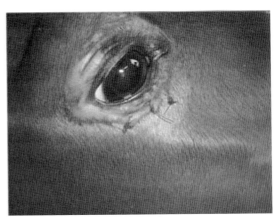

Figure 6.8. Surgical correction of entropion. Courtesy of DeeAnn Wilfong.

of entropion, frequent manual eversion of the eyelid may resolve the problem. Another technique for short-term results is to inject procaine penicillin into the lower eyelid to correct entropion. It may be necessary to repeat the injection after 24 hours. If any of these procedures do not work surgical correction may be needed.

Surgical Correction of Entropion

For surgical correction of entropion the following materials will be needed: nonabsorbable suture 3-0 to 5-0 monofilament nylon or silk, lidocaine, needle holders, and sedation. The foal is adequately sedated and restrained. Lidocaine is used to block the area where the sutures are to be placed. Three to four vertical mattress-tacking sutures per eyelid are usually adequate to evert the eyelid, although more maybe needed. The first suture is passed in the center of the eyelid, beginning 1 mm to 2 mm away from the eyelid margin perpendicular to the eyelid. The next step is to take an additional bite of skin distal to the original bite. The distance between the two bites will determine the amount of eversion of the eyelids that will occur after tying the sutures. The knots should be directed away from the cornea with the end of the suture nearest the cornea cut short and the opposite end cut longer to make removal of the suture easier (Figure 6.8). The sutures are left in place for 1 to 4 weeks. Topical ophthalmic ointment, either for lubrication or to treat a corneal ulcer, is administered several times a day after entropion repair.

A complication that may occur with surgical correction of entropion is accidental abrasion of the cornea if the suture penetrates the inside of the eyelid and scratches the cornea. Care must be taken to avoid overcorrection of the entropion because the foal will not blink properly leading to further corneal damage.

Cardiopulmonary Resuscitation in Foals

Cardiopulmonary resuscitation (CPR) is universally accepted in human medicine and has been applied to many veterinary species. In adult horses, the mass of the animal makes CPR insufficient for sustaining life. However, CPR is technically possible and has been successful in foals. The success of CPR in foals depends on the cause of arrest and early intervention. Anticipation of which foals may require resuscitation and adequate training and preparation of staff are crucial for maximizing chances of a successful outcome.

Indications

CPR is indicated in cases of cardiopulmonary arrest, defined as sudden cessation of spontaneous and effective respiration and heartbeat.

Newborn foals are at risk of arrest during the immediate peripartum period because they may fail to make the physiological transition from fetal to neonatal life. Respiratory arrest almost always occurs first and results in cardiac arrest. Common clinical scenarios resulting in arrest include dystocia, premature delivery, premature placental separation, and delivery by caesarean section. In some cases, the foal may have already arrested before birth. Arrest in foals can also occur outside of the immediate postnatal period secondary to a systemic disease, which results in respiratory or cardiac failure. Perinatal hypoxia can damage the areas of the brain that control respiration, resulting in hypoventilation. Septic shock can alter the oxygen content of the blood and cardiac output, resulting in cardiopulmonary arrest. Primary lung disease, airway obstruction, and failure of respiratory muscles (diaphragm and intercostal), can result in progressive respiratory failure. Although the foal may initially have an increased respiratory rate and effort, these signs may precede respiratory arrest as the muscles fatigue and respiratory acidosis develops due to high carbon dioxide levels in the blood.

Cardiac arrest can occur due to pulseless, non-perfusing arrhythmias, including ventricular fibrillation, ventricular tachycardia, asystole, or pulseless electrical activity. Primary cardiac failure is uncommon in neonatal foals, whereas secondary cardiac failure can be secondary to congenital cardiac defects, hypoxic-ischemic damage, and inflammatory disease.

Although CPR may successfully revive the patient, their ultimate survival depends on identifying and correcting the cause of arrest. Otherwise, they are likely to arrest again, with subsequent resuscitations becoming less likely to succeed. It is also important to keep in mind that if the underlying problem cannot be corrected, such as a foal with congenital defects, CPR is not indicated.

Preparation

There are few situations in which "time" is as important as during an arrest. Being prepared with a specific plan and well-organized, easily accessible supplies is crucial to a successful outcome. The needed supplies will partially depend on whether you will be working in a farm or hospital situation, but the basics are the same. All supplies should be organized in a dedicated, easily accessible, and easily portable container or "crash cart" (Table 6.3). It is often helpful to keep an easily readable, laminated copy of a CPR flow chart and emergency drug doses on the crash cart (Figure 6.9).

Performing CPR

A: Assessment and Airway

A rapid initial assessment of the foal should be made in the first seconds after birth. After a few initial gasps, a normal foal should be breathing regularly with a respiratory rate of 60 to 80 beats per minute within 30 seconds. The heart rate should be regular, with a rate of 60 to 70 beats per minute. Some normal foals have arrhythmias for up to 15 minutes that do not require treatment. Foals that continue gasping for more than 30 seconds or are not breathing, have a heart rate less than 50 beats per minute or absent heart beat, require immediate resuscitation.

After a normal delivery, the foal can simply be observed for the first 20 seconds to ensure it is breathing spontaneously. Following a dystocia or caesarian section, the foal should be dried vigorously and a clear airway should be established by clearing the fetal membranes and fluid from the

Table 6.3. Resuscitation kit supplies.

Essential	Optional
Nasotracheal tubes (7–10 mm × 55 cm)	Oxygen tank and flowmeter
Air syringe	Other drugs
Self-inflating resuscitation bag (Ambu bag)	Heat lamp
Bulb syringe	ECG monitor
Pen light	ETCO$_2$ monitor
Epinephrine	Electrical defibrillator
Syringes and needles	Mask resuscitator
Intravenous catheters (14 to 16 gauge)	
Fluids	
PE tubing or red rubber catheter (>55 cm in length)	

ECG, electrocardiogram; ETCO$_2$, end-tidal carbon dioxide; PE, pediatric.

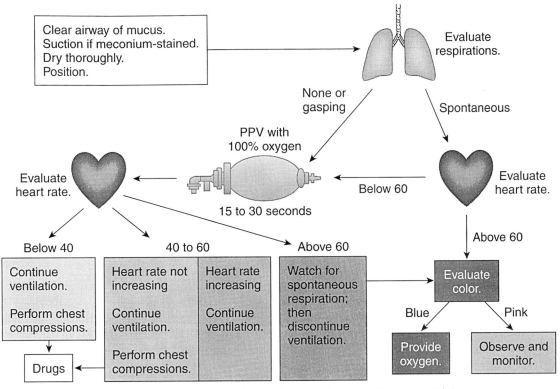

Figure 6.9. A flowchart illustrating the decision making in resuscitation of the newborn foal. PPV, positive pressure ventilation. Courtesy of W.B. Saunders, *Current therapy in equine practice.* 5th ed.

nose and mouth. Drying the foal with the head lowered can aide in clearing fluid from the airways. If meconium staining is evident, the airways should be suctioned with a bulb syringe or mechanical suction unit. If a mechanical unit is used, suctioning should not be performed for more than 5 to 10 seconds at a time because there is a risk of stimulation of the vagus nerve, which can cause bradycardia.

Intubation is the best way to provide a patent airway. Nasotracheal intubation is preferable to orotracheal intubation because there is less chance the tube will be damaged as the foal wakes up. To intubate, the foal should be in sternal or lateral recumbency. Lateral recumbency may be preferable because chest compressions can be started during intubation. With the neck extended to make a straight line from the nasopahrynx into the trachea,

the tube should be held with the curve downward and pushed with one hand ventromedially ("ventral and central") into the ventral meatus while the other hand advances the tube. Once the tip is in the nasopharynx, it can be rotated and advanced slowly through the arytenoids and into the trachea. If the tube is placed correctly, expired air should be felt at the proximal tube while the chest is compressed and the first breath should expand the chest. The cranial ventral neck, just behind the throat latch, should be palpated because the tube is easily palpable if it is in the esophagus. Applying gentle lateral pressure in this region while passing the tube can help prevent it from entering the esophagus. Once the tube is in place, it should be advanced as far as possible to decrease dead space ventilation. The cuff should then be inflated and the tube secured in place. If nasotracheal intubation is unsuccessful after the first few attempts, orotracheal intubation should be attempted.

Mask resuscitators are inferior to intubation because there is a risk of aerophagia, and it is more difficult to effectively ventilate the patient. However, they are a good alternative if trained personnel are not available to intubate the foal.

B: Breathing

Once the foal is intubated, a self-inflating resuscitation bag, such as an Ambu bag, should be attached to the nasotracheal tube. Oxygen should be used if it is available, though room air is often sufficient. Placing the foal on a firm, dry, surface with the bag on the ground allows the person ventilating to use their upper body and the floor to their advantage to squeeze the bag.

The ideal rate of ventilation for foals is unknown, but rates of 20 to 30 breaths per minute are typically effective. Each breath should visibly expand the chest. It is possible to damage the lungs with too much volume or pressure of air, so care should be taken not to be too aggressive.

C: Circulation

Chest compressions are not required in all cases of cardiopulmonary arrest. After 30 seconds of ventilation, the foal should be reassessed to determine if chest compressions are necessary. If there is no heart beat, the heart beat is less than 40 beats per minute, less than 60 beats per minute and not increasing, or a nonperfusing rhythm is present, chest compressions are indicated. The ideal rate of compressions is not known but rates of 80 to 120 per minute are typical. The resuscitator will quickly become fatigued at this rate and should be relieved every 2 to 3 minutes. Ventilation should be continued throughout the compressions. If there is only one person attempting to both ventilate the foal and perform compressions, one breath can be given for every 10 chest compressions.

With the foal on a firm, dry surface, the resuscitator should be positioned at the foal's spine, kneeling or standing. The hands should be placed on top of each other just behind the foal's triceps at the highest point of the thorax. With the shoulders directly over the foal and the elbows locked, the entire upper body can be used to compress the thorax (Figure 6.10). Keep in mind that the goal is to compress the entire thorax, not just the heart. Rolled towels or sandbags should be placed under the foal to support the thorax and aid in compressions. If the foal has palpable broken ribs on one side, that side should be placed down. Though there is a risk of fracturing ribs during the procedure or lacerating the lungs with previously fractured ribs, this is not a reason to avoid performing chest compressions.

D: Drugs

Ventilation and thoracic compressions should always be the first steps during CPR. If there is no heart beat after 1 minute of thoracic compressions and ventilation, epinephrine can be given. Epinephrine is an endogenous catecholamine that causes vasoconstriction, promoting return of blood to the heart. In combination with thoracic compressions, this can promote blood flow to the heart (coronary perfusion), which is essential for a normal heart rhythm.

If vascular access is available, epinephrine should be given intravenously at a dose of 0.01 to 0.02 mg/kg. Epinephrine is supplied as 1 mg/ml;

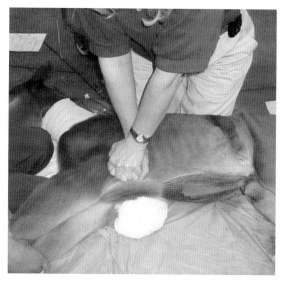

Figure 6.10. Proper positioning for cardiac compression for cardiopulmonary resuscitation.
Courtesy of Dr. Steeve Giguère.

therefore the dose for a typical 50-kg foal is 0.5 to 1 ml. Because epinephrine has a short half-life, if there is no response after the first dose, additional doses can be given every 3 minutes.

If intravenous access is not available, epinephrine can be given intratracheally. With the nasotracheal tube in place, the syringe can be attached to a long red rubber catheter or pediatric tubing and placed down the tube. Higher doses (0.05–0.1 mg/kg of epinephrine) must be used for intratracheal administration due to the lower absorption. Regardless of the route of administration, the drug must circulate to have an effect. Therefore, chest compressions should be continued to try to promote circulation.

Many other drugs have been used during CPR of humans and veterinary species and some may be indicated under specific circumstances. However, there is no strong evidence in humans that there are better alternatives to epinephrine during resuscitation, and some are detrimental, making it difficult to recommend them in horses without more research.

Determining the Efficacy of Cardiopulmonary Resuscitation and Deciding When to Stop

Frequent reevaluation of the patient during CPR can help modify the techniques being used and determine when CPR can safely be stopped. Palpation of pulses is an indication of cardiac output and can help monitor efficacy of chest compressions. However, the degree of forward flow of blood cannot be judged by the pulse and the pulse is not a good indicator of coronary perfusion. The heart beat, if present, can be used to decide when to stop thoracic compression. An electrocardiogram (ECG) is useful during CPR to monitor the cardiac rhythm. However, the ECG is only a reflection of the electrical activity of the heart, which can be present without an effective contraction of the heart muscle (pulseless electrical activity). ECG is therefore not adequate for determining the efficacy of CPR.

Pupil size and response to light is a reflection of blood flow to the brain and is a rapid and easy way to assess effective blood flow. If the person performing thoracic compression has a pen light, they can periodically check the foal's papillary light response. When blood flow is inadequate, the pupils

are fixed and dilated. With adequate blood flow, the pupils become a more normal size and respond to light by constricting.

In a hospital setting, an end-tidal carbon dioxide (ETCO$_2$) monitor (capnograph) can be a useful tool during CPR. The expired tension of carbon dioxide (CO$_2$) is a reflection of the amount of CO$_2$ transported to the lungs by the blood and ventilated and therefore reflects the adequacy of resuscitation. During resuscitation, ETCO$_2$ values below 10 mm Hg reflect inadequate resuscitation.

Sometimes it can be difficult to know how long to continue CPR and when to stop. If CPR has been continued for 15 minutes with no response, success is unlikely and CPR should be stopped. If the foal is responding, CPR should be continued. Once the foal has a regular heart beat greater than 60 beats per minute, chest compressions can be stopped. Ventilation can be stopped once the foal is breathing spontaneously with a regular rate of 16 beats per minute or more and a regular heart rate above 60 beats per minute. The foal may gasp for the first few breaths when initially disconnected from the bag but should then regain a regular rate and pattern.

Postresuscitation Care

After successful resuscitation, foals require intensive care and monitoring because they have suffered a hypoxic event and may arrest again. Monitoring of body temperature, glucose levels, hydration status, and oxygenation of blood and tissues with appropriate treatment is warranted. The cause of arrest should be determined and treated once the foal is stabilized to help prevent repeated cardiopulmonary arrest.

Common Foal Diseases

Sepsis

Sepsis is a common problem in neonatal foals. Sepsis is defined as an infectious process that triggers an associated systemic inflammatory response syndrome (SIRS). This condition is caused by pathogenic bacteria circulating in the blood stream. Clinical signs of sepsis include fever and elevated heart rate or respiratory rate. The foal can rapidly deteriorate and become dehydrated, recumbent, hypothermic, and hypoglycemic. The infectious process can result in pneumonia, diarrhea, infected joints, or an infected physis.

The major risk factors for developing sepsis are failure of passive transfer (IgG <800 mg/dl) of immunoglobulins, improper umbilical care, poor sanitation, and maternal illness such as placentitis. A definitive diagnosis is made by obtaining a positive blood culture. The most common bacteria isolated is *Escherichia coli*. Treatment consists of intensive nursing care, immunoglobulin therapy, and antimicrobial treatment.

Perinatal Asphyxia

A lack of oxygen before or during parturition can result in hypoxia and ischemia in the neonatal foal. The brain, kidney, and gastrointestinal tract are the common areas affected. When the damage is isolated to the brain it is called hypoxic-ischemic encephalopathy (HIE). This condition has also been known as *neonatal maladjustment syndrome* or *dummy foal syndrome*. The foal will appear normal after birth but within 48 hours the foal may lose the affinity for the mare, become unable to suckle, wander aimlessly, and potentially develop seizures. These clinical signs correspond with cerebral edema and ischemia and necrosis of the brain. Treatment consists of supportive care including feeding through a nasogastric tube, intravenous fluid support, and anticonvulsant treatment. If the foal is septic it will require antimicrobial therapy. The prognosis for survival is good if the foal does not seizure. If the foal is septic and develops HIE the prognosis is not as favorable and depends on the severity of the infection.

Prematurity

The normal gestational age for a Thoroughbred foal is between 320 and 365 days with an average of 341 days. Some have defined prematurity as foals with a gestational age of equal or less to 320 days, and although this definition may hold true for some foals it is inadequate for others. For example, a 340-

Table 6.4. Physical characteristics of prematurity.

- Low birth weight.
- Weakness.
- Short and silky hair coat.
- Increased range of joint motion.
- Rear limb flexural laxity.
- Incomplete skeletal ossification (as assessed radiographically).
- Premature foals will often take longer than normal to stand (>60 minutes) and nurse from the mare (>120 minutes).
- The suckle reflex may lack vigor.
- Prominent or domed forehead.
- Floppy ears.

day-old fetus may possess many characteristics of immaturity if its normal or expected gestational length is 360 days. The physical characteristics of premature foals are listed in Table 6.4.

To establish a prognosis for survival several factors must be considered such as the reason for premature delivery, assessment of gestational age and the degree of physical immaturity, the factors in the perinatal period, laboratory data, and the resources available for care. Although all premature foals are at risk for development of complications, particularly of their pulmonary and skeletal systems, the exposure to chronic in utero stress appears to be the most important determinant of survival during the neonatal period. For example, a foal born early to a mare with chronic placentitis and premature lactation will likely stand a much better chance of survival in the extra-uterine environment then a foal that is taken by Cesarean section or induced before complete maturation.

Neonatal Diarrhea

Diarrhea is one of the most common ailments of newborn foals. In addition to primary causes of diarrhea, many septicemic foals can develop diarrhea. Searching for a specific pathogen in the feces of these foals is often unrewarding. Taking a thorough history is important to rule out age-linked causes of diarrhea such as foal heat diarrhea, as well as to rule out other less common causes such as sand ingestion. Frequency of the diarrhea, suckling activity of the foal, and whether or not any other foals are affected on the premises are all pertinent

Table 6.5. Differential diagnosis of diarrhea in foals younger than 30 days of age.

- Foal heat diarrhea (5–12 days of age).
- Rotavirus.
- Coronavirus.
- Septicemia.
- *Salmonella.*
- *Clostridium difficile.*
- *Clostridium perfringes.*
- *Strongyloides westerii.*
- Cryptosporidia.
- Lactose intolerance.

Table 6.6. Differences in physical examination findings specific to the neonate.

- *Cough* is rarely observed in newborn foals with respiratory disease.
- *Nasal discharge* is an uncommon finding in foals with lower respiratory tract disease.
- Absence of *fever* in neonatal foals is common despite having a significant infection.
- *Respiratory rate and rhythm* of ventilation can be an unreliable indicator of respiratory tract disease. An elevated rate is associated with a variety of extrapulmonary conditions including excitement, pain, fever, and anemia and as a consequence to some metabolic derangements, such as acidemia.
- *Mucous membrane color* will usually fail to reflect mild to moderate pulmonary disease as distinct membrane cyanosis does not occur in newborn foals until the arterial partial pressure of oxygen (PaO_2) is very low (about 40 mm Hg).
- *Thoracic auscultation* can be misleading in neonatal foals. Minute ventilation (frequency × tidal volume) is increased in the healthy neonate resulting in easily heard bronchovesicular sounds. Foals with respiratory disease will frequently have abnormal lung sounds, such as crackles and wheezes, but neonates with even severe pulmonary disease will occasionally have little detectable abnormality during auscultation.

questions. The causes of neonatal diarrhea are listed in Table 6.5. Treatment may consist of antimicrobials, intravenous fluid therapy, plasma, withdrawal of milk, analgesics, probiotics, and intestinal protectants.

Respiratory Disease in the Neonatal Foal

The transition from the fluid-filled lung of the foal to an organ that is responsible for efficient gas exchange is both rapid and complex. The process can be complicated by a number of factors, including prematurity or dysmaturity, aspiration of meconium or milk, and bacterial or viral infection.

The detection of respiratory disease in the newborn foal can be challenging. Clinical signs that are often associated with pulmonary tract disease in older foals and adult horses are frequently lacking in the sick neonatal foal (Table 6.6). In the absence of arterial blood gas data or radiographic information, the clinician must rely on vague signs, such as restlessness and agitation, increased respiratory rate, or respiratory distress. Historical information may also aid in diagnosis. This should include an estimation of gestational age, recognition of any maternal problems, the presence or absence of meconium staining of amniotic fluid, and an assessment of IgG status.

Diagnostic tools used to evaluate the respiratory system include thoracic radiography, arterial blood

Table 6.7. Respiratory diseases specific to the neonate.

- Bacterial pneumonia.
- Viral pneumonia.
- Fungal pneumonia.
- Meconium aspiration syndrome.
- Milk aspiration.
- Acute respiratory distress syndrome (ARDS).
- Persistent pulmonary hypertension (PPH).
- Idiopathic or transient tachypnea.
- Fractured ribs.
- Pneumothorax.
- Pleural effusion.

gas analysis, pulse oximetry, and thoracic ultrasonography. The most common cause of respiratory problems is listed in Table 6.7. Treatment includes antimicrobial therapy, oxygen therapy, and in rare cases, mechanical ventilation.

References and Further Reading

Buechner-Maxwell, V. A. 2005. Nutritional support for neonatal foals. *Vet Clin North Am Equine Pract* 21:487–510.

Corley, K. T. T., and J. E. Axon. 2005. Resuscitation and emergency management. *Vet Clin North Am Equine Pract* 21:450–52.

Corley, K. T. T. 2004. Wake up, darn you! CPR for the foal. *Proceedings of the International Veterinary Emergency and Critical Care Symposium.*

Corley, K. T. T., and M. O. Furr. 2003. Cardiopulmonary resuscitation of the newborn foal. In *Current Therapy in Equine Medicine.* 5th ed., 650–55, ed. N. E. Robinson. St. Louis: Saunders.

Fenger, C. K. 1998. Diseases of foals, neonatal and perinatal diseases. In *Equine Internal Medicine,* ed. S. Reed and W. Bayly, pp. 941–42. Philadelphia: W.B. Saunders Co.

Gilger, B. C., and R. Stoppini. 2005. Diseases of the eyelids, conjunctiva, and nasolacrimal system. In *Equine Ophthalmology,* ed. B. C. Gilger, 107–56. Philadelphia: Elsevier Saunders.

Koterba, A. M., W. H. Drummond, and P. C. Kosch. 1990. *Equine Clinical Neonatology.* Philadelphia: Lea & Febiger.

Krause, J. B., and H. C. McKenzie III. 2007. Parental nutrition in foals: a retrospective study of 45 cases (2000–2004). *Equine Vet J* 39(1):74–78.

McKenzie, III, H. C., and R. J. Geor. 2007. How to provide nutritional support of sick neonatal foals. *Am Assoc Equine Pract* 53:202–8.

n. a. 1996. The cardiovascular system. In *The textbook of Veterinary Anatomy,* 2nd ed., ed. K. M. Dyce, W. O. Sack, and C. J. G. Wensing, 248–50. Philadelphia: W.B. Saunders Co.

n. a. 2004. Routine management and clinical examination. In *Equine Neonatology Medicine and Surgery,* ed. D. C. Knottenbelt, N. Holdstock, and J. E. Madigan. Philadelphia: W.B. Saunders Co.

Palmer, J. E. 2005. Ventilatory support. *Vet Clin North Am Equine Pract* 21:458–62.

Palmer, J. E. 2007. Neonatal foal resuscitation. *Vet Clin North Am Equine Pract* 23:159–82.

Pusterla, N., K. G. Magdesian, K. Maleski, S. J. Spier, and J. E. Madigan. 2004. Retrospective evaluation of the use of acetylcysteine enemas in the treatment of meconium retention in foals: 44 cases (1987–2002). *Equine Vet Educ* 6(3):170–74.

Reef, V. B. and C. Collatos. 1988. Ultrasonography of umbilical structures in clinically normal foals. *Am J Vet Res* 49(12):2143–46.

Reef, V. B., C. Collatos, P. A. Spencer, J. A. Orsini, and L. M. Sepesy. 1989. Clinical, ultrasonographic, and surgical findings in foals with umbilical remnant infections. *J Am Vet Med Assoc* 195(1):69–72.

Rooney, D. K. Clinical nutrition. 1998. In *Equine Internal Medicine,* ed. S. Reed and W. Bayly, 226–250. Philadelphia: W.B. Saunders Co.

Turner, A. G. 2004. Ocular conditions of neonatal foals. In *Veterinary Clinics of North America Equine Practice: Updates in Ophthalmology,* ed. T. Cutler, pp. 429–40. Philadelphia: Elsevier Saunders.

CHAPTER 7

Equine Pharmacology

Jennifer L. Davis

Introduction

Pharmacology in the equine patient can be a challenging field. There are relatively few drugs approved for use in horses, and because of this, there is a distinct lack of data available for determining the safety, efficacy, and appropriate dosing regimen for use in the equine patient. Many of the drugs used in practice are selected based on their efficacy in other species, or data published based on studies done in a small number of healthy horses. This chapter will attempt to review the basics of pharmacology and describe common drugs and drug groups frequently used in equine medicine.

Pharmacokinetics and Pharmacodynamics

Dosing regimens in equine medicine are based on the pharmacokinetics (PK) or pharmacodynamics of a drug. PK is the study of what the body does to a drug. This includes drug absorption, distribution, metabolism, and excretion. There are several key concepts in PK that should be understood when trying to interpret PK studies or develop dosing regimens. The first concept is that of *half-life*, which is defined as the time it takes for plasma concentrations of a drug to decrease by 50%. Drugs with a short half-life often require frequent dosing to maintain therapeutic drug levels. Alternatively, drugs with long half-lives require less frequent dosing. If a drug with a long half-life is given too

frequently, it will accumulate in the blood and toxic concentrations may be reached. The half-life of a drug also affects the time it takes for a drug to reach a steady state in the patient. Steady state is defined as the point where drug elimination equals drug intake. As a general rule, it takes five half-lives for a drug to reach steady-state concentrations. The half-life of a drug is influenced by the drug's volume of distribution and its clearance.

The *volume of distribution* is used as a measure of drug distribution into the tissues. A drug with a high volume of distribution (>1 L/kg) is expected to distribute into the plasma and extracellular fluids, but a high proportion of the drug may concentrate intracellularly, or within certain tissues like skin, fat, and bone. A drug with a small volume of distribution (0.2–0.3 L/kg) would be confined mainly to the plasma and the extracellular fluids. The volume of the plasma and extracellular fluid is variable with age; however in neonatal animals (<2 weeks of age), this volume will be higher (0.5–0.6 L/kg). This translates into higher drug doses necessary for neonates for low volume of distribution drugs. For example, the dose of amikacin in a foal is 25 mg/kg, whereas the recommended dose for adults is 7.5 mg/kg. The volume of distribution is often influenced by a drug's solubility characteristics (water soluble versus lipid soluble), its molecular weight, and its ability to bind to plasma proteins.

The *clearance* of a drug is a measure of the amount of drug excreted from the body. The majority of

165

drugs are excreted via the kidneys following metabolism by the liver. Drugs with high clearances are quickly excreted from the body and typically have short half-lives. Clearance can be affected by kidney or liver disease, and some drugs may need to have dose adjustments made in animals with severe disease to prevent drug accumulation and toxicity.

Bioavailability is another important PK concept to understand. It is a measure of the rate and extent of drug absorption following administration by an extravascular route. This is particularly important in horses because the oral bioavailability of many drugs is lower than in other companion animal species, which can lead to treatment failures and an increased risk of gastrointestinal toxicity. Bioavailability is mainly influenced by factors of the drug itself, in particular, the drug's solubility and its ability to penetrate biological membranes, such as those found in the intestine. Bioavailability can also be influenced by individual horse factors, such as feeding status, other concurrent medications, and illnesses.

Pharmacodynamics is the study of what a drug does to the body. This is most frequently related to a therapeutic end point, such as the concentration of an antimicrobial necessary to treat an infection, or the concentration of a drug necessary for an analgesic or anti-inflammatory effect. The pharmacodynamic end point of a drug is usually similar among classes of drugs but drugs within each class will vary in their ability to achieve the end point due to differences in efficacy and potency. For many drug classes in equine medicine, these end points have not been well described. The exceptions are antibiotics and nonsteroidal anti-inflammatory drugs (NSAIDs). Specific pharmacodynamic parameters will be discussed with each drug class when applicable.

Routes of Administration

How and where a drug is administered can greatly influence its effectiveness. Intravenous (IV) drug administration is preferred in many instances when treating critically ill horses because it achieves the highest drug concentrations quickly, and the entire dose of the drug is available to the animal without being influenced by bioavailability. However, there are some drawbacks to this approach. Because drug concentrations are highest with this method of administration, it carries the greatest risk of drug toxicity. It is also technically the most difficult route by which to administer drugs. If done incorrectly the drug may inadvertently be administered into the carotid artery. If this happens the drug is immediately delivered at high concentrations to the brain and may cause signs of central nervous system (CNS) toxicity. To avoid this, it is preferred to give the injection in the upper one-third of the neck where the jugular vein and the carotid artery are furthest apart. It is also best to use an 18-gauge 1 1/2-inch needle that is inserted into the vein all the way up to the hub of the needle unattached from the syringe. If the blood slowly drips from the needle it is in the vein, however, if it pulses through the needle it is most likely in the artery. When administering drugs intravenously it is possible that some drug will go perivascularly. This is not as significant a problem as administering the drug in the carotid artery; however if the drug is highly irritating such as phenylbutazone injection, it may cause some tissue sloughing in the area. There are many structures that can then be affected, particularly if the injection was given in the left side of the neck. These include the jugular vein itself, the carotid artery, the esophagus, and the left recurrent laryngeal nerve. Additionally, repeated IV injections can be irritating to the vein and may lead to vein thrombosis and scarring. If the jugular veins become unusable, drugs can be administered in the cephalic vein in the forelimbs or the lateral thoracic veins on either side of the chest. If multiple repeated injections are to be given, an IV catheter should be used to prevent the aforementioned complications.

Intramuscular (IM) injections can be used in the horse for relatively large volumes of drugs. For many drugs the absorption after IM administration is almost complete compared with IV administration. Absorption may be prolonged, however, and maximum drug concentrations may be lower as a result. IM injections in horses can be made in the neck, the pectoral muscles, and the semimembranous or semitendinous muscles. Small volumes of drug can also be injected in the triceps muscles. The gluteal muscles are not recommended because if an abscess forms in this area it is difficult to drain and treat. Abscesses at the injection site are one complication of IM injections. In some instances these can become infected with a bacterium called *Clostridium*, which can lead to a severe infection within the muscles known as clostridial myositis (see Figure 7.1a and 7.1b). This disease can be fatal if not treated early and aggressively. IM injections can also be painful for the horse, making them potentially dangerous for horse owners and veterinary professionals to administer.

Subcutaneous injections are rarely performed in the horse because they have a relatively small amount of subcutaneous space when compared to other animals. If they are used, they are most commonly administered in front of the shoulder blade. Only small volumes should be administered by this route. Absorption from subcutaneous administration can be erratic, particularly in horses that are dehydrated or hypotensive.

Oral drug administration to horses can be difficult due to the low bioavailability of many drugs and the variability of absorption based on factors such as feeding status and gastrointestinal motility. It is also possible that a significant amount of drug may be lost during administration by this route, particularly in an uncooperative patient. Drugs administered as a top-dressing on feed may bind to the feed particles, thereby further reducing bioavailability. Because of the potential variability in drug absorption following oral administration, this route should not be used in critically ill patients. It is worth noting that oral drug bioavailability is often increased in neonates and young foals, when compared to adults. There are several potential reasons for this, including differences in diet, increased permeability of the intestinal membrane, and differences in gastric pH, which may affect drug solubility and absorption.

IV, IM, and oral drug administrations are the most commonly used routes of administration in the horse. However, there are some other alternative methods that can be used. Inhalant drug therapies are often used in horses with respiratory

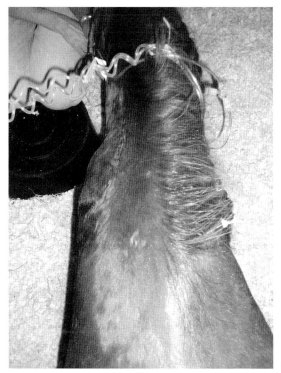

a

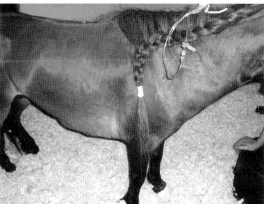

b

Figure 7.1. Severe injection site swelling *(A)* and dependent edema *(B)* with associated clostridial myositis occurring after intramuscular administration of a single dose of flunixin meglumine to a miniature horse mare.

disease to deliver drug directly to the site of the problem. This route does require specialized equipment, however, and some horses do not tolerate it well. Systemic absorption can occur after administration via inhalation; therefore it is possible that drug-related side effects may be seen. Topical therapies are also frequently used particularly for skin and ocular surface diseases. Systemic absorption should be minimal after topical application and the effect is localized at the area to which the drug is applied. This is not to be confused with transdermal drug administration in which the drug is applied to the skin, but systemic absorption and effects are expected. This route of administration is seldom used in horses because it produces highly variable drug concentrations. Rectal administration has been tried with some drugs in horses. This route is useful if the horse has problems with gastric emptying or if the drug would otherwise be quickly metabolized by the liver following oral administration (known as the first-pass effect). However, overall bioavailability via this route is often quite low. Intrauterine or intra-articular drug administration can also be used to deliver high levels of drugs to those areas; however, some systemic absorption is expected to result from these routes and adverse effects may also occur.

Drug Incompatibilities

Pharmacologic interactions occur as a result of inactivation of a drug by another drug or admixture. This can occur by mixing two incompatible drugs in a syringe or vial before administration, often resulting in visible precipitation. Notable examples of this are mixtures of flunixin meglumine and gentamicin or acepromazine and romifidine (see Figure 7.2).

Some drug combinations can inactivate each other without causing a visible precipitate to form. An example of this is potassium penicillin and amikacin. Inactivated drugs will result in therapeutic failure. This is particularly important with antibiotics because decreases in active concentrations can lead to excessive bacterial growth or the development of resistant bacteria.

Another mechanism by which pharmacologic inactivation can occur is through interactions of the drug with the vehicle in which the drug is diluted or mixed. Lactated Ringer's solution (LRS) is a commonly administered fluid in companion animals. This solution contains cations, including calcium. Cations can chelate (bind) and inactivate several

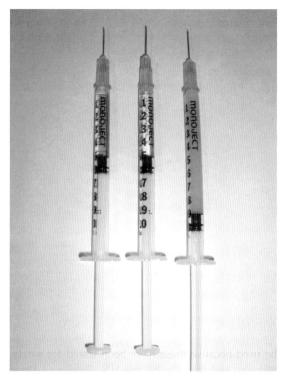

Figure 7.2. Photograph depicting acepromazine *(left)*, romifidine *(middle)*, and a combination of acepromazine and romifidine *(right)*. Note the precipitates that have formed when the two drugs are combined in the same syringe.

classes of drugs including the fluoroquinolone antibiotics (i.e., enrofloxacin) and the tetracycline antibiotics (i.e., oxytetracycline). Compounding of drugs is also a common practice in veterinary medicine; however, some of the vehicles used to mix the drugs may have deleterious effects on drug stability. Again, the fluoroquinolones are a good example of this. Vehicles containing cations will chelate and inactivate fluoroquinolone antibiotics reducing the effective concentration by as much as 50%.

Drug Compounding

Many veterinarians use drug compounding pharmacies to formulate drugs into more convenient and palatable forms for horses. Not all drugs are amenable to compounding. Some drugs require special formulations for absorption to occur. An example of this would be omeprazole, a drug used to treat gastric ulceration. Omeprazole gets degraded by stomach acids before absorption unless it is administered in a special formulation such as Gastrogard paste. Other drugs are not stable in the vehicles that they are mixed with. A good example of this is pergolide, a drug used to treat equine Cushing disease. Pergolide degrades when mixed with water resulting in a lower than expected dose of the drug being administered. Still other drugs, such as tetracyclines, are sensitive to light, oxygen, and temperature and require special containers and storage conditions to prevent degradation. It is important to have a good working relationship with the compounding pharmacy being used and to discuss the stability and efficacy factors related to each drug being compounded. Storage conditions and the vehicles that are used in the formulations are important factors to consider in achieving therapeutic success. Whenever possible, commercially available formulations should be used because these have been tested for safety, efficacy, and stability by the U.S. Food and Drug Administration (FDA).

Drug Dosage Determination

To calculate how much drug to give an individual animal one must know the dose rate of the drug (typically in mg/kg), the animal's weight and the concentration of the drug in the formulation to be given. The total dose can then be determined using the following equation:

$$\frac{\text{Formula Total}}{\text{dose (mg)}} = \frac{\text{Dose (mg)}}{\text{(kg)}} \times \frac{\text{body weight}}{\text{(kg)}}$$

Once the total milligrams necessary for dosing has been determined, the total volume of a solution or the total number of tablets to be given can be determined based on the formulation to be used by dividing the total dose by the mg/ml or the mg/tablet. For example, if we use a dose for drug X of 5 mg/kg in a 500-kg horse, the total milligrams to be administered is 2,500 mg. If this is an injection at a concentration of 100 mg/ml, the total volume of drug to be administered is 25 ml. Alternatively, if drug X is a tablet that contains

100 mg of drug per tablet, 25 tablets would be administered.

Some drugs are administered as a constant rate infusion (CRI) so that the horse is exposed to small amounts of the drug continuously through an IV catheter. To calculate the infusion rate for these drugs similar information is needed, although the dose rate is typically given in mg per kg per min. For example, if a drug Y needs to be given at 0.01 mg per kg per min in a 500-kg horse, we would need to deliver 5 mg/min. This translates to 300 mg/hr or 7,200 mg/day. To deliver this amount of drug, 7,200 mg into 24 liters of fluids would be diluted and then the fluids would be administered at a rate of 1 L/hr. If this is too high of a volume of fluids, the total dose could be diluted in a smaller volume and delivered at a lower rate.

Scheduled (Controlled) Drugs

The Drug Enforcement Agency (DEA) classifies some drugs as scheduled or controlled, based on their potential to become drugs of abuse in humans. These classifications and related information are based on the Controlled Substances Act of 1970. Scheduled drugs must be handled and stored in a special manner, and they require additional book keeping and documentation of their use. The DEA also requires that anyone who administers, prescribes, or dispenses a controlled substance be registered with the DEA.

There are five schedules defined by the DEA. These definitions are listed, along with some examples (see Table 7.1). When attempting to determine if a drug is a controlled substance, the simplest method is to look on the product container for a large capital C with a corresponding Roman numeral inscribed within the C. For example, containers of butorphanol should have a CIV on the label indicating that they are a Schedule IV controlled substance. Should one need to determine the scheduling of a drug without access to a product container the easiest method is to visit the DEA Web site at www.dea.gov/pubs/scheduling.html and search for the drug by generic name.

The Controlled Substance Act requires that complete and accurate records be kept of all quantities

Table 7.1. List of the five categories of scheduled drug substances, as defined by the Drug Enforcement Agency.

Schedule	Definition	Examples
I	Drugs that have medical use in the United States and a high potential for abuse	Heroin, LSD, marijuana
II	Drugs that have defined medical uses and a high potential for abuse	Morphine, pentobarbital, fentanyl
III	Drugs that have a defined medical use and less potential for abuse than Schedule I and II drugs	Euthanasia solution, boldenone, tiletamine
IV	Drugs that have a defined medical use and less potential for abuse than Schedule I–III	Phenobarbital, diazepam, midazolam
V	Drugs that have a defined medical use, less potential for abuse than Schedule I–IV and contain limited quantities of narcotic or stimulant drugs	Cough medicines containing codeine

of controlled substances manufactured, purchased, and sold. Each substance must be inventoried on receipt and every 2 years after receipt. Records for Schedule I and II drugs must be kept separate from all other records of the handler. Records for Schedule III, IV, and V substances must be kept in a readily available form. A sample record keeping form showing the required information is shown in Table 7.2.

Storage of controlled substances is an important issue. As mandated by the DEA, controlled substances must be stored in a securely locked, substantially constructed cabinet or safe. Although double-locking of such safes is not required by law it is considered by most DEA inspectors to be an indicator of a good faith effort to prevent diversion of controlled substances. If controlled substances are stored in a locking toolbox or other such portable storage device the container must be securely affixed to an immovable object such as a wall.

Table 7.2. Sample record keeping log sheets for controlled substances.

Perpetual Log Inventory/Unique Identifier Numbers
Drug: Butorphanol 10 mg/ml injection 10-ml vials

Date	Amount received	Amount disposed	Bottle nos.	Dispensed to	By whom	Received by	Balance
6-4-04	5 × 10 ml		06040401		J. Doe		5 vials
			06040402				
			06040403				
			06040404				
			06040405				
6-8-04		1 vial	06040401	Ambulatory truck 1	J. Doe	J. Miller	4 vials
6-10-04		1 vial	06040402	Intensive care unit lockbox	A. Davis	B. Fox	3 vials

Unique Identifier Log Sheet for Individual Bottles
Drug: Butorphanol 10 mg/ml injection 10-ml vial, bottle number: 06040401
Date Dispensed: 6-8-04 Received by: J. Miller

Date	Patient	Record no.	Amount given	Given by	Amount disposed	Where disposed	Witness	Balance
								10 ml
6-8-04	Sparky Redfield	123596	3 ml	P. Smith				7 ml
6-10-04	Bandit Jones	369556	1 ml	S. Jones	1 ml	Sink	J. Miller	5 ml
6-10-04	Scruffy Jones	369557	2 ml	S. Jones				3 ml

Controlled substances used on ambulatory vehicles should be stored in a secure, unobtrusive location that can be securely locked when not supervised.

In the last decade many veterinary practices have begun to store and dispense controlled substances from automated dispensing machines accessible only by individual computerized passwords and identification numbers. This system allows for individual accountability and is favored by the DEA for large practices using large volumes of controlled substances.

Access to controlled substances in veterinary medicine for the relief of pain and suffering should be viewed as a special privilege and thus protected with due diligence. Awareness of all state and federal DEA requirements, as well as, perpetual evaluation of controlled substance disposition systems will ensure that veterinarians have uninterrupted access to these valuable therapeutic agents.

Specific Drug Classes

It is beyond the scope of this chapter to discuss all of the drugs used in equine medicine. However, the remainder of the chapter will be dedicated to describing the major classes of drugs used in horses and detail when and why they are used, as well as, the adverse effects associated with them.

Antimicrobials

Antimicrobials are one of the most frequently used classes of drugs in veterinary medicine. The following discussion will include drugs that are commonly used for the treatment of bacterial and fungal infections in the horse.

Drugs to Treat Bacterial Infections

These drugs are commonly called *antibiotics*. For antibiotics, the pharmacodynamic parameters necessary for therapeutic success are related to the concentration necessary to inhibit the growth of the causative bacteria also known as the minimum inhibitory concentration (MIC). Antibiotics vary as to whether treatment success is related to the time

(T) that drug concentrations in the plasma or tissue is greater than the MIC (T > MIC) or whether the ratio of the maximum concentration (Cmax) or the total amount of drug measured over time (the area under the concentration [AUC]) that is greater than the MIC (Cmax/MIC or AUC/MIC ratios). Those drugs that use T > MIC as a pharmacodynamic parameter are classified as time dependent antibiotics, whereas those that use Cmax/MIC or AUC/MIC ratios are classified as concentration dependent antibiotics.

Antibiotics can be classified based on their spectrum of activity against certain bacteria. Bacteria are labeled as gram-negative or gram-positive based on properties in their cell wall that causes differential staining. Antibiotics typically have a predictable spectrum of activity against either gram-positive or gram-negative bacteria although some antibiotics are classified as "broad spectrum" in that they are effective against both classifications. Bacteria can be labeled anaerobic, meaning that they require an environment without oxygen to survive. Because some antibiotics do not work in the absence of oxygen, their activity against anaerobic bacteria can be predicted. A further classification of antibiotics involves whether or not they kill bacteria (bactericidal antibiotics) or whether they just inhibit the growth of the bacteria (bacteriostatic antibiotics) so that the host's immune system can then take over and clear the infection.

From the preceding discussion it is evident that the correct choice of antibiotic is going to depend heavily on isolating the bacteria causing the infection. This requires appropriate culture and sensitivity techniques. Culturing the wrong bacterium and culturing the wrong site of infection are two very good reasons for treatment failures that may occur with antibiotic therapy. Other causes for treatment failures include use of antibiotics for the treatment of fever or untreatable disease (i.e., viral), treatment without appropriate surgical intervention, use of irrational antibiotic combinations, using a drug at an incorrect dose, route or frequency of administration, immunocompromised patients, poor owner compliance, development of drug resistance, presence of a foreign body, and PK or pharmacologic antagonism. Additional PK problems can be associated with therapeutic failure such as poor oral absorption and intestinal metabolism of the drug. Therapeutic success relies on a complex interaction of factors attributed to the host, the drug, and the bacteria. The goal of antibiotic therapy is to administer the appropriate drug in sufficient doses with sufficient frequency to maintain concentrations that will eliminate the bacteria at the site of the infection. A summary of the antibiotics most commonly used in horses is found in Table 7.3.

β-Lactam Antibiotics

The β-lactam antibiotics are a large group of drugs that share a similar β-lactam ring structure. They can be further divided into penicillins, cephalosporins, and carbapenems. They work on the cell wall of susceptible bacteria binding to proteins within the cell wall, which creates small pores allowing fluid into the cell. This leads to cell swelling, bursting, and death. They are considered bactericidal and time dependent. In general, they are excellent choices for gram-positive (particularly streptococci) and anaerobic bacteria. However, they may not be effective against staphylococci or *Bacteroides* because these bacteria may produce an enzyme called β-lactamase, which inactivates the antibiotic. For this reason, some of these drugs are given combined with another drug that inhibits β-lactamase, such as clavulanic acid. In horses, oral absorption of β-lactam antibiotics is poor, making them only suitable for IV or IM use. The exception to this is in foals that may have an increased absorption of these drugs up to several months of age.

Penicillins. Penicillin G is the β-lactam drug used most frequently in veterinary medicine. It can be given intravenously as a potassium salt. This formulation should be given slowly, to prevent potential collapse, over a period of 5 to 10 minutes. Diarrhea and an increased heart rate is frequently seen immediately following administration of this drug and should be transient. Potassium penicillin G has a short half-life and must be given frequently to maintain plasma concentrations above the intended MIC for at least 50% of the dosing interval. There is an IM formulation of penicillin G, complexed with procaine, a local anesthetic drug that is used to decrease the pain of the penicillin injection. Reactions to procaine can occur particularly if the drug is accidentally administered into a vein or artery. These reactions include signs of CNS excitement, twitching, muscle tremors, and potential collapse and seizures. These reactions should be transient and last less than 30 to 45 minutes. Some horses may have a decreased ability to metabolize procaine and adverse reactions may be more severe in those animals (Olsen, et al., 2007). Certain horses may exhibit allergic reactions to either penicillin formulation. These may be mild at first with the horse exhibiting transient hives and pruritus (itching). On subsequent exposure, reactions will be more severe and may result in anaphylactic shock. Horses that exhibit signs of allergic reaction to penicillin should not be administered any penicillin drug again.

Ampicillin is another penicillin drug that is used occasionally in equine medicine. The only advantage it has over potassium penicillin G is a slightly increased activity against gram-negative bacteria, although resistance is common. Ticarcillin is also used occasionally in horses, but it is usually reserved for resistant infections, particularly those caused by *Pseudomonas*. It is available in a formulation that is complexed with clavulanic acid, which is suitable for treating staphylococcal infections. Its use is limited in horses due to cost. It is probably most frequently used as an intrauterine infusion.

Cephalosporins. The cephalosporin antibiotics are classified as first-, second-, third-, or fourth-generation, depending on their spectrum of activity. In general, first-generation cephalosporins have a greater activity against gram-positive bacteria and anaerobes. Higher generation cephalosporins have increasing activity against gram-negative bacteria. There are many drugs in this group. Only a few of them are used in horses. Cefazolin is a first-generation drug that is sometimes used preoperatively to prevent bacterial infections occurring during or after surgery. Cephalexin is another first-generation drug that has been studied in horses but it is only available in the United States as an oral formulation, and bioavailability is low (<5%) in

Table 7.3. Summary of the most commonly used antibiotics in equine medicine.

Drug class	Drugs commonly used	Doses	Indications	Contraindications	Adverse effects
Penicillins	Potassium penicillin G, procaine penicillin G	22,000 IU/kg IV q6 h (potassium penicillin G) or 22,000 IU/kg IM q12 h (procaine penicillin G)	Bacterial infections caused by gram-positive or anaerobic organisms	Do not use in patients with a known allergy to penicillins	Allergic reactions; transient diarrhea and elevated heart rate with potassium penicillin G; neurologic disease with procaine penicillin G
Cephalosporins	Ceftiofur	2.2–5 mg/kg IV or IM q12 h	Bacterial infections caused by gram-positive or gram-negative organisms (higher doses)	Do not use in patients with a known allergy to cephalosporins	Allergic reactions; potential antibiotic induced diarrhea
Carbapenems	Imipenem	5–10 mg/kg IV q8–12 h	Bacterial infections with documented resistance to other antibiotics	Do not use in patients with a history of seizures; use with caution in patients with renal disease	Allergic reactions; seizures with rapid IV bolus; nephrotoxicity (risk is reduced when combined with cilastatin)
Aminoglycosides	Gentamicin, amikacin	Gentamicin: 6.6 mg/kg IV or IM q24 h; Amikacin: 25 mg/kg IV q24 h (foals); 7.5–10 mg/kg IV q24 h (adults)	Bacterial infections caused by gram-negative organisms and staphylococci	Do not use in patients with renal disease or botulism	Nephrotoxicity; ototoxicity; neuromuscular blockade
Trimethoprim-sulfonamide combinations	Trimethoprim, sulfadiazine, sulfamethoxazole	25–30 mg/kg PO q12 h	Bacterial infections caused by susceptible gram-positive and gram-negative organisms; protozoal infections (e.g., equine protozoal myeloencephalitis)	Use with caution in pregnant mares during early gestation	Anemia, pancytopenia, congenital defects
Fluoroquinolones	Enrofloxacin, orbifloxacin, marbofloxacin	Enrofloxacin: 5–7.5 mg/kg PO or IV q24 h; Orbifloxacin: 5 mg/kg PO q24 h; Marbofloxacin: 2.5–5 mg/kg PO q24 h	Bacterial infections caused by gram-negative organisms and staphylococci	Do not use in animals less than 2 years old	Cartilage damage in young animals

(Continued)

Table 7.3. *Continued*

Drug class	Drugs commonly used	Doses	Indications	Contraindications	Adverse effects
Macrolides	Erythromycin, clarithromycin, and azithromycin	Erythromycin: 25–37.5 mg/kg PO q6–12 h Clarithromycin: 7.5 mg/kg PO q12 h Azithromycin: 10 mg/kg PO q24–48 h	Bacterial infections caused by gram-positive or intracellular organisms, particularly *Rhodococcus equi* and *Lawsonia intracellularis*	Use with caution in adult animals	Severe diarrhea
Tetracyclines	Oxytetracycline, doxycycline	Oxytetracycline: 10 mg/kg IV q24 h Doxycycline: 10 mg/kg PO q12 h or 20 mg/kg PO q24 h	Bacterial infections caused by gram-positive and gram-negative and intracellular organisms	Use with caution in young animals	Nephrotoxicity; diarrhea; teeth discoloration; collapse; death (IV doxycycline)
Chloramphenicol	Chloramphenicol	35–50 mg/kg PO q6–8 h	Bacterial infections caused by gram-positive and gram-negative and anaerobic organisms	Caution required by people handling the drug and the animal	Anorexia; anemia; aplastic anemia in humans
Nitroimidazoles	Metronidazole	15–20 mg/kg PO q6–8 h	Bacterial infections caused by anaerobic organisms (particularly *Bacteroides fragilis*) and some protozoa	None	Anorexia; neurologic symptoms at high doses or when given intravenously

h, hour; IM, intramuscular; IU, intrauterine; IV, intravenous; q, every.

horses (Davis, Salmon, and Papich 2005). Cefadroxil may be used in foals less than 3 months of age as an oral antibiotic. Cefpodoxime proxetil is an oral third-generation antibiotic that has been studied in horses (Carillo, et al. 2005), and it must be administered several times a day. The plasma concentrations are low, making it of questionable efficacy. The most commonly used cephalosporin in equine medicine is ceftiofur sodium (Naxcel). Ceftiofur sodium is labeled for use in horses for the treatment of respiratory infection caused by streptococci. It can be used for broad-spectrum treatment of non-streptococcal infections, but higher doses (two to four times the label dose) and higher frequency of administration are necessary. It can be given intravenously or intramuscularly.

Adverse effects of cephalosporins are rare in horses. Allergic reactions may occur, although these drugs can sometimes be used in horses that are known to be allergic to penicillins without problem. Diarrhea following administration of ceftiofur has been reported although this occurs infrequently.

Carbapenems. The carbapenems are a newer class of drugs that have a broad spectrum of activity. They are reserved for resistant infections in human medicine, and their use is not recommended in horses, unless a severely resistant infection has been documented. Their use in horses is also limited by cost. Foals with severe septicemia are sometimes treated with a drug in this class called imipenem.

Aminoglycoside Antibiotics

The aminoglycoside antibiotics have excellent activity against gram-negative bacteria and some staphylococci. They have limited activity against other gram-positive organisms and no activity against anaerobes. For this reason they are often given combined with a penicillin or a cephalosporin. They are considered to be bactericidal due to an irreversible inhibition of protein synthesis in the bacterium and are considered to be concentration dependent. The most commonly used drugs in this group are gentamicin and amikacin. Gentamicin is used more frequently in adult horses because of cost considerations. Amikacin is preferred in foals because it has higher activity against some bacteria. They can be administered intravenously or intramuscularly. Aminoglycosides should be used with caution in dehydrated animals because of the potential for nephrotoxicity (kidney damage). To avoid nephrotoxicity, it is recommended that doses be given only once a day. Other potential adverse effects include ototoxicity (damage to the ear canal) and neuromuscular blockade. Ototoxicity has not been reported in horses. The neuromuscular blockade that can occur with aminoglycoside antibiotics is typically not a problem unless they are administered with other neuromuscular-blocking drugs (such as succinylcholine or other anesthetics) or when they are given to horses with diseases of the neuromuscular junction (such as botulism).

Trimethoprim-Sulfonamide Antibiotics

Trimethoprim is almost always administered in combination with a sulfonamide antibiotic because they have a synergistic effect against bacteria when administered together. They work on different steps in the pathway of folic acid synthesis within bacteria, and together they are considered to be bactericidal and time dependent. The combination is broad spectrum with activity against gram-positive and gram-negative bacteria, as well as, some protozoa. Unfortunately, due to their long use in human and veterinary medicine, resistance is fairly common among bacteria, which limits the usefulness of these antibiotics. One major advantage of trimethoprim-sulfonamide combinations is

that they are well absorbed after oral administration in the horse (van Duijkeren, et al. 1994). They are available in generic formulations making them quite cost effective and an excellent choice for long-term antibiotic therapy. These antibiotics may not be as effective as expected in treating abscesses because the necrotic debris found in the center of the abscess may inactivate the sulfonamide component. They are less effective in anaerobic situations. Some sulfonamides have been shown to bind to feed, which may decrease their bioavailability. This can occur when the drug is administered as a top-dressing on grain or to a horse with a full stomach (van Duijkeren, et al., 1996). Adverse effects are rare, although diarrhea has been seen. With prolonged periods of administration, anemia and decreased white blood cell production have been reported. These combinations may result in congenital defects (i.e., skin lesions, decreased red and white blood cell production, and electrolyte disturbances) in the fetus if administered long term to pregnant mares, presumably because of the development of folic acid deficiency in the foal (Toribio, et al. 1998).

Fluoroquinolone Antibiotics

The fluoroquinolone antibiotics are effective against gram-negative bacteria and staphylococci and are ineffective against streptococci and anaerobic bacteria. They can be combined with penicillin or a cephalosporin for broad-spectrum coverage. They are considered to be bactericidal and concentration dependent. They work by inhibiting an enzyme necessary for producing the coiled structure of bacterial DNA, known as DNA gyrase. The fluoroquinolone antibiotics that can be used in horses include enrofloxacin, marbofloxacin, and orbifloxacin. These drugs have a good oral bioavailability, but it can be decreased if they are coadministered with drugs supplements or other vehicles that contain cations, such as calcium or magnesium. This would include things such as molasses, antacids, or iron supplements. Ciprofloxacin, another fluoroquinolone antibiotic that is frequently used in humans and dogs, is not well absorbed in the horse and has been associated with the development of severe diarrhea. Enrofloxacin is the drug most commonly used in horses in this class. It is available as an injectable solution for cattle. This formulation can be safely given to horses intravenously over 5 to 10 minutes. When injected intramuscularly it may be irritating and cause muscle swelling and pain at the injection site. If this formulation is given orally, it can result in erratic absorption and oral ulceration because of the high pH of the formulation. For oral administration, commercially available tablet forms are recommended, but they can be prohibitively expensive. The main adverse effect of fluoroquinolone antibiotics is cartilage damage in young horses. These drugs can bind the magnesium in the joint cartilage, creating defects in cartilage formation, joint effusion, and lameness. The effects are age dependent, and the risk of developing lesions is increased with weight bearing and increased activity.

Macrolide Antibiotics

The macrolide antibiotics are another class of antibiotics that can be used in equine medicine, although their use is typically limited due to their narrow spectrum of activity and the risk of side effects. Their use is limited to the treatment of gram-positive intracellular organisms including streptococci, *Rhodococcus equi*, and *Lawsonia intracellularis* in foals. This is because they concentrate heavily within white blood cells where these bacteria may reside (Davis, et al. 2002). They concentrate in lung tissue, making them good choices for the treatment of pneumonia. They are classified as bacteriostatic and time dependent. The mechanism of action involves inhibition of protein synthesis in the bacteria. Drugs in this class include erythromycin, azithromycin, and clarithromycin. They are often given in combination with rifampin, another antibiotic, to increase penetration into abscesses and prevent the development of resistance. Oral absorption is good, and these drugs are typically administered via this route. Unfortunately, drugs in this class are associated with the development of severe diarrhea in weanlings, adult horses, and even in mares that are stalled with foals that are being treated with a macrolide antibiotic. This may be due to a disruption of the normal bacterial population in the horse's large colon, or it may be due to the fact that these drugs may increase gastrointestinal motility as has been shown with erythromycin.

Tetracycline Antibiotics

The tetracycline antibiotics are considered broad spectrum due to their activity against gram-positive and gram-negative bacteria. Additionally, they have activity against atypical pathogens, such as rickettsial organisms (the causative agents of Potomac horse fever and equine granulocytic ehrlichiosis) and spirochetes (associated with equine recurrent uveitis or "moon blindness"). They are typically classified as bacteriostatic and time dependent. The mechanism of action involves inhibition of protein synthesis in the bacteria. Drugs in this class commonly used in horses include oxytetracycline and doxycycline. Oxytetracycline can be given intravenously or orally. Oral administration has been associated with an increased risk and increased shedding of *Salmonella* species (Owen, Fullerton, and Barnum 1983), so it is typically given intravenously. IV administration carries a risk of some adverse effects. If it is administered too quickly, the animal may collapse, and it may even be fatal in some instances. This is thought to be because of the vehicle that the drug is prepared in or the drug's ability to rapidly bind calcium and cause severe muscle weakness or cardiac arrhythmias. Therefore, oxytetracycline is typically administered intravenously to horses and foals over a period of 10 to 15 minutes. The ability of oxytetracycline to bind calcium has been used clinically. Foals with flexural limb deformities can be given oxytetracycline to cause relaxation of the muscles in the upper limbs, which then causes relaxation of the associated tendons in the lower limbs that are causing the hyperflexion.

Doxycycline is only administered orally to horses. Intravenous administration of doxycycline results in cardiac arrhythmias, collapse, and death (Riond, et al. 1992). The mechanism of these adverse effects is not currently known. In horses, doxycycline is most effective for pathogens that reside intracellularly because it has been shown to concentrate within white blood cells (Davis, Salmon, and Papich 2006). Therefore, it can be used for the treatment of *R. equi*, *L. intracellularis* (proliferative enteropathy), and rickettsial disease. It has been rarely associated with the development of diarrhea in adult horses. More recently, low doses of doxycycline have been used in horses with corneal disease or joint disease not because of its antibiotic effect but because it has an anti-inflammatory effect.

Tetracyclines may cause renal disease if given in large doses. Teeth discoloration may occur in young animals although this is less likely to occur with doxycycline than with oxytetracycline. Injectable or compounded formulations of tetracycline antibiotics may undergo an oxidation reaction when exposed to air or light. This results in a brown discoloration in the formulation, which has been associated with degradation of the drug. Discolored formulations should not be used in animals.

Chloramphenicol

Chloramphenicol is a truly broad-spectrum antibiotic because it has activity against gram-positive, gram-negative, anaerobic, and atypical bacteria. It is bacteriostatic and time dependent. Chloramphenicol's mechanism of action involves inhibition of protein synthesis in the bacteria. It works at the same site as the macrolides antibiotics; therefore these antibiotics should not be coadministered. Chloramphenicol reaches high concentrations in the tissues and in abscesses. It penetrates well into protected sites such as the CNS and the eye. It is most commonly administered orally to horses. IV administration is possible but is usually cost prohibitive. The drawbacks to using chloramphenicol include a short half-life, which requires frequent dosing, and a bad taste, which may cause some horses to resent treatment and become anorexic. Additionally, there are some risks to the person administering the drug. In susceptible humans chloramphenicol can rarely cause an idiosyncratic (unpredictable) aplastic anemia even after exposure to small amounts of the drug. Therefore, when administering chloramphenicol, it is important that gloves are worn and that the tablets are dissolved

not ground or crushed to prevent accidental exposure.

Nitroimidazole Antibiotics

Metronidazole is the only nitroimidazole commonly used in horses in the United States. It has a limited spectrum of activity, which includes anaerobic bacteria and some protozoa. It is considered to be bactericidal and time dependent. Metronidazole works by being metabolized within susceptible bacteria into toxic substances that will then kill the bacteria. In equine medicine, it is mostly used to treat anaerobic infections caused by *Clostridium* and *Bacteroides fragilis*. It can be administered intravenously; however, there is an increased risk of adverse effects, including CNS excitement and seizures, via this route. It is most commonly administered orally and is well absorbed via this route. Unfortunately, because of its taste oral administration often results in anorexia. To prevent this, rectal administration of the drug has been studied (Steinman, et al. 2000). This is a feasible option; however, the absorption is lower by this route and higher doses or frequency of dosing is necessary.

Metronidazole is a good choice of antibiotic for horses with diarrhea because it has been shown to have anti-inflammatory properties in the gastrointestinal tract in other species. It is quite effective against *C. difficile*, a relatively common cause of diarrhea in horses. Metronidazole is frequently administered along with a β-lactam and an aminoglycoside for broad-spectrum coverage in critically ill patients in which the bacterium being treated is unknown.

Drugs to Treat Fungal Infections

The drugs available to treat fungal infections are much more limited in the horse than those used to treat bacterial infections. Many drugs are either too expensive to use, are not absorbed orally, or are not effective against the fungi that commonly infect horses.

Griseofulvin is labeled for use in horses for the treatment of dermatophytes (ringworm). It is useful for this purpose but is ineffective against other types of fungi. Griseofulvin has been reported to cause birth defects in foals when mares are administered the drug early in pregnancy (Schutte and van den Ingh 1997).

Fluconazole, itraconazole, and voriconazole are triazole antifungal drugs that have all been studied in the horse. Fluconazole is well absorbed after oral administration, has no reported adverse effects, and is affordable when given as the generic preparation. Unfortunately, it is not effective against *Aspergillus* or *Fusarium*. It is effective against yeasts, dermatophytes, and *Cryptococcus* organisms. Itraconazole and voriconazole are more effective against *Aspergillus* and *Fusarium*; however, the cost of treatment at this point in time is typically several hundred dollars a day and not practical in many situations. To overcome the high cost of treatment, several compounded formulations of itraconazole have been used. Testing of these formulations has shown that they are not absorbed orally, most likely because of insolubility in the vehicle. Therefore, compounded formulations of itraconazole are not recommended for use in the horse.

Amphotericin B is a fairly broad-spectrum antifungal drug that has been used occasionally in the horse for the treatment of severe systemic fungal infections. Its use is limited by the high potential for nephrotoxicity and cost.

Sodium or potassium iodide is also used as an antifungal drug in horses. Its mechanism of action against fungi is not known; however, it has been used as a successful treatment for nasal fungal infections when combined with surgical resection.

Drugs for the Treatment of Pain and Inflammation

Nonsteroidal Anti-Inflammatory Drugs

The NSAIDs most commonly used in horses include flunixin meglumine (Banamine), phenylbutazone (Butazolidin), and ketoprofen (Ketofen). They are considered nonselective inhibitors of the enzyme cyclooxygenase (COX), which is responsible for producing substances related to pain and inflammation. Newer drugs such as carprofen (Rimadyl), meloxicam (Metacam), and firocoxib (Equioxx) are known as COX-2-selective inhibitors. COX-2 is thought to be mostly responsible for the adverse

effects associated with inflammation. Inhibiting COX-2 enzyme specifically without affecting COX-1 would theoretically be safer. COX-2 is involved in many of the repair processes in the gastrointestinal tract and is needed for healing of gastric or colonic ulceration. Thus, blocking COX-2 may not have all the advantages as previously thought. Drugs licensed for use in horses in the United States are summarized in Table 7.4.

Although these drugs are used in thousands of horses each day and are readily available to horse owners, they should not be used indiscriminately. NSAIDs have been associated with gastric ulceration, particularly in the glandular portion of the stomach. This can lead to anorexia, lethargy, pain, and colic. In severe cases, the ulcer can rupture and cause sudden death. Ulceration can also occur in the colon, causing a syndrome known as right dorsal colitis. Severe diarrhea, toxemia, and hypoproteinemia (low blood protein levels) accompany this disease. The horse often shows signs of colic and weight loss as well. If not treated appropriately, the ulceration in the colon can rupture. Even with appropriate treatment, the horse may become chronically affected because the colon can scar (stricture) causing an intestinal blockage. Ulceration is less frequently reported in other areas of the gastrointestinal tract, including the mouth, gums, tongue, and esophagus. The kidneys can be affected as well. NSAIDs cause a condition known as renal papillary necrosis, which often leads to decreased ability to concentrate urine, dehydration, and electrolyte imbalances. Acute and chronic renal failure may result.

The route of administration of the NSAID can cause adverse effects. Repeated doses of flunixin meglumine in the muscle may cause muscle necrosis, abscessation or infection with a bacteria called *Clostridium*. Clostridial myositis is rare, but it can be a fatal disease and requires immediate aggressive treatment. If phenylbutazone is injected outside of the vein, it can cause severe necrosis and sloughing of the tissues. If it is administered on the left side of the neck, several nerves and the esophagus may all be affected. If the only form of the drug you have available is the injectable formulation, it can be given orally with good bioavailability and less

Table 7.4. Nonsteroidal anti-inflammatory drugs labeled for use in horses in the United States.

Drug	Doses	Cyclooxygenase selectivity	Preferred uses
Phenylbutazone	2.2–4.4 mg/kg IV or PO q12 h	Nonselective	Typically used for musculoskeletal pain. Higher doses will prolong the effect of phenylbutazone but will not increase the efficacy. Higher doses are also associated with an increased risk of adverse effects. Should be used with caution in horses that are anorexic or dehydrated.
Flunixin meglumine	0.25 mg/kg IV q6 h; 1.1 mg/kg IV or PO q12 h	Nonselective	Typically used for colic or systemic inflammatory diseases. Higher doses are also associated with an increased risk of adverse effects. Should be used with caution in horses that are anorexic or dehydrated.
Ketoprofen	2.2 mg/kg IV or IM q12 h	Nonselective	Typically used in foals due to a slightly decreased risk of adverse effects. Can also be used in cases of fever non-responsive to flunixin or phenylbutazone. Less effective for musculoskeletal and colic pain than flunixin or phenylbutazone.
Diclofenac	5-inch strip of cream applied over affected joints	Nonselective	Used as a topical treatment for joint inflammation associated with arthritis. Available as a 1% cream.
Firocoxib	0.3 mg/kg PO loading dose followed by 0.1 mg/kg PO q24 h	COX-2 selective	Used as a treatment for joint inflammation associated with arthritis. May carry a decreased risk of adverse effects if used as the initial therapy. Should not be combined with other NSAIDs or steroids.

COX, cyclooxygenase; h, hour; IM, intramuscular; IV, intravenous; NSAIDs, nonsteroidal anti-inflammatory drugs; PO, by mouth; q, every.

risk of musculoskeletal adverse effects. NSAIDs should not be combined because coadministration of these drugs may increase the risk of developing side effects. The risk of adverse effects is greatly increased when horses are not eating or drinking properly as is the case with most horses with colic. These drugs should never be given to neonatal foals (<2 weeks old) without the supervision of a veterinarian because the doses for adult horses are not equivalent and the foal is at a greater risk of developing the adverse effects previously listed (Baggot 1994).

Nonselective Cyclooxygenase Inhibitors

Acetylsalicylic Acid. Acetylsalicylic acid (aspirin) has been used for almost a century for the treatment of pain and inflammation. At anti-inflammatory doses it can cause severe gastrointestinal side effects in the horse. Its main use is as an antithrombotic through its inhibition of platelet TxA2 production. This may be beneficial in cases of laminitis, disseminated intravascular coagulopathy (DIC), or as a preventative for thrombosis in severe cases of pneumonia or colitis. Doses of 12 mg/kg given

orally have been shown to prolong bleeding times for up to 48 hours.

Flunixin Meglumine. Flunixin meglumine (Finadyne or Banamine) is frequently used in horses for the treatment of colic and endotoxemia. It has not historically been used for treating lameness because of a perceived inferiority to phenylbutazone for musculoskeletal pain. Comparative studies in horses with naturally occurring navicular disease have shown no significant differences in the analgesic effects of flunixin and phenylbutazone. Both flunixin and phenylbutazone have been shown to block endotoxin-induced prostanoid production and inflammation. The real benefit of flunixin in treating endotoxemia or colic may therefore lie in the availability of and ease of injection of flunixin.

Flunixin is absorbed well orally. PK studies of powder and paste formulations show a rapid absorption with peak plasma concentrations occurring at approximately 30 minutes and an oral bioavailability of 86%. Many people use flunixin intramuscularly, particularly owners. This practice should be discouraged because flunixin is highly irritating, and there are reports of abscessation and clostridial myositis secondary to IM administration. As an alternative to IM injections, a recent study examined the oral bioavailability of the injectable formulation. Bioavailability of this preparation was approximately 72%, with similar PKs to the commercially available oral preparations (Pellegrini-Masini, Poppenga, and Sweeney 2004). This may provide a safer alternative to IM injection for horse owners.

There are two commonly used doses of flunixin. The anti-inflammatory and analgesic dose is reported to be 1.1 mg/kg by mouth or IV every 12 hours. This dose has been shown to produce a maximum effect in animal models. Lower doses (0.25 mg/kg IV every 8 hours) have been shown to be effective in preventing the inflammation associated with endotoxin challenge, with presumably fewer side effects and without masking the signs of colic (Semrad, et al. 1987). The flunixin was given pre-challenge in those instances, and the efficacy of this dose in clinic cases is often challenged. It has been shown that using this dose in experimental horses that are repeatedly challenged with endotoxin is not as effective.

Caution should be used when administering flunixin to newborn foals due to differences in PKs and an increased risk for gastric and duodenal ulceration. Area under the curve, clearance, and half-life of flunixin are significantly greater in newborn foals compared to adult horses. The half-life increases from 1 to 2 hours in adults to 6 to 8 hours in foals (Semrad, Sams, and Ashcraft 1993). Dosing intervals should be longer in foals to prevent toxicity of flunixin.

Phenylbutazone. Phenylbutazone is another popular NSAID used in horses. It is cheap and quite effective for treatment of musculoskeletal conditions, including navicular, laminitis, and other causes of lameness. It has been shown to be effective in preventing inflammation after endotoxin challenge; however, it is not as effective as flunixin in preventing the cardiovascular changes associated with endotoxin. Phenylbutazone has a beneficial effect on gut motility and gastric emptying in an endotoxin challenge model.

Oral bioavailability approaches 91%. Similar to the study using flunixin, injectable products of phenylbutazone have good oral bioavailability as well. The time to peak plasma concentration is greatly affected by feeding particularly with a hay diet. The PKs of phenylbutazone are dose dependent with higher elimination half-lives reported after higher dosing. As with flunixin, phenylbutazone PKs are altered in newborn foals and should therefore be used with caution.

Phenylbutazone has a higher incidence of adverse events in the horse when compared to flunixin and ketoprofen (MacAllister, et al. 1993). In instances of gastric ulceration, this may be related to a direct cytotoxic effect after oral administration. The toxic effects are greatly amplified in horses that are anorexic or dehydrated.

Ketoprofen. Unlike flunixin and phenylbutazone, ketoprofen is not absorbed orally or rectally, therefore IV or IM administration is necessary. It is less irritating than flunixin or phenylbutazone, thus repeated IM injections rarely cause problems. Ketoprofen has a higher therapeutic index than either flunixin or phenylbutazone, with fewer adverse effects noted when used at the label dose. Ketoprofen is not as effective in reducing lameness scores in animals with navicular disease. Clinical efficacy in endotoxemia and other inflammatory syndromes is similar, but higher doses may be required to get a comparable effect.

Diclofenac. Diclofenac is a nonspecific COX inhibitor. There are no reports of the use of diclofenac as a systemic anti-inflammatory agent in equine medicine. Topical preparations are available. An 1% liposomal cream is available in the United States for topical treatment of joint inflammation. It has good effects on pain and lameness scores with minimal systemic absorption and minimal adverse effects (Caldwell, et al. 2004). A topical ophthalmic preparation is available.

COX-2-Selective Inhibitors

Meloxicam and Piroxicam. Meloxicam is a COX-2-selective inhibitor labeled for use as an anti-inflammatory drug in the horse in European countries but not in the United States. It is typically given as an injection, but oral bioavailability is nearly complete and absorption is not affected by feeding. Maximum effects are reached at a daily dose of 0.6 mg/kg. This dose has proven effective in lameness models, as well as, experimental models of colic and abdominal pain (Toutain and Cester 2004).

Another NSAID in this group, piroxicam, has recently received some attention in equine medicine, not for treatment of lameness or colic, but for the treatment of squamous cell carcinomas (SCC). These have been shown to produce COX-2. Treatment with piroxicam has produced long-term remissions of SCC in the bladder, urethra, and periocular structures (Moore, et al. 2003). Adverse effects have been noted even at the low doses used (0.2 mg/kg by mouth every 24 hours) and include diarrhea and abdominal pain. It is not known at this time whether or not meloxicam would have a similar effect, with a higher safety profile.

Etodolac. Etodolac is a relatively selective COX-2 inhibitor in the horse. It has been used clinically in horses with a previous history of gastric or colonic ulceration and in a few horses with active gastrointestinal disease with apparent benefits. The optimum dose to use is still questionable at this time. Originally, 20 mg/kg by mouth every 12 hours was used. More recently 20 mg/kg by mouth every 24 hours was shown to be just as effective in treatment of navicular disease (Symonds, et al. 2006). It is possible even lower doses may be used. This would be beneficial because in vitro testing shows that etodolac is a potent COX inhibitor in the horse, and although it is selective at lower concentrations, this selectivity may be lost at the doses that have been previously reported.

Carprofen. Carprofen is generally considered to be a drug that is selective for COX-2 or sparing for COX-1 with a higher safety profile than other commonly available NSAIDs. The exact mechanism of action of carprofen still receives some debate because of its weak effects on COX-2-specific

prostaglandin E2 production in vitro. In horses, its peripheral effects on prostanoid production are much less than either flunixin or phenylbutazone, but its analgesic effects are similar.

Deracoxib and Firocoxib. These drugs have not been studied extensively in equine medicine. Preliminary PKs of deracoxib show that absorption is slow, but the plasma concentrations persist for long periods of time. At this point it is not known what plasma concentrations are necessary for effects, and there is still a need for clinical studies.

Firocoxib is a drug introduced in the United States in 2005 and labeled for use in the horse as a paste preparation for oral administration at a dose of 0.1 mg/kg. Efficacy testing has shown a similar response to phenylbutazone in naturally occurring lameness. In safety studies, oral ulcers were detected at three and five times the label dose; however, no other adverse effects were noted. Firocoxib is highly COX-2 selective and may be a safer alternative to use in horses. Clinical evidence of this is lacking at this time, however.

Steroids

Steroids are powerful anti-inflammatory drugs. As such, they are used in horses to treat allergic conditions (e.g., heaves, hives, or anaphylactic reactions), immune-mediated diseases, and joint diseases. They work at the cellular level to inhibit the genes that produce inflammatory mediators. Aside from their anti-inflammatory effects, steroids have many metabolic and physiologic effects that often limit their use as therapeutic anti-inflammatory agents in the horse.

Steroids are classified on the basis of their potency (as compared to hydrocortisone), their specificity or lack of mineralocorticoid action, and their duration of action based on the duration of adrenal suppression following administration. Table 7.5 classifies some of the commonly used steroids in equine medicine.

Many different routes of administration of steroids have been tried to help minimize the systemic effects, while providing good anti-

Drug	Route	Glucocorticoid potency	Mineralocorticoid potency	Duration of action
Hydrocortisone (cortisol)		1	1	<12 hours
Prednisolone sodium succinate	IV or IM	4	0.8	<24 hours
Dexamethasone	IV or IM	25–30	0	4–7 days
Methylprednisolone	IA	5	0.5	10 days
Triamcinolone acetonide	IM	5	5	14 days
Prednisolone acetate	IM	4	0.8	21 days

Table 7.5. Classification of steroids.

IA, intra-articular; IM, intramuscular; IV, intravenous.

inflammatory activity. Parenteral administration (IV or IM) attains the highest plasma concentrations and has the most potential for side effects. Oral administration is commonly used for long-term treatment of allergic or immune-mediated diseases. The bioavailability of oral prednisolone and dexamethasone is good, and these drugs are often successful in treating inflammatory diseases. Oral prednisone has not been proven to be effective in the horse because of the low oral absorption and a poor conversion to its active metabolite (prednisolone).

Chronic respiratory diseases, such as heaves, can be treated with inhaled steroids using specialized equipment. There is still some systemic absorption using this route; however, the systemic effects are minimized and higher doses are delivered directly to the site of action (the lungs). Beclomethasone dipropionate and fluticasone propionate are commonly administered via this route.

Intra-articular injections of steroids have been shown to reduce capsule swelling, decrease the duration of lameness, and decrease heat in arthritic joints. Unfortunately, they can cause progressive degeneration within the joint due to deleterious effects on the cartilage, and thus, they cannot be used too frequently. Despite the detrimental effects this route is often used in horses with degenerative joint disease particularly in low motion joints such as the distal hock joints. Commonly used drugs (listed in order of increasing potency) include methylprednisolone, triamcinolone, betamethasone, isoflupredone, and flumethasone.

As previously stated, steroids can have some pronounced systemic effects; some of which can be quite harmful. There is an association between corticosteroid administration and the development of laminitis in horses. The incidence of laminitis in horses given normal doses of commonly used steroids is probably extremely low. It is still a concern if the horse requires high doses for treatment or if there is already underlying pathology in the foot. Other adverse effects of steroids include development of metabolic derangements such as hyper- or hypoadrenocorticism and increases in liver enzyme values. Because their profound affects on the immune system, immunosuppression is possible, even at clinically used doses (Harkins, et al. 1993).

Most steroids are used as anti-inflammatory medications. There is another class of steroids that is sometimes used in equine medicine. The anabolic steroid class includes drugs such as boldenone (Equipoise) and stanazolol (Winstrol). Unlike the steroids previously described, these drugs are used to promote appetite and increase muscle mass in ill or severely debilitated animals. These drugs are often used illegally to enhance performance and increase growth in young animals. When used for these purposes, they can cause premature closure of growth plates, impaired fertility, and increased aggressiveness and uncontrollable behavior.

α_2-Agonists

α_2-Agonists are commonly used for sedation and pain relief in horses. They include xylazine

(Rompun), detomidine (Dormosedan), and romifidine (Sedivet). These drugs can be used to facilitate examinations or perform minor surgical procedures. They are also excellent at providing pain relief in horses with colic. Xylazine is the least potent of the three and requires a higher dose with more frequent dosing to achieve the desired effect. Detomidine is the most potent and longest lasting.

Unfortunately, α_2-agonists also have side effects associated with them, and they can only be used short-term pain relief. These drugs cause a decrease in gastrointestinal motility, which is contraindicated in horse with colic because they already have an altered motility. In addition, they have many effects on blood pressure and heart function (Yamashita, et al. 2000). They can cause a heart arrhythmia known as second-degree atrioventricular block in horses, particularly in those already predisposed. Oversedation can lead to severe ataxia and "wobbliness" in the patient, and some horses may even fall down causing injury to themselves and others. Care must be taken when administering these drugs because they can cause severe respiratory depression in humans, decreasing their ability to breathe and sometime necessitating mechanical ventilation after accidental injection.

Opiates

Opiate drugs are derivatives of morphine. The opiates most frequently used in horses include butorphanol (Torbugesic) and fentanyl (Duragesic). tramadol (Ultram) is currently being studied. These drugs provide pain relief with minimal sedation at commonly used doses and no anti-inflammatory effects. At high doses, they can actually cause an excitation reaction resulting in the horse twitching, circling, and vocalizing. These drugs can inhibit gastrointestinal motility, although butorphanol is less likely to produce this effect. Duragesic is a transdermal delivery system, which means that the drug is applied to the skin using a specially developed patch. The drug must then be absorbed through the skin and reach the circulation where it produces an effect. Unfortunately, this system produces variable results because highly variable drug absorption (Orsini, et al. 2006). Opiates are considered scheduled drugs meaning they are regulated by the FDA because they are known to be drugs of abuse in humans. These drugs should not be given without a veterinarian's supervision.

Antispasmodics

N-Butylscopolammonium bromide (Buscopan) has recently been approved for use in horses with spasmodic colic, flatulent colic, and simple impaction colics. It works by shutting down gastrointestinal motility for a short period of time, thereby blocking the pain caused by intestinal spasms. As previously stated, decreasing gastrointestinal motility is often contraindicated in cases of colic; so if one dose of Buscopan does not cure the horse, it should be considered that the colic is coming from something other than those conditions previously listed, and a second dose should only be administered with caution. Buscopan causes an elevation in heart rate for at least 30 minutes following administration.

Drugs for the Treatment of Gastric Ulceration

Antacids

Antacids can reduce gastric acid production, but they require large volumes and frequent administration to be effective. In a study examining administration of 180 ml Maalox, gastric pH was increased for at most 45 minutes (Murray and Grodinsky, 1992). In another study, 240 ml Maalox TC increased gastric pH for 2 hours (Clark, et al. 1996). Antacids produce symptomatic relief but are not efficient in healing gastric ulceration. An exception may be antacids containing aluminum, which may have some effect on healing of gastric glandular lesions. Aluminum hydroxide has been shown to enhance gastric mucosal nitric oxide, which should promote mucosal blood flow.

Mucosal Protectants

Sucralfate is the major mucosal protectant used for treatment of ulcers in horses. The mechanism of action likely involves adherence to ulcerated mucosa, stimulation of mucus secretion, enhanced mucosal blood flow, and enhanced prostaglandin E synthesis. These are all factors relevant to glandular mucosa, and it is doubtful that sucralfate is effective in treating ulcers in the squamous mucosa. In fact, lesions in the squamous mucosa can develop while a horse is being treated with sucralfate. Additionally, administration of sucralfate with other drugs that are known to be chelated by cations, such as fluoroquinolones and tetracyclines, and may decrease bioavailability of those drugs.

H_2 antagonists

These include such drugs as ranitidine, cimetidine, and famotidine. Ranitidine is most commonly used in horses because of a more consistent oral absorption and a demonstrated effect on increasing gastric pH. Ranitidine at 6.6 mg/kg orally every 8 hours provides adequate suppression of acidity in the greatest percentage of horses. Effective dosages of cimetidine have not been examined as extensively as those of ranitidine, but an effective oral dose may be as high as 50 mg/kg/day. Treatment with cimetidine or ranitidine should continue for at least 21 days but may take as long as 3 to 4 months. It would appear that the effect on gastric acidity of oral administration of 3.3 mg/kg famotidine is similar to that with 6.6 mg/kg ranitidine. Formulations for IV administration of H_2 antagonists are available but are expensive. Ranitidine should be given intravenously at 1 to 1.5 mg/kg every 8 hours and cimetidine at 6.6 mg/kg three to four times daily.

Proton Pump Inhibitors

Omeprazole blocks gastric acid secretion by inhibiting the parietal cell H^+-K^+-ATPase (proton pump) that secretes hydrochloric acid. Omeprazole is a potent inhibitor of gastric acidity in horses. Because of its potency once daily treatment is feasible. The drug is unstable at low pH, so specialized formulations have been developed for use in the horse. This drug is quite effective in treating gastric ulceration; however, it may take several days before there is a noticeable clinical effect. Doses range from 1 to 2 mg/kg for prevention to 4 mg/kg by mouth 24 hours for treatment of severe disease.

References and Further Reading

Baggot, J. D. 1994. Drug therapy in the neonatal foal. *Vet Clin North Am Equine Pract* 10(1):87–107.

Caldwell, F. J., P. O. Mueller, R. C. Lynn, and S. C. Budsberg. 2004. Effect of topical application of diclofenac liposomal suspension on experimentally induced subcutaneous inflammation in horses. *Am J Vet Res* 65(3):271–76.

Carrillo, N. A., S. Giguère, R. R. Gronwall, M. P. Brown, K. A. Merritt, and J. J. O'Kelley. 2005. Disposition of orally administered cefpodoxime proxetil in foals and adult horses and minimum inhibitory concentration of the drug against common bacterial pathogens of horses. *Am J Vet Res* 66(1):30–35.

Clark, C. K., A. M. Merritt, J. A. Burrow, and C. K. Steible. 1996. Effect of aluminum hydroxide/magnesium hydroxide antacid and bismuth subsalicylate on gastric pH in horses. *J Am Vet Med Assoc* 208(10):1687–91.

Davis, J. L., S. Y. Gardner, S. L. Jones, B. A. Schwabenton, and M. G. Papich. 2002. Pharmacokinetics of azithromycin in foals after i.v. and oral dose and disposition into phagocytes. *J Vet Pharmacol Ther* 25(2):99–104.

Davis, J. L., J. H. Salmon, and M. G. Papich. 2005. Pharmacokinetics and tissue fluid distribution of cephalexin in the horse after oral and i.v. administration. *J Vet Pharmacol Ther* 28(5):425–31.

———. 2006. Pharmacokinetics and tissue distribution of doxycycline after oral administration of single and multiple doses in horses. *Am J Vet Res* 67(2):310–16.

Giguere, S., J. F. Prescott, J. D. Baggot, R. D. Walker, and P. M. Dowling. 2006. *Antimicrobial Therapy in Veterinary Medicine*, 4th ed. Ames IA: Blackwell Publishers.

Harkins, J. D., J. M. Carney, and T. Tobin. 1993. Clinical use and characteristics of the corticosteroids. *Vet Clin North Am Equine Pract* 9:543–62.

MacAllister, C. G., S. J. Morgan, A. T. Borne, and R. A. Pollet. 1993. Comparison of adverse effects of phenylbutazone, flunixin meglumine, and ketoprofen in horses. *J Am Vet Med Assoc* 202(1):71–77.

Moore, A. S., S. L. Beam, K. M. Rassnick, and R. Provost. Long-term control of mucocutaneous squamous cell carcinoma and metastases in a horse using piroxicam. *Equine Vet J* 35(7):715–18.

Murray, M. J., and C. Grodinsky. 1992. The effects of famotidine, ranitidine and magnesium hydroxide/aluminium hydroxide on gastric fluid pH in adult horses. *Equine Vet J Suppl.* 1992 Feb; (11):52–55.

Olsén, L., C. Ingvast-Larsson, H. Broström, P. Larsson, and H. Tjälve. 2007. Clinical signs and etiology of adverse reactions to procaine benzylpenicillin and sodium/potassium benzylpenicillin in horses. *J Vet Pharmacol Ther* 30(3):201–7.

Orsini, J. A., P. J. Moate, K. Kuersten, L. R. Soma, and R. C. Boston. 2006. Pharmacokinetics of fentanyl delivered transdermally in healthy adult horses—variability among horses and its clinical implications. *J Vet Pharmacol Ther* 29(6):539–46.

Owen, R. A., J. Fullerton, and D. A. Barnum. 1983. Effects of transportation, surgery, and antibiotic therapy in ponies infected with Salmonella. *Am J Vet Res* 44(1):46–50.

Pellegrini-Masini, A., R. H. Poppenga, and R. W. Sweeney. 2004. Disposition of flunixin meglumine injectable preparation administered orally to healthy horses. *J Vet Pharmacol Ther* 27(3):183–86.

Plumb, D. C. 2008. *Veterinary Drug Handbook,* 6th ed. Ames, IA: Blackwell Publishers.

Riond, J. L., J. E. Riviere, W. M. Duckett, C. E. Atkins, A. D. Jernigan, Y. Rikihisa, and S. L. Spurlock. 1992. Cardiovascular effects and fatalities associated with intravenous administration of doxycycline to horses and ponies. *Equine Vet J* 24(1):41–45.

Schutte, J. G., and T. S. van den Ingh. 1997. Microphthalmia, brachygnathia superior, and palatocheiloschisis in a foal associated with griseofulvin administration to the mare during early pregnancy. *Vet Q* 19(2):58–60.

Semrad, S. D., G. E. Hardee, M. M. Hardee, and J. N. Moore. 1987. Low dose flunixin meglumine: effects on eicosanoid production and clinical signs induced by experimental endotoxaemia in horses. *Equine Vet J* 19(3):201–6.

Semrad, S. D., R. A. Sams, and S. M. Ashcraft. 1993. Pharmacokinetics of and serum thromboxane suppression by flunixin meglumine in healthy foals during the first month of life. *Am J Vet Res* 54(12):2083–87.

Steinman, A., M. Gips, E. Lavy, I. Sinay, and S. Soback. 2000. Pharmacokinetics of metronidazole in horses after intravenous, rectal and oral administration. *J Vet Pharmacol Ther* 23(6):353–57.

Symonds, K. D., C. G. MacAllister, R. S. Erkert, and M. E. Payton. 2006. Use of force plate analysis to assess the analgesic effects of etodolac in horses with navicular syndrome. *Am J Vet Res* 67(4):557–61.

Toribio, R. E., F. T. Bain, D. R. Mrad, N. T. Messer 4th, R. S. Sellers, and K. W. Hinchcliff. 1998. Congenital defects in newborn foals of mares treated for equine protozoal myeloencephalitis during pregnancy. *J Am Vet Med Assoc* 212(5):697–701.

Toutain, P. L., and C. C. Cester. 2004. Pharmacokinetic-pharmacodynamic relationships and dose response to meloxicam in horses with induced arthritis in the right carpal joint. *Am J Vet Res* 65(11):1533–41.

van Duijkeren, E., A. G. Vulto, M. M. Sloet van Oldruitenborghhoosterbaan, D. J. Mevius, B. G. Kessels, H. J. Breukink, and A. S. van Miert. 1994. A comparative study of the pharmacokinetics of intravenous and oral trimethoprim/sulfadiazine formulations in the horse. *J Vet Pharmacol Ther* 17(6):440–46.

van Duijkeren, E., B. G. Kessels, M. M. Sloet van Oldruitenborgh-Oosterbaan, J. J. Breukink, A. G. Vulto, and A. S. van Miert. 1996. In vitro and in vivo binding of trimethoprim and sulphachlorpyridazine to equine food and digesta and their stability in caecale contents. *J Vet Pharmacol Ther* 19(4):281–87.

Yamashita, K., S. Tsubakishita, S. Futaok, I. Ueda, H. Hamaguchi, T. Seno, S. Katoh, Y. Izumisawa, T. Kotani, and W. W. Muir. 2000. Cardiovascular effects of medetomidine, detomidine and xylazine in horses. *J Vet Med Sci* 62(10):1025–32.

Laboratory Diagnosis in Equine Practice

Craig F. Shoemaker

Laboratory Use and Safety

General Laboratory Safety

A full understanding of the proper use and care of laboratory equipment is essential. A good working knowledge of procedures for use, care, and maintenance of equipment is necessary to ensure that personnel performing laboratory tests are safe and that results generated are as accurate as possible. Laboratory personnel should be thoroughly trained in the operation of all laboratory equipment and regular review of these procedures should be mandatory.

Laboratory Apparatus

In-house diagnostic equipment routinely found in equine veterinary practice laboratories may include the following: hematology/blood chemistry analyzer(s), electrolyte analyzer, blood gas analyzer, microscope, centrifuge, and incubator. Additional equipment specific for practice type and needs may also be present. Proper training in the use and care of laboratory equipment is critical to ensure that results obtained are accurate and useful in assessing the medical status of patients.

Sample Preparation and Submission Protocol

Veterinarians have several options available to them regarding analyses of laboratory samples. Samples can be analyzed using in-house diagnostic equipment, or they may be sent to a commercial veterinary laboratory. The advantages of in-house laboratory testing include rapid turn-around time and the ability to run samples immediately after collection; in addition, in-house laboratory equipment offers an economic advantage for many practices. Disadvantages of in-house laboratory testing include the cost of equipment and the need for technical operator expertise. The major advantage of commercial laboratories is that there is no investment in equipment, and they provide a full complement of testing services, technical expertise, and oversight of procedures. One of the major disadvantages of commercial laboratories is the delay in receiving results, which can impact clinical decisions.

Many samples collected in equine practice require special handling to ensure that results obtained are meaningful and useful to the practitioner. Collection techniques and sample preparation are determined by sample type. A few examples of sample types include blood, body fluids, aspirates, tissue biopsies, and scrapings. It is necessary to know in advance the type of tests that are to be run so that samples can be properly prepared and submitted in a timely fashion. The proper preparation and submission of samples minimizes the deleterious effects of aging and resultant sample deterioration. Even mild sample deterioration can negatively influence test results.

Deterioration of samples can result from the following:

Autolysis is the normal process of cell membrane breakdown, which results in cell lysis and destruction. Although all samples undergo this process, autolysis is accelerated by increased ambient temperature and humidity. The use of preservatives and cooling during shipment slows the rate of sample autolysis.

Hemolysis is the dissolution or destruction of red blood cells (RBCs). As a result, hemoglobin is liberated into the medium in which the RBCs are suspended causing a discoloration of the serum or plasma. This discoloration may distort any subsequent colorimetric or photometric analysis. Increases in temperature and physical shock are common causes of sample hemolysis. Damage to RBCs often occurs from forceful pushing of blood samples through a needle into a collection tube; care should be taken when transferring blood samples in this manner. Efforts should be made to harvest serum or plasma soon after collection and before shipping samples.

Necrosis is the process of cell death and lysis. Necrosis occurs in tissues after death or in tissue samples after they have been harvested for analysis. The process of necrosis begins immediately; high temperatures are responsible for accelerated sample necrosis. Fresh tissue samples should immediately be placed in an appropriate fixative (10% formalin) before shipping. Samples that are to be submitted to reference laboratories should be placed in an appropriate preservative before transport. Shipment of samples over a weekend should be avoided at all costs.

All samples submitted must be identifiable. Information required for every sample submitted includes:

- Owner information.
- Animal information (i.e., age, gender, breed, tattoo number, name).
- Detail of sample collection.
- Relevant clinical history of patient.
- List of numbers and types of samples being submitted.
- Details of samples and collection sites.
- Types of tests requested.

Proper packaging of all biological samples before shipment is essential to ensure that they arrive safely and undamaged. In addition, packaging should prevent any leakage of contents should a container break during handling. Sound packaging also serves to protect those handling the package while in transit. All packages containing biological samples should meet the following criteria:

- Samples should be placed in a primary leakproof container, which is then placed within a secondary leakproof container. Containers can be made of glass, metal, or plastic.
- Samples should be placed in containers using leakproof seals, or alternatively, screw caps reinforced with waterproof tape.
- The primary container should have suitable padding and adequate absorbent material capable of absorbing the entire contents.
- A secondary container made of durable, waterproof, lightweight material should be used to contain primary container.
- A comprehensive itemized list of contents should be attached to the secondary container. This list should include all contact numbers and any additional paperwork that is required.
- The secondary container and all attachments are placed into an outer shipping package.
- The outer shipping package should protect the contents from external damage, provide information as to who is sending and receiving the package, provide specific details and contact numbers and clearly display all appropriate hazard designations.

- Specific information regarding packaging requirements can best be obtained from the laboratory to which the samples are being sent.

Samples that are to be sent to an outside reference laboratory should be sent either first class mail or by a carrier, which provides overnight delivery. All packages should be clearly labeled "Pathological Specimen—Fragile—Handle with Care." Primary containers should be securely sealed and have a maximum volume of 50 ml.

Hematology

Blood is classified as one of the connective tissues and comprises approximately 10% of body weight. Blood consists of cellular components suspended in a complex solution called *plasma*. Plasma is the liquid component of blood, accounting for about one-half of its total volume. Once clotting has occurred and the fluid is separated from the cellular components of blood, the liquid portion is referred to as serum (plasma absent clotting factors).

Cellular Components of Blood

The cellular components of blood consist of erythrocytes (RBCs), leukocytes (white blood cells), and thrombocytes (platelets). Erythrocytes and thrombocytes are anucleated cells (lacking a nucleus) performing most of their functions within the blood. Leukocytes (i.e., lymphocytes, neutrophils, monocytes, eosinophils and basophils) are nucleated cells that migrate out of postcapillary venules into connective tissue or lymphatic tissue. They perform their functions both within and outside the bloodstream. The examination of a well-prepared blood film is essential when examining the size, shape, and maturity of blood cells. Blood films are also useful in determining the relative number of each type of white blood cell.

Plasma

Plasma is a solution of nutrients and various proteins, mainly albumin and various globulins, including immunoglobulins, which are responsible for much of the body's defense against infection. The following is a list of the various components of plasma:

- Water.
- Plasma proteins (i.e., albumin, globulin, fibrinogen, prothrombin).
- Mineral salts.
- Nutrients (i.e., amino acids, carbohydrates, fatty acids).
- Gases (i.e., carbon dioxide and oxygen to a lesser degree are free gases in solution).
- Waste products (i.e., urea and creatinine).
- Hormones.
- Enzymes.
- Antibodies.
- Antioxidants.

Functions of Blood

Cells are continuously adding waste products, secretions, and metabolites to blood while taking from it vital nutrients, oxygen, hormones, and other substances. Overall, blood performs many different functions

Blood Is Used to Transport
- Oxygen to and carbon dioxide away from tissues.
- Digested nutrients to tissues.
- Waste products from tissues to kidneys and liver for excretion.
- Water to tissues.
- Hormones and enzymes throughout the body.

Blood Is Used to Regulate
- Maintain body temperature by heat distribution.
- Control hemorrhage via clotting mechanisms.
- Maintain acid-base balance.
- Regulate water and electrolytes.
- Protect against infection through the actions of white blood cells.
- Protect against infection via antibodies and antitoxins it transports.

Packed Cell Volume

Packed cell volume (PCV) or hematocrit (Hct) is an estimate of the percentage of cells within the blood. RBCs make up the largest percentage of cells numbering 6 to 12 million/ml as compared to white blood cells which number 6 to 12 thousand/ml. Normal PCV values vary depending on age, fitness, and breed of the horse. PCV is used to assess dehydration and anemia. Optimum PCV values are close to 40%, with levels below 35% and above 45% possible indicators of a problem. Excitement or stress can increase the estimation of PCV by increasing the numbers of circulating RBCs via splenic contraction. In the equine athlete, PCV values may continue to rise as fitness levels increase; however, in many cases, rising PCV is indicative of problems secondary to work-related issues. Neonates have a PCV of 40% to 52%, decreasing to 29% to 41% by 6 months of age; therefore, interpretation of samples from foals must take this into account.

An increased PCV may be as a result of:

- Dehydration.
- Stress and excitement (splenic contraction).
- Endotoxic shock.

A decreased PCV may be due to:

- Blood loss anemia (i.e. hemorrhage).
- Hemolytic anemia, (i.e., infectious piroplasmosis, and equine infectious anemia), immune-mediated hemolysis (neonatal isoerythrolysis), oxidative injury (i.e., red maple leaf, onion), toxicities (i.e., clostridial organisms and intravenous dimethyl sulfoxide [DMSO]), and iatrogenic hemolysis (hypertonic saline).
- Decreased erythrocyte production (i.e., secondary to chronic inflammatory disease, nutritional deficiency, neoplasia, or toxicity).

Collection of Blood

The collection of blood from horses is most commonly achieved by venipuncture. Samples can be obtained from a number of anatomical sites, including:

- Jugular vein—the most common collection site in the horse as it is readily available in adults and foals.
- Cephalic vein on forelimb.
- Saphenous vein on hind limb.
- Transverse facial vein (small volumes only).

Blood is easily collected using a Vacutainer tube with a needle and needle holder; however, an ordinary hypodermic needle and syringe can also be used. There are a number of different Vacutainer tubes available:

- Red top: plain draw tube—no anticoagulant.
- Purple top: ethylenediaminetetraacetic acid (EDTA).
- Green top: heparin.
- Blue top: sodium citrate—required for coagulation studies.
- Grey top: oxalate fluoride—used when assessing glucose concentration.
- Yellow top: acid citrate dextrose—required for cross matching or blood typing.

Arterial blood sampling is commonly used to assess acid-base status. Common sites for arterial blood collection include:

- Facial artery (heavily sedated or anesthetized horse).
- Transverse facial artery (heavily sedated or anesthetized horse).
- Dorsal metatarsal artery (recumbent foals).
- Carotid artery (conscious horse).
- Median artery (sedated or anesthetized horse).

Red Blood Cells

The normal ranges for RBC-related parameters, like those for PCV, vary according to the type of horse. When assessing the RBC count, refer to the range provided by the laboratory used.

Red Blood Cell Production

Erythropoiesis (*erythro* = RBC and *poiesis* = to make) is the term used to describe the formation or production of RBCs. The organ responsible for regulating RBC production is the kidney. The kidneys

Table 8.1. How to collect blood from jugular vein.

To collect jugular blood sample:
  Properly restrain horse before sampling.
  Adult horses should always be in a halter or bridle while collecting sample regardless of their demeanor.
  Foals must be held properly around head and body (ear and tail hold).
  Have collection materials ready (i.e., Vacutainer tube, needle, and holder assembled).
  Raise vein by applying gentle pressure at base of neck (usually left side).
  Clip hair over vein one-third of the way down the neck. Clipper blade should be directed perpendicular to the vein. The carotid artery is not as
    superficial in this location and should be avoided.
  Clean sample site with alcohol swab.
  Gently sink needle into skin over vein until a lack of resistance is felt. Blood should drip from other end of needle.
  Attach vacutainer tube to the needle and hold steady. If collecting more than one tube collect ethylenediaminetetraacetic acid (EDTA) sample first.
  Remove needle from neck and apply pressure while inverting tube.

Adapted from Coumbe 2001. *The Equine Veterinary Nursing Manual*, Oxford: Blackwell Science, Ltd.

release the hormone erythropoietin in response to low oxygen levels in the circulating blood. The effect of erythropoietin on the bone marrow is to cause an increase in the production of RBCs from stem cells within the bone marrow. These cells divide and begin synthesizing hemoglobin, which is stored within the cell's cytoplasm. On completion of hemoglobin synthesis, the nucleus is extruded from the RBC and cells become known as reticulocytes or immature erythrocytes. Reticulocytes do not usually leave the bone marrow in horses and are rarely seen in the peripheral circulation except in cases of severe anemia. Once equine red cell maturation is complete, cells are released into the peripheral circulation where their average life span is 140 to 150 days.

Red Blood Cell Morphology

Most mammalian erythrocytes are round and somewhat biconcave-disc shaped. Equine erythrocytes, as compared to canine, are smaller, have less concavity and lack central pallor (see Figure 8.1). Equine erythrocytes demonstrate a tendency for marked rouleaux formation (aligning like stacked coins; Figure 8.2. Rouleaux formation causes erythrocytes to separate rapidly from plasma, resulting in a high erythrocyte sedimentation rate in this species. This characteristic necessitates thorough

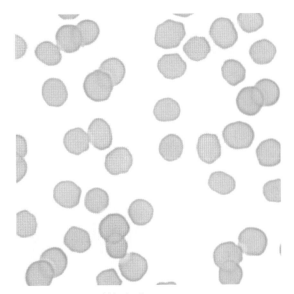

Figure 8.1. Equine red blood cells.
Courtesy of IDEXX and Dr. Dennis DeNicola.

mixing of blood samples before analysis. Rouleaux formation must also be differentiated from autoagglutination (Figure 8.3), which can be observed grossly or microscopically in cases of immune-mediated hemolytic anemia. Both rouleaux formation and autoagglutination, which is sometimes

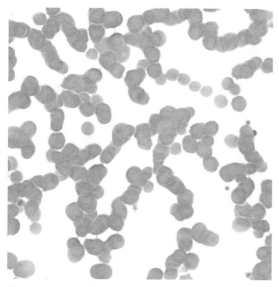

Figure 8.2. Rouleax formation.
Courtesy of IDEXX and Dr. Dennis DeNicola.

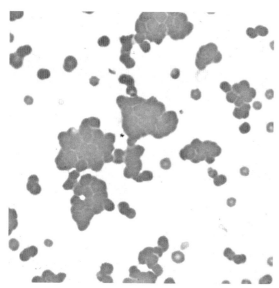

Figure 8.3. Red blood cell agglutination.
Courtesy of IDEXX and Dr. Dennis DeNicola.

observed during severe inflammatory disease, are dispersed by saline dilution; whereas, autoagglutination associated with immune-mediated anemia is not. The direct antiglobulin or Coombs' test detects immunoglobulin or complement on the surface of erythrocytes and is used to diagnose immune-mediated hemolytic anemia in the horse.

A number of textbooks provide excellent information and pictures identifying the normal and abnormal RBC morphology of the horse. Morphologic terms and cell types include:

Anisocytosis is the variability in the size of erythrocytes usually due to an increased RBC diameter at distribution.

Microcytosis are abnormally small RBCs; a normal finding in foals up to 1 year in age, attributable to a physiologic iron deficiency.

Poikilocyte is any abnormally shaped erythrocyte. This is a descriptive term usually reserved for RBCs that exhibit a variety of morphologies.

Spherocytes are spherical erythrocytes sometimes observed in horses with immune-mediated hemolysis.

Echinocyte is a burr cell with short, regularly spaced spicules extending from the surface of RBC; it may be associated with uremia.

Acanthocyte is a spur cell with irregularly spaced spicules extending form the RBC surface; it may be associated with liver disease or gastrointestinal malabsorption.

Elliptocytes are oval erythrocytes found in cases of iron deficiency or myelophthisic anemia (e.g., replacement of bone marrow by tumor, fibrosis, or granulomatous processes).

Leptocyte is a thin, flat RBC frequently associated with hepatic disease or iron deficiency.

Codocyte is a target cell with a dense central area of hemoglobin surrounded by a pale zone, associated with hypochromic anemia (e.g., cell deficient in hemoglobin and iron content) or hepatic disease.

Howell-Jolly bodies are basophilic nuclear remnants seen in cytoplasm of erythrocytes, occasionally observed in blood smears from healthy horses. Approximately 10 in 10,000 erythrocytes contain Howell-Jolly bodies in the normal horse.

Heinz bodies are oxidized precipitated hemoglobin indicating oxidative damage to RBCs, associated with intravascular or extravascular hemolysis (Figure 8.4).

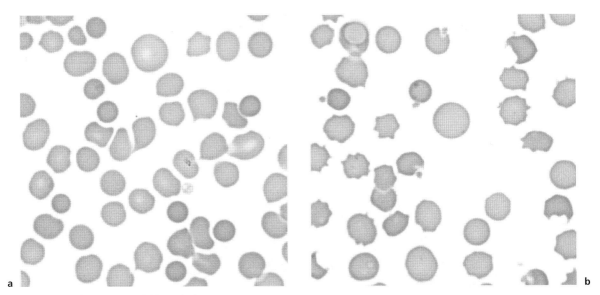

Figure 8.4. *(A)* Anisocytosis and *(B)* Heinz bodies. Courtesy of IDEXX and Dr. Dennis DeNicola.

White Blood Cells

White blood cells, or leukocytes, are cells of the immune system, which defend the body against infectious disease and foreign materials. Several different and diverse types of leukocytes exist, all of which are produced from a pluripotent cell in the bone marrow known as the hematopoietic stem cell. Leukocytes are found throughout the body including the blood and lymphatic system. One of the primary techniques used to identify the different types of leukocytes is to look for the presence of granules, resulting in the differentiation of cells into those containing granules (granulocytes) and those lacking granules (agranulocytes).

Granulocytes are leukocytes characterized by the presence of differently staining granules within their cytoplasm when viewed under light microscopy. These granules are membrane-bound enzymes that function primarily in the digestion of endocytosed or engulfed particles. There are three types of granulocytes named according to their specific staining properties: neutrophils, eosinophils, and basophils. Agranulocytes are white blood cells lacking granules and include lymphocytes, monocytes, and macrophages.

White Blood Cell Types and Function

Neutrophils serve as the primary defense against invasion of tissues by microorganisms, and they total about 60% of the total white blood cell count. Neutrophils kill bacteria and can also damage or participate in the destruction of mycotic agents, algae, and viruses. Neutrophilia, an increase in the absolute numbers of circulating neutrophils, can result from inflammation, stress, or corticosteroid administration. Neutropenia, a decrease in the absolute number of circulating neutrophils, often results from an increased tissue demand. Band cells are immature neutrophils released from the bone marrow in times of increased demand.

Lymphocytes are white blood cells present in the blood, lymph, and lymphoid tissues. The two major classes of lymphocytes include B-cells and T-cells. During infection, B-cells mature into plasma cells, which produce antibodies against specific antigens; this is known as humoral immunity. T-cells are thymus-derived lymphocytes that participate in a variety of cell-mediated immune responses, including defense against intracellular bacteria, virus infected cells, and tumor cells.

Monocytes and macrophages represent the second major branch of the circulating phagocyte system. Monocytes, after migrating from the bloodstream into tissues, develop into macrophages, the specific phagocytosing cells within the tissues. Chronic inflammation results in monocytosis or an increase in the numbers of circulating monocytes.

Eosinophils are large and covered with red staining granules. Eosinophils participate as a major component of systemic hypersensitivity reactions. Eosinophilia, or an increase in the absolute eosinophil count, suggests allergic or parasitic infection, fungi, or foreign bodies resulting in granulomatous inflammation and occasionally, neoplastic disease such as lymphoma.

Basophils are covered with blue staining granules. Basophils contain large amounts of histamine, as well as other mediators of inflammation. Basophilia, an increase in the absolute basophil count, may be seen in response to systemic allergic reactions and the invasion of tissues by parasites. Basophils are of limited value in the evaluation of equine blood (Figure 8.5).

Platelets in mammals are anucleate cells (lacking a nucleus) that contain small pink-red granules. Platelets are shed into the bloodstream from large precursor cells (megakaryocytes) located in the bone marrow; they are key players in the hemostatic process. Equine platelets tend to be uniform in size and shape with granules, which stain very lightly with routine hematology stains, making the platelets faint and sometimes difficult to see at lower magnifications. Platelet counts in horses are often lower than those observed in other species, with 6 to 20 platelets per high-magnification (oil immersion) field an adequate count (Figure 8.6).

Blood Film

Examination of a well-prepared blood film is an integral part of the hemogram, allowing for the quantification of the different types of leukocytes (differential cell count), estimation of the platelet count, and the detection of morphologic abnormalities. It is important to note that although many of the automated hematology analyzers provide a differential cell count, this does not fully substitute for

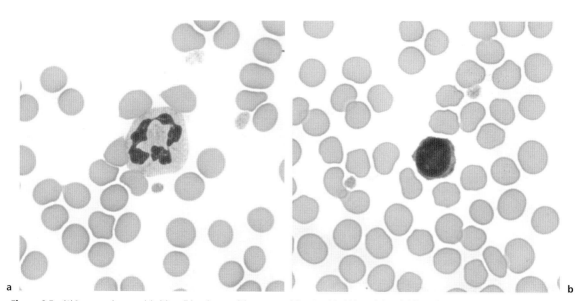

a   b

Figure 8.5. *(A)* Segmented neutrophil; *(B)* small lymphocyte; *(C)* monocyte; *(D)* eosinophil; *(E)* basophil; and *(F)* large lymphocyte. Courtesy of Wiley-Blackwell, *Veterinary hematology: atlas of common domestic species*.

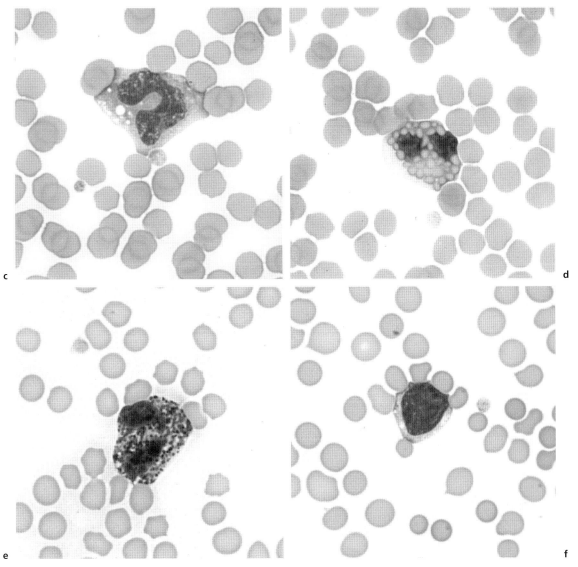

Figure 8.5. *Continued*

microscopic examination of a blood film by an experienced laboratory technician.

How to Make a Blood Film

The proper preparation of a blood film is prerequisite to an accurate assessment of the hemogram. To prepare a proper blood film:

- Use only new, clean microscope slides.
- Place a small drop of well mixed EDTA/whole blood near the frosted end of slide.
- Place another slide in front of the blood drop at approximately a 30-degree angle to the first; draw back until slide touches blood drop in the acute angle between slides.
- After blood has spread to within 2 to 3 mm of the edge of slide push the second slide

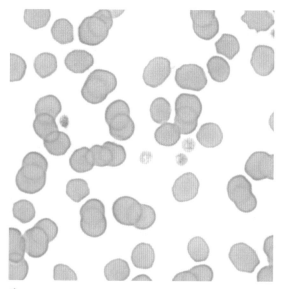

Figure 8.6. Equine platelets.
Courtesy of IDEXX and Dr. Dennis DeNicola.

Figure 8.7. Blood film preparation.
Courtesy of IDEXX and Dr. Dennis DeNicola.

quickly and smoothly across the full length of the first.

• A well-formed smear has a flame shape.
• Prepare several slides for each patient.
• Air-dry the prepared blood films quickly, and store at room temperature until processed.
• Do not blot or wipe dry as this introduces scratches.
• Do not refrigerate; condensation forms on cold slides and can lyse or rupture cells.
• Keep away from formalin.
• Do not fix slides until ready to stain.
• Most common stains are Romanowsky stains (i.e., Wright, Giemsa and modified quick stains) because they afford best overall morphologic assessment.
  • These stains contain both acid stain (usually eosin) and basic stain (such as new methylene blue).
  • Structures rich in basic compounds, such as eosinophil granules, bind the acidic dye and are stained red.
  • Acidic structures, such as DNA/RNA or basophilic granules, are stained blue by the basic stain.

Common faults and artifacts of blood smears include:

• Thickness: a smear that is too thick makes evaluation of individual cells difficult; too thin and cell numbers are insufficient.
• Unequal distribution of cells.
• Crenation (shrinkage) due to too slow air-drying.
• Streaks and smears which make interpretation difficult.
• Improper staining.
  • Overstaining—all cells are deeply colored; this can obscure important cells.
  • Understaining—cellular details of leukocytes are barely distinguishable and red cells are very faint. This should not be confused with hypochromia (abnormal hemoglobin content in erythrocytes).

Blood films should be evaluated using the "battlement technique" in which the slide is examined microscopically by repeatedly moving two fields up, two fields over, and two fields down until 100 cells have been counted yielding a percentage of each leukocyte cell type. This percentage can then be multiplied by the total white cell count to obtain an absolute cell count (Figure 8.7).

Laboratory Evaluation of Blood Samples

Hematologic Evaluation

A complete blood count (CBC) is an integral component of any diagnostic workup of the horse. This includes every sick patient, preanesthetic examination and screening, wellness profiles, and geriatric monitoring. The CBC can be used to assess the general health of patients and provide insight into underlying disease. Reference laboratories continue to play a major role for many equine practitioners, especially smaller or predominantly ambulatory practices. Many referral hospitals and larger practices use in-house hematology analyzers. In-house diagnostic equipment allows veterinarians to obtain information quickly, allowing for prompt medical intervention. In many instances, this information can mean the difference between treatment success and failure. In-house instrumentation represents a substantial investment for the equine practitioner. For this reason, it is essential that there is a good understanding of the available technologies and their capabilities so that decisions made best serve the practice. Hematology analyzers have greatly improved over the years and now offer more accurate results with automated two-, three-, or five-part differential counts. In addition, newer analyzers have fewer maintenance requirements and require less technical expertise to operate.

In-house hematology units can be grouped according to technology:

- Qualitative buffy coat (QBC).
- Impedance counters.
- Laser flow cytometers.

Qualitative Buffy Coat

The QBC analyzers classify cells based on density and staining properties of cellular components. High speed centrifugation is used to separate blood into plasma, buffy coat (white blood cells and platelets), and RBCs (Figure 8.8).

QBC analyzers work well and are extremely efficient at screening normal hematology. These analyzers are easy to use, economical, and require little to no maintenance. One distinct disadvantage of this type of analyzer is that it does not provide a full five-par differential. Lymphocytes and monocytes are grouped together, and in equine samples, it is not possible to differentiate eosinophils from other granulocytes. One advantage of the QBC in clinical practice is that it does provide a means of assessing fibrinogen in the equine patient.

Impedance Counters

Based on the Coulter principle, these analyzers size and count particles based on the resistance of par-

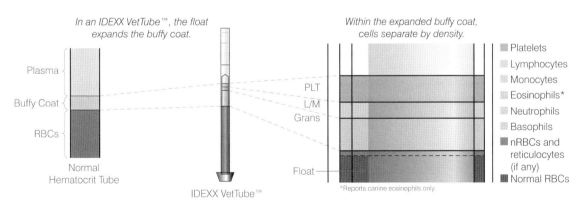

Figure 8.8. Veterinarian autoread tube. Courtesy of IDEXX.

ticles as they pass through a small aperture between two electrodes. Disadvantages of this technology include difficulty in differentiating between different types of white blood cells because cells are classified by size alone. In addition, nucleated RBCs and clumped platelets are similar in size when compared to leukocytes and may be misclassified as white blood cells. Large platelets or small clumps of platelets may also be misclassified as erythrocytes. Impedance-based systems also require the use of reagent fluids for normal instrument cycling and involve a considerable amount of maintenance and cleaning, which increases the per test price. Moderately priced, these analyzers provide rapid results; however, they do not provide an accurate five-par differential count.

Laser Flow Cytometry

The method most often used by reference laboratories, and the newest and most accurate automated cell analyzer technology, is laser flow cytometry. This technology analyzes individual cells as they pass through a laser beam because each cell creates a specific pattern of light scatter as it passes through the beam. The scatter pattern is then analyzed and interpreted based on cell size, nuclear characteristics, and cytoplasmic contents.

Laser flow cytometry provides practitioners with a true five-par differential, which is a more accurate assessment of the hematologic parameters (Figure 8.9).

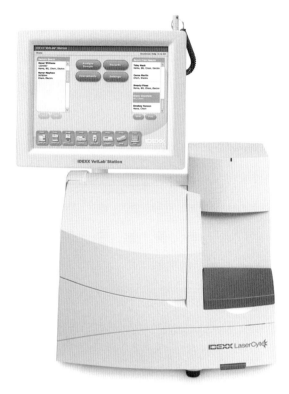

Figure 8.9. Lasercyte.
Courtesy of IDEXX.

Clinical Chemistry

Clinical chemistry, also known as clinical biochemistry, is the area of pathology concerned with the analysis of bodily fluids. Unlike hematology, which is the examination and measurement of the cellular components of blood, clinical chemistry focuses on the noncellular components of blood, blood serum, and plasma.

Serum Proteins

The combined concentration of albumin and globulin (g/L) provide the total serum protein concentra-

tion. Albumin is the most abundant plasma protein in mammals and is essential for maintaining the osmotic pressure required for the proper distribution of fluids between intravascular compartments and tissues. Measurement of total protein, albumin, globulins, and fibrinogen provides an index of hydration status, as well as, indices of infection, inflammation, increased protein loss, or decreased protein production.

The total globulin count is comprised of α-globulins and γ-globulins. α-Globulins are acute-phase reactant proteins produced by the liver in response to inflammation and include fibrinogen and haptaglobulin. These proteins are increased in concentration during active inflammation and are useful in the assessment of the inflammatory response. γ-Globulins include the immunoglobulins, or antibodies. Specific measurement of antibody levels, such as immunoglobulin G (IgG), can be useful in determining the immune status of an animal. IgG is commonly used to assess the efficacy of maternal transfer of immunity to foals (Figure 8.10). Serum proteins may be estimated by automated machines using colorimetry or the total serum concentration may be estimated manually using a refractometer. Quantification of the individual components of the total globulins may be obtained using serum protein electrophoresis. Quantifying these fractions is useful when the total globulin concentration is abnormal (Table 8.2).

Electrolytes

Electrolytes are a critical element in cellular metabolism, muscle contraction, nerve transmission, and enzymatic reactions. Mild alterations can have a negative impact on performance, whereas more serious imbalances or deficits may lead to metabolic disruptions that threaten life or result in death. Although the body closely regulates electrolytes, they are frequently lost in sweat, urine, feces, and through exercise and illness. Therefore, it is important to monitor electrolyte status in athletic horses and in all cases of illness.

Acid-Base Balance

Optimal enzyme system function in the body requires maintenance of a narrow pH range, the result of critical acid-base balance. In the normal horse, blood is slightly alkaline or basic (pH 7.35–7.45). Decreased pH is termed acidosis and is caused by an increase in the concentration of hydrogen ions ($[H^+]$). Increased pH is termed alkalosis and results from an overall decrease in the $[H^+]$.

Buffer systems that maintain the normal pH include bicarbonate, phosphates, and proteins. Bicarbonate $[HCO_3^-]$ is the most important extracellular buffer, whereas phosphates and proteins contribute mostly to intracellular acid-base balance. Bicarbonate is the only buffer measured when calculating the acid-base status. The bicarbonate system is represented by the following equation: $CO_2 + H_2O \leftrightarrow H_2CO_3 \leftrightarrow H^+ + HCO_3^-$. Acid-base disturbances are listed in Table 8.3.

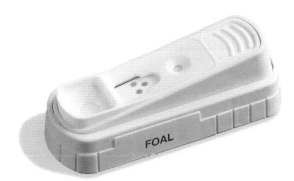

Figure 8.10. SNAP foal immunoglobulin G test. Courtesy of IDEXX.

Table 8.2. Normal serum protein values and abnormalities.

	Total serum protein	Albumin	Globulin
Normal value	60–70 g/L	25–40 g/L	20–35 g/L
Increased value	Dehydration	Dehydration	Dehydration
	Secondary to increased globulins		Acute inflammation
			Chronic inflammation
			Parasitism
			Liver failure
Decreased value	Secondary to decreased albumin	Protein losing enteropathy	Immune dysfunction
		Massive exudate production	
		Protein losing nephropathy	
		Liver failure	

Adapted from Coumbe 2001. *The Equine Veterinary Nursing Manual*, Oxford: Blackwell Science, Ltd.

Table 8.3. Acid-base disturbances.

Acid-base disturbances	Acidosis	Alkalosis
Respiratory	↑ carbon dioxide, ↓ pH	↓ carbon dioxide, ↑ pH
Metabolic	↓ bicarbonate, ↓ pH	↑ bicarbonate, ↑ pH

Muscle Enzymes

Levels of specific enzymes detected in the blood may help indicate the presence of muscle injury or disease. Monitoring these enzymes may aid in determining the severity and progression of the injury. The two important enzymes indicative of muscle damage are:

- *Creatine kinase (CK):* highest concentrations of this enzyme are found in skeletal muscle, cardiac muscle, and brain tissue. There is no apparent exchange of CK between the cerebrospinal fluid and plasma; therefore, in the absence of clinical cardiac disease, elevations in CK can be attributed primarily to skeletal muscle.
- *Aspartate aminotransferase (AST):* AST is not tissue specific, but it is found primarily in skeletal muscle, cardiac muscle, and liver, although activity is present in several other tissues.

Although not entirely specific, elevation of these enzymes is commonly associated with injury to skeletal muscle resulting from:

- Exertional rhabdomyolysis (e.g., azoturia, myositis, and tying up).
- Nutritional myodegeneration (e.g., selenium or vitamin E deficiency).
- Postanesthetic myopathies.
- Postendurance multisystemic disease.

The level and extent of muscle injury can be evaluated using plasma levels and half-life differences of these enzymes. Plasma levels of CK peak within 6 hours and decline rapidly, whereas AST plasma concentrations peak at 24 hours and remain high for 7 to 10 days.

Liver Enzymes

Acute damage to the liver can result in leakage of various soluble enzymes normally found within the cytoplasm of hepatocytes. Increased blood activity of these enzymes may indicate active hepatic disease. Hepatic enzymes include:

Sorbitol Dehydrogenase

Sorbitol dehydrogenase (SDH) is liver specific and is widely used in the evaluation of acute liver disease. A short half-life makes SDH ideal for evaluating acute, ongoing hepatic disease. Values usually return to baseline within 3 to 5 days after transient hepatic insult. The short half-life of SDH necessitates analysis within hours of collection. Normal blood activity of SDH in horses is less than 8 units/L. Foals 2 to 4 weeks of age may have SDH activity slightly higher than adults. Prolonged halothane anesthesia can elevate SDH levels. Elevation in SDH may indicate:

- Active hepatic necrosis.
- Obstructive or strangulating gastrointestinal disease.
- Acute toxic enteritis (bacterial toxins).

Glutamate Dehydrogenase

Glutamate dehydrogenase (GLDH) has the highest tissue activity in liver and increases in this enzyme can be considered specific for acute liver disease. The half-life GLDH is 14 hours.

Aspartate Aminotransferase

Aspartate aminotransferase (AST) was formerly known as glutamic oxaloacetic transaminase (GOT). All cells contain AST, but the highest concentrations are found in liver and skeletal muscle. Cardiac muscle, erythrocytes, intestinal cells, and kidney are also sources of AST. Increases are most commonly associated with muscle damage but may occur following acute hepatic necrosis. Hemolysis and lipemia falsely increase AST values. The half-life of AST is typically more than 2 weeks. Evaluation of AST is most useful when analyzed with other tissue-specific enzymes, such as CK, in muscle-related injury or disease. Serum AST activity in the adult horse ranges from 98 to 278 units/L.

Alanine Aminotransferase

Formerly known as glutamic pyruvic transaminase (GPT), alanine aminotransferase (ALT) is not specific to liver. Increases in ALT may be evident with acute liver disease, but myositis also results in increased blood levels; therefore ALT is not considered to be useful for predicting liver disease in horses.

Alkaline Phosphatase

Alkaline phosphatase (ALP) is not specific to liver. Tissues including bone, intestine, kidney, placenta, as well as leukocytes contain ALP. Cholestasis and certain drugs including glucocorticoids induce the production and release of ALP. Foals have ALP values that are two to three times higher than adult values due to increased osteoblastic activity. Increases in ALP may also be seen with pregnancy, hemolysis, and gastrointestinal disease.

Lactate Dehydrogenase

Five isoenzymes of lactate dehydrogenase (LDH) exist and are specific to liver, muscle, erythrocytes, intestinal cells and renal tissue, respectively. An increase in LDH is not useful unless the isoenzyme is identified. Isoenzyme-5 (LDH-5) is useful in evaluating acute hepatocellular disease in horses. LDH-5 levels typically return to normal within 4 days after transient insult to the liver. LDH-5 is also found in muscle and is therefore only specific for liver disease if other indicators of muscle damage, such as creatine kinase, are normal. LDH-5 is stable at room temperature for 36 hours.

Gamma Glutamyl Transferase

Gamma glutamyl transferase (GGT) is found in cells of the liver, renal tubules, and pancreas. Although not liver specific, some consider GGT levels to have the highest sensitivity for evaluating horses for evidence of liver disease, given that pancreatic disease is rare in horses and GGT contained within renal tubule cells is released into urine not the blood. The half-life of GGT is approximately 3 days. GGT is stable in serum for 2 days at room temperature or 30 days if serum is frozen. Normal values for adult horses typically don't exceed 30 units/L. GGT values for foals 2 weeks to 1 month of age are generally higher than adult values. Healthy donkeys, mules, and asses may have GGT values two to three times greater than adult horses.

Bilirubin

Serum bilirubin concentration is not a sensitive indicator of liver disease in horses. Total bilirubin concentration is comprised of both unconjugated and conjugated bilirubin. Increases in the unconjugated or prehepatic bilirubin may occur in the absence of hepatic disease. Anorexia in the horse results in an increase in unconjugated bilirubin. Hemolysis, intestinal obstruction, cardiac insufficiency, and the administration of certain drugs (e.g., steroids, heparin, and halothane anesthesia) may also result in increased unconjugated bilirubin. An increase in the conjugated bilirubin concentration is a more reliable indicator of hepatic disease.

Renal Function

Evaluation of the kidney, especially glomerular filtration rate (GFR), is most commonly accomplished by examining blood urea nitrogen (BUN) and serum creatinine (Cr) concentrations. *Azotemia* is the term that describes an elevation in BUN and Cr. Observable increases in BUN and Cr do not occur until 75% of nephrons are non-functional. These indices are of little value in evaluating early or minor changes in GFR; however, once elevated, minor increases are a sensitive indicator of ongoing renal deterioration. Dehydration, diseases of tissue catabolism, and high protein diets are often associated with small increases in BUN and Cr. Increases in Cr have been associated with acute severe myopathies.

Renal disease should be suspected if both BUN and Cr are significantly increased.

Intestinal Function

Assessment of intestinal function can be made by measuring increases in cellular enzymes released from damaged enterocytes in the face of disease. Enzymes typically measured in the clinical assessment of intestinal disease are:

- ALP: Intestinal ALP is the gut specific isoenzyme and is released following damage to intestinal epithelium.
- LDH: this specific isoenzyme is released secondary to intestinal injury.
- Parasites (i.e., small strongyles) or cellular infiltrates (i.e., lymphosarcoma or eosinophilic enteritis) invade the intestinal mucosa and result in increased serum concentrations of these gut specific isoenzymes.

The uptake of glucose from the small intestine into the blood can be measured by the oral glucose tolerance test. This test can be used to assess intestinal function; malabsorption, or disruption in glucose absorption, results from many conditions affecting the small intestine.

Blood Glucose

Glucose concentrations are measurable in serum or whole blood. The normal range for blood glucose in the adult horse is 70 to 110 mg/dl. Glucose concentration can be measured by:

- Dipsticks provide estimation of glucose concentration.
- Glucometers point of use devices that can measure glucose in whole blood with or without anticoagulants.
- Automated chemistry analyzers are most accurate assessment of glucose concentration.
- Transient increases in glucose levels are often associated with:
  - Excitement/stress.
  - Pregnancy.
  - Obesity.
  - Breeds (i.e., Shetland ponies).

Hyperglycemia in horses can be caused by:

- Excitement/stress.
- Acute severe colic.
- Cushing syndrome (pituitary pars intermedia dysfunction).
- Glucocorticoid administration.
- Administration of α_2-agonist (xylazine).

Hypoglycemia is rarely observed in adult horses but can be caused by:

- Pregnancy toxemia.
- Endotoxic shock.
- Liver failure.
- Inappetence in foals.

Foals have increased blood glucose concentration when compared to adults. Values for neonates can range from 108 to 190 mg/dl, with values decreasing to 105 to 165 mg/dl by 12 months of age. Monitoring glucose levels in sick foals is extremely important.

Serum Biochemistry Analysis

Veterinarians use clinical chemistry, as well as other laboratory tests to diagnose disease, monitor disease progression or response to therapy, and to screen for the presence of disease in apparently healthy animals. A wide variety of chemistry tests are offered by clinical pathology laboratories for this purpose. Laboratories differ on the combination of selected tests (or panels) that they offer to help veterinarians evaluate for disease in most body systems. Specialized chemistry tests not included in the normal panel may be useful in the diagnosis of specific disease processes. Veterinarians must be aware of the availability and purpose of these specialized tests to maximize the usefulness of the clinical chemistry laboratory for the diagnosis of specific disease.

In-house chemistry analyzers can provide additional advantages to practitioners over reference laboratory testing. Advantages include:

- Providing better medicine: in-clinic testing provides clients with immediate results and diagnosis, allowing prompt treatment and management of disease.

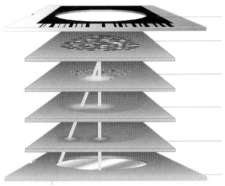

Patient sample is applied to
the top of the spreading layer

Spreading layer
Sample is distributed evenly

Filtering layer
Filters out substances that interfere with results

Reagent layer
Reagent reacts with sample

Indicator layer
Reacted sample collects for spectral analysis

Support layer
Optical interface

Figure 8.11. Veterinarian test dry slide filtering.
Courtesy of IDEXX.

• Better time management for clients: allows veterinarians to examine the patient, perform laboratory work, discuss results and prescribe treatment during a single visit. In-house diagnostics save time and maximize client satisfaction.

Immediate results build immediate value; an in-clinic laboratory allows veterinarians to provide information within minutes, reinforcing the value of their services to their clients.

A number of chemistry analyzers are available for in-clinic use. Three basic technologies are available: absorbance spectrophotometry (wet systems), top-read reflectance spectrophotometry (dry reagent strips), and bottom-read reflectance spectrophotometry (dry slides). Dry slide chemistry technology, which was introduced in 1978, is considered to be the gold standard in human health care. Dry slide chemistry slides are designed with a unique filtering layer that minimizes the affects of interfering substances such as those found in hemolyzed, icteric and lipemic samples (Figure 8.11). Absorbance and top-read reflectance spectrophotometric technologies do not allow for the separation of the sample from these interfering substances; consequently, sample results are often negatively impacted. An example of an analyzer that utilizes dry slide technology is the IDEXX Vet Test Chemistry Analyzer (Figure 8.12).

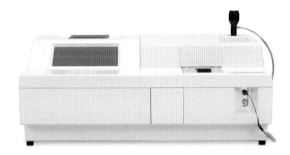

Figure 8.12. Veterinarian test.
Courtesy of IDEXX.

Urinalysis

Urine Collection

A urinalysis should be performed when urinary tract infection or renal disease is suspected. Collection of urine can be accomplished by methods including:

• Midstream catch during micturition.
• Catheterization of bladder.
• Cystocentesis in foals.

Collection of urine via catheterization is more appropriate for bacterial examination because contamination from the external genitalia is minimized. Catheterized samples often have increased

RBC, transitional epithelial cell, and protein concentrations.

Urine samples should be collected in a sterile container and analyzed immediately after collection for color, clarity, odor, turbidity, and specific gravity.

Urine Appearance

Normal equine urine is pale yellow to deep tan in color, and it is often turbid due to the presence of large amounts of calcium carbonate and mucus. Terms used to describe urine include:

Hematuria is a red discoloration due to the presence of RBCs, which will settle if the sample is allowed to stand for a period of time. Microscopic examination confirms the presence of RBCs.

Hemoglobinuria is a pink to red discoloration due to the presence of hemoglobin. Color will not settle to bottom if sample is left to stand; this distinguishes hemoglobinuria from hematuria. Plasma will usually have an abnormal orange/red discoloration.

Myoglobinuria is a brown to red/black discoloration due to the presence of myoglobin. Myoglobinuria can be distinguished from hemoglobinuria because it does not typically discolor plasma.

Urine color can also vary depending on hydration status or the administration of certain drugs. Two drugs associated with discoloration of urine in horses are rifampin and nitazoxanide. Rifampin, used to treat *Rhodococcus equi* infections in foals, often turns urine orange in color. Nitazoxanide, the active drug in Navigator Antiprotozoal Oral Paste, a treatment for equine protozoal myeloencephalitis (EPM), often turns urine a bright yellow.

Specific Gravity

Urine specific gravity is a measure of the concentration or amount (total weight) of substances dissolved in urine and is a useful estimate of the renal tubules to either concentrate or dilute urine. A refractometer can provide a quick and easy assessment of urine specific gravity; however, urine spe-

cific gravity is often overestimated due to the presence of larger molecules in urine, such as glucose or proteins. For this reason, the urine osmolality provides the most accurate estimate of urine concentration. Urine specific gravity is used to separate urine concentration into three categories:

- Urine more dilute than serum (hyposthenuric): Specific gravity <1.008; osmolality <260 mOsm/kg.
- Urine and serum similar in osmolality (isosthenuric): Specific gravity of 1.008 to 1.014; osmolality 260 to 300 mOsm/kg.
- Urine more concentrated than serum (hypersthenuric): Specific gravity >1.014; osmolality >300 mOsm/kg.
- Normal equine urine is often concentrated, having a specific gravity of 1.025 to 1.050 and an osmolality of 900 to 1200 mOsm/kg.

Urine pH

The pH of normal equine urine is usually alkaline (7.0–9.0). Acidic pH in the horse is sometimes observed after vigorous exercise or in the presence of urinary tract infection. The feeding of concentrates generally decreases the urinary pH toward a neutral (7.0) value.

Chemical Tests

A variety of biochemical tests may be performed on equine urine (Table 8.4). Reagent strip (dipstick) analysis is commonly used because of ease of measurement.

Urine Sediment

Examination of urine sediment is a useful diagnostic technique in the evaluation of urinary tract disorders in horses. Sediment should be examined within 60 minutes after collection of urine. To perform sediment examination:

- Centrifuge 10 ml of fresh urine in a conical plastic tube at 1,000 rpm for 3 to 5 minutes.
- Discard supernatant (this can be used for quantification of protein content).

Table 8.4. Biochemical tests on equine urine.

Test	Normal range	Disease that may cause abnormal finding
pH	7.0–9.0	Acidic with concentrate feeding or metabolic acidosis
Protein	<100 mg%	Massive concentrations seen with glomerular disease; slight increases with lower urinary tract inflammation
Glucose	None usually present	Glucosuria can be seen with hyperadrenocorticism, stress, or excess glucose administration
Ketones	None usually present	Ketosis is rarely observed in horses
Bilirubin	None usually present	Bilirubinuria rare; seen with obstructive jaundice or hemolysis
Hemoglobin	None usually present	Hemoglobinuria seen with severe intravascular hemolysis
Myoglobin	None usually present	Myoglobinuria seen with extensive muscle cell degeneration

Adapted from Coumbe 2001. *The Equine Veterinary Nursing Manual,* Oxford: Blackwell Science, Ltd.

Table 8.5. Examination of equine urine sediment.

Content	Normal finding	Disease that may cause abnormal result
Red blood cells	None usually present	May indicate inflammation, trauma, or neoplasia; also seen postcatheterization or cystocentesis
White blood cells	None usually present	Marked numbers associated with inflammation
Transitional/ epithelial cells	Few usually present	Inflammation, trauma, or neoplasia of bladder
Bacteria	None usually present	Presence significant if accompanied by inflammatory cells
Crystals (distinguished by morphologic appearance)	Calcium carbonate crystals commonly seen; phosphate and calcium oxalate crystals rare	Increased numbers of phosphate crystals may indicate infection
Casts	Cellular casts rarely seen; hyaline (protein) casts occasionally seen	Increased numbers of cellular casts may indicate tubular damage

Adapted from Coumbe 2001. *The Equine Veterinary Nursing Manual,* Oxford: Blackwell Science, Ltd.

- Resuspend pellet at bottom of tube with a wooden applicator stick.
- Transfer a drop of sediment to glass slide and apply coverslip.
- Stain slide.
- Examine sediment at low power for casts.
- Examine sediment at high power for erythrocytes, leukocytes, epithelial cells, bacteria, and parasites.

Urine sediment includes:

Casts represent the normal turnover of renal tubular epithelial cells and are a rare finding in normal equine urine but may be observed with inflammatory and infectious processes. Examination should be prompt as casts are unstable in alkaline urine.

RBCs may be a normal finding if sample is collected via catheterization or cystocentesis, otherwise less than 5 RBCs per high-powered field should be observed. Increased numbers of RBCs can be associated with inflammation, infection, toxemia, neoplasia, and exercise.

White blood cells in numbers greater than 10 per high-powered field are often associated with infection or inflammatory disorders.

Bacteria are not normal in equine urine. The absence of bacteria on sediment examination, however, does not rule out their presence. Bacterial cultures should be performed on urine collected by catheterization or cystocentesis (foals).

Crystals of calcium carbonate of variable size are a common finding in normal equine urine, as are calcium phosphate crystals and occasionally calcium oxalate crystals (Table 8.5).

- A few drops of 10% acetic acid solution will dissolve crystals and allow for an accurate assessment of urine sediment.

Collection of Body Fluids

Many types of body fluids can be collected and analyzed for diagnostic purposes. When collecting samples it is important that proper technique is used, including aseptic preparation of the surgical site and the use of sterile gloves and instruments. The use of proper physical and chemical restraint is also extremely important when collecting samples.

Samples should be collected in sterile containers and split into both anticoagulant (EDTA) collection tubes (for cytology) and collection tubes without anticoagulant (for biochemistry, bacteriology, and limited cytology). Additional types of collection tubes may be required for specific tests. Physical properties of collected fluids should be noted, such as volume, color, transparency, clot formation (if not in EDTA), and odor.

Peritoneal Fluid

Collection and analysis of peritoneal fluid (PF) is a common diagnostic technique performed on many equine patients with gastrointestinal disease. PF analysis can help determine a specific diagnosis or may indicate inflammatory, vascular, or ischemic disease of the intestine. Increased protein concentration in the PF indicates acute vascular compromise, and protein concentrations and cellular components (RBCs and white blood cells) in the PF increase because vascular compromise of the intestine is prolonged. Severe inflammation results in the presence of large quantities of protein and white blood cells, primarily neutrophils, in the PF. The presence of bacteria is indicative of intestinal mucosal barrier breakdown and when combined with ingesta, and degenerate neutrophils indicate intestinal rupture.

Synovial Fluid

The collection of synovial fluid from joints (arthrocentesis) is indicated whenever joint inflammation or hemorrhage is suspected. Normal joint fluid is clear to yellow in color, viscous in nature, and should contain less than 2,500 nucleated cells/dl. The cellular ratio should be 50% neutrophils and 50% lymphocytes/monocytes. The protein content in normal joint fluid should be less than 2.5 mg/dl. Infection should be considered if the total cell count exceeds 10,000 cells/dl or in cases with nucleated cell counts between 2,500 and 10,000 cells/dl when greater than 90% of the cells are neutrophils. In many cases treatment decisions must be made quickly. In-house evaluation of joint fluid can provide a quick assessment of protein content (refractometer), white blood cell count (hemocytometer), and the presence of neutrophils and bacteria (differential stain). If additional information is required, the sample can be sent to a reference laboratory for further analysis. If infection is suspected, prompt treatment is recommended in an effort to minimize the destructive nature of bacteria and the products of inflammation.

Cerebrospinal Fluid

Collection and analysis of cerebrospinal fluid (CSF) is of diagnostic importance when evaluating neurological disease in the horse. Two different sites from which CSF may be collected include the lumbosacral space and the atlantooccipital (cisterna magna) space. Regardless of the collection site, the use of sterile technique when collecting CSF is extremely important. Proper sedation is required when acquiring CSF from the lumbosacral site and general anesthesia is necessary when the CSF sample is obtained from the cisterna magna.

CSF samples should be visually evaluated following collection for clarity and clotting. Normal CSF is clear and does not clot. Clots may represent the presence of fibrinogen secondary to inflammation. The turbidity of CSF increases with increased cell counts (RBCs and white blood cells), epidural fat, bacteria, fungal, or amoebic organisms. Cytology and culture are helpful in determining the cause of CSF turbidity. In most cases, CSF samples are sent to an outside laboratory for analysis. Normal protein values range from 20 to 124 mg/dl depending on the measurement technique. Total protein concentration is higher in CSF taps acquired from the lumbosacral space as compared to those acquired from the atlantooccipital space. CSF

Table 8.6. Normal features of fluid samples.

Feature	Peritoneal fluid	Pleural fluid	Synovial fluid	Cerebrospinal fluid
Color	Pale yellow/yellow	Yellow	Pale yellow	Colorless
Turbidity	Clear	Clear	Clear	Clear
Viscosity	Not tacky	Not tacky	Tacky	Not tacky
Nucleated cell count	$<5 \times 10^9$ cells/L	$<10 \times 10^9$ cells/L	$<0.5 \times 10^9$ cells/L	$<0.01 \times 10^9$ cells/L
Predominant cells present	Large mononuclear cells/neutrophils	Large mononuclear cells/neutrophils	Mononuclear cells	Mononuclear cells
Protein concentration	<20 g/L	<40 g/L	<15 g/L	<1.0 g/L
Other				CPK: < 25 IU/L Glucose 1.7–4.2 mmol/L

Adapted from Coumbe 2001. *The Equine Veterinary Nursing Manual*, Oxford: Blackwell Science, Ltd.

enzyme activity, such as CK and aspartate amino-transferase, may be increased in certain diseases such as EPM, polyneuritis equi, equine degenerative myopathy, and equine motor neuron disease. An increase in CSF lactate concentration may also serve as a nonspecific indicator of neurological disease in the horse (Table 8.6).

Pleural Fluid

Pleural fluid is collected by placement of a needle through an intercostal space (thoracocentesis). Normally, only small amounts of fluid are present; however, in cases of pleural disease, large amounts of fluid can accumulate. Ultrasonography is useful for identifying fluid and for assisting in proper needle placement. Normal pleural fluid contains less than 10,000 nucleated cells/μl and less than 2.5 g/dl of protein. Aerobic and anaerobic cultures should be submitted. A putrid odor often indicates the presence of anaerobic bacteria, which may worsen the prognosis. Therapeutic drainage of the pleural space is commonly required if large amounts of fluid are present.

Tissue Biopsy

Histopathological examination of tissue biopsies may often result in definitive diagnosis of disease. Other techniques, such as fine-needle aspirates and smears, are often more limited in the information they can provide. Tissue biopsies should be placed in an appropriate transport solution such as 10% formalin for transport to a diagnostic or reference laboratory for histologic evaluation. Various tissues can be biopsied in the equine patient including:

Skin Biopsy

The site selected for a skin biopsy should not be aseptically prepped because shaving and scrubbing removes crusts and epithelial tissue that may be important in determining a diagnosis. The use of local anesthetics is usually sufficient for obtaining most skin biopsies; however, in some cases sedation is necessary.

Four surgical techniques can be used to biopsy the skin: excisional, wedge, punch, or elliptic. The ideal technique for removal of a single nodule is excisional, which allows for the removal of the lesion at the time of histologic diagnosis. When the lesion is a tumor that is too large to excise, a wedge biopsy should be performed. Most lesions can be successfully biopsied using the punch technique. The exception to this would be vesicular, bullous, or ulcerative lesions.

Muscle Biopsy

Muscle biopsies can be useful in providing insight into particular manifestations of neuromuscular disease. Biopsies should be taken from both diseased or abnormal and normal muscle for comparative purposes. Percutaneous needle biopsy and open incisional biopsy performed under local anesthesia both provide diagnostic samples. Fixation of muscle tissue depends on the type of analysis. Routine histopathologic samples can be placed in formalin. Samples that are to undergo histochemical analysis require special fixation to ensure rapid freezing while minimizing freezing artifacts. Special fixatives may be required if other histopathologic techniques are required.

Liver Biopsy

A liver biopsy can provide important diagnostic, prognostic, and therapeutic information. Samples should be immediately placed into formalin for histopathologic evaluation and in transport media for culture of microorganisms. Complications associated with this technique include hemorrhage, pneumothorax, peritonitis from bile leakage, colon or abscess puncture, and spread of infection from infectious hepatitis. These complications can be reduced by performing a hemostatic profile to assess the risk of hemorrhage and by using ultrasonography to guide needle placement.

Endometrial Biopsy

An endometrial biopsy is considered to be a routine component of a general breeding soundness examination in the mare and will provide information that may assist in predicting the likelihood of a mare's ability to carry a foal to term and in determining appropriate treatment for infertility. Endometrial biopsies can reveal the degree of inflammatory change and the presence of degenerative changes, such as periglandular fibrosis and enlarged or dilated lymphatics, which may indicate a uterine clearance problem. Biopsy findings must be assessed in conjunction with the physical examination findings and other diagnostics, such as ultrasonographic examination of the uterus when determining the breeding soundness of mares.

Endometrial biopsies are classified into four categories (I, IIA, IIB, and III).

Renal Biopsy

Renal biopsy can be a useful diagnostic tool in the horse for identifying the affected region of the kidney and the type, chronicity, and severity of lesions. Renal biopsy is performed with the horse sedated and restrained in stocks. A Tru-cut biopsy needle or a triggered biopsy device is guided into the renal parenchyma; ultrasonographic guidance is helpful and reduces the risk of hemorrhage and rupture of the bowel. Collected tissue should be placed in formalin for histopathologic and electron microscopic evaluation and additional samples can be used for bacterial culture and immunofluorescence testing. Renal biopsy results have most commonly been used to document the presence of chronic disease in horses even though the inciting cause cannot often be determined because significant renal disease develops before the onset of azotemia (elevated BUN and Cr). Pathologic lesions are widespread by this point and often merely reflect end stage renal disease. In some instances, renal biopsy can help differentiate between infectious (pyelonephritis) and congenital (renal dysplasia) kidney disease. One must consider the limitations and the risks of renal biopsy before performing this technique in the horse.

Pulmonary Biopsy

Percutaneous lung biopsy has been used to further investigate radiographic and ultrasonographic findings that are consistent with pulmonary neoplasia or granuloma.

This procedure should not be performed if the patient is tachypnic (rapid respiration), in respiratory distress, exhibiting excessive coughing, or is known to have a bleeding disorder. Pulmonary biopsy is not indicated in cases of pneumonia, pleuropneumonia, or pulmonary abscessation. Complications that may occur following pulmonary biopsy include epistaxis, pulmonary hemorrhage, tachypnea, respiratory distress, and in rare instances, the development of hemothorax (blood within the thoracic cavity).

Intestinal Biopsy

Histopathological examination of tissues obtained from the intestines is often used to diagnose chronic inflammatory, infiltrative, or neoplastic conditions and can be useful in assessing the degree of damage following obstructive or ischemic events. Rectal mucosal biopsies are collected in a similar fashion to endometrial biopsy; tissue is easily collected and there are few complications. Full thickness intestinal biopsies require a surgical approach either through a flank incision or ventral midline approach. Laparoscopy offers a safe approach for visualization of the large intestine and other abdominal structures and biopsy of masses, lymph nodes, mesentery, or intestinal serosa. Endoscopy offers a safe approach to tissue collection from the upper gastrointestinal tract.

Skin and Hair Analysis

Dermatological problems are common in horses. In most instances, analysis of skin and hair samples allows for a diagnosis of the underlying problem. A number of different collection techniques are available for identifying the causative agent.

Hair Plucks

These useful in identifying dermatophyte (ringworm) infections. Preparation of skin before sampling includes wiping the affected area with 70% isopropyl alcohol to reduce the level of contaminants and allowing skin to dry. Sterile forceps should be used to collect hair plucks. Samples should be obtained from the edge of suspected lesion (i.e., hairless region) and placed in a sterile container. Diagnosis of ringworm infections (dermatophytosis) is often made by placing hair plucks on fungal specific media; dermatophytes are allowed to grow over a period of days permitting identification. In most cases, ringworm infections

are successfully treated before obtaining fungal growth results.

Hair Brushings

These also useful in investigating dermatophytosis in horses.

Acetate Tape Preparations

These preparations are useful in identifying *Oxyuris equi* (pinworm) infections (Figure 8.13). This technique can also be useful in identifying mites or lice. Materials required include acetate (nonfrosted) tape, mineral oil, and glass microscope slides. The procedure includes pressing the acetate tape over several areas in the anal and perianal region when looking for *O. equi* eggs. When attempting to identify Chorioptes mites, the suspect area should be lightly clipped and sampled in a similar manner. The tape is then applied (adhesive side down) to a glass microscope slide that has been coated with mineral oil (mineral oil aids in clearing debris and facilitates examination of the slide). Identification of parasites can be made by examining the slide with a 10× objective.

Skin Scrapings

These scrapings used primarily to demonstrate microscopic ectoparasites, specifically mites. Materials necessary for skin scraping are a sterile container, mineral oil, a #10 scalpel blade, glass slides, and coverslips. Superficial skin scrapings provide information about the surface of the epidermis. Deep skin scrapings collect material from within the hair follicle. Capillary bleeding indicates that scrapings were deep enough. Material collected from the scrapings should be placed in a sterile container until further examination is possible. Microscopic examination beginning with 10× magnification of the sample placed in a small amount of mineral oil beneath a cover slip. Significant findings can then be examined using the 40× objective. Photographs of biting lice (*Damalinia equi*), sucking lice (*Hematopinus asini*), and mites (*Chorioptes equi*) are found in Figure 8.14.

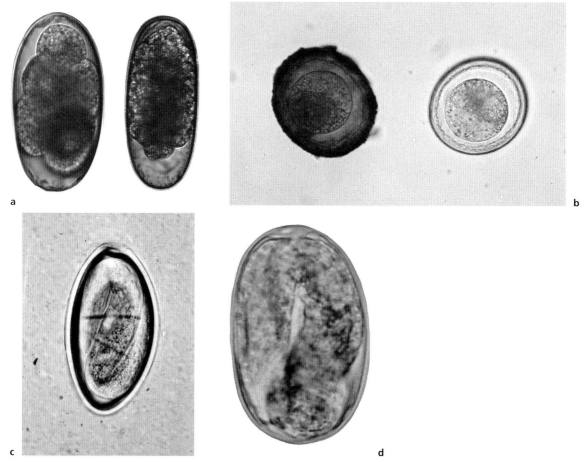

Figure 8.13. Common equine parasite eggs. a) Strongyle, b) Parascaris, c) Oxyuris, and d) Strongyloides westeri. Courtesy of Dr. Dwight D. Bowman, Cornell University.

Cytology

Cytology can be useful when lesions are pustules, vesicles, nodules, tumors, or swellings. Cytological testing can quickly determine the presence or absence of an infectious organism and provide an assessment of the cell type (neoplastic versus inflammatory) present in the lesion. The surface of the lesion(s) should be cleaned with an antiseptic preparation and allowed to dry. Pustules and vesicles can be easily sampled by gently opening an intact lesion with the tip of a sterile #15 scalpel blade and collecting the contents on a glass micro-scope slide. After the slide is allowed to air-dry it can be heat fixed, Giemsa- or Wright-stained, and examined microscopically.

Evaluation of nodules, tumors and swellings is best accomplished using fine-needle aspiration with a 22- to 25-gauge needle on a 12-ml syringe. The needle is introduced into the mass and negative pressure applied. The needle can then be removed from the syringe, the syringe filled with air, and the needle reattached. The contents of the syringe can then be expressed onto a glass microscope slide, which is then dried, fixed, and stained as previously described.

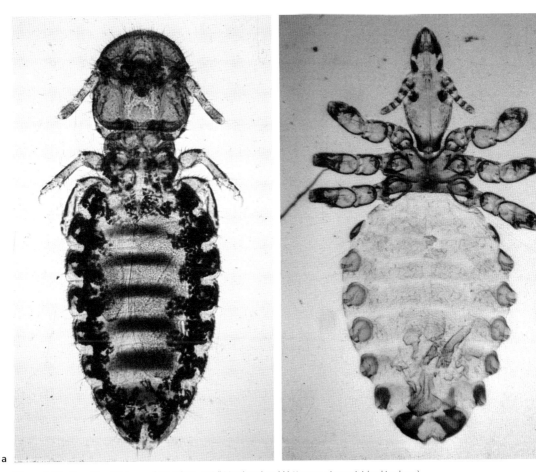

a

b

Figure 8.14. Lice of the U.S. horse. a) Damalinia equi (biting louse) and b) Haematopinus asini (sucking louse). Courtesy of Dr. Dwight D. Bowman, Cornell University.

Fecal Analysis

Feces collected for analysis should be fresh to ensure accurate results. When collecting samples directly from the horse, it is extremely important to use proper restraint and care because there are risks to both the horse and personnel. A minimum of 10 g of feces should be collected. Samples that are more than 2 hours old should be stored at 4°C until examined to prevent the further development of parasitic stages. If samples are to be shipped to a laboratory for analysis they can be cooled to 4°C and then packed with ice for shipment. Fecal samples are best stored and shipped in WhirlPak bags, small plastic bags, plastic containers, disposable laboratory gloves, or rectal palpation gloves turned inside out. All samples should be clearly labeled using a black indelible marker; information should include animal identification, date of sample collection, and the name of the person responsible for the sample.

Equine fecal samples can be assessed in clinic for number and type of parasite ova using a number of fecal flotation methods. These tests concentrate eggs and oocysts present in the feces into a drop of solution for easy identification and counting. Important comparative factors in the fecal flotation techniques are the specific gravity of the flotation solution, the viscosity or type of solution used, and the rate of shrinkage or contraction caused by the solution. A specific gravity that is too low will not float many of the parasitic stages, whereas a solution with a specific gravity too high makes identification difficult because of cell shrinkage. Higher specific gravity solutions can also decrease test efficiency by increasing the amount of debris visible during microscopic examination. Most parasitic stages float efficiently at a specific gravity of 1.2.

Procedures for Fecal Floatation

Parasite eggs may be floated using a centrifuge or using gravity alone if large numbers of parasite eggs are present. When small numbers of parasite eggs are present, then centrifugation is a superior method of analysis.

Fecal Analysis by Gravity Floatation

Take approximately 3 g (a tablespoon full) of feces and mix with enough floatation solution to form a slurry. Strain through metal strainer (standard kitchen strainer or a tea strainer) or a layer of cheesecloth. Discard the solids and place the remaining fecal solution into a test tube or similar vessel. Fill it to top and place a coverslip on top. Set the laboratory timer for 10 minutes. After 10 minutes, remove the slide or coverslip, place it on a microscope slide and examine under the microscope.

Fecal Analysis by Centrifugation

Prepare the feces as described for gravity floatation. Place the remaining fecal solution into a centrifuge tube. If the centrifuge has swinging buckets, then place a coverslip on top. If the centrifuge has a fixed angle, then leave the coverslip off. Spin the tubes at 800 to 1,000 rpm for 5 to 7 minutes. Remove the cloverslip (or if fixed angle, take a drop off the top of the tube) and examine under the microscope.

Examination by Microscope

The microscope used for fecal examination should have 4×, 10×, and 40× objectives (thus providing 40×, 100×, and 400× magnification with a 10× eyepiece). It is also helpful to have an eyepiece micrometer for measurement of unusual parasite ova. Because the fecal solutions are hostile to precision optical instruments, most veterinary laboratories have a microscope that is dedicated to fecal analysis and save the better microscopes for examination of other clinical materials.

When examining fecal preparations it is important to examine the entire surface of the coverslip. The mechanical stage makes it easy to the move the slide from side to side and top to bottom. The most common parasite ova found in U.S. horses include the large and small strongyles and the roundworms *Parascaris equoroum* and *O. equi*. There are many species of strongyles and their ova look alike under the microscope. With the exception of *Nematodirus*, it is only possible to determine the exact species by using special methods that involve hatching the ova and examining the resulting larvae. Less common are the ova from the tapeworm *Anoplocephala perfoliata*, the intestinal threadworm *Strongyloides westeri*, and oocysts from the coccidian *Eimeria leuckarti*. Photographs of these parasite ova are found in Figures 8.15 and 8.16.

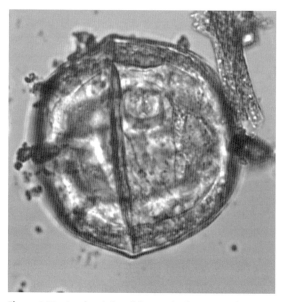

Figure 8.15. *Anoplocephala perfoliata* egg (equine tapeworm). Courtesy of Dr. Dwight D. Bowman, Cornell University.

212

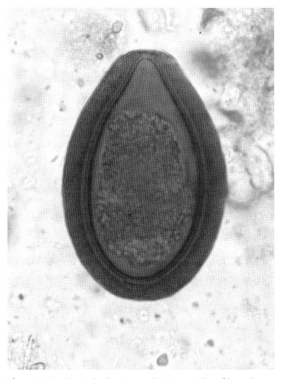

Figure 8.16. *Eimeria leuckarti* oocysts (enteric coccidian of horses). Courtesy of Dr. Dwight D. Bowman, Cornell University.

Virology

Viral infections are responsible for some of the most important diseases of horses including equine influenza, equine herpes virus (EHV), equine infectious anemia (EIA), various encephalitis viruses and more recently, West Nile virus. Treatment of viral disease remains challenging because few antiviral drugs are available and their use is often ineffective, impractical, and cost prohibitive in the horse. Primary treatment of viral disease includes supportive care and control of secondary complications such as bacterial infections.

Diagnosis of Viral Disease

The diagnosis of viral disease has most often relied on the detection of antibodies, viral antigens, and the demonstration of virus itself. Methods of detection include:

- Viral isolation (VI): direct demonstration of virus in living cells or laboratory animals.
- Viral antigens (AG): techniques include enzyme-linked immunosorbent assay (ELISA), polymerase chain reaction (PCR), immunofluorescence (IF), or radioimmunoassay (RIA).
- Antibody titer (AB): the agar gel immunodiffusion (AGID) test or the Coggins test as it is known, if EIA is suspected.

Advances in molecular biology have improved viral diagnostics in the horse. Recombinant viral proteins or peptides for use in serologic testing have greatly increased the sensitivity and specificity of antibody testing. The ability to isolate viruses in clinical samples has also improved in recent years. Immunohistochemistry and the polymerase chain reaction (PCR) are now routine tests, which are sensitive, specific, and provide rapid identification of viruses.

Sample Submission

Detection of viruses can be accomplished by submission of swabs (i.e., nasal), blood, body fluids, or tissues. Samples should be collected early in the course of disease and transferred to a special transport medium that provides viral support while inhibiting bacterial growth. Samples should be shipped on ice immediately after collection. Contacting the reference laboratory before collection and shipment of samples is an important step that can improve detection rates. Serial sampling may be required to demonstrate rising antibody titers (Table 8.7).

Microbiology

Microorganisms, or microbes, are living organisms that are too small to be seen by the naked eye. They are single celled or unicellular in nature and include bacteria, fungi, and protozoa.

Bacterial Morphology

The basic morphologic forms of bacteria include:

- Bacilli (rod shaped).
- Cocci (spherical).

- Spirilla (spiral shaped).
- Vibrios (curved).

Bacterial Classification

Bacteria can further be classified by their staining characteristics, which are dependent on characteristics of the cell wall. Examples include:

- Gram stain positive: *Clostridium* species.
- Gram stain negative: *Salmonella* species.
- Acid-fast bacilli: *Mycobacterium*.

Bacteria can also be classified as aerobic or anaerobic in nature. Aerobic bacteria, such as those found on the skin of horses, require the presence of oxygen

for survival. Anaerobic bacteria can be grouped into obligate and facultative anaerobes. Obligate anaerobes cannot withstand oxygen in the environment, whereas facultative anaerobes will grow and replicate with or without oxygen.

Bacterial Culture

Bacteria can be grown in a clinic laboratory for purposes of identification. Providing the required nutrients and growth environment (i.e., pH, temperature) is necessary for bacterial growth. Specific culture media provide the nutrients required for growth of a particular bacterial species. Both solid and liquid media are used depending on the type of bacteria suspected. A number of different growth media available for use in veterinary practice are listed in Table 8.8.

Once the appropriate culture plate has been selected, the bacterial sample must be applied to or "plated" onto the medium. Correct "plating" allows the sample to grow thinly on the medium making identification possible. The "streaking method" used to apply the sample to culture media is described in Table 8.9.

Samples can be prepared and examined within a practice setting, or they can be sent to a reference laboratory. Certain bacterial samples (i.e., contagious equine metritis swabs [CEM]) usually require a trained laboratory technician.

Table 8.7. Viral samples and tests.

Sample type	Types of virus isolated	Isolation technique
Blood	Equine influenza virus	Virus isolation
	Equine herpes virus	Viral antigens
		Antibody titer
Tissues	Fetal tissues for equine herpes virus	Viral antigens
		Viral isolation
Swabs	Nasopharyngeal swabs for equine influenza, conjunctival swabs for equine arteritis virus	Viral isolation
Body fluids	Semen for equine arteritis virus	Viral isolation

Adapted from Coumbe 2001. *The Equine Veterinary Nursing Manual*, Oxford: Blackwell Science, Ltd.

Table 8.8. Media commonly used in veterinary practice.

Medium	Plate(P) or broth(B)	Type	Bacteria grown
Nutrient agar	P	Simple (basal)	Any
Chocolate agar	P	Enriched	Certain pathogens
Blood agar	P	Enriched	Most pathogens
MacConkey's agar	P	Selective (enteric species) and differential	Enteric species; lactose fermenters versus non lactose fermenters
Deoxycholate citrate agar	P	Selective	*Salmonella* species
Sabouraud's agar	P	Selective	Fungi
Nutrient broth	B	Simple (basal)	Any
MacConkey's broth	B	Selective	*Enteric* species
Selenite broth	B	Enrichment	*Salmonella* species

Adapted from Coumbe 2001. *The Equine Veterinary Nursing Manual*, Oxford: Blackwell Science, Ltd.

Table 8.9. How to plate bacteria.

- How to plate bacteria:
- Place a small sample of culture (i.e., one drop) onto the medium at the edge of the plate.
- Flame a platinum bacterial loop until it is red hot. After loop is allowed to cool touch onto agar somewhere distant from the sample.
- Streak from the sample in a zigzag across one-third of the plate.
- Use a hooded Bunsen flame to heat the loop again until red hot.
- Cool loop and repeat streaking, going from the zigzags already present to form a new patch over another one third of the plate.
- Repeat again to cover the last one third of the plate and lid the plate before incubating.

Adapted from Coumbe 2001. *The Equine Veterinary Nursing Manual*, Oxford: Blackwell Science, Ltd.

Smears of bacterial cultures are prepared for staining and identification. A properly prepared smear accomplishes two things: It causes bacteria to adhere to a slide so that they can be stained and observed; it also kills the bacteria, rendering pathogenic bacteria safe for handling. In the preparation of bacterial smears it is important to learn to recognize the correct density of bacteria on the slide surface. Identification is complicated by overlapping of bacteria when the sample is too dense; locating and identifying bacteria is made difficult if the sample is applied too thinly. Bacterial smears may be prepared by the following methods:

- Directly from a swab that is then rolled onto a clean microscope slide. Examples include swabs obtained from a wound or vesicle.
- Transfer of a liquid using a wire loop or pipette. One drop is applied to a slide. An example of this would be abscess contents.
- Transfer of a bacterial colony from an agar plate using a sterile loop. The colony is placed in one drop of sterile water on a microscope slide and mixed.
- Slides are allowed to air-dry; they are then passed through a flame (two to three quick passes is sufficient) to kill bacteria and cause them to adhere.
- After the slide cools the staining procedure is conducted.

Staining Techniques

Gram Stain

The Gram stain is routinely used as an initial procedure in the identification of an unknown bacterial species. Bacteria bear a slight negative charge and usually bind positively charged dyes, such as methylene blue and crystal violet. Bacterial species can be classified as gram-positive, gram-negative, or gram-variable, depending on the ability of cells to retain the blue dye. Gram-negative bacteria do not retain the dark blue color, but they can be counterstained a light red and observed using bright field microscopy. Gram staining is also referred to as "differential staining" because two different dyes are used to identify bacteria.

Acid-Fast Stain

The property of acid fastness, detected by use of an acid-fast stain, is primarily of clinical application to detect members of the genus Mycobacterium. *M. tuberculosis*, the etiologic agent of tuberculosis, is the most common pathogen in this group. Other microorganisms, particularly the Nocardia, can be identified by their acid-fast characteristics. The term *acid fast* is derived from the resistance displayed by acid-fast bacteria to decolorization by acid once they have been stained by another dye.

Methylene Blue Stain

This stain is considered to be a simple stain in comparison to the Gram stain or acid-fast stain, both of which require a counterstaining step. Methylene blue stain is especially useful for observing metachromasia (multiple colors with single dye) in bacterial species such as *Corynebacteria*.

Acquiring Swabs

In equine practice it is common to take swabs from a number of sites. It is important to remember that bacterial swabs must be processed quickly to maximize the chances of identifying the bacteria involved. It is also important to obtain samples aseptically avoiding contamination. Sites commonly sampled in horses include:

- Nasopharyngeal swabs—suspected *Streptococcus equi* (strangles) infection.
- Uterine swabs—infectious endometritis cases.
- Abscesses and wounds.
- Clitoral sinus swabs—to detect *Taylorella equigenitalis*, the causative organism in CEM.
- Surgical sites—suspected areas of infection.
- Conjunctival swabs.

Sensitivity Testing

Selection of the appropriate antibiotic for treatment of bacterial infections is important given the incidence of resistant bacterial organisms. In some cases, a diagnosis can be made based on the clinical experience of the veterinarian and appropriate antimicrobial therapy initiated. In cases involving infections from unknown causes, samples should be submitted to the appropriate laboratory for isolation and identification so that effective antimicrobial agents can be selected. Tests such as the Kirby-Bauer, E test, or minimum inhibitory concentration (MIC) method should be used if the identified organism has unpredictable susceptibility patterns. Serologic demonstration of rising antibodies can be used for the identification of certain pathogens (i.e., ehrlichiosis, leptospirosis, and Brucellosis).

References and Further Readings

Bowman, D. D. 2003. *Georgis' Parasitology for Veterinarians.* 8th ed. St. Louis: Saunders.

Benjamin, M. M. 1978. *Outline of Veterinary Clinical Pathology.* 3rd ed. Ames: Iowa State University Press.

Carter, G. R., and M. M. Chengappa. 1991. *Essentials of Veterinary Bacteriology and Mycology.* 4th ed. Malvern: Lea & Febiger.

Foreyt, W. J. 1994. *Veterinary Parasitology Reference Manual,* 3rd ed. Pullman: Washington State University.

Hodgson, D. R., and R. J. Rose. 1994. *The Athletic Horse: Principles and Practice of Equine Medicine.* Philadelphia: W.B. Saunders.

McKinnon, A. O., and J. L. Voss. 1993. *Equine Reproduction.* Malvern: Lea & Febiger.

Reagan, W. J., T. G. Sanders, and D. B. DeNicola. 1998. *Veterinary Hematology: Atlas of Common Domestic Species.* Ames: Iowa State University Press.

Reed, S. M., W. M. Bayly, and D. C. Sellon. 2004. *Equine Internal Medicine.* 2nd ed. St. Louis: Elsevier.

Smith, B. P. 1996. *Large Animal Internal Medicine,* 2nd ed. St. Louis: Mosby-Year Book.

Thrall, M. A. 2006. *Veterinary Hematology and Clinical Chemistry.* Ames: Blackwell Publishers.

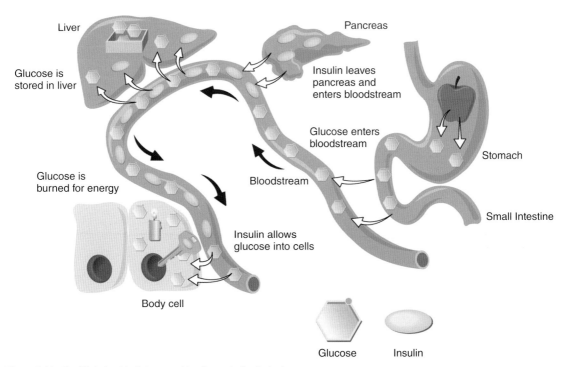

Figure 2.11. Simplified pictorial of glucose and insulin metabolism in the horse.

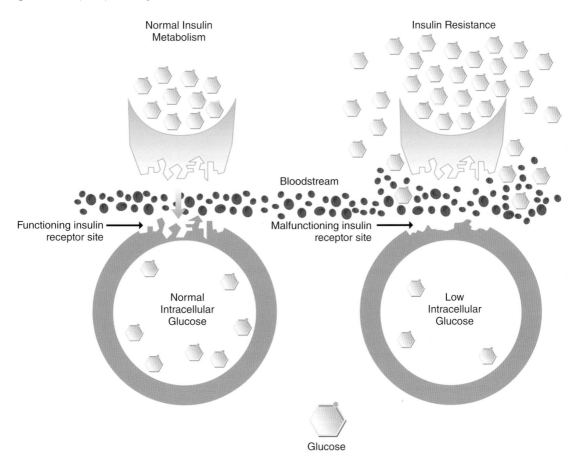

Figure 2.12. Potential theory of causative factor related to insulin resistance, involving damaged insulin receptors.

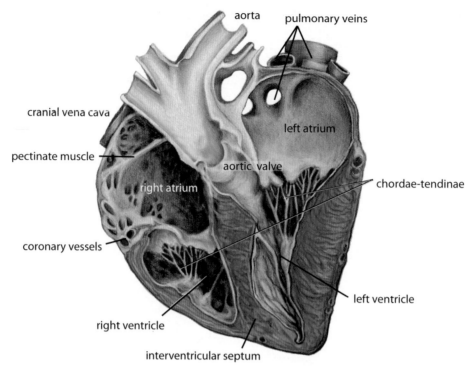

Figure 3.2. Longitudinal section anatomy of the equine heart.
Courtesy of Dr. Robin Peterson.

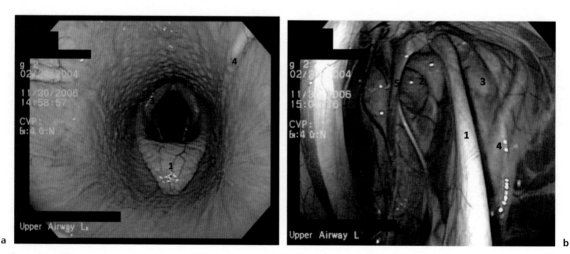

Figure 3.6. *(A)* Endoscopic view of the larynx. 1, epiglottis; 2, vocal folds; 3, arytenoid cartilages; 4, pharyngeal openings to the guttural pouches. *(B)* Endoscopic view of the left guttural pouch. 1, stylohyoid bone; 2, medial compartment; 3, lateral compartment; 4, external carotid artery; 5, internal carotid artery.
Courtesy of Dr. L. M. Riggs.

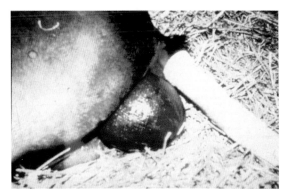

Figure 4.5. A red velvety bag will protrude out of the vulva when the chorioallantois separates prematurely from the endometrium during labor. It must be cut and the foal delivered immediately.
Courtesy Dr. LeBlanc.

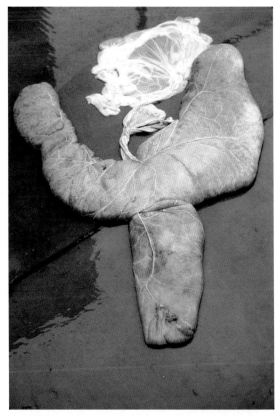

Figure 4.6. Fetal membranes. The chorioallantois, a large blue-tinged sac, is attached to the endometrium. Fetal side is shown in picture. The smaller white tissue is the amnion. It surrounds the fetus during pregnancy.
Courtesy Dr. LeBlanc.

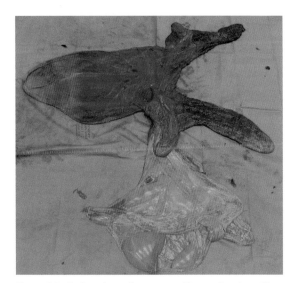

Figure 4.7. Fetal membranes from a mare with ascending placentitis. Note the brown, granular appearance of the maternal side of the chorioallantois in the area of the cervical star.
Courtesy Dr. LeBlanc.

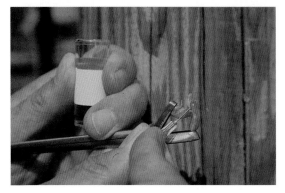

Figure 4.14. Endometrial tissue sample collected for histological evaluation needs to be lifted gently out of the basket and then placed in Bouin's solution.
Courtesy Dr. LeBlanc.

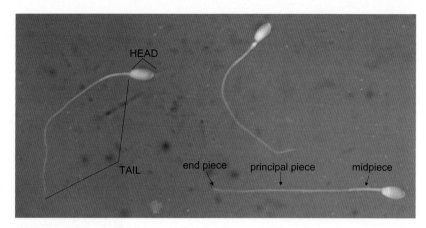

Figure 4.17. Spermatozoa fixed with eosin-nigrosin stain (1,000×). Courtesy of Dr. Kelleman.

HEAD

TAIL

end piece   principal piece   midpiece

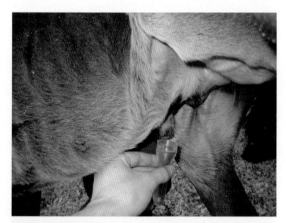

Figure 6.2. Dipping the umbilicus with chlorhexidine. Courtesy of Dr. Steeve Giguere.

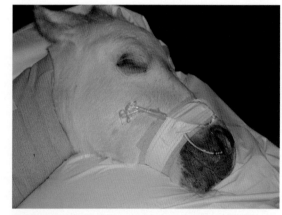

Figure 6.3. Nasogastric tube secured with a Chinese finger snare. Courtesy Dr. Dana Zimmel.

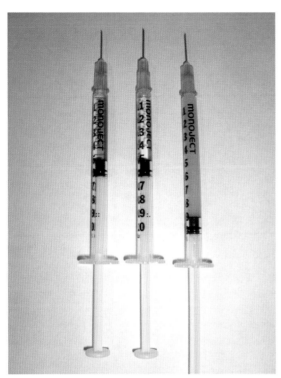

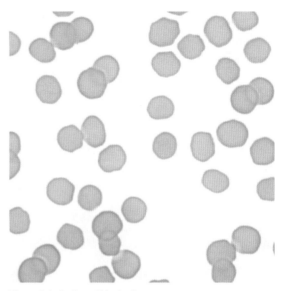

Figure 8.1. Equine red blood cells.
Courtesy of IDEXX and Dr. Dennis DeNicola.

Figure 7.2. Photograph depicting acepromazine *(left)*, romifidine *(middle)*, and a combination of acepromazine and romifidine *(right)*. Note the precipitates that have formed when the two drugs are combined in the same syringe.

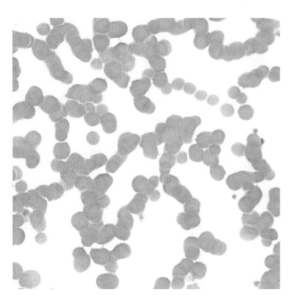

Figure 8.2. Rouleax formation.
Courtesy of IDEXX and Dr. Dennis DeNicola.

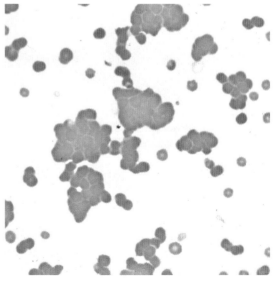

Figure 8.3. Red blood cell agglutination.
Courtesy of IDEXX and Dr. Dennis DeNicola.

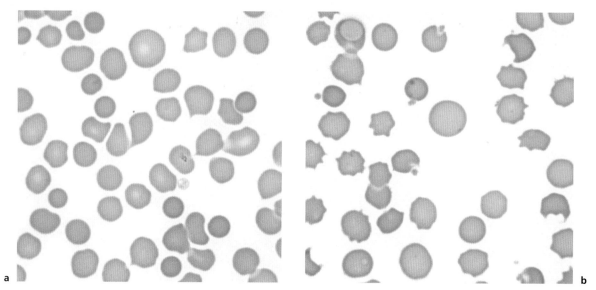

Figure 8.4. *(A)* Anisocytosis and *(B)* Heinz bodies.
Courtesy of IDEXX and Dr. Dennis DeNicola.

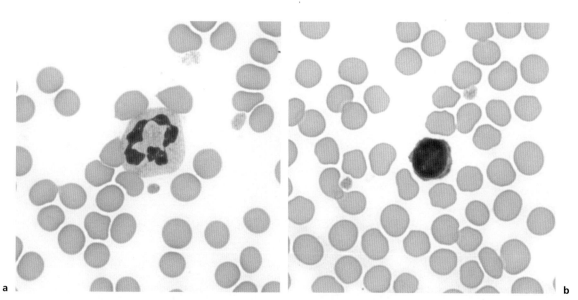

Figure 8.5. *(A)* Segmented neutrophil; *(B)* small lymphocyte; *(C)* monocyte; *(D)* eosinophil; *(E)* basophil; and *(F)* large lymphocyte.
Courtesy of Wiley-Blackwell, *Veterinary hematology: atlas of common domestic species.*

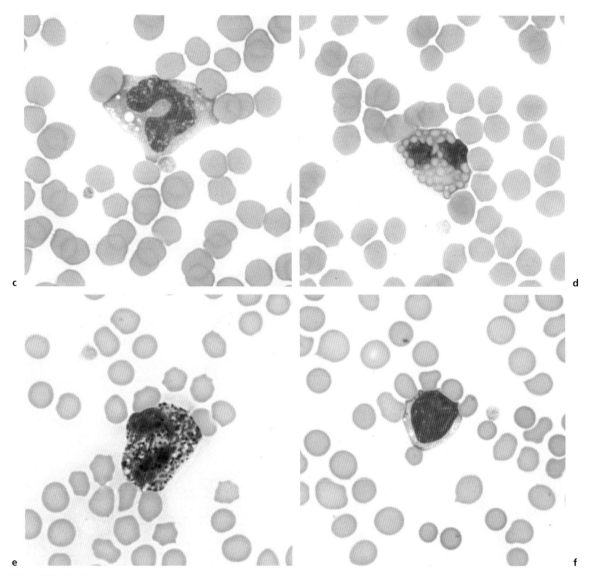

c

d

e

f

Figure 8.5. *Continued*.

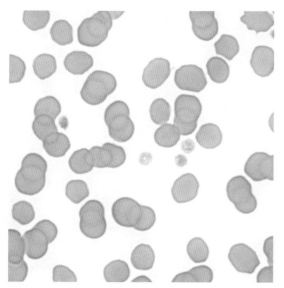

Figure 8.6. Equine platelets.
Courtesy of IDEXX and Dr. Dennis DeNicola.

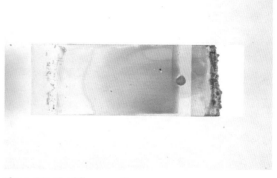

Figure 8.7. Blood film preparation.
Courtesy of IDEXX and Dr. Dennis DeNicola.

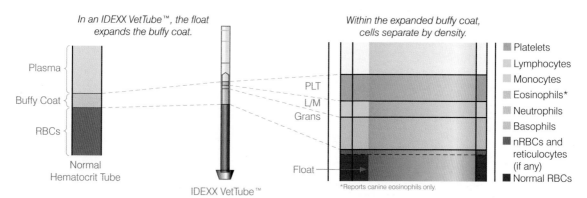

Figure 8.8. Veterinarian autoread tube.
Courtesy of IDEXX.

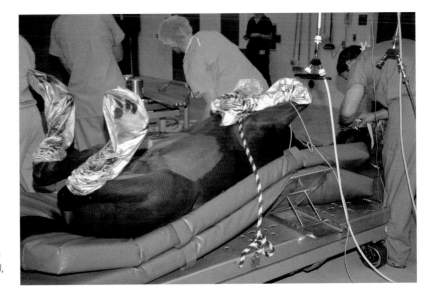

Figure 9.5. Horse positioned in dorsal recumbency on operating room table (symmetrical with legs in natural, flexed position).

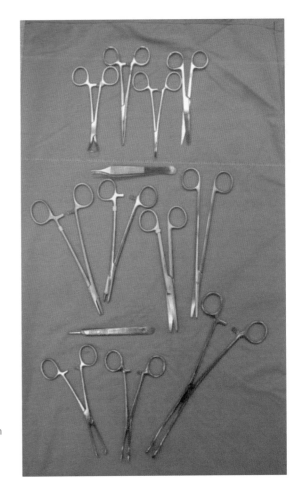

Figure 10.1. Common Instruments.
Top row from left to right: penetrating towel clamps, Kelly Haemostatic forceps, mosquito forceps, and sharp/blunts operating scissors. *Under top row:* Brown Adson tissue forceps. *Middle from left to right:* Mayo-Hegar needle holder, Olsen-Hegar needle holder, Mayo scissors, and Metzenbaum scissors. *Under middle row:* scalpel handle.
Bottom from left to right: Allis tissue forceps, Babcock tissue forceps, and sponge forceps.

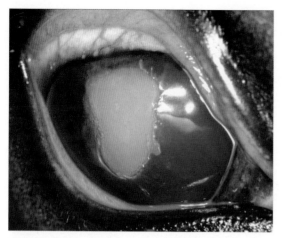

Figure 11.7. Fluorescein dye used to detect a corneal ulcer. Courtesy of Dr. Dennis Brooks.

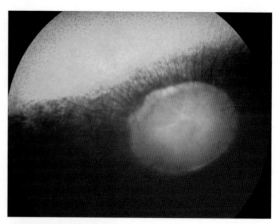

Figure 11.10. Retina and optic nerve. Courtesy of Dr. Dennis Brooks.

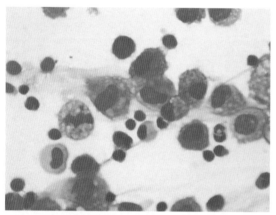

Figure 12.9. Cytologic appearance of normal bronchoalveolar lavage fluid. Note that the majority of cells are macrophages or lymphocytes. Courtesy Dr. Elizabeth Welles, Auburn University, AL.

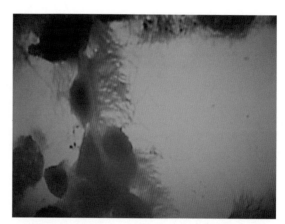

Figure 12.13. Cytologic examination of a transtracheal wash obtained from a normal horse. Most of the cells present are ciliated, columnar respiratory epithelial cells.

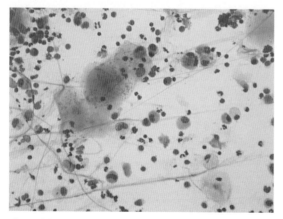

Figure 12.14. Bacterial contamination in a transtracheal wash sample. Courtesy Dr. Elizabeth Welles, Auburn University, AL.

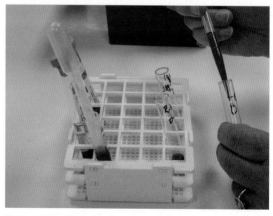

Figure 12.15. Washing erythrocytes.

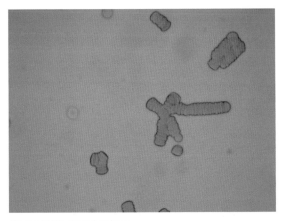

Figure 12.16. Normal rouleaux.

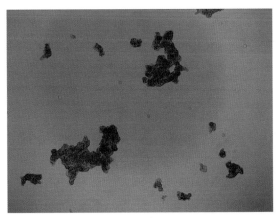

Figure 12.17. Incompatibility agglutination.

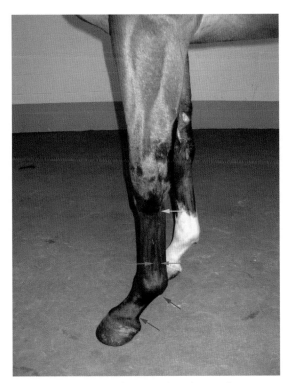

Figure 13.1. Injection sites for perineural anesthesia. *Red arrow:* palmar digital. *Blue arrow:* abaxial sesamoid. *Green arrows:* low four-point suspensory. *Yellow arrow:* high four-point/high suspensory.

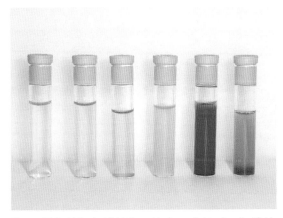

Figure 14.3. Abdominal fluid. Normal is clear to light yellow. Red fluid represents increased red blood cells from ischemic bowel or blood contamination during the procedure.
Courtesy Dr. Michael Porter.

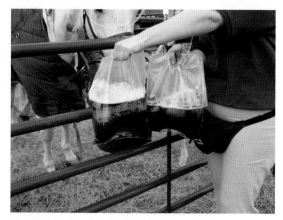

Figure 14.4. Urine from an endurance horse that is dehydrated and "tying up." The red color of the urine is due to myoglobin. Courtesy Dr. Michael Porter.

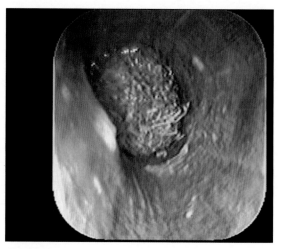

Figure 14.5. Endoscopic view of esophageal choke. Courtesy Dr. Guy Lester.

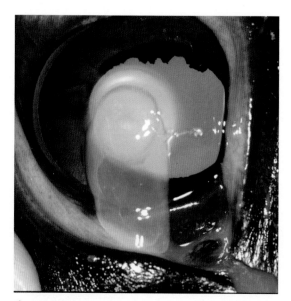

Figure 14.13. Rupture of the cornea due to severe corneal ulcer. Courtesy of Dr. Michael Porter.

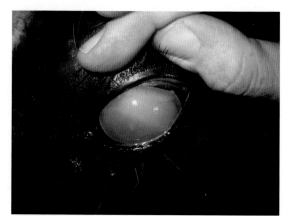

Figure 14.14. Diffuse corneal edema of a horse's eye. Courtesy of Dr. Michael Porter.

Equine Anesthesia

Erin M. McNally and Luisito S. Pablo

Preanesthetic Assessment

History

The anesthetist should obtain a full and current history on each patient. They should determine the present problem and any previous problems the horse may have encountered. If the horse has had anesthesia previously it may be useful to obtain the old anesthesia record because this may aid in choosing an appropriate anesthetic regime. The anesthetist should determine if the horse has known allergies or any other preexisting conditions that could complicate the anesthetic period. These may include hyperkalemic periodic paralysis (HYPP), heaves, pneumonia, diarrhea, anemia, hypoproteinemia, or an upper airway condition.

Physical Examination

A complete physical examination should be conducted before each anesthetic episode. Evaluate the cardiovascular system by auscultation of the heart, palpation of pulses, observing mucous membrane color, and checking for jugular pulses. If a murmur or arrhythmia is ausculted, a cardiac workup should be considered. Evaluate the respiratory system by auscultation of the lungs and checking for nasal discharge. If there is a question as to the status of the horse's respiratory system, a rebreathing examination should be performed. This forces the horse to take deeper breaths, allowing for more sensitive auscultation of respiratory sounds. If crackles or wheezes are heard, thoracic ultrasound or radiographs may be needed before anesthesia to fully evaluate the patient. The horse's temperature should be taken before anesthesia because this may be an indication of infection. To properly assess the anesthetic risks, hydration status of the horse should be determined. If abnormalities are found on the physical examination, having the horse undergo anesthesia for an elective procedure should be considered carefully.

Laboratory

Every hospital has its own requirement for blood work for general anesthesia, often dependent on the age of the horse and the problem or the procedure being performed. At the very least a complete blood count (CBC) be performed. A CBC includes packed cell volume (PCV), total solids (TS), fibrinogen, and white blood cell (WBC) count. A PCV and TS will reveal if the patient is anemic, hypoproteinemic, or hypovolemic. Fibrinogen and WBC count may indicate active inflammation or infection. Again, any abnormal values, although not precluding anesthesia, should be taken into consideration, especially if the procedure is an elective one.

A chemistry panel is not always essential for elective procedures, although, it should be performed for horses with certain conditions such as colic, diarrhea, or horses on medications that may cause systemic toxicities. A blood gas may be useful to evaluate acid-base status and lactate values, especially in a horse with compromising disease such as colic.

Airway

Another part of preanesthetic assessment is consideration for airway management. Communication with the surgeon is important. It is vital that the anesthetist knows the status of the horse's airway before induction of anesthesia in the event that a tracheostomy or endoscopic-guided intubation is needed.

Anesthetic Preparation

Fasting

Withholding all food for 12 hours before anesthesia is no longer routine at all veterinary hospitals. Recently, it has become more common to let horses continue to have free choice hay and water. This decreases stress and is feasible as long as the anesthetist is aware that ventilation may be compromised more in these horses because of a more distended gastrointestinal (GI) tract.

Further Preparation

An intravenous (IV) catheter should be aseptically placed (14 gauge, 5.5 in.) in the right or left jugular vein. The horse's coat should be groomed and feet cleaned so that dirt and bedding are not brought into the operating room. Immediately before induction of anesthesia, the horse's mouth should be thoroughly rinsed with a hose or an oral dosing syringe (Figure 9.1) to remove feed impacted in the horse's mouth, which may otherwise be dragged into the horse's airway during intubation.

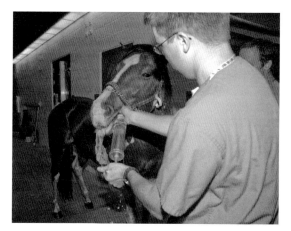

Figure 9.1. Rinsing horse's mouth with water using oral dosing syringe.

The horse should be weighed. In the absence of a scale, a weight tape can be used to estimate the horse's weight.

Premedication and Sedation

Most horses need to be premedicated before induction of anesthesia. Advantages to premedication include increased muscle relaxation, decreased stress, analgesia, and a reduction in the amount of induction agent necessary. Choice of premedication depends on the horse's personality and disease process. Premedications can be given intramuscularly, intravenously, or orally. Most horses tolerate placement of an IV catheter with no sedation, so the majority of horses are premedicated intravenously through an IV catheter. If placement of an IV catheter or an IV injection is not possible, an intramuscular (IM) injection can be performed. IM injections should be made in the lateral neck or the semimembranous or semitendinous muscles. In horses that are aggressive or fractious, detomidine (an α_2-agonist) can be given orally for sedation.

Commonly, a horse's premedication is chosen from one or a combination of three categories: phenothiazines, α_2-agonists, and opioids, with the final goal being sedation, muscle relaxation, and analgesia (Tables 9.1 and 9.2). The α_2-agonists provide excellent muscle relaxation, excellent sedation, and good analgesia, so this category tends to be the

Table 9.1. Characteristics of the three classes of premedicants.

Premedicant class	Sedation	Muscle relaxation	Analgesia
α₂-Agonists	+++	+++	++
Phenothiazine	+	+	−
Opioids	+/−	+	+++

Table 9.2. Common premedicants and their dosages and routes of administration.

Premedicant		Dosage and route of administration
Phenothiazine	Acepromazine	0.01–0.04 mg/kg IV (not to exceed 25 mg)
		0.08 mg/kg IM
α₂-Agonists	Xylazine	0.3–0.6 mg/kg IV
		1.0–2.0 mg/kg IM
	Detomidine	5–10 µg/kg IV or IM
		60 µg/kg oral (mucosal)
	Medetomidine	5–7 µg/kg IV (deep sedation, with severe ataxia)
		10 µg/kg IV (recumbency)
		10 µg/kg IM (moderate sedation within 20 minutes)
	Romifidine	0.03–0.06 mg/kg IV, IM
Opioids	Butorphanol	0.02–0.05 mg/kg IV
		0.05–1.0 mg/kg IM
	Morphine	0.1 mg/kg IV
		0.2–0.25 mg/kg IM

IM, intramuscularly; IV, intravenously; µg, micrograms.

most commonly used premedicant with the option of adding an opioid, for increased analgesia, or acepromazine, for increased sedation and muscle relaxation. Signs of good sedation include lowered head, drooping lower lip, and a broad-based stance (Figure 9.2).

Phenothiazines

Phenothiazines are one class of premedicants, of which acepromazine is the primary drug used in horses. Its mode of action is incompletely understood but probably involves blockage of dopamine receptors in the brain. In low doses, acepromazine produces tranquilization or a calming effect, whereas higher doses are needed for sedation. One recent paper found that sedation only occurs in 60% to 70% of horses. Acepromazine produces a decreased response to environmental stimuli, but horses retain auditory and visual acuity. They will still respond to loud sound and rapid movement. The horse should be left in a quiet area to achieve maximum effect. Peak effect takes about 20 minutes. One method of using acepromazine is to give the drug intramuscularly while the horse is still in its stall, 30 to 45 minutes before leading the horse to the induction area. Alternatively, an IV injection can be given 15 to 30 minutes before bringing the horse to the induction stall. The duration of effect varies from horse to horse but may last from 1 to 4 hours. Acepromazine is metabolized by the liver and excreted in urine.

Acepromazine is a α-adrenergic blocker. It produces peripheral vasodilation, which may cause hypotension, especially in hypovolemic animals. It produces a significant decrease in mean arterial pressure (MAP), central venous pressure (CVP), and respiratory rate (RR); an insignificant decrease in heart rate (HR) and cardiac output (CO); and no change in arterial blood gases. It also stabilizes the heart during halothane anesthesia so that higher levels of epinephrine are required to induce arrhythmias and ventricular fibrillation. In fact, acepromazine has been associated with a lower mortality rate in equine anesthesia.

There are disadvantages to using acepromazine as a premedication, most importantly hypotension as a result of vasodilation. The hypotension is not clinically significant at low doses and responds well to fluid loading. Regardless, it may be best to avoid acepromazine in debilitated or hypovolemic patients. Additionally, in mature stallions, recently castrated males, or geldings, acepromazine may paralyze the penis in a relaxed, extended state (paraphimosis or priapism). In this position, the penis is vulnerable to blunt trauma and to the effects of gravity (i.e., swelling and blood pooling). As a precautionary measure, it is best to avoid acepromazine in a breeding stallion (because of possible legal action). If it is used, it should be used at a lower dose. A final disadvantage to

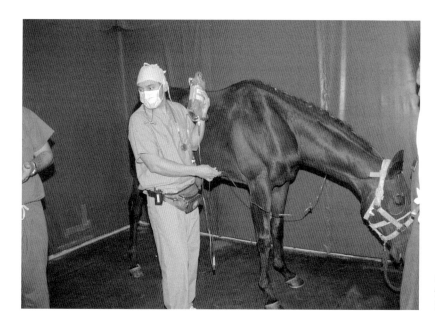

Figure 9.2. Horse after premedication and before induction; note lowered head and drooping lower lip.

acepromazine as a premedication is that it provides no analgesia.

Dose and administration: 0.01 to 0.04 mg/kg intravenously (not to exceed 25 mg) or 0.08 mg/kg intramuscularly

α_2-Agonists

The α_2-agonists stimulate the central α_2-adrenoceptors leading to central nervous system (CNS) depression. They are potent nonnarcotic sedatives and analgesics. As a group, α_2-agonists have the following effects on the cardiovascular system: hypertension from vasoconstriction, reflex bradycardia, and then hypotension. They decrease CO, increase CVP, and cause transient dysrhythmias, including second degree atrioventricular block, especially when given intravenously. They have minimal respiratory effects in healthy animals. Other side effects include sweating, hyperglycemia, and increased urine production. As with acepromazine, the maximum effect is best reached when administered in a quiet environment. Horses can still respond by kicking or biting if stimulated and they remain sensitive to touch. Each α_2-agonist has a slightly different effect and duration of action

(Table 9.3). Increasing dosages tend to not increase degree of sedation but will increase duration of effect. α_2-Agonists are metabolized by the liver and excreted in the urine.

Reversal of α_2-Agonists

The sedative effects of α_2-agonists are reversible by α_2-antagonists. This is rarely necessary in horses but may be considered if a horse is having a prolonged recovery, and it was known to have received a large dose of an α_2-agonist. Yohimbine (Yobine; 0.15–0.25 mg/kg intravenously) has weak antagonistic activity because it is not specific for α_2-receptors. Tolazoline (Priscoline) is another α_2-antagonist that is no longer commonly used because it has the least specificity for α_2-receptors of all the α_2-antagonists. It has also been associated with GI bleeding in humans, as well as abdominal pain, nausea, and diarrhea. Atipamezole (Antisedan) is much more specific for α_2-receptors. It is the reversal agent of choice for medetomidine but can also be used for the other α_2-agonists. It is usually given intramuscularly at an equal volume to the amount of medetomidine used (ml for ml). The dose range is variable from 0.02 to 0.15 mg/kg. Caution must

Table 9.3. α_2-agonists characteristics.

Xylazine (Rompun, Anased)
Dosage and administration
0.3–0.6 mg/kg IV
1.0–2.0 mg/kg IM

Onset of action
1–2 minutes IV
10–15 minutes IM

Duration of action
For analgesia 15–30 minutes
For sedation 40–60 minutes

Detomidine
Considered to have a more predictable effect than xylazine
Dosage and administration
5–20 μg/kg IV or IM

Duration of sedation
90–100 minutes
Oral or buccal absorption of detomidine (60 μg/kg) produces sedation in
    45 minutes (not to be swallowed)

Medetomidine (Domitor)
Has higher α_2-agonist selectivity than xylazine, detomidine, and
    romifidine

Dosage and Administration
5–7 μg/kg IV (deep sedation with severe ataxia)
10 μg/kg IV (may result in recumbency)
10 μg/kg IM (moderate sedation within 20 minutes)

Duration of sedation
60–90 minutes

Romifidine (Sedivet)
Similar to α_2-agonists mentioned above but is advertised to produce less
    ataxia and instability

Dosage and Administration
0.03–0.06 mg/kg IV, IM

Duration of sedation
Up to 2 hours

IM, intramuscularly; IV, intravenously; μg, micrograms.

be used when administering the α_2-antagonists intravenously as severe hypotension can result. For this reason, it is most common to administer the antagonist intramuscularly. Atipamazole has rapid absorption from the muscle and arousal is usually seen within 5 to 10 minutes.

Opioids

Advantages of using opioids as a premedicant for horses include analgesia and mild sedation with minimal cardiovascular effects. Typically, opioids are given in combination with an α_2-agonist or acepromazine. The use of opioids alone as a premedication results in little sedation. Especially in higher doses and when used alone, opioids may cause excitement or dysphoria.

There are three primary opioid receptors: μ, κ, and δ, of which the δ receptor has no available therapeutic agent acting on it. Commonly used opioids are classified as μ-receptor agonists (e.g., morphine, meperidine, fentanyl, and methadone), mixed agonist-antagonists (butorphanol), partial agonists (buprenorphine), and pure opioid antagonists (e.g., naloxone, nalmefene, and naltrexone). Opioids are primarily metabolized in the liver and excreted in the urine.

Butorphanol

Butorphanol is a κ-agonist and μ-antagonist. It seems to potentiate the sedative effect of α_2-Agonists. It provides mild, short-lasting analgesia (approximately 1 hour). Butorphanol can also be used to partially reverse the effects of μ-agonists.

Dosage and administration: 0.02 to 0.05 mg/kg intravenously or 0.05–0.1 mg/kg intramuscularly.

Morphine

Morphine is a full μ-agonist. It also potentiates the sedative effects of α_2-agonists. IM administration may reduce the likelihood of excitement and may have a longer lasting effect. Another option is to give a different sedative (acepromazine or an α_2-agonist) first, followed by IV morphine after the horse has become sedate.

Dosage and administration: 0.1 mg/kg intravenously or 0.25 mg/kg intramuscularly.

Duration of analgesia is 4 to 6 hours.

Disadvantages of opioids, as previously mentioned, include possible excitement (increased locomotor activity), which can be avoided by concurrent use with another sedative and with using lower doses. Additionally, opioids may decrease GI motility, especially with repeated use.

221

Table 9.4. Dosage and route of administration of nonsteroidal anti-inflammatory drugs used in horses.

Nonsteroidal anti-inflammatory drug	Dosage and route of administration
Flunixin meglumine	0.25–1.1 IV, IM, or PO q 8–24 hours
Carprofen	0.7 mg/kg IV or PO q 24 hours
Phenylbutazone	2.2–4.4 mg/kg IV or PO q 12–24 hours
Firocoxib	0.1 mg/kg PO q 24 hours

IM, intramuscularly; IV, intravenously; PO, by mouth; q, every.

GI motility should be closely monitored. In the future it may be possible to decrease slowed GI motility without reversing analgesia by administration of a peripheral opioid antagonist. Methylnaltrexone is one such drug that is being used in human medicine to reduce ileus for human patients receiving opioids.

Nonsteroidal Anti-Inflammatory Drugs

Nonsteroidal anti-inflammatory drugs (NSAIDs) are commonly used as premedication in horses for reducing postoperative inflammation and pain (Table 9.4). They offer no additional sedation but should be considered in the premedication as part of a multimodal plan for analgesia. NSAIDs work by blocking the enzymes that are required for the conversion of arachidonic acid to inflammatory mediators (i.e., prostaglandins primarily). The primary enzyme is cyclooxygenase (COX) of which there are two main isoforms, COX-1 and COX-2. Prostaglandins do not directly induce pain, but they do sensitize nerve endings to chemical mediators ("inflammatory soup"). Examples of NSAIDs are flunixin meglumine, phenylbutazone, carprofen, and firocoxib.

Because some of the products of arachidonic acid do have physiologic purposes, blocking their production does have consequences. NSAIDs have several known toxic side effects of which damage to the GI tract and kidney are most common. Gastric ulceration and right dorsal colitis are usually the

result of the use of NSAIDs. This effect may arise from disruption of the mucosal barrier, interference with mucosal blood flow, and an effect on acid secretion.

Especially in hypotensive states, NSAIDs may cause renal toxicity, again related to inhibition of prostaglandin synthesis. Prostaglandins are involved in regulation of renal blood flow, especially under low-flow situations (i.e., shock and anesthesia-induced hypotension). The horse seems to be less susceptible to renal damage than other species.

Finally, NSAIDs have been known to prolong bleeding times via platelet inhibition. Again, this does not seem to be a significant problem in the horse.

Analgesia in Horses

Pain is an unpleasant sensory and emotional experience associated with actual or potential tissue damage or described in terms of such damage. This is the accepted definition of pain as described by the International Association for the Study of Pain. Animal caretakers have an ethical and moral obligation to treat pain in equine patients, but besides this, there are negative effects of pain. Pain causes metabolic and hormonal changes, which include catabolism, weight loss, and behavioral changes. Pain may lead to delayed recovery and increased morbidity, as well as, cause immunosuppression. By using preemptive analgesia, that is providing analgesia before the onset of the noxious stimulus, wind-up pain may be decreased, which can lead to a hyperalgesic state. In hyperalgesic states, horses react to normal, nonpainful stimulus, such as touch, in a painful way. We have the ability to treat pain at many levels by using therapies that work at different receptors and at different places in the nervous system. Nociception, which is the detection of tissue damage by the nervous system without conscious perception of the damage, can be blocked or reduced at the level of the peripheral nerve, the spinal cord, and the brain. The main categories of analgesics that we have are local anesthetics, opioids, NSAIDs

α_2-agonists, and *N*-methyl-D-aspartate (NMDA) antagonists.

Local Anesthetics

Local anesthetics used in horses include bupivacaine, lidocaine, and mepivacaine. Local anesthetics can be used in topical preparations, for infiltration, in peripheral nerve blocks, and in the epidural space. Local anesthetics are sodium channel blockers; they work by preventing the conduction of nerve impulses.

Topical anesthesia can be done with eutectic mixtures of lidocaine and prilocaine (EMLA cream) applied directly to the skin. Applications for this include numbing the skin for IV catheter placement or epidural. Infiltrative anesthesia involves infiltrating the tissues around a wound or mass to be resected without directly blocking a specific nerve. For instance, local anesthetic can be infiltrated into the testicle before castration or directly into the spermatic cord. Peripheral nerve blocks involve blocking specific nerves in the periphery that carry sensory information from the site of interest. Examples of this include retrobulbar nerve block, mandibular or maxillary nerve block, and various nerve blocks of the legs. Epidural analgesia involves depositing local anesthetic, an opioid, an α_2-agonist, or a combination of these three drugs into the epidural space. In horses this is typically done at the sacrococcygeal space for perineal procedures or caudal abdominal procedures. Caution must be used because an improper concentration or volume of local anesthetic could cause a horse to become recumbent. Lidocaine can also be used as a constant rate infusion during anesthesia to provide analgesia, as well as, to spare the effects of minimum alveolar concentration (MAC) (see Partial Intravenous Anesthesia section).

Opioids

As previously discussed, opioids are another option for providing analgesia to horses. Butorphanol and morphine are the opioids most commonly used in horses. Caution must be used with repeat dosing of opioids due to the GI side effects. Opioids work by modulating pain fibers (primarily C and A-delta fibers) to transmission. They do not block transmission by these fibers but make the transmission less intense. Opioid receptors are present spinally and supraspinally. Opioids can act at several locations, including epidurally and in the joints.

α_2-Agonists

Besides sedation, α_2-agonists provide some analgesia. Analgesia is provided through modulation of pain fibers, similar to the method for opioids. α_2-agonist can also be used epidurally.

N-Methyl-D-Aspartate Antagonists

The primary NMDA antagonist used in equine medicine is ketamine. Ketamine is not analgesic used by itself, but it does decrease "wind-up" pain by acting at the NMDA receptor. Ketamine can be given as a constant rate infusion during anesthesia (See Total Intravenous Anesthesia and Partial Intravenous Anesthesia sections).

Nonsteroidal Anti-Inflammatory Drugs

NSAIDS are part of a multimodal approach to pain management (see previous section on NSAIDs).

Induction

The method of induction is slightly different at every hospital. The safest induction method is the one with which the staff is most comfortable.

Tilt Table Induction

A tilt table induction involves strapping the horse to a tilting table after sedation. The induction drugs are given after the horse has been strapped to the table. The table is tilted as the horse relaxes until the horse is in a lateral position. If the members of the staff are familiar with this method of induction, it is smooth and easy. To make it a safe induction,

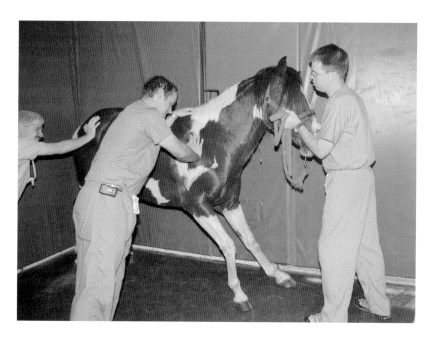

Figure 9.3. Induction of horse in padded induction stall.

it requires a team effort of people who know what to expect.

Padded Induction Stall

Another method of induction is within a padded induction stall with the horse being directed into recumbency by a team of humans (Figure 9.3). One person holds the head by a strong halter, while the remaining people (one to three) put gentle pressure along the horse's side with the horse against one of the four walls of the room. After the induction drugs are given the horse ideally will sit first on its haunches followed by its front legs. Once it is in sternal recumbency it is pulled over on its side. This is a safe method of induction with experienced handlers who are familiar with the course of events. The person on the head should have the most experience. If the horse becomes excited during induction, all personnel should leave the room.

Alternatively, a crush door can be used in place of the humans along the side of the horse, thereby eliminating the need for people to be in the room for induction.

After the horse has obtained lateral recumbency and is intubated, leg straps are placed around the horse's fetlocks, and a hoist is used to lift the horse onto the operating table.

Field Anesthesia (Free Fall)

In the field, induction is done with the free-standing horse. After good sedation is achieved, the induction drug or drugs are given. The horse should be directed into recumbency with one person holding the halter. In most cases this simply means steadying the horse by the halter as it lies down (Figure 9. 4). Lifting the horse's head up and to the right will direct it into left lateral recumbency, whereas lifting up and to the left will direct it into right lateral recumbency.

Induction Drugs

Numerous drug combinations are available for induction. The ultimate goal is to combine unconsciousness with muscle relaxation with minimal cardiorespiratory effects.

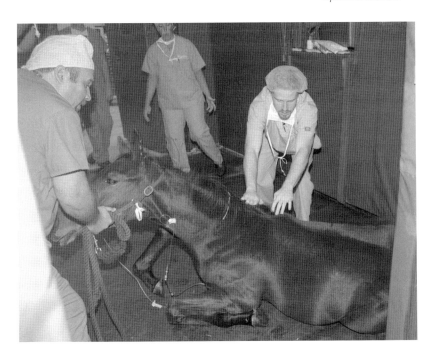

Figure 9.4. Horse in free fall induction within padded recovery stall.

Muscle Relaxants

Two main drugs are used for muscle relaxation: guaifenesin and benzodiazepenes (diazepam or midazolam).

Guaifenesin

Guaifenesin is primarily used in anesthesia as a muscle relaxant. It does not produce unconsciousness. It is a centrally acting muscle relaxant (i.e., brain stem and spinal cord). It does not act at the neuromuscular junction. It causes skeletal muscle relaxation with minimal respiratory depression or cardiovascular depression. Concentrations greater than 10% can cause hemolysis, and the typical formulation used in horses is 5%. Guaifenesin provides no sedation or analgesia. It is metabolized by the liver and excreted in the urine. A typical dose is 30 to 50 mg/kg if the horse is well sedated beforehand. A higher dose (50–100 mg/kg) may be required if lower doses of sedatives are used before induction. It is infused rapidly until signs of incoordination are evident. Guaifenesin is sometimes used in "triple drip" (i.e., guaifenesin, xylazine, and ketamine) for total intravenous anesthesia (TIVA). With long duration infusions, guaifenesin may contribute to ataxia in recovery.

Benzodiazepenes

Diazepam is the benzodiazepine most commonly used in induction of horses, usually combined with ketamine. Benzodiazepenes work by potentiating gamma-aminobutyric acid (GABA) responses at the $GABA_A$ receptor by allosterically modulating GABA binding. Diazepam causes muscle relaxation, minimal cardiovascular and respiratory effects, and no analgesia. Diazepam is not water soluble and therefore precipitates with most other solutions. It does not precipitate, however, with ketamine. It is metabolized primarily in the liver and excreted in urine. Benzodiazepenes can be antagonized with flumazenil (0.04 mg/kg intravenously).

Drugs that Produce Unconsciousness

Ketamine

Ketamine is considered a dissociative anesthetic, wherein there is a dissociation between the thala-

225

mocortical system and the limbic system in the brain. It does this through antagonism of NMDA receptors. It causes analgesia, amnesia, and a cataleptic state, which describes lack of response to external stimuli and muscular rigidity.

Ketamine produces analgesia by antagonism of the NMDA receptor at spinal and supraspinal sites. It also reduces the MAC of inhalant anesthetic. By indirect sympathetic stimulation it increases HR, blood pressure and CO. It is metabolized in the liver and excreted in the kidneys.

Ketamine can be used alone or with a muscle relaxant. If used alone, it is recommended to premedicate with a higher dose of α_2-agonist to achieve good muscle relaxation. If the sedative effect of the α_2-agonist is not adequate, do not give ketamine alone because muscle tremors or seizures may occur. If not followed by inhalant anesthesia, the duration of anesthesia with ketamine induction is 5 to 10 minutes. Anesthesia could be prolonged if necessary by intermittent boluses of ketamine at one-fourth to one-half the initial dose of ketamine. In addition ketamine can be used as a constant rate infusion to reduce the MAC of inhalant anesthesia or for analgesia (See Total Intravenous Anesthesia and Partial Intravenous Anesthesia sections).

Ketamine is not recommended in situations in which increased intracranial pressure (ICP) or intraocular pressures (IOP) are concerns. Increased ICP may occur due to increased cerebral blood flow caused by the cerebral vasodilating property of ketamine. IOP may occur due to rigidity of intraocular muscles caused by ketamine. This effect may be negated by good premedication or concurrent use with a muscle relaxant.

Thiopental
Thiopental is a barbiturate anesthetic specifically a thiobarbiturate. Barbiturates directly activate the $GABA_A$ receptor mediating chlorine influx. Thiopental has a short duration of action due to redistribution from high blood flow organs (brain) to low blood flow organs (fat). The initial redistribution is to muscle. Thiopental is not a good option for continuous rate infusions because once all compartments are saturated, recovery is related to the half-life of the drug. Thiopental has a long terminal half-life. Ultimate elimination is by hepatic metabolism.

Like ketamine, thiopental is typically given with other drugs for induction. Its overall effects depend on dose and what drugs it is administered with. Hypotension is typically seen as a result of venodilation. Myocardial depression does occur but it is insignificant at low doses. Thiopental sensitizes the heart to catecholamines. At high doses respiratory depression occurs. Thiopental offers no analgesia.

Without sedation large doses of thiopental are needed for induction (10 mg/kg). Higher doses have more side effects. Thiopental can be given by itself (3–5 mg/kg) after good sedation with an α_2-agonist. It is a more common to administer thiopental after or with guaifenesin after sedation with an α_2-agonist. Thiopental has largely been replaced by ketamine in most practices but is still a good induction drug, especially in situations in which increased ICP or IOP are potential concerns. Care must be taken to avoid perivascular injections of thiopental. Because of the very basic nature (pH about 11) of the drug, a perivascular injection will cause irritation and possible tissue sloughing.

Propofol
Propofol is an induction agent commonly used in dogs and cats. It is not as commonly used in horses, mainly because of the large volume required and the associated cost. However, it can be used for foals or smaller horses (<100 kg) in which the volume could be bolused in a reasonable amount of time.

Propofol works by having a direct effect on both spinal supraspinal $GABA_A$ receptors. It causes anesthesia with no analgesia. Disadvantages include hypotension and respiratory depression or apnea. Its primary metabolism is via the liver, but it is believed that some extrahepatic metabolism does occur. Return to consciousness occurs by redistribution from areas of high blood flow (brain) to areas of lower blood flow (muscles, fat).

Propofol is formulated as an oil/water emulsion containing soybean, egg lecithin, and glycerol. It serves as an excellent medium for microbial growth, so typically an opened vial should be discarded after 6 hours.

The dose range of propofol is 2 to 8 mg/kg, and this should only be given after good sedation is achieved. Propofol may cause myoclonus and limb paddling after induction. Propofol be used as a TIVA in an adult horse; however, a large volume would be required (see Total Intravenous Anesthesia section).

Induction Drug Combinations

Guaifenesin-Thiopental. Guaifenesin prolongs the effect of thiopental, improves muscle relaxation, and improves recovery if not given excessively (Tables 9.5 and 9.6). There are less severe cardiovascular and respiratory effects due to using a lower dose of thiopental. More concentrated guaifenesin results in a quicker induction, and a faster infusion results in a quicker induction and a less total volume required. Guaifenesin can be used as a mixture with thiopental or given separately.

Mixture: 3 g thiopental can be added to 1 L 5% guaifenesin. This mixture is administered intravenously in a fast bolus to effect. The calculated dose is 2.2 ml/kg. Most horses become recumbent with about two-thirds of the calculated dose of this mixture.

Separate: Alternatively, 5% guaifenesin can be administered separately until the horse is ataxic and then a bolus of thiopental (5 mg/kg) is given. The usual dose of guaifenesin needed is about 55 mg/kg. Some horses may go down on this combination but still be too light for hoisting, requiring additional thiopental and guaifenesin. Some anesthetists continue the guaifenesin at a slower rate until the horse is situated on the table and started on inhalant.

Guaifenesin-Ketamine. Ketamine is substituted for the barbiturate in this combination. It is somewhat more difficult to assess anesthetic depth with ketamine than thiopental because ketamine maintains good ocular reflexes. Also, it has a slightly longer induction phase than guaifenesin-thiopental. As with guaifenesin-thiopental, this can be given as a mixture or separately:

Mixture: Combine 1 g ketamine with 1 L of 5% guaifenesin. Administer intravenously in a fast bolus to effect. Typically, 2.2 mg/kg of ketamine is needed.

Separate: Administer 5% guaifenesin separately until the horse is ataxic and follow with 1.5 to 2.2 mg/kg ketamine as a bolus.

Xylazine-Ketamine. Xylazine can be given at a higher than normal premedication dose (1.1 mg/kg intravenously), and this can be followed by ketamine alone at 2.2 mg/kg. At least 3 to 5 minutes

Table 9.5. Anesthesia protocol for healthy young horse.

Premedication (Wait at least 5 minutes for sedation)	1. α_2-Agonist 2. α_2-Agonist + opioid 3. α_2-Agonist + opioid + acepromazine 4. α_2-Agonist + acepromazine
Induction	1. 5% Guaifenesin: Administer rapidly to effect 50–100 mg/kg IV Ketamine 1.5–2.2 mg/kg IV OR 10% Thiopental* 4–6 mg/kg IV 2. Diazepam or midazolam 0.02–0.1 mg/kg IV Ketamine 1.5–2.2 mg/kg IV 3. Ketamine 2.2 mg/kg IV If full dose of xylazine was used as premedication

*For healthy older horse use same protocol but lower dosages.
IV, intravenously.

Table 9.6. Anesthesia protocol: Exploratory laparotomy with acute abdominal disease (colic).

Premedication: May not need Use lowest dose possible	1. α_2-Agonist 2. α_2-Agonist + opioid Avoid acepromazine in hypovolemic animals
Induction	1. 5% Guaifenesin: Administer rapidly to effect 50–100 mg/kg IV Ketamine 1.5–2.2 mg/kg IV 2. Diazepam or Midazolam 0.02–0.1 mg/kg IV Ketamine 1.5–2.2 mg/kg IV

IV, intravenously.

should be given for the xylazine to take effect before giving the ketamine. This method should not be used if good sedation with xylazine is not achieved.

Diazepam-Ketamine. After sedation, ketamine at 2.2 mg/kg is mixed with the same volume of diazepam (0.1 mg/kg). This mixture is given as an IV bolus. Some anesthetists may choose to use half the volume of diazepam (0.05 mg/kg) if sedation is good. Additionally, the diazepam can be given separately before the ketamine. This method should be reserved for more experienced anesthetists because the horse may become excited with administration of diazepam separately.

Inhalant Induction
Foals can be induced with inhalant anesthetic following nasotracheal intubation. Isoflurane or sevoflurane can be used. If the foal is healthy, the maximum vaporizer setting is used. In a sick foal, the vaporizer setting is slowly increased until the foal is anesthetized. To minimize the concentration of inhalant anesthesia needed the foal may be premedicated with diazepam and an opioid. (See Anesthesia and Sedation in Foals section.)

Intubation

Following induction of anesthesia, the horse needs to be intubated if it is to be maintained on inhalant anesthesia. For brief field procedures such as castrations, horses are not usually intubated. For the majority of procedures done in a hospital setting, the horses are intubated to protect the airway even if TIVA is being used.

Orotracheal Intubation

Endotracheal tube sizes in adult horses (about 450 kg) range from 20- to 30-mm internal diameter (ID), with the average horse requiring a width 26-mm ID. For orotracheal intubation, a mouth gag is inserted between the horse's upper and lower incisors to avoid tearing of the tube as it is passed between the teeth. The tongue is pulled outside of the mouth and the horse's neck is extended. The tube is passed beyond the base of the tongue and should slide easily between the arytenoids through the larynx into the trachea. If resistance is encountered, the tube is backed out slightly, rotated 90 degrees and passed again. Sometimes this process needs to be repeated several times before the tube is successfully passed. The tube should never be forced, so if it does not seem to be advancing the next tube size down should be tried. If several minutes have passed and the horse is still not successfully intubated, an endoscopically guided intubation should be considered.

After intubation the cuff of the tube should be inflated. To avoid damage to the tracheal mucosa, as little air as possible should be used to inflate the cuff. Inflation of the cuff is necessary to avoid leakage of anesthetic gases during positive pressure ventilation. The horse should be attached to an anesthetic machine and a normal tidal volume breath should be administered while someone is listening for a leak or feeling the horse's ventral neck for vibrations. Air should be added to the cuff until the leak is corrected.

Nasotracheal Intubation

Certain procedures (e.g., tooth repulsion) may require nasotracheal rather than orotracheal intubation. This should be discussed with the surgeon ahead of time. Smaller tubes are used for nasotracheal intubation. The size range is 16-mm to 22-mm ID for adult horses. A well-lubricated tube is inserted through the nostril into the ventromedial meatus while the horse's neck is extended. This should only be done by an experienced anesthetist. The tube should never be forced. Damage to the nasal soft tissues may result in bleeding.

Positioning on the Operating Room Table

Correct positioning on the operating room (OR) table is important to prevent myopathies and neuropathies, which are serious postanesthetic complications in horses that could result in euthanasia.

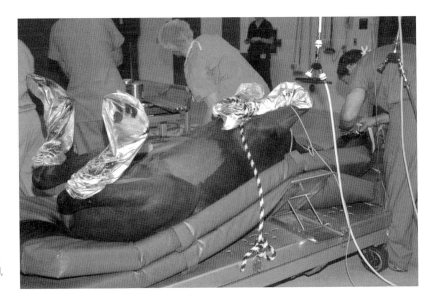

Figure 9.5. Horse positioned in dorsal recumbency on operating room table (symmetrical with legs in natural, flexed position).

(See Complications section.) The horse's halter should be removed. The ears and tail should be in a natural position. If the horse is in dorsal recumbency the front and hind legs should be in a natural, flexed position (Figure 9.5). If the front legs are tied down, make sure the ropes are not too tight. The hind legs should not be overextended. Extension of the hind legs or leg may be required for certain surgical procedures, but the surgeon should be aware that the horse should not be in such a position for too long. The horse's body should be symmetrical on the table with the head not turned toward one side. If the horse is in lateral recumbency the lower leg should be pulled forward relative to the upper leg (Figure 9.6). A pad should be placed between the upper and lower legs (hind and front). No part of the horse should be hanging off the table. For horses greater than 600 kg, double padding of the table may be considered.

Maintenance

Options for maintaining anesthesia include inhalant anesthesia, TIVA, and partial intravenous anesthesia (PIVA). Besides keeping the horse anes-

thetized, further things to consider are ventilation, monitoring, and supportive care.

Inhalant Anesthesia

Inhalation anesthesia is the most common method for maintaining anesthesia in a hospital setting. Inhalants are administered with 100% oxygen as the carrier gas. The typical oxygen flow rate is 10 ml/kg/min, but usually higher rates are used for the first 10 minutes of anesthesia. This helps to denitrogenate the system, as well as, to shorten the time until equilibrium between the concentration set on the vaporizer and the concentration of inhalant that the horse is receiving.

There are two main choices for inhalants: sevoflurane and isoflurane. A third inhalant, halothane, was widely used for horses until recently. Halothane is no longer manufactured in the United States, so this discussion will be limited to sevoflurane and isoflurane.

Sevoflurane and isoflurane have similar systemic effects. They both decrease systemic blood pressure and vascular resistance in a dose-dependent manner. CO decreases due to decreased contractility of the heart. They may sensitize the

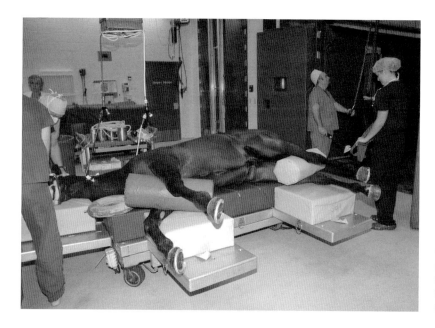

Figure 9.6. Horse in lateral recumbency on operating room table (lower front leg pulled forward, pad between upper and lower legs in front and back).

heart to catecholamines; although, halothane is known to be more arrhythmogenic than sevoflurane and isoflurane. They both produce dose-dependent respiratory depression and renal and hepatic blood flows are decreased. Both inhalants provide excellent muscle relaxation and neither inhalant is analgesic, requiring the use of an analgesic drug as a premedicant and during anesthetic maintenance.

The amount of inhalant needed to produce a surgical plane of anesthesia is described in terms of MAC. This is the end-tidal concentration of inhalant agent necessary to prevent purposeful movement in response to noxious stimulus in 50% of test subjects. MAC is a measure of potency and can be used to compare different anesthetics. To prevent movement in surgical procedures, it is usually necessary to maintain an end-tidal concentration of anesthetic that is 1.3 times MAC. The MAC of sevoflurane is 2.31, whereas the MAC of isoflurane is 1.31.

After attaching a horse to an anesthetic machine, it takes time for the inhalant concentration in the blood to equilibrate to the setting on the vaporizer. Both the volume of the anesthetic equipment and the large volume of the horse itself need to be considered in the time taken to saturate the tissues. Using a higher flow rate for the first 10 to 20 minutes of anesthesia and setting the vaporizer at a higher concentration speeds the times to equilibration. The brain concentration is what determines whether or not the horse is anesthetized, and it takes time for the brain concentration to approach the delivered concentration of anesthetic. Certain physical properties of the inhalants, such as solubility in the blood, affect the time it takes to get to a higher brain concentration. With low solubility in blood, sevoflurane has a faster onset time than isoflurane and a more rapid recovery than isoflurane. Additionally, the cardiovascular status of the horse effects the time it takes for the brain to achieve the necessary concentration of inhalant. A horse with a higher CO takes longer to achieve equilibration than a horse with a lower CO.

Certain factors can decrease and increase MAC of inhalants (Table 9.7). Hypothermia, old age, sedatives and analgesics, pregnancy, and endotoxemia may decrease MAC. Hyperthermia and CNS stimulants may increase MAC.

Table 9.7. Drugs that decrease minimum alveolar concentration.

1. Acepromazine
2. α_2-Agonists
3. Ketamine
4. Opioids (variable—may cause central nervous system excitation and increase minimum alveolar concentration [MAC])
5. Benzodiazepenes
6. Lidocaine
7. Nitrous oxide

Systems for Delivering Inhalant Anesthesia

Oxygen is the primary gas used to deliver inhalant anesthesia in equine anesthesia. The anesthesia machine is designed to deliver a precise mixture of inhalant and oxygen based on the operator's setting. Components of the anesthesia machine include sources, regulators, and flow meters, plus one or more vaporizers.

Gas Sources

Oxygen may be supplied by a pipeline from a liquid oxygen source or from a cylinder attached to the machine. Cylinders are designated alphabetically—A being the smallest. Cylinders are color coded. In the United States, green is for oxygen and blue is for nitrous oxide. Some hospitals use primarily pipeline oxygen with cylinders as back up. The two main types of oxygen cylinders are E tanks and larger H tanks. Oxygen in cylinders is primarily in the gaseous form, so pressure is proportional to its contents. The volume of oxygen in an E cylinder can be estimated by multiplying the pressure (pounds per square inch [psi]) by 0.3. A full E cylinder has a volume of 600 L (0.3 × 2000 psi). The volume of oxygen in an H tank can be estimated by multiplying psi by 3. A full H tank contains 6,900 L.

Pressure Regulators

The anesthetic machine regulates the oxygen leaving the cylinder or the pipeline to maintain a constant flow. A pressure-reducing valve placed downstream from the cylinder reduces the pressure to about 45 psi. Pipeline oxygen pressure is about 50 psi to ensure preferential delivery of gases from the pipeline. Pressures in gas cylinders are high and must be reduced and regulated to provide safe, efficient supplies of gases to the flow meters. A regulator provides a constant pressure and flow to the flow meter despite the continual drop in pressure as the gas in the cylinder is depleted.

Most machines are equipped with an oxygen flush valve that bypasses the flow meter and the vaporizer. The flush valve delivers a high, unmetered flow (35–75 L/min) of oxygen for refilling the circle system quickly in emergencies.

Flow Meters

Flow meters measure and indicate the rate of the flow to the common gas outlet. Flow rate is indicated by a small metal ball or a rotating bobbin. Indicators are read at the top, except for ball-shaped indicators, which are read in the center. The control knobs for flow meters should be not tightened excessively.

Vaporizers

Vaporizers are designed to change the liquid anesthetic into vapor, which describes the gaseous state of agents that are liquids at room temperatures. Vaporizers are designed to add a controlled amount of anesthetic to the flow of gases going to the patient.

Classification of Vaporizers. Most modern vaporizers are of the variable bypass design. Fresh gas entering the vaporizer is split into two streams: a small carrier portion passes through the vaporizer, whereas a larger bypass portion exits the vaporizer without contacting the anesthetic. The streams mix after exiting to deliver the concentration set on the dial. Most modern vaporizers are of the flowover design. The carrier gas enters a vaporizing chamber and becomes saturated with anesthetic.

Vaporizers can be classified by where they are in the circuit. Most modern vaporizers are out of circuit. In contrast to vaporizers located within the breathing circuit, out-of-circuit vaporizers are less affected by changes in ventilation and flow. Most modern vaporizers are temperature compensated and single agent specific. Variable bypass, concentration-calibrated vaporizers (most modern vaporizers) should be serviced and recalibrated periodically by a qualified technician.

Breathing Systems

After the vaporizer, the common gas outlet is next encountered. The mixture of anesthetic gases and oxygen exits the anesthesia machine through the common gas outlet. It then enters the fresh gas inlet of the breathing system.

The circuit delivers oxygen and anesthetic and removes carbon dioxide (CO_2). There are three circuits available: circle systems (rebreathing), to and fro systems (rebreathing), and nonrebreathing systems. Of these, circle systems are used almost exclusively in horses with nonrebreathing systems being impractical due to the high fresh gas flow (approximately 100 ml/kg/minute) needed to remove CO_2.

Circle Systems

Circle systems (Figure 9.7) are called rebreathing systems because all or part of the expired gases

(after removal of CO_2) are recirculated to the patient. The main components of a circle system are the fresh gas inflow, inspiratory and expiratory unidirectional valves, two corrugated tubes forming the inspiratory and expiratory limbs, a Y piece connecting the corrugated tubes to the endotracheal tube, a reservoir bag, a pop-off valve, and a soda lime canister and carbon dioxide absorbent.

- *Fresh gas inlet:* located on inspiratory side of circle between CO_2 absorbent and inspiratory one-way valve.
- *Inspiratory one-way valve:* promotes flow of gases in single direction in circle; opens during inspiration, closes during expiration.
- *Inspiratory breathing hose:* conducts gases from one-way valve to Y piece.
- *Y piece:* connects inspiratory and expiratory tubes to endotracheal tube; the only mechanical dead space in a properly functioning circle.
- *Expiratory breathing hose:* conducts gases from Y piece to expiratory one-way valve.

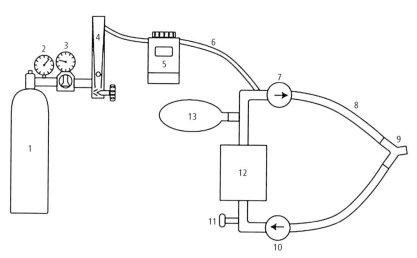

Figure 9.7. Diagram of circle system for delivering inhalant anesthetic.

1. Oxygen supply
2. Oxygen pressure gauge
3. Pressure regulator
4. Flow meter
5. Vaporizer
6. Common gas outlet
7. Inspiratory one-way valve
8. Breathing hoses
9. Y piece
10. Expiratory one-way valve
11. Pop-off valve
12. Carbon dioxide absorber (canister)
13. Reservoir bag

- *Expiratory one-way valve:* opens on expiration, closes on inspiration.
- *Pop-off:* safety feature to vent excess gas and prevent development of excessive pressure; should be open except during intentional positive pressure application to the system.
- *Reservoir bag:* provides for patient's tidal volume and minute volume during spontaneous ventilation; Guideline: 6 × tidal volume (6 × 10 ml/kg × BW_{kg})
- *Canister:* should have volume approximately twice patient's tidal volume because gas space around granules of absorbent is about one-half the volume of the canister.

Carbon Dioxide Absorption. CO_2 is removed from the circuit by a chemical reaction with soda lime or baralyme (barium hydroxide lime). Soda lime is more efficient in absorbing CO_2. Heat and water are byproducts of this reaction. Indicators are added to the absorbent and change color as the absorbent becomes exhausted. Absorbent is soft when functional and becomes hard when consumed. Absorbents should be changed regularly, usually when half to two-thirds of the canister has been consumed. The immediate color change fades away over time, so absorbent that appears unchanged in color may in fact be consumed. For this reason it is important to keep track of hours of use of a canister and change it regularly.

Scavenging. A scavenging system should be attached to the circle system to eliminate waste from the OR environment. Potential health hazards associated with exposure to inhalants in the short term are headaches, fatigue, lethargy, depression, pruritus, decreased performance, and mental activity. Potential side effects of long-term exposure are spontaneous abortions, congenital abnormalities, neoplasia, hepatic disease, and renal disease.

The scavenging system is connected to the exit portal of the pop-off valve through corrugated tubing. Gas can be disposed of actively via a vacuum system or passively. Venting gases to the floor is not effective. A conduit through an outside wall is effective but will pollute the outside environment. Active charcoal canisters are also effective but should be changed every 8 hours and cannot handle high oxygen flow rates.

To-and-Fro-System

The to-and-fro system is different from the circle system in that it has no unidirectional valves or breathing tubes. The endotracheal tube is connected directly to the system, close to the soda lime canister. The fresh gas flow enters between the canister and the endotracheal tube. Exhaled gas moves through the soda lime into the rebreathing bag and from the rebreathing bag back through the soda lime to the horse on inspiration. The advantage of this system is that it is portable. The disadvantages are that the canister is located close to the endotracheal tube making it difficult to position and support and increasing the risk of inhaling soda lime dust.

Ventilation

After induction, intubation, and positioning the horse on the OR table, the horse should be connected to the breathing circuit by the Y piece (if using circle system). There are essentially two modes of ventilation in anesthetized horses: spontaneous ventilation and intermittent positive pressure ventilation (IPPV). The decision of whether or not to artificially ventilate should be based on the comfort level of the anesthetist and arterial blood gases, looking at partial pressure of carbon dioxide in blood ($PaCO_2$) and partial pressure of oxygen in blood (PaO_2). General anesthesia alters respiratory function via action of anesthetic drugs, as well as, positioning. In the anesthetized recumbent horse, PaO_2 can markedly decrease and $PaCO_2$ increase. A $PaCO_2$ of 60 to 75 mm Hg is common during general anesthesia in horses (normal 35–45 mm Hg).

There is dose-dependent respiratory depression with inhalant anesthesia so monitoring respiration and adjusting delivered inhalant anesthetic to the horse during spontaneous ventilation can be used as a way to titrate delivered inhalant to the appropriate depth of anesthesia. In most cases horses do not respond to painful stimuli during light planes of anesthesia by changing respiration; a horse will show nystagmus or move on the table without altering its respiratory pattern. A high $PaCO_2$ causes respiratory acidosis (pH < 7.4). A pH less than 7.4

Table 9.8. Advantages and disadvantages of intermittent positive pressure ventilation.

Advantages	Disadvantages
1. Inhalant anesthetic administered predictably	1. Cardiac output reduced by 30%
2. Hypoventilation prevented	2. Decreased $PaCO_2$ results in loss of cardiovascular stimulation from increased $PaCO_2$
3. Higher PaO_2 maintained (not always; IPPV alone does not eliminate or prevent hypoxemia)	

IPVV, intermittent positive pressure ventilation; PaO_2, partial pressure of oxygen in blood; $PaCO_2$, partial pressure of carbon dioxide in blood.

but greater than 7.2 stimulates the cardiovascular system, whereas a pH below 7.2 results in cardiovascular depression and may predispose the anesthetized patient to arrhythmias.

Intermittent Positive Pressure Ventilation

Criteria for when and whether or not to start IPPV varies from hospital to hospital. One can start the horse on spontaneous ventilation, check a blood gas, and decide whether or not to ventilate based on the results of the blood gas or begin IPPV immediately. The reason for the controversy is that IPPV has advantages and disadvantages (Table 9.8).

Most modern anesthetic machines for adult horses have a ventilator built into the design so it is easy to switch between the two methods. Ventilators may be driven by electricity, compressed gas, or both. Before starting a horse on a ventilator it is important to become familiar with how the ventilator works and how ventilator settings can be adjusted. Typically the tidal volume delivered is 10 to 20 ml/kg, and the peak inspiratory pressure is between 20 and 30 cm H_2O with 5 to 8 breaths per minutes. Final ventilator settings should be made based on results of arterial blood gases. Increasing tidal volume or breaths per minute will decrease $PaCO_2$, whereas decreasing tidal volume or breaths per minutes will increase $PaCO_2$.

Total Intravenous Anesthesia

An alternative to inhalant anesthesia that is especially useful for short field procedures or to facili-

tate transport from one area to another is TIVA. One option for TIVA is a mixture of ketamine, guaifenesin, and xylazine, also known as triple drip. Ketamine (1–2 g) and 500 mg of xylazine are added to 1 L of 5.0% guaifenesin. This solution is administered at 2 to 3 ml/kg/hour. Other options for TIVA include propofol at 150 to 500 µg/kg/minute, propofol with ketamine (150 µg/kg/minute and 50 µg/kg/minute, respectively) or ketamine with an α_2-agonist. Ketamine with an α_2-agonist provides poor muscle relaxation, which is why guaifenesin is added, as in triple drip.

The horse should still be monitored as for inhalant anesthesia and if respiratory depression or apnea occurs, the horse should be intubated and ventilated.

Partial Intravenous Anesthesia

PIVA describes a combination of inhalational and injectable anesthetic techniques, the goal being to achieve "balanced" anesthesia, using less of each.

PIVA can be achieved with a ketamine constant rate infusion (50 µg/kg/minute) or medetomidine or xylazine constant rate infusion (3.5–5 µg/kg/hour and 1 mg/kg/hour, respectively). Ketamine and an α_2-agonist can also be used together.

Lidocaine can be infused intravenously at 50 to 100 µg/kg/minute alone or with ketamine or an α_2-agonist. The constant rate infusion is usually started after a loading dose. The lidocaine loading dose is 1 to 2 mg/kg. If the ketamine infusion is started after induction, the induction dose of ketamine can be considered the loading dose; otherwise, 0.25 to 0.5 mg/kg can be used as the loading dose.

All anesthesiologists and anesthetists have their own method of using PIVA, but in most cases, constant rate infusions of lidocaine and ketamine are slowed or discontinued within an hour of the expected end of the procedure.

Monitoring

Minimal monitoring parameters should include RR, HR, pulse strength, mucous membrane color, and depth of anesthesia. Ideally, additional monitoring should include electrocardiogram (ECG), direct blood pressure, and blood gases. Capnography and pulse oximetry are also useful tools for monitoring. Regular monitoring allows early recognition of intraoperative problems, allowing prompt treatment and usually correction of the problem.

Normal HR in an adult horse is 28 to 40 beats per minute. Athletic animals tend to have slower heart rates than nonathletic ones. Additionally, administration of certain drugs will cause a lower than normal heart rate, primarily α_2-agonists. Treatment of bradycardia is not essential in every case, especially if arterial blood pressures are good.

Pulse strength will give the anesthetist a general idea about systemic blood pressure, although having good pulses is not a guarantee of good blood pressure. Pulse pressure is determined by the difference between systolic and diastolic pressures. A large difference between these two will result in good pulse pressure, even if both numbers individually are lower than normal. Hence, direct blood pressure monitoring is essential if accurate blood pressure values are needed.

RR can be determined by watching chest excursions or bag movement. Normal respiratory rate is 4 to 10 breaths per minute.

Mucous membrane color should generally be pink. Pink mucous membranes usually indicate adequate oxygenation but not necessarily that arterial oxygenation is optimal. When 100% oxygen is being delivered PaO_2 should be 400 to 600 mm Hg, but animals with lower values will still have normal looking mucous membranes. Cyanosis (blue mucous membranes) results from hypoxemia and usually only after PaO_2 is less than 60 mm Hg. The color of mucous membranes depends on perfusion (heart function) and is influenced by drug-induced factors such as vasoconstriction (α_2-agonists).

Depth of Anesthesia

Maintaining the horse in an adequate plane of anesthesia is obviously important because too deep a plane may result in hypotension, whereas

Table 9.9. Monitoring depth of anesthesia

Sign	Interpretation
Palpebral reflex	Slight or slow response with injectable anesthesia Present or absent under inhalant anesthesia; disappears with time
Corneal reflex	Should always be present in surgical planes of anesthesia; absent if horse is too deep
Changing eye position	Insensitive—eye may change position throughout anesthesia
Nystagmus	Horse is too light—movement may occur
Lacrimation	Light plane of anesthesia
Anal tone	Insensitive—brisk contraction horse may be too light; absence of contraction horse may be too deep
Movement	Light plane of anesthesia

too light a plane may result in movement or the horse feeling pain (Table 9.9). The palpebral eye reflex and eye movement are two important factors that help the anesthetist to determine depth of anesthesia. The palpebral reflex is elicited by gently brushing the eyelashes or tapping the medial canthus of the eye. Under injectable anesthetics the palpebral reflex is usually present and a slow closure of the eyelid can be elicited. With inhalants it can be present or absent but tends to disappear as the anesthesia time and depth of anesthesia increases. Horses in dorsal recumbency tend to lose the palpebral reflex due to edema in the periocular region.

Eye position is not a reliable indicator of depth in horses. Eye position may be central or ventromedial. The position of both eyes interchanges during anesthesia. *Lateral nystagmus*, which is rapid side to side movement of the eye, is an indication that the horse is awakening and may move imminently. Some horses may move before rapid nystagmus is seen. The *corneal reflex*, which is closing of the eyelid resulting from pressure on the cornea, should always be present. To prevent damage to the cornea the eyelid should be lightly pressed against the cornea when checking for this reflex. *Lacrimation* or tearing is common during light planes of anesthesia but is reduced or absent at a surgical plane of

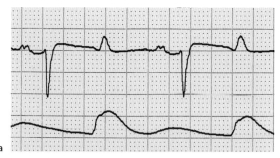

a

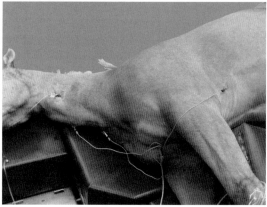

b

Figure 9.8. *(A)* Lead II electrocardiogram with corresponding arterial blood pressure wave. *(B)* Placement of electrocardiogram.

anesthesia. *Movement* of the horse indicates an inadequate plane of anesthesia.

If access to the eye is limited, anal tone can be used as a subjective measure of depth of anesthesia. Stimulation of the anus should cause reflex contraction of the anal sphincter. A brisk contraction may indicate too light a plane of anesthesia, whereas complete absence may indicate too deep a plane of anesthesia.

Electrocardiogram

The ECG is a useful tool in recognizing arrhythmias and changes in HR (Figures 9.8A and B). It does not give information on how efficiently the heart is ejecting blood because it only indicates electrical activity.

Because the size of horses, the electrodes are usually placed in the cranial thoracic region and neck, making sure they surround the heart to obtain

waves of appropriate size. Leads I, II, and III are all useful.

Blood Pressure

Blood pressure is an indirect indicator of hemodynamic status in the horse. Blood pressure can be low if vascular resistance is low without any change in CO. It can be high if vascular resistance is high and CO is low, thus it is not a perfect indicator for CO. Until CO monitoring is more available in a clinical setting, it is the best tool for estimating CO. Blood pressure can be measured noninvasively (indirect) or invasively (direct). Direct blood pressures are the preferred method and the standard of care for anesthetized horses in an OR setting.

Indirect blood pressures can be measured by the Doppler method or the oscillometric method. The Doppler method uses the return to flow principle and detects systolic pressure. A cuff is placed around the tail and a Doppler probe placed over the coccygeal artery. The flow of blood through the artery is detected by the probe and converted to an audible signal. The cuff is inflated with an aneroid manometer and the flow prevented. The audible signal stops. The pressure on the cuff is slowly released until the audible signal is heard again. The pressure at which the audible signal is heard corresponds to the systolic pressure. Cuff size can be the limiting factor in obtaining an accurate systolic blood pressure. The cuff width should be 40% of the circumference of the tail.

The oscillometric method involves placing a cuff around the tail or limb. The machine detects changes in the intercuff pressure (caused by the pulse wave) from which systolic, diastolic, and mean blood pressures are calculated. This method is more reliable in a foal than an adult horse. Some machines are designed to detect heart rates only greater than 30 to 40 beats per minute. Inaccurate readings will result from incorrect cuff size.

Direct blood pressure measurement involves catheterizing a peripheral artery. Typical arteries used are the lateral metatarsal, facial, transverse facial, and coccygeal artery. Catheter sizes may range from 22 to 20 gauge with a 20-gauge catheter being appropriate for most adult horses. The catheter is then connected to a transducer and amplifier that display readings on an oscilloscope. Systolic, diastolic, and MAPs, as well as the pulse waveform are displayed. The transducer must be zeroed and placed at the level of the heart. Normal values are systolic from 90 to 120 mm Hg, diastolic from 40 to 70 mm Hg, and MAP from 60 to 85 mm Hg. Most clinics aim to keep MAP above 60 mm Hg, using changes in the depth of anesthesia, fluids, and inotropic support to achieve this. Blood pressure is dependent not only on CO but on systemic vascular resistance. Blood pressure should be interpreted in light of drugs given that may have an effect on systemic vascular resistance. The α_2-agonists increase systemic vascular resistance. Horses that have received a bolus of or are on a constant rate infusion of α_2-agonists will usually have good blood pressure but this does not necessarily mean that CO is normal.

Making Changes to Depth of Anesthesia

Should movement occur, immediate action must be taken to avoid injury to the horse and OR personnel. A typical course of action would be to bolus a small amount of the induction agent (10%–20% of the induction dose, 100–200 mg thiopental for an adult horse or 0.1–0.2 mg/kg ketamine). This should be followed by increasing the delivered concentration of inhalant by turning up the vaporizer setting. Changing the setting on the vaporizer will result in an increased depth of anesthesia, but it may take 15 to 20 minutes for equilibration to occur. Increasing the oxygen flow rate if possible, as well as ,turning up the vaporizer to a higher than necessary concentration for a brief period will increase the rate at which equilibration occurs. When turning up the vaporizer to higher settings, it is important to monitor the depth of anesthesia closely because it is easy to overshoot and make the depth of anesthesia too deep.

If it is observed that the horse is getting light (i.e., nystagmus, lacrimation) there are several options to address the situation; the vaporizer can be turned up, administer a small bolus of α_2-agonist, ketamine, an opioid, or consider starting the horse on a constant rate infusion of α_2-agonist

(if the horse is cardiovascularly stable), ketamine, or lidocaine.

Supportive Care

Supportive care is necessary while the horse is under anesthesia to decrease intraoperative complications and morbidity. Survival alone is not the goal of a good anesthetist; the goal should be to make the anesthetic period as safe as possible.

Fluids

To support CO, it is standard of care to administer replacement fluids to horses under anesthesia. The standard is 10 ml/kg/hour. In an uncomplicated surgery on a healthy horse, crystalloids are used for fluids. Examples of crystalloids include lactated Ringer's solution, Normosol-R, Plasmalyte-R, and 0.9% sodium chloride. The fastest the fluids can be administered without pressure through a 14-gauge catheter is 5 L/hr. If additional fluid boluses are necessary, a second or third catheter should be placed or the fluids can be given under pressure in a pressure bag.

If the horse is hypoproteinemic or the anesthetist is struggling to keep MAP above 60 mm Hg, colloids may be considered. Colloids include hetastarch and dextrans. Boluses of 5 to 10 ml/kg can be used. To administer the bolus as quickly as possible and to continue giving crystalloids at the same time, a second catheter should be placed.

An additional use for colloids is in a situation in which whole blood is needed. The colloid can be given to support blood pressure until whole blood arrives. The typical rule is to transfuse whole blood if greater than 20% of the horse's blood volume has been lost. The blood volume of most horses in liters is equal to 8% of the body weight in kilograms. For example the blood volume in a 500-kg horse is 0.08×500 kg $= 40$ L. If 20% of the blood volume is lost (0.2×40 L $= 8$ L), a transfusion is needed. If the horse has a low blood volume before blood loss it may be prudent to transfuse earlier (before 20% blood loss).

There are several methods for quantitating blood loss. One method is to quantify the number of blood soaked 4×4-gauze sponges and laparotomy pads. Normally a soaked 4×4 gauze will hold 10 ml of blood and a laparotomy pad will hold 50 ml. There may be differences based on brand, but these are rough rules of thumb. Frequently during bloody surgery, blood accumulates on the floor and forms a clot. Another method for quantifying blood loss is to weigh these clots. One kilogram of weight is approximately equal to 1 L blood. Finally, if suction is being used, the PCV of the suction fluid should be measured. Multiplying this by the volume of the suction fluid and dividing by the PCV of the animal, estimates the volume of blood in the suction fluid.

Blood volume in suction fluid (ml)

$$= \frac{\text{PCV suction fluid} \times \text{volume suction fluid (ml)}}{\text{PCV patient}}$$

Another option for fluid, especially when blood is being lost rapidly or in a severely hypovolemic animal is hypertonic saline (7.5% sodium chloride). Hypertonic saline can be given at 2 to 5 ml/kg to rapid expand the intravascular volume. Hypertonic saline pulls fluid in from interstitial spaces by osmosis so it is important to give crystalloids concurrently to replace what is drawn from the interstitial spaces.

Blood Pressure Support

The minimal acceptable MAP is 60 mm Hg. The anesthetist has several options for maintaining blood pressure. The first is to ensure adequate depth of anesthesia. A deep plane of anesthesia will decrease blood pressure. If the animal is hypotensive and thought to be too deep, the first course of action is to decrease the delivered concentration of anesthetic by turning down the vaporizer setting. Secondly, administer fluids. Fluids should be administered at 10 ml/kg/hour. If it is thought that the horse is hypotensive because of hypovolemia, a second catheter should be placed. Crystalloids, colloids, or blood can be infused rapidly through the second catheter if necessary. Before a second catheter is placed the anesthetist should administer a positive inotrope (see Table 9.9). Ephedrine, dobu-

tamine, and dopamine are examples of positive inotropes that can be administered. Ephedrine is given as an IV bolus (0.05–0.2 mg/kg). It is an indirect sympathomimetic that will also tend to increase heart rate. It only has short-term effects. Dobutamine is a β_1-agonist that is cardioselective. It is usually given as a constant rate infusion at a rate of 0.5 to 5 μg/kg/minute. Higher rates in some horses will cause tachycardia. Some horses are more sensitive than others to the tachycardic effects. If a horse becomes tachycardic, it is best to slow or stop the constant rate infusion because severe tachycardia can contribute to further decrease in CO. Dopamine is a noncardioselective positive inotrope. Its effect varies according to the range over which it is infused. At lower doses (0.5–5 μg/kg/minute), the β_1 effects are primarily seen with increased myocardial contractility and some increased HR (Table 9.10). At higher doses (>5 μg/kg/minute) dopamine causes vasoconstriction and tachycardia. The preferred positive inotrope is dobutamine.

Neuromuscular Blockers

Certain procedures, particularly ophthalmologic procedures, require neuromuscular blockade intraoperatively. For ophthalmologic surgery, the purpose is to achieve a central globe. Neuromuscular blockade should only be done by an experienced anesthetist or anesthesiologist. Controlled ventilation is required for these procedures and the depth of neuromuscular blockade should be monitored with a peripheral nerve stimulator.

Drugs for neuromuscular blockade include depolarizing and nondepolarizing neuromuscular

Table 9.10. Positive inotropes used in large animal anesthesia.

Drugs	Mechanism of action	Dose/Rate
Ephedrine	Indirect sympathomimetic (β_1- and α_1-agonist)	0.05–0.2 mg/kg
Dobutamine	β_1-agonist	0.5–5 μg/kg/min
Dopamine	β_1-agonist-lower doses	0.5–5 μg/kg/min
	α_1-agonist-higher doses	>5 μg/kg/min

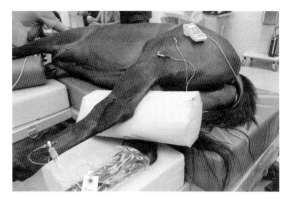

Figure 9.9. Peripheral nerve stimulator on superficial peroneal nerve.

blockers. Succinylcholine is the primary depolarizing neuromuscular blocker and is not commonly used in veterinary medicine. The most common nondepolarizing neuromuscular blocker used in veterinary medicine is atracurium with an onset time of about 5 minutes and a duration of 20 to 30 minutes. Other nondepolarizing neuromuscular blockers include pancuronium and vecuronium. Neuromuscular blockers are reversed with acetylcholinesterase inhibitors. Neostigmine and edrophonium are the two primary reversal agents used in veterinary medicine, with edrophonium being the more common option for horses. It has less muscarinic effect (less bradycardia) and as such, the use of atropine or glycopyrrolate in conjunction with its use is not necessary. Edrophonium must be administered slowly because it can cause hypotension if given too quickly. Additionally, reversal agents should only be given after at least one twitch has returned on the peripheral nerve stimulator.

The peripheral nerve stimulator is typically placed on the superficial peroneal nerve (Figure 9.9). The peripheral nerve stimulator delivers four pulses at a set current (usually 20 mA) in 2 seconds. A train of four twitches is indicative of no to minimal neuromuscular blockade. The goal is to have one of four twitches for optimal blockade. Two or three of four twitches may be acceptable if the patient's eye is not moving and the horse does not have spontaneous breaths during controlled ventilation. The degree of blockade is evaluated by comparing strength of the fourth twitch to that of the first.

Recovery

Most facilities use a padded stall for recovery, the dimensions of which may vary. If the box is too large, the horse may be able to get too much momentum as it is trying to get up, and in this way injure itself. If the box is too small, the horse may get stuck in corners easily and it may be more dangerous for someone to go in and assist the horse.

There are various methods of recovering a horse safely. First, the monitoring equipment is removed. If the horse was unstable during the procedure, it may be necessary to leave on certain pieces of monitoring equipment, such as the ECG or direct blood pressure. Leaving an arterial line in during recovery is especially risky because if the catheter were to come out, a large hematoma could result or if it comes uncapped the horse may lose blood before it is able to be recapped. Ideally an arterial line should be removed and held off for 3 to 5 minutes.

It is the anesthetist's option to wean off the ventilator or not, if a demand valve is available in recovery. A demand valve is a device for delivering a breath from wall outlet oxygen. Most demand valves will deliver at a flow rate of about 150 L/min. A breath can be delivered two to three times per minute until the horse is breathing adequately on its own. Alternatively, the horse can be weaned off the ventilator by decreasing breaths per minute and tidal volume as the procedure is coming to an end. (The anesthetist should be aware that decreasing tidal volume during weaning may possibly lead worsening of alveolar collapse.) If no demand valve is available, the horse should stay attached to or nearby an anesthetic machine until it is spontaneously breathing.

After removing monitoring equipment, the horse is placed on pads in the recovery stall. If the horse was in lateral during the procedure, it should be placed in the same lateral position for recovery. If the horse was in dorsal, either lateral position can be used. If the horse had an orthopedic procedure performed, it will have an easier time standing and

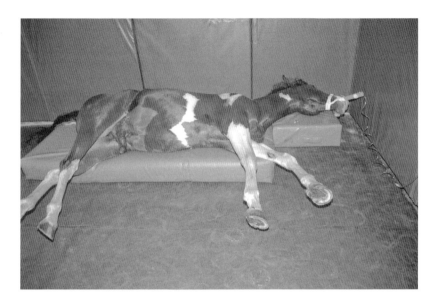

Figure 9.10. Horse on foam mats in padded recovery stall; intubated with oxygen insufflation; lower front leg pulled forward relative to upper front leg.

reduce its chance of fracture if the affected leg is up. The lower front leg should be pulled forward to help avoid a triceps myopathy or radial nerve neuropathy (Figure 9.10).

Leaving the endotracheal tube in place until the animal is standing or chewing on the tube is recommended. The tube is taped around the horse's nose or lower jaw. Oxygen is insufflated via plastic tubing inserted into the endotracheal tube with a flow rate of 10 to 15 L/minute.

After removing the horse from inhalant, most horses will attempt to stand within 30 minutes to 1 hour. In an ideal recovery a horse will roll into sternal, remain in sternal for a brief period, and then stand in one attempt with minimal weakness and ataxia. An important factor affecting the quality of recovery is the disposition of the horse. Horses with quiet demeanor tend to have smoother recoveries than horses that are nervous and flighty. The quality of recovery depends on how ready a horse is to stand when it first tries to stand. As inhalant leaves the brain, the horse may become conscious of its surroundings and try to stand but be too weak and uncoordinated to stand successfully. A goal of recovery is to get the horse to remain recumbent during this phase. The recovery stall should be dark and quiet to help facilitate this.

Most recovery stalls are equipped with dimmer lights but alternatively a towel can be placed over the horse's eye.

Recovery Options

If the horse is small, it can be physically held down until the anesthetist deems it is ready to stand. This is done by applying pressure with the knee to the horse's lateral neck area and lifting the horse's nose off the mat. The horse is usually ready to stand when it no longer has nystagmus and has made two or three strong attempts at lifting its head. This method works better for foals and small ponies. It is physically impossible for an average 500-kg horse.

The more common alternative is to use chemical sedation to sedate the horse during this awakening phase. An α_2-agonist, typically xylazine (0.1–0.2 mg/kg) or romifidine (0.01–0.02 mg/kg), is used to achieve this sedation. Xylazine may be used if a shorter sedation period is desired, whereas romifidine produces longer lasting sedation with potentially less instability and ataxia.

Another option for recovery that should be seriously considered, especially if the horse has had a fracture repaired, is a head and tail rope recovery. This consists of placing a specially designed halter on the horse and attaching a rope to the halter and the tail. A recovery stall with rings or bars is necessary for this type of recovery. The ropes are placed through the rings or over the bars. One person usually controls the horse by applying pressure to its neck, as with a hand recovery, until it is ascertained that the horse is ready to attempt to stand (no nystagmus). As the horse tries to stand, it is assisted by one person pulling on the head rope and one on the tail rope. The ropes are pulled down through the rings or over the bars, and in this way, they guide the horse on its way up. Care must be taken not to put too much pressure on the head rope; if the horse's head is lifted too high it may flip over backward or the horse may become disoriented.

Some institutions have alternative methods for recovery including pools, pool/raft systems, and inflatable recovery mattresses. Pool recoveries are usually reserved for high-risk orthopedic fractures and require experience staff to ensure the horse's safety.

Most institutions have a recovery scoring system to record the quality of recovery in a standardized way. The scoring systems usually take into account the horse's attitude, sternal phase, move to stand, number of attempts to stand, stability after standing, strength, and whether or not an accident occurred.

Anesthesia and Sedation in Foals

Potential reasons for anesthesia in foals include umbilical hernia repair, umbilical abscess resection, septic joint arthroscopy or flushing, patent urachus repair, ruptured bladder repair, colic, and various orthopedic procedures (Tables 9.11, 9.12, and 9.13). In most cases, the foal should be stabilized before anesthesia is attempted. The neonatal foal should be allowed to nurse up to the time of induction. Older foals on solid food may have food withheld for 4 to 6 hours.

Physiologic Considerations

The anesthetic requirement of foals is similar to adults. Foals have slightly different cardiovascular physiology than adult horse. Foals younger than 3

Table 9.11. Anesthetic protocol for healthy foals younger than 6 weeks of age.

Premedication (Wait at least 5 minutes for sedation)	1. Xylazine 0.2–1.0 IV, IM
	2. Diazepam 0.05–0.1 IV
	3. Butorphanol/diazepam 0.10/0.10 IV
Induction	1. Isoflurane or Sevoflurane (nasotracheal or mask)
	2. Ketamine 2–3 mg/kg IV

IM, intramuscularly; IV, intravenously.

Table 9.12. Anesthetic protocol for sick foal.

Premedication* (Wait at least 5 minutes for sedation)	1. Butorphanol 0.05–0.1 IV
	+/– Diazepam 0.10–0.2 IV
Induction	1. Isoflurane or sevoflurane (nasotracheal or mask)
	2. Ketamine 2–3 mg/kg IV

*May not be necessary
IV, intravenously.

Table 9.13. Anesthetic protocol for healthy foal older than 6 weeks.

Premedication (Wait at least 5 minutes for sedation)	1. Xylazine 0.2–1.0 mg/kg IV, IM
	2. Xylazine/butorphanol 0.3/0.02 mg/kg IV
Induction	1. 5% Guaifenesin: Administer by gravity to effect 50–100 mg/kg IV
	Ketamine 1.5–2.2 mg/kg IV
	OR
	10% Thiopental* 4–6 mg/kg IV
	2. Diazepam or midazolam 0.02–0.1 mg/kg IV
	Ketamine 1.5–2.2 mg/kg IV
	3. Ketamine 2.2 mg/kg IV
	If full dose of xylazine was used as premedication

*For healthy older horse use same protocol but lower dosages.
IM, intramuscularly; IV, intravenously.

to 5 days may have a patent ductus arteriosus or a patent foramen ovale. With changes due to anesthetic drugs, vascular shunts may worsen. For this reason, anesthesia should be avoided in foals younger than 3 to 5 days.

The CO of foals is dependent on HR, and generally foals have a higher cardiac index than adults. Despite this, they tend to have lower systemic blood pressure than adults possibly as a result of an immature sympathetic nervous system. These differences are most obvious in foals between 1 and 6 weeks of age. By 1 month of age, cardiac index is lower but blood pressure is higher, probably because of an increased systemic vascular resistance. Often foals need inotropic support under anesthesia. Based on research, it does seem that they respond to dobutamine, dopamine, and ephedrine. The response may be more obvious in increased heart rate than increased blood pressure.

Foals are less tolerant of hemorrhage or dehydration. It must be kept in mind that they are less able to increase stroke volume in response to volume loading due to a less compliant heart. If blood is needed whole blood from the mare can be used, preferably with a cross-match.

The respiratory system of foals is also different than adults. They have a higher minute ventilation mainly due to a higher respiratory rate. This results in a rapid rise in the alveolar concentration of inhalation anesthetics. Foals tend to have a rapid induction and recovery from inhalation anesthetics. Up to about 6 weeks of age they are more susceptible to alveolar collapse and hypoxemia. For this reason, IPPV should be used judiciously in foals in the same way that it is used in adult horses. If a foal is excessively hypoventilating or hypoxic, positive pressure ventilation should be considered.

Foals are more susceptible to hypothermia than adult horses. They have a large surface area-to-body mass ratio and a small amount of subcutaneous fat. A forced-air warming device and warm-water blankets should be used when possible in foals younger than 6 weeks of age. After 6 weeks, they may not need heat supplementation unless they are sick or have a wet hair coat.

With their high metabolic rate, foals are more susceptible to hypoglycemia, especially if sick or fasted. Glucose should be monitored carefully (every 30–60 minutes) and supplemented if needed.

Whether or not a foal is hypoproteinemic should be considered. Hypoproteinemic foals may have enhanced responses to highly protein bound anesthetic agents such as diazepam. A greater portion of CO in foals is delivered to the brain so they may have a more profound response to the same dose of drug. For nonprotein-bound drugs, foals may display an apparent resistance to the first IV bolus due to a larger volume of distribution.

By 1 to 2 weeks of age, hepatic function is well developed, so metabolism of drugs is not as much of an issue especially when only a single bolus is given. Renal function may take several weeks to reach adult levels. By 1 month of age, foals should be able to metabolize and excrete at a rate similar to adults.

Anesthetic Preparation of Foals

Preanesthetic assessment should be the same as for adult horses. If respiratory function is in question, an arterial blood gas should be performed. The blood glucose concentration should be measured before induction. Foals in respiratory distress or with pneumonia should be preoxygenated. This can be done via a face mask or nasal insufflation.

Mare
The mare is typically kept present during induction and must be sedated. Sedation should include a drug of relatively long duration of action. Acepromazine is given either intramuscularly or intravenously for its longer lasting effects with an α_2-agonist for its more immediate and potent sedative effects.

Premedication
Sedation of sick foals is generally not necessary. Sedation with low doses of diazepam (0.05–0.1 mg/kg) or low doses of xylazine (0.3–0.5 mg/kg) may be used if necessary.

Induction
Induction may be achieved with an inhalant agent via a nasotracheal tube or mask or with parenteral drugs. After induction with a nasotracheal tube or mask a tube should be passed orotracheally.

Especially for larger foals (>100–150 kg) inhalant induction may be impractical due to inability to restrain the foal. In these cases, parenteral inductions can be used similar to those used in adult horses. Propofol may be considered as an induction agent. A smaller volume would be needed than for an adult horse making it an affordable option. If guaifenesin is used care must be taken not to go over the toxic dose (300 mg/kg).

Maintenance

Maintenance of anesthesia is similar to that for adult horses, and monitoring should be similar as well. Due to differences in metabolism and excretion it may be best to avoid parenteral infusions in foals younger than 1 month of age. Direct arterial catheterization may be more difficult in foals due to smaller and more fragile and mobile arteries.

Recovery

Foals should be kept warm into recovery. Premature or sick foals should be placed in a sternal position as soon as possible. In most cases, an assisted or "hand" recovery is feasible and recommended. This involves physically restraining the foal until he or she is deemed ready to stand and then assisting standing by holding the head and tail (one person on head and one on tail). The mare should be kept away until the foal is standing.

Complications

Airway Obstruction

The status of the horse's upper airway should be assessed before induction. If a problem is anticipated, an endoscope should be readily available and a tracheostomy kit prepared. In some cases it may even be prudent to preclip and scrub for a tracheostomy. Having endotracheal tubes one or two sizes smaller than that you would expect to use would also be a good idea saving time from scrambling for one in an emergency. If a tracheostomy is performed, a cuffed endotracheal tube should be inserted and 100% oxygen insufflated.

A severe complication of airway obstruction is postobstructive pulmonary edema. This can develop very quickly after only a brief period of obstruction and should be monitored for after an obstruction is thought to have occurred. A blood gas should be conducted to evaluate oxygen level. If frothy, pink liquid (pulmonary edema) begins to come out of the endotracheal tube or the horse is tachypneic or dyspneic after the obstruction is relieved, then postobstructive pulmonary edema should be suspected. Furosemide can be administered at 0.5 to 1 mg/kg intravenously. If the airway obstruction has occurred preoperatively, it must be left up to the surgeon or anesthesiologist whether to continue with the procedure. If the animal is not hypoxic and has not developed pulmonary edema then, it may be possible to continue the procedure, especially if the procedure will improve the obstruction. If the animal is hypoxic or has developed pulmonary edema, the animal should be recovered with the endotracheal tube cuff inflated and left in place.

Hypoxemia

Hypoxemia is defined as PaO_2 less than 60 mm Hg. Horses can survive with PaO_2 less than 60 mm Hg, but all practical methods to correct hypoxemia should be employed regardless to decrease morbidity. Clinical signs of hypoxemia are hard to appreciate under anesthesia. Cyanosis, tachycardia, hypertension, and bucking the ventilator or gasping breaths may be observed. The primary cause of hypoxemia in horses is a mismatch of ventilation (V) and perfusion (Q) in the lungs (V/Q mismatch) and shunting (this essentially means that some deoxygenated blood completely bypasses the lungs and goes straight to systemic circulation). These occur due to the compression of the lung by the weight of abdominal viscera on the diaphragm. The disturbance is usually worse in horses in dorsal versus lateral position and can be worsened by abdominal organ distension or pregnancy. Additional causes of hypoxemia that should be ruled out are decreased inspired oxygen fraction (check flow meter), improperly placed endotracheal tube (in esophagus), and hypoventilation.

243

Hypoventilation alone should not cause a PaO_2 less than 60 mm Hg if 100% oxygen is being breathed. A checklist for the management of hypoxemia is as follows:

1. Ensure fraction of inspired oxygen (FiO_2) of 100%.
2. Correct hypoventilation if animal has high $PaCO_2$—provide IPPV.
3. Optimize inspiratory-to-expiratory ratio (1:1 ratio may be considered).
4. Increase CO by use of fluids and positive inotropes; ensure that animal is not in a deep plane of anesthesia.
5. Provide positive pressure ventilation with positive end-expiratory pressure (not routine due to decrease in CO).
6. Give bronchodilator (albuterol, 2 µg/kg) endotracheally—method of action not understood.

Oxygen should be insufflated postoperatively to help avoid or decrease amount of hypoxemia in recovery, especially because oxygen levels are not routinely monitored in recovery.

Hypotension

Arterial hypotension is defined as a MAP of less than 60 mm Hg (foals < 50 mm Hg). Hypotension is probably the most common complication in large animal anesthesia and almost every horse will develop hypotension without intervention. Possible causes of hypotension are hypovolemia, vasodilation (from drugs, endotoxemia, shock), poor CO, decreased myocardial contractility due to anesthetic agents, and inappropriate depth of anesthesia. Correction of hypotension depends on the cause. The following checklist can be used:

1. Check depth of anesthesia: if too deep, lighten plane by turning down vaporizer setting; may consider balancing anesthetic technique by using PIVA.
2. Administer fluids at 10 ml/kg/hour. This should already be done in most cases but if hypotension is a problem, check that fluids are actually running; consider putting in second or third IV catheter to bolus additional fluids, colloids, or blood.

3. Administer positive inotrope; dobutamine is the preferred positive inotrope at 0.5 to 5 µg/kg/min. Consider giving bolus of ephedrine 0.0 to −0.2 mg/kg (short acting).
4. Check blood gas and electrolytes. Optimize ventilation. If pH is less than 7.2, cardiac contractility is reduced. Maintaining pH between 7.2 and 7.4 via permissive hypercapnia may provide cardiovascular stimulation; correct electrolytes if necessary. Calcium is often low in horses with colic, administer 10 to 20 mg/kg if ionized calcium is less than 1.2 mmol/L.
5. Other options for increasing blood pressure, especially if vasodilation due to shock or endotoxemia is suspected, are vasopressors (phenylephrine and vasopressin).

Generally, blood pressure can be maintained above 60 mm Hg with supportive care in elective cases. Even with these supportive measures, blood pressure can be difficult to maintain in some emergency cases.

Hypercapnia

Hypercapnia is a $PaCO_2$ above normal (>45 mm Hg). This is common during general anesthesia due to the depressant effects of drugs on the respiratory center. Hypercapnia generally results from hypoventilation. Other less common causes are malignant hyperthermia and hyperkalemic periodic paralysis (HYPP). Alternatively, hypercapnia may precipitate HYPP.

Hypercapnia up to a point causes sympathetic stimulation and increased CO. More severe hypercapnia can increase cardiac instability and decrease pH. When pH is less than 7.2, cardiac contractility, and therefore, CO are decreased.

If the cause for the hypercapnia is hypoventilation, controlled ventilation can be started at the anesthetist's discretion. If the horse is already on controlled ventilation, tidal volume and breaths per minute should be optimized to reduce CO_2. Additionally, it may be prudent to ascertain that rebreathing of CO_2 is not a cause of the increased $PaCO_2$. Rebreathing may occur if CO_2 absorbent is depleted or due to the presence of a faulty expiratory valve. It may not be possible to check for the presence of inspired CO_2 without a capnometer or capnograph.

Arrhythmias

Arrhythmias can be tachycardias, bradycardias, and ventricular or atrial in origin. Ventricular arrhythmias are quite unusual in horses. Intermittent premature ventricular contractions (PVCs) need not be treated if blood pressure is maintained and they are unifocal. Ventricular tachycardia (HR > 100) or multiple PVCs affecting blood pressure should be treated. Use lidocaine at 0.5 to 1.5 mg/kg intravenously for immediate control. The underlying cause should also be treated. Possible underlying causes are heart disease, severe toxemia, colic, sepsis, electrolyte disturbance (potassium, magnesium, or calcium), and viral or bacterial infections. Under anesthesia, electrolytes may be the only immediately correctable cause. Electrolytes should be checked at the first sign of ventricular arrhythmias and corrected if necessary.

Atrial premature contractions (APCs) may be associated with enlarged atria or electrolyte problems (hypokalemia). These are not usually treated unless clinical signs are present.

Atrial fibrillation is fibrillation of the atria with some impulses passing through the atrioventricular node to cause ventricular contraction. Atrial fibrillation may be tachycardic or not. It may be associated with heart disease or could be incidental. If atrial fibrillation is detected before anesthesia, the horse should have a complete workup before being anesthetized and stabilized before anesthesia.

Sinus bradycardia is a heart rate of less than 26 beats per minutes. This is usually associated with increased vagal tone in a fit horse or due to drugs given for anesthesia and is not usually treated with an anticholinergic, especially is blood pressure is normal. Sinus arrest is a long pause on the ECG that may be followed by an escape beat. This is due to increased vagal tone in a fit horse or due to anesthetic drugs. If the patient is compromised it may be treated with atropine or a β_1-agonist.

Second-degree atrioventricular block is when there are p-waves on the ECG with no associated QRS complex. This usually occurs due to increased vagal tone and from anesthetic drugs, especially α_2-agonists.

Metabolic Problems

Hyperkalemia

The most common electrolyte derangements involve potassium and calcium. Hyperkalemia can cause arrhythmias and may be fatal if not treated. Hyperkalemia can be caused by ruptured bladder (foals) or HYPP. Quarter horses or quarter horse crosses with certain lineages are predisposed to HYPP, and this association should be determined before anesthesia. If potassium is greater than 5.5 mmol/L before anesthesia, general anesthesia will be risky, and the patient should be stabilized first. Signs of an HYPP episode under general anesthesia may include the following:

1. Muscle fasciculation.
2. ECG changes.
3. Tachycardia.
4. Tachypnea.
5. Hypercapnia.
6. Hyperthermia.

Fluids should be switched to a fluid not containing potassium (sodium chloride). Calcium gluconate should be administered (0.2–0.4 ml/kg intravenously) to protect against the cardiotoxic effects of hyperkalemia (this will not lower potassium). Acidemia should be treated by administering sodium bicarbonate (1–2 mEq/kg intravenously) and controlling respiratory acidosis. Insulin can also be used to shift potassium into the cells, but an appropriate dosage is not established for horses. In horses with known HYPP, blood gases and serum electrolytes should be closely monitored, as well as ECG. ECG changes are often the first signs seen. These changes include increasing amplitude of T waves, bradycardia, decreasing amplitude of p waves, and widening of QRS complexes.

Prolonged recovery is the most common complication from general anesthesia of HYPP patients. Horses should recover in a quiet, darkened stall with oxygen supplementation. If a horse is having difficulty in recovery and HYPP is a possibility, electrolytes should be checked.

Hypocalcemia

Most commonly hypocalcemia is seen in horses with colic and endotoxemia. Hypocalcemia should be corrected if ionized calcium is less than 1.2 mmol/L. Calcium at 10 to 20 mg/kg is administered intravenously.

Postanesthetic Myopathies and Neuropathies

It is difficult to tell the difference between myopathies and neuropathies, and they can be concurrent problems. Myopathies are painful and associated with muscle swelling or hardness. Myopathies result in characteristic increases in muscle enzymes on bloodwork. Myopathies are thought to be the result of an ischemic injury to muscles because of decreased perfusion and increased intracompartmental muscle pressure. A neuropathy might result from prolonged pressure on a particular nerve. Myopathies can affect a single muscle group or be generalized, and they can occur on either the dependent or nondependent side. Most of the time the myopathy or neuropathy will not become apparent until recovery. The animal may have difficult in recovery, be lame, have swollen and hard muscles, seem painful, and be sweating.

There are numerous risk factors for myopathies and neuropathies none of which have been identified as the primary cause. Myopathies can occur after seemingly uneventful anesthetic episodes in which blood pressure was maintained, positioning seemed adequate, padding was used, and the procedure was short. The risk factors include a period of hypotension, heavier horses, longer procedures, and poor positioning. For these reasons, it is always a goal to minimize hypotension, position the horse adequately, and minimize anesthesia time.

Treatment of myopathies and neuropathies involve assisting to stand, slinging, splinting the foreleg (for triceps myopathy/radial nerve neuropathy), maintaining hydration, and administering analgesia, acepromazine, and dimethyl sulfoxide (DMSO).

Cardiac Arrest

Cardiac arrest rarely occurs in elective procedures unless due to overdose of anesthetic or after administration of a certain drug. The prognosis is poor if cardiac arrest does occur due to the difficulty in performing cardiopulmonary resuscitation in horses. Administration of inhalant and any TIVA or PIVA should be stopped and 100% oxygen should be continued. If the horse is not intubated, the horse should be intubated and ventilated at a rate of 6 to 10 breaths per minute. Chest compressions should be started if no pulse is palpable. This involves someone delivering a blow with the knee behind the horse's elbow area. Compressions should be administered at 40 to 80 per minute. Epinephrine can be given at 0.02 mg/kg to cause vasoconstriction. Atropine can be administered at 0.01 to 0.02 mg/kg. If spontaneous circulation returns, drugs with specific cardiac and vasoactive effects should be used to stabilize CO and blood pressure (dobutamine). If ventricular fibrillation occurs, defibrillation is indicated although unlikely to be successful in an adult horse.

Problems with Recovery

Problems that may occur during recovery include nasal edema, trauma, limb fracture, myopathies or neuropathies, and laryngospasm.

Nasal edema is quite common post-anesthesia, especially after long procedures and in horses that were in dorsal recumbency. Phenylephrine nasal spray may be sprayed into the horse's nostrils before it recovers, if nasal edema is a concern, or this can be done after the horse is extubated. Usually nasal edema will not be a problem but may cause noisy breathing after the horse is extubated.

Minor *traumas* such as skin abrasions and bitten lips or tongues are relatively common and not a cause for concern.

Limb fractures most likely occur in horses that have had a limb fracture repaired. The fracture usually occurs at the surgery site or at a fulcrum point of the cast. A head and tail recovery may be considered for a horse with a repaired fracture or recovering with a cast.

Laryngospasm may occur at extubation causing an upper airway obstruction. After the horse is extubated flow through the nostrils should be checked. If respiratory obstruction is strongly suspected, the horse should be nasotracheally intubated or a tracheostomy done if intubation is not possible.

References and Further Reading

Doherty, T., and A. Valverde. 2006. *Manual of Equine Anesthesia and Analgesia.* Ames, IA: Blackwell Publishers.

Tranquilli, W. J., J. C. Thurmon, and K. A. Grimm. 2007. Anesthesia, analgesia and immobilization of selected species: Horses. In *Lumb and Jones' Veterinary Anesthesia.* 4th ed., ed. J. C. Thurmon, W. J. Tranquilli, G. J. Benson, and W. V. Lumb, 717–29. Ames, IA: Blackwell Publishers.

CHAPTER 10

Surgical Assistance

Gail Broussard, Elizabeth Hinton, and Tracy McArthur

The Preoperative Operating Room

The operating room (OR) should be equipped pre-operatively. Before entering the OR, proper attire including disposable cap, mask, and shoe covers should be donned. In the ideal situation, the gowning surface would be located in a low traffic area in the OR to prevent a break in gowning technique. The instrument table should be placed in close proximity to where the surgeon will be standing for the procedure. Any ancillary equipment that will be used for the procedure should be checked and ready for use. Portable suction units, electro-cautery units, and some form of fluid pump for flushing joints or for use during arthroscopies for joint distention are common pieces of ancillary equipment used. However, some ORs are quite small and require the patient to be in place before equipment can be set up in the area of operation.

Patient Induction and Preparation

After the OR has been prepared properly, then induction and preparation of the patient can proceed. An equine hospital with surgical facilities usually has an area, or separate room, to accommodate induction and preparation of the surgical site. This is preferred because the preparation procedure on horses can include dirt, hair, and dander that can aerosolize during preparation. There are facilities in which induction, prep, surgery, and recovery use the same room. In this situation it would be prudent to perform as much patient clipping and gross preparation of the surgical site before induction as possible, and the sterile items in the OR should not be opened and set up until the surgical site is fully prepared.

Patient Positioning and Preparation

Surgical tables are available that can accommodate all three positions routinely used for horses under anesthesia. Some patient tables are designed with a hydraulic lift system, which can raise or lower or tilt the table to accommodate the surgeon's preference.

In dorsal recumbency the patient is positioned on its back with all four legs supported in an upright position. Proper padding, in this case beneath the patient, and support will be discussed later. In right or left lateral recumbency, with the patient on its side, leg supports with appropriate padding, in addition to padding beneath the body, are required.

Proper and adequate support of the patient is of the utmost importance to avoid serious and potentially fatal complications that can occur. Postanes-thetic myopathy, resulting from lack of adequate profusion and oxygenation of muscle mass, can be

249

caused by inadequate support or improper positioning and is of special concern in the draft breeds because of their size and weight. Postanesthetic neuropathy, secondary to excessive pressure on nerve bundles or inadequate perfusion, can produce similar muscle dysfunction during recovery, making it difficult, if not impossible for the patient to return to a stable standing position. Myopathy and neuropathy can either be temporary or permanent; in the latter case, humane destruction may be necessary. Postoperative therapy of these conditions usually includes anti-inflammatory medications, intravenous fluids, and appropriate physical support such as slinging.

To ensure that the patient is receiving adequate support, the padding should be made of industrial grade foam covered in a nonabsorbent material such as vinyl. Most companies that manufacture equine surgical tables also produce customized padding for use in the various recumbent positions. Thickness of the pads varies; for instance, a lateral pad might be 7 inches thick, whereas a dorsal pad might be 10 inches thick.

Limb positioning and support is also critical. In lateral recumbency, the "down" legs (both front and hind) should be pulled well forward and supported parallel to the body, and the "up" legs should be well supported in a position parallel to the body so as to diminish pressure on the down legs and optimize perfusion. Most equine surgical tables have customized leg supports that will facilitate both positioning and support; however, if these are unavailable, other support structures such as separate cushions or garbage cans with cushions can suffice.

A horse in dorsal recumbency requires adequate padding beneath its body. Padded shoulder supports are supplied with most tables that will maintain the horse in dorsal recumbency. The limbs can then be positioned according to the surgery to be performed. Vertical poles with rings, which can be mounted on the table, can support the limbs in varying degrees of extension. Alternatively, the forelimbs can be restrained in a flexed position with hobbles or cotton ropes affixed to the table. The hind legs are best supported in mild extension, attached to leg poles, so as to improve perfusion.

Preparation of Patient

Once the patient is induced and positioned, aseptic preparation of the surgical site must be completed. Clipping with a number 40 blade of an area extending approximately 10 cm from the incision site should be performed while a shop vacuum is used simultaneously to remove loose hair, dander, and debris from the patient and surrounding area. The patient is now ready for the surgical scrub.

Rough Preparation and Bucket Preparation

The first in a two-step preparation is considered the "rough prep," often referred to as a "bucket prep."

Equipment:

3-gallon stainless steel bucket.
Small (500 ml) stainless steel container with a handle.
Stainless container containing 4 × 4 gauze sponges soaked in a 70% alcohol can be useful.
Squeeze bottle filled with povidone-iodine scrub.
Nonsterile 4 × 4 gauze sponges.
Nonsterile examination gloves.
Povidone-iodine scrub or chlorhexidine gluconate.
10% povidone-iodine solution.
70% alcohol in a spray or squeeze bottle.

To begin, examination gloves should be worn during the first step in the preparation process.

Fill the 3-gallon stainless bucket with warm tap water, and add enough povidone-iodine solution to turn the water into a light tea color.

Place one handful of nonsterile 4 × 4 gauze sponges into the bucket along with the smaller stainless steel container.

During this preparation, the dominate hand of the technician should be designated as the "scrubbing hand" (sometimes referred to as the "dirty hand") and will come into contact with the patient's skin. The nondominate hand will be used to reach into the preparation bucket to retrieve gauze sponges and pass them to the dominate scrubbing hand. It is imperative that the scrubbing hand not contaminate the passing hand or the bucket. Likewise the "clean" hand should never make contact with the patient's skin, so as to prevent cross-contamination from patient to solution.

After the gauze has been passed, with the clean hand, scrub should be applied to the entire clipped area and to the gauze. Starting at the incision site, scrubbing should progress in a circular motion to the periphery of the clipped area. A helpful suggestion is to imagine a bull's-eye at the surgical site and work from that spot outward. Make sure that the povidone-iodine scrub is leaving a yellow lather; this indicates the correct concentration of scrub. Multiple gauze sponges will be required to complete this task; always starting at the center of the bull's-eye and progressing outward. Then, with the clean hand reach into the bucket, take the stainless graduated cylinder and rinse the entire clipped area. Do not pour in a fashion that will allow the rinse solution to run over the clipped area from the hairline. Repeat this step at least two more times; do it more often if the area is especially contaminated. Alcohol from the spray or squeeze bottle should be used as the final rinse. Alternatively, alcohol soaked sponges may be used to wipe away soap lather, using the same clean/contaminated hand technique.

The rough bucket prep should always be the first step and may be the only preparation used for some surgeries such as standing castrations. Contact time, dilution, and friction are the factors that produce an effective preparation of the surgical site. Contact time, that is, the amount of time the antimicrobial agent stays in contact with the skin, must be at least 5 minutes. If only a rough prep is used, then alcohol should be the final rinse, followed by an application of sterile preparation solution either with sterile sponges or a squeeze or spray bottle. Sterile disposable applicators, which resemble a soap dispensing scrub wand for dishwashing, that contain sterile surgical prep solution (iodine povacrylex and a 74% isopropyl alcohol) are available in individual peel packages. Apply the final preparation solution in a circular motion starting at the surgical site and paint a layer of solution on the clipped area in progressively larger circles. The label should be referred to for safety precautions. This prepping solution leaves a film barrier around

the surgical site that may provide some sustained antimicrobial effects.

Aseptic Prepping

An aseptic preparation should be used as the final preparation in most surgical procedures to minimize the possibility of postoperative infection.

Equipment:

Sterile surgical gloves.
Povidone-iodine scrub (chlorhexidine can be used in place of povidone-iodine scrub; however, alcohol cannot be used with chlorhexidine because it will deactivate it.)
70% alcohol.
1,000-ml bottle of sterile water or saline.
Sterile preparation pack containing two small basins, sponge forceps, approximately fifty 4×4 gauze sponges placed inside each basin and two cloth huck towels.
An instrument table or cart on which to open the prep pack for use.

It is most efficient to keep all preparation items available in a central location because some of the same items are also used for rough prepping.

Unwrap the sterile prep pack. Handle the wrap by the corners only to ensure proper aseptic technique. Open the 70% alcohol, povidone-iodine scrub, and saline. Open gloves, and glove only the dominate hand at this time. With the sterile gloved hand remove the sterile 4×4 sponges from the basins and set them on the sterile field. Pick up the povidone-iodine scrub with the nongloved hand and fill a basin one-fourth full. Fill the other basin three-fourths full with alcohol. Top off each basin with saline. When pouring, hold the containers at least 6 inches above the sterile field.

The second sterile glove can now be donned and 4×4 sponges placed into each basin. The same technique is applied to the aseptic scrub as was used in the bucket scrub. It is important to designate a clean hand and a dirty (usually the dominant one) hand. Take the sponge forceps in the clean hand, and retrieve a povidone-iodine scrub sponge and the gauze in the palm of that the scrubbing hand. Be careful not to contaminate the tips of the sponge forceps or the clean hand with the dirty hand. Using a povidone-iodine scrub soaked sponge, begin scrubbing in the same circular pattern working from the primary site toward the clipped edge. The lather should again be yellow. When the sponge starts to dry or the suds lighten to a white, then discard that sponge and replace it with fresh one. Depending on the size of the area, it is possible that several scrub sponges in each pass from center to periphery.

Once the area has been scrubbed and covered thoroughly with the yellow suds and the contact time has equaled 5 or more minutes, the area is wiped with the alcohol sponges. Using the clean hand, or sponge forceps take one alcohol 4 × 4 sponge and drop it into the dirty scrubbing hand. Use this first gauze to clean the glove surface by squeezing the gauze out with the dirty hand away from the sterile field and surgical site, and then discard the sponge. Begin the rinse with a second alcohol-soaked 4 × 4 sponge, starting in the center of the surgical field and working to the periphery in the same fashion as the scrub was applied. Use as many alcohol gauzes as needed until all the soap has been removed.

Scrubbing with povidone-iodine scrub and wiping with alcohol sponges should be repeated twice. This will insure adequate contact time. The total three full scrubs will last at least 10 minutes. *Always* scrub or wipe from the incision site out to the periphery.

Once the aseptic preparation has been completed, one of the sterile cloth towels may be laid over the prepped area to protect it while the horse is moved into surgery or until the surgeon is ready to drape the area. Especially in dorsal recumbency, soap and rinse water or alcohol tend to accumulate in the folds of skin between the abdomen and hind legs. This should be carefully dried with clean towels before the horse is moved or draped.

The Surgical Team

The surgical team may consist of a surgeon, an assistant surgeon or a assisting "scrub" technician, a circulating technician to retrieve and open instruments during surgery, and an anesthesia technician. However, in many instances these roles are filled by a single veterinarian and one technician.

All personnel entering the OR need to be in proper attire. Clean fresh scrubs should be worn for each procedure. Disposable masks, shoe covers, and disposable caps should be worn by everyone entering the OR. The surgeon and scrub technician will need to perform a 10-minute surgical hand scrub with a sterile disposable scrub brush and either a 4.5% chlorhexidine gluconate soap or a 7.5% povidone-iodine soap.

Gowning should be performed in a low-traffic area inside the OR that is equipped with a flat surface on which to open the gown packs in an aseptic manner. Most disposable, presterilized gowns are wrapped and then placed in a peel type pack. Remove the wrapped gown from the peel pack and place it on the flat surface. Open the gown wrapping by handling on the corners. The corners of the wrap will have a tendency to flip back over and contaminate the gown, so be cautious. A sterile towel (for drying hands following scrubbing) and sterile surgical gloves can be opened aseptically onto the gown surface. To ensure asepsis, be especially careful when opening the sterile items so that only the corners of the wrap are handled.

The surgical hand scrub, when performed correctly, will greatly decrease the number of microorganisms on the surgeons' hands, thus minimizing the likelihood of transfer contamination. The technique recommended by Gordon, Puterbaugh, and Davis (2005) in "Scrubbing, Gowning, and Gloving" is as follows:

Open the sterile scrub brush and place it close by for easy access.
Place hands and forearms under running water. The temperature and flow should be adjusted beforehand.
With antimicrobial soap, lather the hands first followed by the forearms to a point 2 inches above the elbow.
Use the finger nail cleaner.

With the sterile scrub brush, start at the finger tips then progress to the fingers, including the webbing in between. Scrub the palms and back of the hand then proceed to the wrist. Continue from the wrist up to 2 inches above the elbow, being sure that all surfaces of the front and back of the hands and forearms are subjected to the friction of the brush and soap.

Transfer the brush to the other hand, and repeat the procedure. Additional soap may need to be applied to maintain adequate lather. Total contact/ scrubbing time should be 10 minutes.

Rinse both hands and arms, from finger tips down the arms holding the hands pointed upwards and proceed into the operating room. Keep hands pointed up and elbows above the waist.

When drying hands, pick up the towel and step back from the sterile gown surface. Use one end of the towel to dry one hand and the other end for the other hand, starting at the fingers and working toward the elbows. Do not use long wiping motions instead creep down the hands and arms. Discard the towel when done.

To don the gown, pick up the folded sterile gown and step back from the surface leaving adequate room to avoid contamination. Hold the gown with both hands by the collar and let it unfold. Once it is unfolded, the armholes will be exposed. Insert one hand inside each sleeve stopping just short of the sleeve cuffs. As a closed gloving technique is preferred, the cuffs should not be touched with the fingers or hands. A circulating technician can assist with adjusting and tying gowns and should only handle the closure on the collar behind the neck and inside the gown at waist level. Inside the gown on the right side at waist level, there will be a tie or snap that will attach to a closure on the inside at the left.

Once both arms are inside the sleeves, gloves may be donned using the closed gloving technique with the hands inside the gown and unexposed.

Take the folded cuff of the left glove with the right hand, which is still enclosed in the gown sleeve, and place the palm of the glove against the palm of the left hand (which is also still enclosed in the gown sleeve) with the fingers pointing up the left arm. Grip the front edge of the cuff with the left hand. Grip the back edge of the cuff with the right

hand and pull it over the left hand. The fingers of the left hand may now be extended into the glove and the right hand can be used to turn the cuff edges down over the cuff and sleeve of the gown. Repeat the same procedure with the right glove using the now gloved left hand. For left-handed surgeons, gloving the right hand first may be more comfortable (Gordon, et al. 2005).

Preparing the Operating Room

It is imperative that proper aseptic technique be employed when opening instrument packs. Only the edges or corners of the packs should be handled by technicians who are not gowned and gloved, and these corners should never touch sterile fields. Peel packs containing sterile items are sterile only inside the sealed borders. Items that are wrapped with draping material, such as large instrument packs, should have at least two, preferably three, layers wrapping them. Disposable drapes will most commonly be wrapped with one drape and placed inside a peel pack.

The instrument table should be prepared in the following manner: first an instrument table cover should be placed over the table top surface. Most table covers can be opened by finding the center of the folds. Unfold the table cover from the center so that the ends of the drape drop over each end of the table. Anything below table top level is considered a nonsterile area. Once the table is draped then the instrument packs, drapes, and ancillary items can be opened. The circulating technician should never walk between sterile fields but should stand behind the instrument table to open additional packs, taking care to avoid holding the packs over the surgical table while opening them.

To open the pack, place it in the nondominant hand with the tail of the outer drape facing the front of the table. With the dominant hand, pull the tail of the wrap and hang it over the nondominant hand, being careful to not to allow it to touch the sterile surface of the table. Then, take one corner of the wrap at a time and unfold each and allow them to hang down the sides. Finally, pull the last corner over the forearm. If there are two wraps left on the pack, then repeat this sequence one more time. One wrap should be left covering the pack when it is either placed on the table or handed to the surgeon.

Gather all the corners of the drapes with the dominant hand in a sweeping motion so that the arm holding the pack is covered with noncontaminated wrap. Be careful to grab the excess at the corners so that noncontaminated wrap covers the nondominate hand and arm. Step toward the table, and gently set the pack on the table top. Do not lean over the instrument table, and always stay 1 foot back from the table and 1 foot above the table when pouring saline or opening single items onto the table.

The small ancillary items such as blades and suture material should be opened next. Preferably they should land on top of the pack. Sharp items could penetrate the table cover. Scalpel blades come packaged in a small peel pack. Again, stand back from the table, and start to peel the blade package open until the blade is exposed right to the tip. Walk up to the table, turn the peel pack upside down and open it the rest of the way with the blade landing on top of the instrument pack. If the surgeon or assistant is available to accept a sterile item, let them lean over the sterile table to reach it.

Drapes are often wrapped the same way as instrument packs and should be opened in the same manner and placed on the table beside the surgical pack containing the towel clamps

Careful observation of the sterile fields, draping techniques and opening of packs must be followed, and any break in sterile technique mentioned immediately. If the patient is moved from a prep area into the OR, it is the responsibility of the circulating technician to ensure that there is absolutely no break in aseptic technique. Nonsterilized people should never pass between sterile fields created by the instrument table, surgeon, and patient. Sterilized people should face the sterile field, keeping hands and arms above waist line, and pass nonsterilized people with their backs to them. Nonsterilized people must maintain a distance of at least 1 foot from a sterile field. Maintenance of sterility is a team effort.

Common Instruments

Common instruments that should be recognized:

Penetrating towel clamps are used to secure drapes directly to the patient and have sharp points. Nonpenetrating towel clamps with blunt tips are used to fasten drape to drape or secure items to a drape.

Blunt tipped operating scissors are used for cutting suture or drapes.

Kelly and mosquito haemostatic forceps are used for clamping off small blood vessels.

Tissue forceps are used for picking up and holding tissue and may be rat-toothed with small teeth at the tips or have less sharp ends, such as the Brown Adson thumb forceps.

Mayo-Hagar needle holders are used for passing and pulling suture needles. Olsen-Hagar needle holders are used the same way but have blades built in for cutting the suture.

Mayo scissors are more substantial than Metzenbaum scissors and are used for cutting heavy thick tissue. Metzenbaum scissors usually have a long handle and short delicate blades and are used for delicate sharp or blunt tissue dissection.

A scalpel handle is used to hold a blade for making incisions.

Allis tissue forceps have short teeth on the ends and are used to retract less delicate tissue such as skin edges.

Babcock forceps are less traumatic and are used to hold delicate tissues such as viscera. Sponge forceps can also be used in the same manner as Babcock forceps or are used to grab and hold sponges or gauze.

Surgical Packs

There are many different ways to customize surgical packs. Three versions will be described. A simple suture pack consists of one Rat Toothed forceps, one Brown Adson thumb forceps, a Mayo-Hagar needle holder, #3 scalpel handle, straight Mayo scissors, Sharp/Blunt operating scissors, straight hemostat forceps, three cutting suture needles, one taper

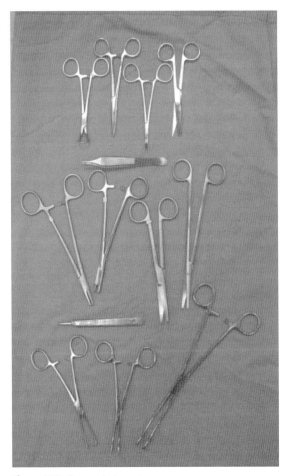

Figure 10.1. Common Instruments.
Top row from left to right: penetrating towel clamps, Kelly Haemostatic forceps, mosquito forceps, and sharp/blunts operating scissors. *Under top row:* Brown Adson tissue forceps. *Middle from left to right:* Mayo-Hegar needle holder, Olsen-Hegar needle holder, Mayo scissors, and Metzenbaum scissors. *Under middle row:* scalpel handle.
Bottom from left to right: Allis tissue forceps, Babcock tissue forceps, and sponge forceps.

needle, and 4 × 4 gauze sponges. This is a convenient pack to use when closing lacerations, debulking granulation tissue, or for an emergency tracheotomy.

A general or soft tissue surgery pack might be used for an exploratory laparotomy, an enucleation, or repair of a deep laceration. This pack could contain one Rat Tooth thumb forceps, one Brown

Adson forceps, one #3 scalpel handle, one #4 scalpel handle, large kidney forceps, large tumor forceps, Vulsellum forceps, Rochester-Carmalt forceps, Olsen-Hagar needle holder, Mayo-Hagar needle holder, sharp/blunt operating scissors, straight Mayo scissors, curved Mayo scissors, curved Metzenbaum scissors, bandage scissors, four Halstead Mosquito forceps, four Allis tissue forceps, six Crile hemostats, four nonperforating towel clamps, eight penetrating towel clamps, and a basin filled with 4 × 4 gauze sponges.

An orthopedic pack might consist of: two Brown Adson thumb forceps, one Rat Tooth thumb forceps, two #3 scalpel handles, two Mayo-Hagar needle holders, one bone rongeur, two Senn retractors, one Gelpi retractor, two bone curettes, two bone gouges, one mallet, two bone chisels, two periosteal elevators, five Crile hemostats, eight Halstead Mosquito hemostats, four Allis tissue forceps, one Vulsellum retractor, one bandage scissors, two Metzenbaum scissors, three Mayo scissors, one sharp/blunt scissors, four nonperforating towel clamps, twelve penetrating towel clamps, and one basin filled with 4 × 4 gauze sponges.

Decontaminating and Sterilizing

Developing a system that will identify instruments intended for one particular pack with improved efficiency during cleaning and sterilizing is a good one and it could use color-coded autoclavable tape.

The process by which instruments, packs, and ancillary items are sterilized varies from place to place. The most common method is steam sterilization, and most veterinary practices will have an autoclave. There are five types of steam sterilizers: gravity displacement, pre-vacuum, flush, pressure, and pulse. Each kind has its own parameters and the manufacturer's guide to operation should be adhered to ensure effective sterilization. Sterilizing indicators inside packs are the most accurate means of assessing sterilization; however, most practices use autoclave tape that undergoes color change based on temperature.

Instruments should be decontaminated before sterilization. Soaking in enzymatic solution will clean visible debris from the surface; use of a soft bristled brush may be necessary to remove material from grooves. Rinsing followed by careful inspection and complete drying before repacking will preserve instrument finish. Certain pneumatic tools require oiling according to manufacturer's direction to ensure function and longevity.

The shelf life of sterile packaged items is dependent on many factors and can be maximized to 6 months by sealing packs in outer plastic wrappings. All sterilized packs should be kept in a dry dust-free closet, out of high traffic areas.

Tissue Injury

Tissue injury requires thorough evaluation before a proper treatment plan can be established.

Initial Assessment and Preparation

The first step in dealing with tissue damage should be to assess the injury, including:

- Is the damage the result of a wound?
- What structures are involved?
- How did it occur?
- When did it occur?
- How has it been treated?

While assessing the injury, the type of wound should be established, including incised wounds, abrasions, lacerations, puncture wounds, complicated wounds, contusions, or burns. An *incised wound* (including a surgical wound) is one in which the skin edges are cleanly cut by a sharp object such as a scalpel, glass, or metal objects. Bleeding will usually occur. An *abrasion* is an area of the body surface denuded of skin or mucous membrane by some unusual or abnormal mechanical process, accompanied by minimal bleeding and some serum or plasma exudate. A *laceration* is a torn, ragged, and often mangled wound. The depth of the wound and degree of damage to surrounding tissues are variable. Hemorrhage is usually minimal unless underlying vessels are involved. These are typically caused by barbed wire. A *puncture wound* is one that is caused by a sharp object that passes through skin into underlying tissues.

The size and depth of the wound are variable. They can be quite small and easily overlooked or be large and deep as from a fence post. *Complicated wounds* are those in which multiple structures are involved including integument, muscle, nerves, vessels, and other organs. Degloving injuries, flap wounds involving muscle, wounds involving synovial structures, and those with exposed bone are examples. *Contusions* are skin injuries that include bruising and occur in horses commonly around the head if an animal is down and thrashing. *Burns* are injuries that result in partial or full thickness dermal injury and can be caused by caustic chemicals, heat, electricity, or friction. First-degree burns affect the epidermis only. Second-degree burns result in damage to the epidermis and varying depths of dermis. With third-degree burns, the full thickness of skin is completely destroyed as are variable depths of subcutaneous tissue (Knottenbelt 2003).

During the assessment phase, it is important to determine the degree of contamination. The National Academy of Science and the National Research Council have developed a classification system for wound contamination that includes four categories: clean, clean-contaminated, contaminated, and dirty/infected. *Clean* wounds are non-traumatic, elective, incisional wounds in which aseptic technique is maintained. Infection rate in clean wounds is usually 1% to 4%. *Clean-contaminated* wounds are those in which a minor break in asepsis occurs. The recorded infection rate in these wounds is 5% to 15%. *Contaminated* wounds are those in which a major break in aseptic technique occurs or the wound was the result of trauma. Areas that are contaminated have bacteria present that are not replicating or causing host injury. The infection rate for wounds of this nature is 16% to 25%. *Dirty/infected* wounds are traumatic injuries in which bacteria have colonized ($>10^5$ organisms/g of tissue or ml of exudate), are replicating and are causing injury to the host (Auer 2006, Hunt 1980).

After assessment, the area should be properly cleansed, which may require sedation and local or regional analgesia or general anesthesia. The following outline provides a suggested course:

l. Apply a sterile water-based gel (K-Y jelly) or sterile gauze to the wound to aid in removal of hair and debris that soil the wound during clipping.

2. Clip the hair around the wound leaving wide margins to allow for debridement and to diminish contamination. Wetting the hair before clipping will help prevent hair and dander from falling into the wound.

3. Aseptically clean the wound and surrounding tissue using povidone-iodine or chlorhexidine scrub and solution. Avoid using hydrogen peroxide because it causes thrombosis of the microvasculature, is cytotoxic to fibroblasts, and has a narrow antimicrobial spectrum. If possible, avoid getting scrub directly in the wound because scrub can be cytotoxic to tissue; however, adequate cleansing of the wound is more important. Avoid using alcohol in an open wound.

In determining which scrub to use, some considerations may include:

a. Chlorhexidine has a better residual antibacterial capacity and continued activity in the presence of serum, blood, and pus as compared to povidone-iodine.
Povidone-iodine is better to use around eyes because chlorhexidine can cause ocular toxicity.

b. Chlorhexidine (0.5%) inhibits epithelialization and granulation tissue formation.

c. Alcohol can be used in the presence of povidone-iodine but reduces the residual affect of chlorhexidine but should not be introduced directly into an open wound.

1. After the initial cleansing, flush or lavage the area with sterile saline, lactated Ringer's solution (LRS), which is less acidic than saline, 0.05% chlorhexidine solution, or 0.1% to 0.5% povidone-iodine solution. Use a 35-ml or 60-ml syringe with an 18-gauge needle to create a pressurized stream, which may help remove debris and contamination. Avoid using excessive pressure because this could drive contamination deeper into the tissue. Apply the lavage solution at an angle rather than directly into the tissue to drive the debris away from the area rather than into the wound.

2. Debride the area of any grossly contaminated and devitalized tissue. It is important to assess the viability of all tissue and leave any questionable tissue attached. Devitalized tissue will be white or black, lack pain sensation, may be cold, and will lack blood supply. Tissue viability may need to be reassessed later and further debridement performed in stages.

Closure

Once the wound had been cleaned and debrided, wound closure is the next step in wound management. The different methods of wound closure include:

- *Primary closure* is performed if the injury is recent and only mild contamination and tissue damage are present.
- *Delayed primary closure* is performed 3 to 5 days postinjury when there has been mild to moderate contamination or exudates.
- *Second intention healing* is used in wounds that are grossly contaminated or infected. The wound is allowed to heal by contraction, granulation tissue formation, and epithelialization.
- *Secondary closure* is performed after the formation of granulation tissue and may be performed several weeks after injury if contraction and epithelialization fails or is disfiguring.

During the closure process, some wounds may require a drain. Drains are indicated in areas that may have fluid accumulation within dead space. The most common drain used is the Penrose drain, which allows fluid to drain around it rather than through it. The drain should be placed away from the primary suture line and exit the skin at the most dependent area of the wound. When possible, the area should be bandaged to help prevent ascending infection.

Phases of Healing

Regardless of the method of closure, all wound healing progresses through defined phases. These phases include the inflammatory and debridement phase, the proliferative or repair phase, and the maturation phase. The *inflammatory phase* begins immediately after the wound is created and lasts 1 to 3 days. Immediate hemorrhage generally occurs assisting cleansing of the wound and providing for an influx of cells that help in debridement. Vasodilation usually occurs within 5 to 10 minutes of the injury. During this time, fibrinogen and other clotting elements appear. These reactions result in heat and redness. A fibrin clot forms which helps with hemostasis and provides a framework for repair. Neutrophils and macrophages enter the area that attack extracellular bacteria and facilitate breakdown of necrotic material and removal of debris.

The second phase is the *proliferative* or repair phase. This phase usually begins 3 days post-injury and lasts 1 to 3 weeks. During this phase, fibroblasts begin to appear which synthesize collagen to give the wound strength. Capillary ingrowth and epithelialization begin to occur as well. Granulation tissue will start to appear 4 to 6 days post-injury as a result of the fibroblasts, collagen, and new capillaries. The granulation tissue provides a surface over which epithelial cells migrate, provides resistance to infection, assists in wound contraction, and contains blood vessels that bring in oxygen, nutrients, mediators, and cells. However, if granulation tissue becomes excessive, it will retard wound healing because it prevents contraction and epithelialization. Factors that impede epithelialization include infection, excessive granulation tissue, repeated dressing changes, and reduction of oxygen tension. Factors that promote epithelialization include growth factors, topical antimicrobials, and semiocclusive dressings (Telfa).

The final stage is the *maturation* phase. During this time, epithelialization and contraction continue. This phase usually begins about 3 weeks post-injury and may last several months. Fibroblast numbers decrease, the capillary network increases, collagen fibers cross-link and reorient along the lines of tension resulting in an increase in tensile strength. The scar tissue that forms is typically 15% to 20% weaker than the surrounding tissue.

Skin Grafting

In some situations, skin grafting may be used to assist in healing by improving the wound healing process, shortening the recuperation time, and improving cosmetics and function. Grafting may also be needed in areas that have full thickness skin defects, where epithelialization is not active or is retarded, or if wound contraction is not occurring.

Grafts are classified as autografts, allografts, and xenografts. *Autografts* are grafts in which the tissue is taken from the animal itself. *Allografts* are grafts in which the tissue is taken from a different animal of the same species. *Xenografts* are those grafts in which the tissue is derived from a different species.

Pedicle grafts are those in which at least one attachment to the donor site is maintained during graft healing. These are also called flap grafts and are commonly used for conjunctival grafting for corneal injuries and ulcerations. *Free grafts* are those in which the donor skin is dependent on nutrients from the recipient. These are further classified according to the thickness of the skin derived from the donor site as full thickness or split thickness grafts. *Split thickness grafts* are comprised of epidermis and various thicknesses of dermal tissue. *Full thickness grafts* include all elements of epidermis and dermis but are devoid of subcutaneous tissue and fascia.

Skin grafts are further classified as mesh grafts, tunnel grafts, and pinch and punch grafts. *Mesh grafts* are used when expansion of the graft size is needed to allow coverage of large areas and drainage of fluid, which is a common reason for graft failure. *Tunnel grafts* are used when the graft bed is less than ideal. The cosmetic effects are not as good as mesh grafting but the technique is more practical. Strips of donor skin are harvested and drawn through tunnels in the recipient granulation tissue. The exposed ends are glued or sutured to the wound margin. *Pinch and punch grafts* are the simplest and most practical but may be less cosmetic. The grafts are taken from the neck or ventral abdomen and implanted into the recipient granulation bed.

Wound Care

Following wound closure, bandaging may be necessary to manage the wound and aid in prevention of contamination, minimization of swelling, obliteration of dead space, limitation of hemorrhage, immobilization, and support.

There are three layers that make up a bandage. The first layer is the primary (contact) layer. This is the layer directly against the wound and serves to protect the wound from contamination and with open wounds; it may be used to facilitate wound debridement. This layer includes various types of dressings depending on its purpose. Nonadherent dressings (Telfa pads) are used over areas of primary closure with little or no drainage or wounds that are in the repair stage with formation of granulation tissue. Adherent dressings are indicated in open wounds that require debridement and include wet-to-wet, wet-to-dry, and dry-to-dry. Dry bandages are used to remove low viscosity exudates from the wound. Wet bandages dilute high viscosity exudates and enhance their absorption. A wet bandage may use saline or 0.05% chlorhexidine solution or sterile gauze with topical ointment (ADAPTIC or ABD pads). Occlusive dressings are indicated for wounds with a healthy granulation bed, advanced contraction, decreased fluid production, and early epithelialization. These dressings interact with the wound fluid to form a gel over the wound surface such as Dermaheal and BioDres.

The second layer of the bandage is the absorptive layer, which keeps blood, serum, exudates, and necrotic debris away from the wound surface. Material used for this layer can include Conform, cast padding, and roll cotton.

The third layer functions to hold the primary and secondary layers in place. Vetrap and Elastikon can be used for this purpose, and if support or immobilization is needed, additional layers may be applied with sheet cotton, Sterirolls, or field bandages.

Certain types of injuries may require special types of bandaging. These include selective pressure bandages, stents, casts, and splints. *Selective pressure bandages* are used in areas where fluid may accumulate or where even surface pressure is difficult to attain. To make a selective pressure bandage, gauze sponges are rolled and placed over the area and held in place with Conform and Elastikon. Areas where these bandages may be indicated include the carpus and the cannon bone. *Stents* are used over areas where circumferential bandaging can be difficult to apply such as the stifle. To make a stent, some type of material such as a huck towel or gauze sponge is rolled and secured to the area with sutures.

Casts are used when complete immobilization is needed such as heel bulb lacerations, for wounds directly over joints, and for fracture repairs. Horses with casts must be confined to stall rest and monitored closely for the presence of heat or discharge through the cast associated with a developing cast sore or swelling above the cast. The cast should also be checked for any wear, especially around the toe. The top of the cast should be sealed with Elastikon to prevent debris from getting inside the cast.

Splints are used in areas that require extra support or immobililzation but to a lesser degree casting. Ready-made splints can be purchased or can be made from PVC piping or wood. When applying splints, it is important to apply adequate padding. Like casts, areas that are splinted should be checked regularly for developing pressure sores.

The frequency of bandage changes may vary During the debridement phase, the bandage may need to be changed on a daily basis and then decreased to every other day until there is little to no exudate. Once the wound has developed a healthy granulation bed and epithelialization is evident, bandage changes can be done less frequently.

In the initial stages of healing, hydrotherapy may be useful in managing open wounds. At the time of bandage changes, hydrotherapy can be performed and should be done for 10 to 15 minutes. Hydrotherapy stimulates formation of granulation tissue and increases blood flow to the area and decreases inflammation. Once the granulation bed has filled in, hydrotherapy should be discontinued to allow for contraction and epithelialization.

Topical ointments may be useful in wound management and include antibacterials, debriding agents, antiseptic ointments, and protectants. The *antibacterials* are silver sulfadiazine (Silvadene), nitrofurazone, povidone-iodine ointment, triple antibiotic ointment, and Panalog. Silvadene is used to stimulate formation of healthy granulation tissue and has antibacterial properties. It is a good choice for open wounds and especially for burns It has been known to cause a transient leucopenia in long-term use or in compromised patients, so it may be necessary to monitor the white cell count. Nitrofurazone is a common topical used to promote granulation tissue formation; however, it does decrease epithelialization. This topical is carcinogenic and has been shown to cause mammary tumors in rats. If used, gloves should be worn during its application. Povidone-iodine ointment is a topical which has antibacterial and antifungal properties. Panalog is an antibiotic/antifungal topical containing a corticosteroid that will decrease granulation tissue and act as an anti-inflammatory and anti-pruritic agent. The *debriding agents* are Granulex, honey, Varidase, and meat tenderizer. Honey acts as a debriding agent and accelerates the healing process by decreasing edema and increasing macrophage migration. *Antiseptic ointments* include Nolvasan Ointment. A good *protectant ointment* is Derma Gel (Swiss Formula), which protects and soothes.

Preparation of the Surgical Patient

Regardless of the procedure that is being performed, consideration should be given to pre-operative and postoperative antibiotics, pain management, surgical preparation, and postoperative care. As a general rule, most surgical patients will receive perioperative antibiotics, the selection of which depends on surgeon preference, the bacterial population the patient is likely to be exposed to, and the procedure to be performed. Common choices include penicillin, which will kill most gram-positive organisms (K-Pen or PPG), and gentamicin, which will kill many gram-negative organisms. These antibiotics are routinely given 30 minutes to 1 hour before surgery unless intraoperative cultures are to be obtained, in which case antibiotics are given after the samples are obtained. Analgesic therapy should be considered and routinely includes phenylbutazone or flunixin meglumine.

Presurgical preparation ideally includes clipping the surgical site and performing an initial surgical scrub before moving the patient to the surgical suite. However, it is important to avoid abrasions of the surgical site, which can predispose to infection, when clipping; therefore, it should be performed immediately before surgery or on the same day followed by a surgical scrub and placement of a light bandage over the area.

Following clipping, either a bucket prep or a sterile prep may be performed. Bucket preps are restricted to surgeries that involve structures that are considered contaminated (e.g., hoof, oral cavity). Sterile preps are performed on areas that involve synovial structures (e.g., joints, tendon sheaths), long bones, implants, and abdominal or thoracic cavities.

Common Orthopedic Procedures

Today, the prognosis for recovery from a severe orthopedic injury is far better than in the past because of advances in surgical techniques. Many of these horses are salvaged and some may have a good prognosis for return to athletic endeavor.

Fracture Repair

Horses with unstable fractures require immediate careful assessment and supportive therapy. Sedation to avoid further trauma during the examination should be considered.

Temporary stabilization of the fracture should be the immediate concern and is imperative before transport. The location of the fracture will dictate the type of splinting or casting that will achieve adequate support. Adequate hydration of the horse with blood loss or dehydration should be accomplished before shipment. Antibiotic therapy may be indicated if an open wound or serious soft tissue trauma is associated with the fracture and analgesic therapy may positively affect the horse's temperament.

Horses should be shipped in confined single stalls that will allow them to use the walls and tail or chest bars for support. Gradual acceleration and deceleration, as well as slow turns are vital and may not be well recognized by some drivers.

If the horse is going to be examined and treated rather than transported, the examination should begin with inspection of the affected limb. Sedation may be necessary to perform the examination. Any lacerations or open draining wounds should be noted. Pulses distal to the fracture should be assessed to ascertain that the blood vessels remain intact. Radiographs should be taken to confirm the presence and configuration of the fracture. In situations in which the fracture is obvious, wound care and limb stabilization are the primary concerns and should be completed before obtaining radiographs. With rare exception, sedation rather than general anesthesia should be used to facilitate the examination and initial stabilization. If surgical repair is elected, the horse should receive appropriate medical therapy, as previously described, before surgery. In many cases, allowing the horse to stabilize before surgery will result in a much improved recovery from anesthesia. A long-term catheter should be placed and the patient started on intravenous fluids, with antibiotics, analgesics, and anti-inflammatory agents administered before surgery.

The surgical technique will be dictated by a combination of factors including location and type of fracture, the value of the horse, and the surgeon's preferences. Small chip fractures can be repaired by arthroscopy, whereas more complex long bone fractures will likely require internal fixation or the application of a transfixation cast or external fixture.

Many factors aside from the fracture configuration can affect the outcome of complicated fracture repairs, including soft tissue injury, age, general health, size, and disposition of the horse.

Anesthetic induction and recovery are major factors affecting the successful repair of complicated fractures and experienced assistance during both phases is critical. Aftercare is equally important and includes protection of the surgical site with appropriate bandaging or casting, perioperative antibiotics, and pain management. Treatment of the contralateral foot to minimize the likelihood of mechanical laminitis is also important. Strict stall rest is indicated until adequate fracture healing has occurred.

Arthroscopy

Arthroscopy in horses has become a common procedure used both as a diagnostic and therapeutic modality for lesions involving synovial structures including joints and tendon sheaths (tenoscopy). The minimally invasive nature of the technique speeds postoperative recovery and allows more complete visualization than that afforded by an arthrotomy. Aseptic technique is essential regardless of whether the procedure is performed in the standing horse with sedation or under general anesthesia. Postoperative bandaging of the site and variable periods of stall rest are determined by the location and severity of the lesion.

Desmotomy and Tenotomy

Transection of a ligament (desmotomy) or tendon (tenotomy) can be performed to correct congenital or acquired flexural deformities and as a treatment of laminitis.

Deep digital flexure contracture, characterized by a club foot appearance, may respond to transaction of the inferior check ligament. In cases in which the superficial digital flexor contracture is present, causing knuckling over at the fetlock, a superior check ligament desmotomy can be performed.

Desmotomy of the medial patellar ligament can be performed on horses that exhibit upward fixation of the patella that cannot be resolved with training and exercise.

Deep digital flexor tenotomy may be indicated for some horses with significant rotation of P3 secondary to laminitis.

Growth Plate Retardation and Periosteal Stripping

Angular limb deformities (ALDs) are commonly encountered in foals and weanlings and are classified as either valgus or varus. A *valgus* deformity is defined as a lateral deviation of the limb distal to the location of the deformity. A *varus* deformity is a medial deviation of the limb distal to the location of the deformity. Treatment varies with the location and severity of the deformity and can range from splinting and corrective hoof trimming to surgical intervention using periosteal stripping or growth plate retardation.

Neurectomy

A neurectomy is transaction of a nerve and may include resection of a portion of the nerve. Neurectomies are generally performed as to alleviate chronic pain.

Soft Tissue Procedures

Castration and Cryptorchid Castration

The most common soft tissue surgical procedure performed on male horses is castration or gelding. When one or both testicles have not descended through the inguinal ring, the individual is described as a cryptorchid or "high flanker."

The surgical procedure and approach will be determined by the location of the testicles, the attitude, size, and age of the horse, and the surgeon's preference. A routine castration with two descended testicles can be accomplished with sedation and local infiltration of anesthetic agents or under general anesthesia. Cryptorchid castrations are routinely performed under general anesthesia and may be laparoscopically assisted.

A rough bucket prep technique is generally used for standing castrations, whereas an aseptic prep is indicated for the other techniques.

Colic

Acute or chronic signs of abdominal pain in a horse of any age, such as pawing, looking back, or biting at the flanks, rolling, restlessness, lack of appetite, and lying down, is frequently described as colic. Some individuals respond to purely medical therapy, whereas others may require surgical intervention. Physical examination should include heart rate (normal = 28–44 beats per minute), respiratory rate (8–20 breaths per minute), temperature (99° F –100.5° F), capillary refill time (<2 seconds), mucus membranes (moist, pale pink), and auscultation of gastrointestinal sounds in all four abdominal quad-

rants. The cecum and large intestine are heard in the upper right quadrant, the large intestine in lower right quadrant, the small intestine in the upper left quadrant, and the large intestine in the lower left quadrant. Gut sounds may be characterized as normal, increased, decreased, or absent.

Nasogastric intubation may be performed to assess gastric contents, alleviate distention, or to instill fluids and lubricants directly into the gastrointestinal tract.

Laboratory evaluations may help to assess hydration (packed cell volume = 32%–48%), electrolyte balance, total protein (5–7g/dl), complete blood count, and acid-base balance. Abdominocentesis (collection of peritoneal fluid by percutaneous aspiration) may assist in determining bowel viability or the development of peritonitis. Evaluation of the abdominal cavity via ultrasonography can be valuable especially in foals.

The surgical approach to the abdomen can include a ventral midline celiotomy, a ventral paramedian approach, a flank or an inguinal incision, and the patient will be positioned on the table accordingly.

If dorsal recumbency is selected , catheterization of the bladder in the male horse will prevent urine contamination of the surgical field during the procedure. The end of the penis should be cleansed well and the catheter passed in an aseptic fashion. Once the urinary catheter in place, the penis is packed into the sheath using 4×4 gauze, and the sheath is sutured closed using a simple continuous pattern. The urinary catheter can be hung off the side of the patient into a bucket.

Postoperative colic patients require careful continuous or frequent observation; fluid and analgesic therapy is routine.

Virtually any horse is susceptible to colic but management can play a key role in prevention. Client education including explanation of factors involved, signs to watch for, and preventative management options can be beneficial.

Neoplasia

Neoplasia in the horse can present in many forms such as squamous cell carcinoma (SCC), sarcoids, lymphosarcoma, and melanoma.

Therapy is dependent on tumor type and responsiveness and can include:

- Cryotherapy: application of extreme cold.
- Radiation: surface irradiation or implantation of iridium "seeds."
- Hyperthermia: application of heat.
  - Chemotherapy: Podophyllum; 5-lururoruracil; Cisplatin.
- Laser therapy: CO_2 diode; Nd:YAG.

Ovariectomy

An ovariectomy is the removal of one or both ovaries and may be used for treatment of ovarian neoplasia, correction of aberrant behavior, or to create "teaser" mares.

Surgical techniques include:

- Colpotomy: using a chain æcraseur through a vaginal approach.
- Flank approach: performed standing.
- Ventral approach: midline or paramedian under general anesthesia.
- Laparoscopy: visual inspection of all structures using a fiberoptic endoscope.

Upper Airway and Guttural Pouches

Examination of the upper airway using a flexible fiberoptic endoscope or video endoscope permits visualization of the nasal cavity, nasopharynx, larynx, guttural pouches, and trachea. Sedation may interfere with the normal function in the larynx.

The pharynx is a musculomembranous tubular structure that is positioned between the nasal septum and the larynx. The trachea lies ventral to the esophagus and attaches to the cricoid cartilage of the larynx and descends to the lungs, branching at the carina to form the major bronchi. Each tracheal ring is comprised of connective tissue, smooth muscle fibers, and cartilage that provides stiffness to the structure. The epiglottis closes against the larynx during swallowing, protecting the trachea and lungs from ingesta, whereas the soft palate serves the same function for the nasal passages.

Commonly diagnosed abnormalities of the pharynx and larynx include collapse of the pharyn-geal vault, dorsal displacement of the soft palate with respect to the epiglottis, aryepiglottic fold entrapment of the epiglottis, subepiglottic cysts, arytenoid chondritis (inflammation of the arytenoid cartilage) and laryngeal hemiplegia ("roaring"). Congenital malformation of the soft palate (cleft palate) can be seen in foals. Adjacent to the pharynx are the guttural pouches, each of which has an opening on the lateral walls of the nasopharynx through which an endoscope can be passed.

Tracheotomy

A tracheotomy is performed by creating a vertical incision along the ventral aspect of the middle of the trachea followed by separation of adjacent tracheal rings by incision of the connective tissue and mucosa between them. A tracheotomy tube is then inserted to provide an open airway, bypassing an obstruction in the upper airway.

Urogenital System

Several conditions can affect the equine bladder that may require surgical intervention, including patent urachus in the neonatal foal, uroperitoneum, urolithiasis (bladder stones), and neoplasia.

Certain procedures can be done under standing intravenous anesthesia. For a perineal urethrostomy, an epidural may be used in conjunction with the intravenous sedation to provide regional analgesia.

Once the epidural is placed, secure the tail out of the field by folding the length of the tail over a long thin rope then wrapping both tail and rope using brown gauze or a palpation sleeve to contain all hair and loose debris. Secure the top of the wrap with tape. Once the tail is completely wrapped, use the rope to secure the tail out of the way by taking it around the horse's neck.

References and Further Reading

Auer, J. A. 2006. *Equine Surgery.* 3rd ed. Philadelphia: Saunders Elsevier.

Ball, M. A. 1999. *Understanding the Equine Eye.* Lexington, KY: Eclipse Press.

Belknap, M. 2004. *Horsewords: The Equine Dictionary: The Ultimate Reference Book.* Rev. 2nd ed. North Pomfret, VT: Trafalgar Square Books.

Bentz, B. G. 2004. *Understanding Equine Colic.* Lexington, KY: Eclipse Press.

Blanchard, T., D. Varner, C. Love, S. Brinsko, S. Rigby, and J. Schumacher. 2002. *Manual of Equine Reproduction.* 2nd ed. St. Louis: Mosby.

Bramlage, L. R. (2003, May 29). *Castration: Creation of a Gelding from a Colt or Stallion.* American Association of Equine Practitioners: Newsroom. Retrieved July 17, 2007, from American Association of Equine Practitioners Web site: www.aaep.org.

Briggs, K. 2007. *Understanding Equine Nutrition.* Rev. dd. Lexington, KY: Eclipse Press.

Coumbe, K. 2001. *Equine Veterinary Nursing Manual.* New York: John Wiley & Sons.

Edwards, G. B., and N. A. White. 1999. *Handbook of equine colic.* Boston: Butterworth-Heinemann.

Gordon, B., S. Puterbaugh, K. Davis. 2005. Scrubbing, gowning, and gloving. *Cine-Med* 5–7.

Hanrath, M., and D. H. Rodgerson. (2002). Laparoscopic cryptorchidectomy using electrosurgical instrumentation in standing horses. *Vet Surg* 31:117–24.

Hayes, C. M, and R. Knightbridge. 2002. *Veterinary Notes for Horse Owners: New Revised Edition of the Standard Work for More Than 100 Years.* New York: Simon & Schuster.

Hunt, T. K. 1980. *Wound Healing and Wound Infection: Theory and Surgical Practice.* New York: Appleton-Century-Crofts.

Johnson, A. M. 1994. *Equine Medical Disorders: Library of Veterinary Practice.* 2nd ed. Hoboken, NJ: John Wiley & Sons.

Knottenbelt, D. C. 2003. *Handbook of Equine Wound Management.* Philadelphia: W. B. Saunders.

Parker, R. 2002. *Equine Science.* 2nd ed. New York: CENGAGE/Delmar Learning

Rush, B., and T. Mair. 2004. *Equine Respiratory Diseases.* Hoboken, NJ: John Wiley & Sons.

Walker, D. F. 1980. *Bovine and Equine Urogenital Surgery.* Philadelphia: Lea & Febiger.

White, N. A. 1990. *Current Practice of Equine Surgery.* Philadelphia: J.B. Lippincott Company.

Nursing Care

Bonnie S. Barr, Dennis Brooks, Laura Javsicas, and Dana Zimmel

Examinations

An important aim of nursing care is to recognize subtle changes or significant trends in the patient's condition. Monitoring the horse's condition begins with a solid understanding of normal parameters and behavior. These basic skills are required for technicians in ambulatory practice, as well as those who work in intensive care units.

Adult and Neonatal Physical Examination

The horse or foal should be observed from a distance to study obvious changes in behavior, posture, or muscle asymmetry.

The basics of the physical examination are temperature, heart rate (HR), and respiratory rate (Table 11.1). A flow chart is used to record the patient's vital signs over time (Figures 11.1 and 11.2). The normal temperature in an adult horse is 99°F to 101.5°F. The normal temperature in a neonatal foal (less than 30 days of age) is slightly higher at 99°F to 102.0°F. Digital thermometers are commonly used today and are safer than working with a glass mercury thermometer. Plastic sleeves that cover the thermometers are available to minimize the chance of spreading contagious diseases.

The HR can be ausculted behind the left or right elbow in the horse (Figure 11.3). The HR is slow in the normal adult ranging from 32 to 40 beats per minute. The neonatal foal has a normal HR of 80 to 120 beats per minute. The facial pulse can be felt on the medial side of the ramus of the mandible in front of the muscular portion of the cheek. The

pulse should be strong and regular. A faint pulse is palpated when the cardiovascular system is compromised (low blood pressure). If a murmur is ausculted, palpating the pulse at the same time can help determine if the murmur is systolic or diastolic. The jugular veins should be palpated to make sure they are smooth and soft. Distended, thickened, or pulsing veins can indicate a problem such as heart disease or a thrombosed vein. Palpation of the ears and limbs is important in sick horses to assess if they are cold, indicating hypovolemia or endotoxic shock.

The respiratory rate can be counted by watching the horse's flank move or listening to breath sounds over the trachea or lungs. The normal respiratory rate in the adult horse is 12 to 24 breaths per minute. In the neonatal foal, the normal respiratory rate is 36 to 40 breaths per minute. A complete evaluation of the respiratory system includes auscultation of the thorax and trachea. The horse has 18 ribs and the lungs extend to the sixteenth rib. The lung field can be identified from the sixteenth rib at the point of the hip drawing a straight line to the elbow (Figure 11.4). To make the horse take deep breaths, a plastic bag is placed over the nose. Time should be spent listening to both sides of the thorax on inspiration and expiration. The nostrils should be examined for evidence of any nasal discharge. Clear serous fluid can be normal after exercise. Thick yellow discharge, green discharge, or feed materials present in the nostrils are abnormal and warrant further investigation. Airflow should be assessed by placing a hand in front of each nostril to feel for the passage of air. Abnormal odors on the breath can indicate anaerobic bacterial infection of the

Date:	5/12/2008						
Weight (kg):	1						
CALL IF	<	>	CALL IF			CALL IF	
TP			pH			Lactate	
PCV			Na			Reflux	
Temp			K			O$_2$ Sat	
Heart Rate			Glu				
Resp Rate			HCO$_3$				

Problem/Diagnosis: _____

Faculty:	
Resident:	

Student (Phone Number) _____

MONITORING PARAMATERS		8	9	10	11	12	1	2	3	4	5	6	7	8	9	10	11	12	1	2	3	4	5	6	7
ICU q 2 4 6 8 12 24	HRS																								
Arterial blood gas	HRS																								
Colic/Comfort Check	HRS																								
PCV/TP	HRS																								
Venous blood gas- catheter vein:	HRS																								
	HRS																								
	HRS																								
	HRS																								
	HRS																								

MEDICATIONS (Drug, Dose/Kg. Amt, Route)		8	9	10	11	12	1	2	3	4	5	6	7	8	9	10	11	12	1	2	3	4	5	6	7
	HRS																								
	HRS																								
	HRS																								
	HRS																								
	HRS																								
	HRS																								
	HRS																								
	HRS																								
FLUSH CATHETHER BOTH PORTS	HRS																								

FLUIDS (Type, mL/hR or bolus amt. freq)		8	9	10	11	12	1	2	3	4	5	6	7	8	9	10	11	12	1	2	3	4	5	6	7
	HRS																								
	HRS																								
	HRS																								
	HRS																								
	HRS																								
	HRS																								
	HRS																								
	HRS																								
	HRS																								

RESPIRATORY THERAPY		8	9	10	11	12	1	2	3	4	5	6	7	8	9	10	11	12	1	2	3	4	5	6	7
Oxygen insufflations	L/MIN																								
Clean nasal insuff tube	HRS																								
Check oxygen supply	Q 24 HRS																								

ADDITIONAL INSTRUCTIONS/EXPLANATIONS

_____

_____

_____

CLINICIAN _____ RESIDENT _____ STUDENT _____

Figure 11.1. Medical treatment sheet.
Courtesy of Dr. Dana Zimmel.

CL: **235811** Patient ID: **209579** 5/12/2008

MONITORING

TIME												
ATTITUDE												
TEMPERATURE												
PAIN SCORE												
HEART RATE												
RESP RATE												
MM Color												
CRT												
DP – Front												
DP – Rear												
GI Left/Right												
FECES (#, consistency)												
URINE												
REFLUX												
APPETITE												
FLUIDS REMAINING												
H20 Intake (record when filled)												
Comments												
Initials												

PCV/TP/BLOOD GAS RESULTS

PCV												
BLOOD GLUCOSE												
Na												
K												
Ca												
pH												
pCO2												
pO2												
HCO3												
BE												
Lactate												
sPO2												

ADDITIONAL Comments

Total Day IV Fluids (L):		Total Water Intake		Total Reflux (L):	

Figure 11.2. Patient flow chart.
Courtesy of Dr. Dana Zimmel.

Table 11.1. Normal vital parameters.

Adult
Temperature = 99°F–101.5°F
Heart rate = 28–44 beats per minute
Respiratory rate = 8–24 breaths per minute

Neonatal foal (less than 2 weeks old)
Temperature = 99.5°F–102°F
Heart rate = 80–120 beats per minute
Respiratory rate = 24–40 breaths per minute

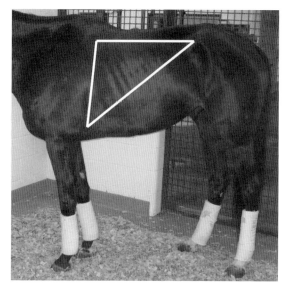

Figure 11.4. Outline of the lung field.
Courtesy of Dr. Dana Zimmel.

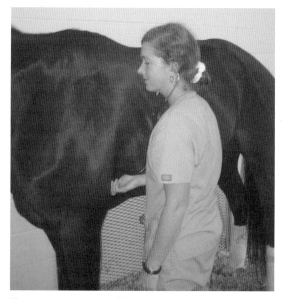

Figure 11.3. Auscultation of the heart behind the left elbow.
Courtesy of Dr. Dana Zimmel.

lungs. The pharynx should be palpated and gently squeezed to see if a cough can be elicited. The lymph nodes under the jaw should be palpated for pain or enlargement.

The mucous membranes of the oral cavity should be pink and moist. The capillary refill time should be less than 2 seconds in a normal horse. The color of the mucous membranes can indicate disease processes and should be noted carefully in the medical record. Yellow mucous membranes can indicate anorexia or severe liver disease. Blanched or white

mucous membranes point toward severe blood loss or decreased cardiac output (CO). Red or purple mucous membranes can reflect endotoxemia or septic shock. Mucous membranes that are speckled with red areas are called *petechia* and are associated with coagulation disorders or abnormalities of the capillary vessels. Brown or chocolate mucous membranes can occur in horses with red maple leaf toxicosis. Prolonged capillary refill time is a reflection of decreased perfusion most likely from dehydration.

The gastrointestinal system can be evaluated by auscultation of four "quadrants" (upper and lower left, upper and lower right) and on the ventral midline. The gut sounds (borborygmi) present on the right side are associated with large colon motility and consist of loud waves of gas moving through liquid ingesta. On the left side, borborygmi are usually more subtle partly because of the presence of the spleen against the left body wall. Auscultation of the ventral abdomen may be useful to detect an accumulation of sand in the large colon. Absence of intestinal sounds indicates decreased intestinal motility and may accompany signs of abdominal discomfort (colic). The quantity and consistency of manure output is important in the assessment of horses with colic. Dry hard feces covered in mucus are consistent in horses with impactions. Loose feces signify diarrhea that could be caused by bacterial, viral, parasite, toxic, or dietary problem.

The examination of the abdomen also includes visual inspection and palpation of the male external genitalia or the mammary gland in mares. These areas should be palpated carefully because some horses resent this procedure. Examination of the male external genitalia involves evaluation of the penis and testicles in intact males. The consistency, size, number, position, and sensitivity of the testicles should be noted. The prepuce and the penis should be evaluated for abnormal swelling or skin lesions. In mares, the mammary gland should be evaluated for symmetry of the two halves, increased firmness, masses, inappropriate lactation, discharge, and excessive sensitivity. Mares that have had several foals may have a more developed udder than mares that never had a foal. The udder may become slightly uneven after several foals. In a neonatal foal, the umbilical stalk should be monitored daily for signs of enlargement, purulent discharge, or leakage of urine. The umbilical stalk should normally dry up and fall off within the first 30 days of life.

Horses prefer to urinate where they are housed whether it is in stall or pasture. They will frequently urinate on returning to their stalls after exercise, examination, or travel. Some horses, which have been on the racetrack, have been trained to urinate when the handler whistles. Horses urinate at rest, not while eating or lying down. A healthy nonexercising horse consumes approximately 1 gallon per 100 pounds of body weight of water a day, produces approximately 1 to 3 gallons of urine a day (3 to 18 ml/kg/day) and urinates four to six times per day. The normal urine specific gravity (USG) should be greater than 1.028. The normal USG of neonatal foal is less than 1.008. Examples of abnormal urination are straining to urinate (stranguria), passing small spurts of urine (pollakiuria), exhibiting pain on urination (dysuria), passing no urine (anuria), and passing large amounts of urine frequently (polyuria). Normal urine can vary from pale to dark yellow and can be clear or quite cloudy. Clear, pale urine is more dilute than the more concentrated dark yellow, cloudy urine. Urine of horses normally contains large amounts of mucus. Red, brown to dark brown urine may indicate the presence of blood or other pigments, like those originating from damaged muscle.

Examination of the limbs starts with an assessment of the conformation. Each leg should then be individually palpated to detect the presence of any swelling, pain, or heat. The range of motion of all the joints should be assessed. The digital pulses should be palpated on all four feet (Figure 11.5).

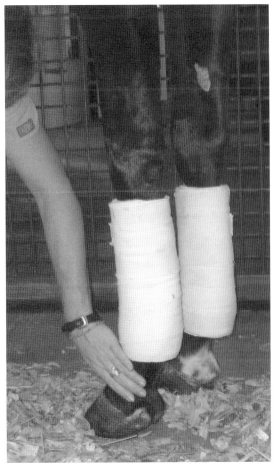

Figure 11.5. Palpation of digital pulses. Courtesy of Dr. Dana Zimmel.

Increased pulse may indicate the presence of inflammation in the foot. Horses with laminitis often have increased digital pulses in the affected limbs. All four feet should be picked up, cleaned, and examined. In neonatal foals, the joints should be monitored closely for any subtle swelling or pain. Infection of the joint or physis is a common complication in foals with septicemia.

Lameness Examination

The lameness examination can be divided into two parts, the passive examination and active examination. The passive examination involves observation of the horse in a stall for obvious signs of limb discomfort and or muscle atrophy. All the limbs are palpated carefully for detection of any heat or swelling associated with the muscles, joints, tendons, or ligaments. The hooves should be cleaned and examined carefully noting the placement of the shoes if present. Hoof testers are applied to the sole, bars, and frog to isolate a potential area of soreness.

The active examination involves watching the horse walk and trot on a hard surface in a straight line. Depending on the degree of lameness the horse may need to be lunged in a small circle on firm ground to evaluate the lameness. Circling the horse will accentuate some types of lameness, and it is helpful to watch the horse at all three gaits in both directions. Some horses may only show lameness with a rider, and those horses must be evaluated under saddle to isolate the lameness.

The next step is to flex each joint individually. Each fetlock and carpi are flexed for 30 to 60 seconds depending on the degree of discomfort the horse exhibits. The hind limb is evaluated similarly by first flexing the fetlock joints for 30 to 60 seconds and then the hock and stifle for 60 to 90 seconds.

Lameness is graded on a scale of 1 to 5. There are various scoring systems used in horses today but the most widely adopted is the American Association of Equine Practitioners (AAEP) scale. Zero means the horse is sound. Grade 1 lameness is often difficult to observe and may not be consistently apparent. Grade 2 lameness is difficult to observe at a walk or trotting a straight line but is consistent when the horse is worked in a circle, on firm ground, or under saddle. Grade 3 lameness is consistently observable at a trot under all circumstances. Grade 4 lameness is obvious lameness with marked nodding, hitching, or short striding. Grade 5 lameness is characterized by minimal weight bearing in motion or at rest and the inability to move.

The basic observations of watching a horse move include identifying a head nod, hip hike, stride length, and fetlock drop. The head nod usually implies forelimb lameness. The horse's head will drop or go "down" on the sound leg. The hip hike can be visualized to the untrained eye by placing tape on the tuber coxae to accentuate the asymmetrical movement of the pelvis. Evaluating lameness is an art, and there are many veterinarians who specialize in only lameness. The next step is to perform diagnostic nerve blocks and image the area isolated. These components of the examination will be covered in other chapters of this book.

Equine Ophthalmic Examination

To perform an ophthalmic examination it is necessary to have a bright focal light source such as a transilluminator or a direct ophthalmoscope. The head is examined for symmetry, globe size, movement and position of the globe, ocular discharge, and blepharospasm. The general appearance of the eyes and adnexa is noted. It can be useful to examine the angle of the eyelashes on the upper lid to the cornea of the two eyes because droopiness of the lashes of the upper lid may well indicate blepharospasm, ptosis, enophthalmos, or exophthalmos. Normally the eyelashes are almost perpendicular to the corneal surface. The first sign of a painful eye often is the eyelashes pointing downward.

Reflex Testing
A crude test of vision is the "menace response." To test the menace response, make a quick threatening

motion toward the eye to cause a blink response or a movement of the head. Care is taken not to create air currents toward the eye when performing this test. Horses have a sensitive menace response. The horse should also quickly squint or "dazzle" when a bright light is abruptly shown close to the eye. The *palpebral reflex* is tested by gently touching the eyelids and observing the blink response. Vision could be further assessed with maze testing with blinkers alternatively covering each eye. The maze tests should be done under dim and light conditions.

The *pupillary light reflex* (PLR), which has direct and indirect components, evaluates the integrity of the retina, optic nerve, midbrain, oculomotor nerve, and iris sphincter muscle. The normal equine pupil responds somewhat sluggishly and incompletely, unless the stimulating light is particularly bright. Stimulation of one eye results in the constriction of both pupils. The PLR is valuable in testing potential retinal function in eyes with severe corneal opacity.

Diagnostic Testing

It is important to approach each eye problem in the horse in an ordered and systematic manner. The majority of cases can be diagnosed by using standard ophthalmic clinical examination techniques. Intravenous sedation, a nose or ear twitch, and supraorbital sensory and auriculopalpebral motor nerve blocks may be necessary to facilitate the examination.

The *auriculopalpebral nerve* (motor nerve to the orbicularis oculi muscle) can be palpated under the skin and blocked with 2 to 3 ml of lidocaine just lateral to the highest point of the zygomatic arch (Figure 11.6). The *frontal or supraorbital nerve* (sensory to the medial two-thirds of the upper lid) can be blocked at the supraorbital foramen. This foramen can be palpated medially at the superior orbital rim where the supraorbital process begins to widen. Line blocks can be used near the orbital rim to desensitize other regions.

Schirmer tear testing is a method to measure reflex tearing and should be used for chronic ulcers and eyes in which the cornea appears dry. The Schirmer

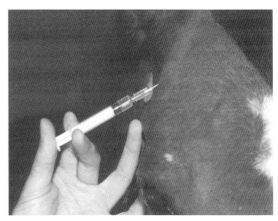

Figure 11.6. Blocking the auriculopalpebral nerve. Courtesy of Dr. Dennis Brooks.

tear test must be done before instillation of any medications into the eye. The test strip is folded at the notch and the notched end inserted over the temporal lower lid margin. The strip is removed after 1 minute and the length of the moist end measured. Strips are frequently saturated in horses after 1 minute, with values ranging from 14- to 34-mm wetting per minute considered normal. Values less than 10-mm wetting per minute are diagnostic for a tear deficiency state.

Corneal cultures using microbiologic culture swabs should be obtained before placing any topical medications in the eye. The swabs should be gently touched to the corneal ulcer. Corneal scrapings to obtain cytology specimens to detect bacteria and deep fungal hyphal elements can be obtained at the edge and base of a corneal lesion with topical anesthesia and the handle end of a sterile scalpel blade. Superficial swabbing cannot be expected to yield the organisms in a high percentage of cases, so removing the superficial debris can be helpful before collecting the sample. Cytology of eyelid and conjunctival masses can also be diagnostic.

The cornea should be clear, smooth, and shiny. Placing *fluorescein dye* (used non-diluted) in the eye to identify corneal ulcers should be routine in every eye examination of the horse (Figure 11.7). Small corneal ulcers will stain that might otherwise be undetected.

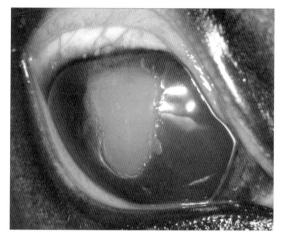

Figure 11.7. Fluorescein dye used to detect a corneal ulcer.
Courtesy of Dr. Dennis Brooks.

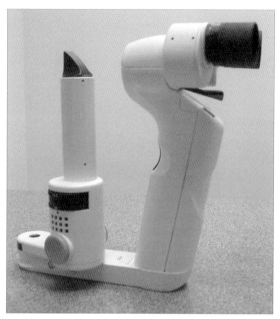

Figure 11.8. Slitlamp, which is used to evaluate the anterior chamber of the eye.
Courtesy of Dr. Dennis Brooks.

Seidel's test: Fluorescein can be used to detect perforated corneas or leaking corneal sutures. Placing fluorescein over a suspected corneal or scleral defect will result in a color change in the dye because the aqueous humor dilutes the fluorescein.

Tear film breakup time (TFBUT): Normal tear film is continuous. Blinking maintains the tear film continuity. The tear film breaks up if blinking does not occur often enough. Dark dry spots will appear under cobalt blue-filtered light as part of normal evaporation and diffusion of tears. Fluorescein dye is placed on the cornea and not flushed off. The lid is manually blinked three times and held open to expose the tear film to evaporation. The time required for a dry spot to appear on the corneal surface after blinking is referred to as the TFBUT. In a normal healthy eye, dry spots start occurring between blinks at about 10 to 12 seconds. A TFBUT of less than 10 seconds is abnormal and probably associated with instability of the mucin layer of the tear film.

Rose bengal dye should be used in selected cases after installation of fluorescein to identify the integrity of the tear film. Rose bengal dye strips are available at www.akorn.com.

To determine the patency of the *nasolacrimal system,* it is best to use irrigation from the nasal

orifice with a nasolacrimal cannula or curved multipurpose syringe, although fluorescein dye penetration through the nasolacrimal system may also indicate patency.

The anterior chamber (AC) is best examined with a handheld or transilluminator mounted *slitlamp* (Figure 11.8). The AC contains optically clear aqueous humor. Increased protein levels in the AC can be noted clinically as *aqueous flare*. White cells in the AC are called *hypopyon*, and red cells in the AC are called *hyphema*. Aqueous flare, hypopyon, and hyphema indicate uveitis.

The *intraocular pressure (IOP)* of horses is 16 to 30 mm Hg with a Tonopen applanation tonometer (Figure 11.9). A mydriatic should be applied to the eye once the pupillary light response has been evaluated. The agent of choice is topical 1% tropicamide, which takes 15 to 20 minutes to produce mydriasis in normal horses and has an action that persists for approximately 8 to 12 hours.

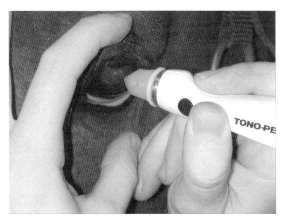

Figure 11.9. Tonopen, which is used to measure intraocular pressure. Courtesy of Dr. Dennis Brooks.

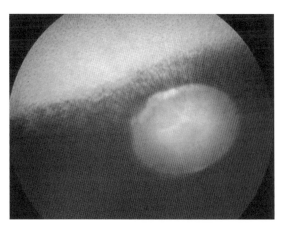

Figure 11.10. Retina and optic nerve. Courtesy of Dr. Dennis Brooks.

Atropine is used for therapeutic mydriasis because it can dilate the normal horse pupil for greater than 2 weeks.

The *lens* should be checked for position and any opacities or cataract. There are a number of lens opacities that may be regarded as normal variations: prominent lens sutures, the point of attachment of the hyaloid vessel, refractive concentric rings, fine dustlike opacities, and sparse vacuoles within the lens substance. Cataracts are lens opacities and are associated with varying degrees of blindness. They can be congenital, secondary to previous uveitis, and be progressive or nonprogressive. In some horse breeds they may be hereditary.

Normal aging of the horse lens will result in cloudiness of the lens nucleus *(nuclear sclerosis)* beginning at 7 to 8 years of age, but this is not a true cataract. The suture lines and the lens capsule may also become slightly opaque as a normal feature of aging.

The adult vitreous should be free of obvious opacities. Vitreal floaters can develop with age or be sequelae to equine recurrent uveitis (ERU). They are generally benign in nature.

The *retina* and *optic nerve* are examined with a direct, Panoptic, or indirect ophthalmoscopes (Figure 11.10). The rotary lens setting of the direct ophthalmoscope should be set to 0 to examine the retina and optic nerve and to a "green" number 20 to focus on the lids and cornea.

Magnification of the fundic image with the direct ophthalmoscope is 7.9× laterally and 84× axially in horses, and with the indirect ophthalmoscope and a 20D lens is 0.79× laterally and 8.4× axially. The Panoptic ophthalmoscope has an intermediate level of magnification between the direct and indirect ophthalmoscopes. The fundus should be examined for any signs of ERU, such as peripapillary depigmentation. The nontapetal region ventral to the optic disc should be carefully examined with a direct ophthalmoscope because this is the area where focal retinal scars are seen. Retinal detachments may be congenital, traumatic, or secondary to ERU and are serious faults due to their association with complete or partial vision loss.

The *electroretinogram* can be useful in evaluating retinal function in horses and can be performed at referral centers.

B-scan ultrasound, computerized tomography (CT), and magnetic resonance imaging (MRI) are important for evaluating intraocular and orbital lesions in the horse.

Neurological Examination

The purpose of a neurological examination is to determine if a neurological abnormality exists and to locate the source (brain versus spinal cord) of the problem. A complete history and physical examination are conducted first. A neurological examination form should be used to record the abnormal findings (Figure 11.11). The tools required to perform a neurological examination include a penlight or ophthalmoscope, hemostat, and a plexometer if the horse or foal is recumbent. The goal of a neurological examination is to localize the lesion to the brain, spinal cord, peripheral nerves, muscles, or the skeleton. The neurological examination begins at the head and evaluates behavior, mental status, head posture, and the cranial nerves. The second component of the examination is to evaluate the gait and posture. To complete the examination the neck, forelimbs, trunk, hind limbs, tail, and anus must be evaluated.

Head

Inappropriate behavior would include head pressing, compulsive walking, constant yawning, or sudden aggressiveness. A horse that compulsively circles tends to circle toward the side of the brain affected. These changes in behavior are typically associated with cerebral disease. Changes in mental status can indicate a problem in the cerebrum or brain stem. Clinical signs of disease affecting this location in the brain can range from coma to lethargy. The position of the head can implicate certain areas of the brain that may be affected. Horses with a head tilt may have a lesion involving the vestibular system. In contrast, horses with a head or neck turn may have a lesion of the cerebrum. Horses that exhibit fine jerky movements of the head (known as tremors) reflect a lesion in the cerebellum.

There are twelve cranial nerves that need to be examined that will assist in localization of the lesion to a certain portion of the brain (Table 11.2). The olfactory nerve (I) is responsible for sense of smell. The optic nerve (II) is responsible for vision and can be tested with the menace response. Neonatal foals have a decreased or absent menace response for the first week of life. The PLR can be used, but it tests both the optic and oculomotor nerves. The oculomotor

Table 11.2. Cranial nerves.

	Cranial nerve	Function
I	Olfactory	Smell
II	Optic	Vision
III	Oculomotor	Eye movement
IV	Trochlear	Eye movement
V	Trigeminal	Motor to muscles of mastication
		Sensation of the head
VI	Abducens	Eye movement
VII	Facial	Motor to muscles of facial expression
VIII	Vestibular	Hearing and balance
IX	Glossopharyngeal	Sensory and motor to pharynx and larynx
X	Vagus	Sensory and motor to pharynx and larynx
XI	Accessory	Motor to muscles of the neck
XII	Hypoglossal	Motor to muscles of the tongue

nerve (III) is responsible for the constrictor muscles of the pupil. The extraocular muscles are controlled by three nerves, the oculomotor, trochelar nerve (IV), and abducens nerve (VI). These nerves are tested by observing eyeball position within the orbit and observing eye movement. The trigeminal nerve (V) supplies motor innervation to the muscles of mastication and sensory nerve fibers to most parts of the head. Loss of motor function of the trigeminal nerve will result in a dropped jaw or the inability to chew. The sensory branches of the trigeminal nerve are tested by light tapping or pricking of the nasal mucosa, lower lip, eyelids, and ear. The facial nerve (VII) is responsible for motor movement of the facial muscles. Damage to the facial nerve can result in a deviated muzzle, drooping lip, ptosis of the upper eyelid, or dropped ear. The vestibuocochlear nerve (VIII) is responsible for hearing and balance. Clinical signs of unilateral vestibular dysfunction include a head tilt, circling to the side of the lesion, and nystagmus (fast phase) away from the side of the lesion. The most common lesions of the vestibulocochler nerve include middle or inner ear infections, head trauma, or temporohyoid osteoarthropathy. The glossopharyngeal nerve (IX) and the vagus nerve (X) provide sensory and motor innervation to the pharynx and larynx. The inability to swallow is the most common clinical sign associated with

NEUROLOGIC EXAMINATION OF LARGE ANIMALS

OUTPATIENT:	STALL NO.:
DATE:	TIME:
CLINICIAN:	CHARGES:
STUDENT:	ACCOUNT:
HISTORY:	

PHYSICAL EXAMINATION:

NEUROLOGIC EXAMINATION:

HEAD:
- Behavior;
- Mental Status:
- Head Posture:
- Head Coordination:

Craniel Nerves:

EYES	LEFT	RIGHT
Ophthalmic Examination:		
Vision; II:		
Menace; II-VII, Cerebellum:		
Pupils, PLR; II-III:		
Horners; Symp:		
Strabismus; III, IV, VI, VIII:		

FACE		
Sensation; Vs, cerebrum:		
Muscle mass, jaw tone; Vm:		
Ear, eye, nose, lip reflex; V-VII:		
Expression; VII:		
Sweating, Symp:		

VESTIBULAR—EAR		
Eye drop:		
Nystagmus; resting:		
positional:		
vestibular:		
Hearing:		
Special vestibular:		

TONGUE		
Tone, mass, fasciculations; XII, cerebrum:		

PHARYNX, LARYNX		
Voice; IX, X:		
Swallow; IX, X:		
Endoscopy:		
Slap test:		

	LEFT		RIGHT	
	FORE	HIND	FORE	HIND
GAIT: Paresis:				
Ataxia:				
Hypometria:				
Hypermetria:				
Total deficit:				
Other:				

NECK & FORELIMBS:	LEFT	RIGHT	TRUNK & HINDLIMBS:	LEFT	RIGHT	TAIL & ANUS:	LEFT	RIGHT
Hoofwear:			Hoofwear:			Strength:		
Posture:			Posture:			Muscle Mass:		
Strength:			Strength:			Tone:		
Muscle Mass:			Muscle Mass:			Reflexes:		
Tone:			Tone:			Sensation:		
Reflexes:			Reflexes:			Rectal:		
Sensation:			Sensation:					
Sweating:			Sweating:					

ASSESSMENT

SITE OF LESION(S): General (circle): cerebrum, brainstem, peripheral cranial nerves, cerebellum, spinal cord, peripheral nerves, muscles, skeleton

Specific:

CAUSE OF LESION(S):

PLAN
- DX:
- RX:
- EX:

SIGNATURE: _____ DATE / /

WHITE—Medical Record; GREEN—Clinician; PINK—Billing Tracer

VMTH—N3B 08/89

Figure 11.11. Neurological examination form.
Courtesy of Dr. Dana Zimmel.

dysfunction of these nerves. The accessory nerve provides motor innervation to the muscles of the neck including the trapezius and the cranial part of the sternocephalicus muscles. The hypoglossal nerve (XII) is responsible for motor control of the tongue. The tongue can be evaluated by gently pulling the tongue out of each side of the mouth. The horse should respond by placing it properly back into the mouth.

Gait and Posture

The next portion of the neurological examination is to evaluate the gait and posture. The purpose of the moving examination is to observe the horse walking in a straight line, circling in both directions, backing, walking up a down a hill, walking over objects, and pulling on the horse's tail when standing and walking (Figure 11.12). Elevating the horse's head when walking up and down an incline and blindfolding the horse are additional procedures that can be performed to evaluate the gait. The goal of the examination is to observe the presence of weakness or ataxia (incoordination). The gait deficits are graded from 0 to 5 depending on the severity. Weakness can be assessed by

observing the horse drag its limbs. Abnormal hoof wear or a low arc to the stride may be present. Pulling on the tail when at rest and when walking can detect weakness of the hindquarters. Ataxia can be further divided into hypometria (stiff gait), hypermetria (overreaching or excessive joint movement), or dysmetria, which incorporates both hypermetria and hypometria. Horses can be observed to sway from side to side, step on themselves, stumble, or circumduct the outside limb when circled.

Additional Procedures to Evaluate Spinal Cord Function

The neck and forelimbs should be observed for muscle symmetry, muscle atrophy, and skeletal defects. The neck should be palpated over each vertebrate to detect pain. The horse should be asked to flex its neck to the elbow in both directions by enticing it with a carrot or hay. Using the same method the horse should be asked to move it head up and down in a vertical plane. A stiff or painful neck can indicate cervical arthritis or stenosis of the cervical vertebrae. The cervicalfacial reflex is tested by tapping the skin from the atlas to the second

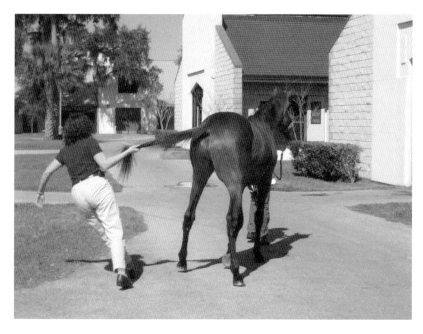

Figure 11.12. Demonstration of the tail pull test.
Courtesy of Dr. Dana Zimmel.

vertebra (C2) just below the jugular groove. The muscles of the neck will contract simultaneously with movement of corners of the mouth and a flick of the ear. The cervical reflex is tested between C2 and the shoulder on the lateral neck by slight pricking of the skin. The cervical musculature and skin should flinch when stimulated. An absence of a response can correspond with a cervical spinal cord lesion. The panniculus reflex of the thorax can be tested by prodding along the body wall between the ribs. The response should be contraction of the cutaneous trunci muscles. If this reflex is absent it indicates a problem in the spinal cord between C8 and S1. Running the tip of a pen over the thoracolumbar area next to the spine should cause the horse to extend the spine. Extending the pen over the hindquarters will cause flexion of the spine. The tail tone can be assessed by gently lifting the tail and detecting any weakness in muscle tone. The perineal reflex is tested by gentle pricking of the perineal skin which causes contraction of the anal sphincter and clamping down of the tail.

Nursing Skills

Blood Collection

The collection of blood for diagnostic testing is an essential tool in equine medicine. Blood can be taken from multiple sites and can be collected into tubes containing different substances depending on the type of test being performed. Some tubes contain anticoagulants, such as ethylenediaminetetraacetic acid (EDTA), for tests requiring whole blood, whereas others contain coagulants to encourage clotting for tests requiring serum (Table 11.3).

Performing Venipuncture

Venipuncture is most often performed using the jugular vein but the cephalic, medial saphenous, lateral thoracic, and the transverse facial venous sinus can be used. Blood can either be collected directly into an evacuated glass or plastic blood tube by using a blood collection needle or aspirated with a needle and syringe and then injected into the tube. Typically a 1-to 1.5-in. 20-gauge needle is used. A plastic needle holder designed for the blood collection needle allows for easy sampling, particularly when multiple tubes are required from one horse. Venipuncture is best performed with one person holding and restraining the horse while another person collects. The vein should be held off and palpated so that it is clearly identified by the collector. The needle is then gradually advanced through the skin and into the vein at approximately a 45-degree angle. The tube is then attached and the vein held off until the tube is fully filled. It is important not to overfill or under fill the tube to ensure the additive is properly diluted. The tube should be disconnected from the needle before the needle is removed from the horse's neck to help prevent a hematoma at the injection site. It typically is not necessary to hold off the vein after venipuncture. However, keeping the horses head elevated for a few minutes following venipuncture will decrease the incidence of hematoma formation.

When collecting blood, it is important to remember that the tube has a vacuum. To prevent losing the vacuum during collection, the needle should

Table 11.3. Commonly used blood collection tubes.

Color	Additive	Action of additive	Sample obtained	Common tests
Purple	Ethylenediaminetetraacetic acid	Anticoagulant	Whole blood	Complete blood count, cross-matching
Red	None (glass) clot activator (plastic)	Clot formation	Serum	Serum chemistry, antibody levels
Red/black stripped	Gel for serum separation and clot activator	Clot formation	Serum	Serum chemistry
Green	Sodium or lithium heparin	Anticoagulant	Plasma	Plasma chemistry
Blue	Citrate	Anticoagulant (reversible)	Whole blood	Coagulation testing, platelet counts

always be inserted into the vein first and then into the tube. If the needle comes out of the vein, the vacuum will be lost. A needle and syringe may be easier in patients that do not remain still during venipuncture, such as foals and fractious animals. Collecting directly into the tube is preferred whenever the platelet count is of concern because the platelet count may be falsely decreased due to adherence to the syringe.

Collecting Blood from the Transverse Facial Venous Sinus

A dilation of the transverse facial vein forms a sinus located approximately 2 cm ventral and parallel to the facial crest. This site provides an excellent alternative to the jugular vein for horses in which frequent venipuncture is required, but they are at risk of, or have active, thrombophlebitis of the jugular vein. Compared to the other veins mentioned, this site often results in less reaction from the horse and may be safer for the person collecting the blood.

The site is located approximately 2 cm below the facial crest, level with the medial canthus of the eye (Figure 11.13). A 1.5-in. 20- to 25-gauge needle with a syringe attached or a blood collection needle is inserted at an upward angle of 60 degrees toward the base of the facial crest, all the way to the bone. Slight crepitation will be felt as the needle hits the bone. The tube or syringe is then attached and blood is aspirated. If no blood flows, the needle can be redirected.

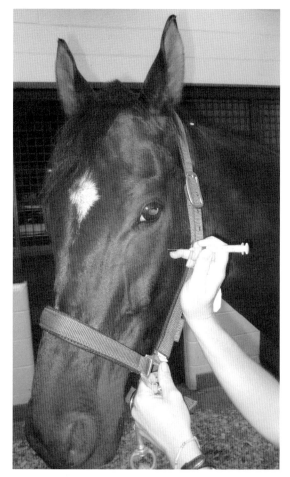

Figure 11.13. Blood collection from the facial sinus. Courtesy of Dr. Dana Zimmel.

Collection of Blood for Culture

Blood cultures may be indicated from any patient that is suspected to be septicemic and are most often taken from neonatal foals. Blood is placed in specifically designed bottles or tubes containing broth and incubated. If the patient has been receiving antibiotics, a special broth containing beads, which help bind the antibiotics, should be used to increase the probability of obtaining a positive culture. Blood cultures must be drawn using strict aseptic technique. Blood cultures can be collected in conjunction with placing an intravenous catheter or through a direct stick of a peripheral vein. If

taking a sample when a catheter is placed, both hands must be kept sterile and the sample should be taken directly from the catheter hub before flushing the catheter or attaching an extension set. If taking a sample by direct stick, sterile gloves, a needle, and syringe opened using sterile technique should be used. A subcutaneous bleb of lidocaine injected near the vein can be helpful to decrease the patient moving and contaminating the field, particularly when collecting a sample from the cephalic or saphenous vein of a foal. The volume of blood taken depends on the culture container to be used but a large volume (7–10 ml) is typical because this increases the probability of isolating bacteria. After obtaining the sample, a new needle should be placed on the syringe before injecting blood into the bottle or tube.

Intravenous Catheters and Catheter Placement

Intravenous catheters allow for the administration of fluids, medications, and anesthetic agents. They can also aide in obtaining serial blood samples without repeat venipuncture. There are many different types of catheters available, and they vary based on the material they are made of, the gauge (diameter), length, and method of insertion. The type of catheter chosen depends on many factors, including the size of the patient and where the catheter will be placed, what it will be used for, how long it will be used, and cost. There is the potential for serious complications associated with the use of catheters and choosing the correct catheter can help decrease the risk of complications. In general, use of the smallest gauge, shortest length, and least reactive catheter suitable for the treatment goals will help prevent thrombophlebitis.

Selection of Catheter Site
The most frequently used site for intravenous catheterization is the jugular vein. Before catheterization, it is important to palpate and hold off all veins to evaluate filling and for evidence of thrombosis or prior vein trauma. If the jugular veins are not appropriate due to thrombosis, lack of access to the down vein in recumbent horses or other causes, alternate sites that can be used include the cephalic, lateral thoracic, and saphenous veins.

Catheter Characteristics

Catheter Materials
The material of the catheter determines how long it can be maintained and the ease of placement (Table 11.4). Catheters made of silicone and polyurethane are quite pliable. These materials are appropriate for long-term use because these materials are minimally reactive in the vessel and therefore are less thrombogenic. Polyvinyl chloride,

Table 11.4. Catheter characteristics.

Material	Reactivity	Rigidity	Example
Teflon	++	++++	Angiocath
Polyurethane	+	++	Mila
Polyvinyl	++++	+++	Tygon
Polypropylene	+++	+++	Polyethylene tubing
Silicone	+	+	Centrasil

polyethylene, and polypropylene are more thrombogenic and are therefore suitable for short-term use. These materials tend to be less flexible, which makes them more likely to kink, but can make them easier to place.

Catheter Size
The gauge of the catheter refers to the external diameter. Catheters with gauges ranging from 10 to 18 are commonly used in equine practice. The gauge of the catheter is inversely proportional to the size, in other words, a 10-gauge catheter has a larger external diameter than an 18-gauge catheter. For routine catheterization of the jugular vein of an adult horse, a 14-gauge catheter is typically used, whereas a 14- or 16-gauge catheter would be suitable for a foal. The larger the diameter of the catheter (the smaller the gauge), the faster fluids can be administered because there will be less resistance to flow. A 10-gauge catheter would be appropriate when rapid hydration is required. It is important to remember that a larger diameter is potentially more irritating to the vein. Therefore, the smallest catheter appropriate for the situation should be used, and large-bore catheters should be removed once the horse is rehydrated. Smaller catheters would be appropriate for placement in veins other than the jugular, such as the cephalic, lateral thoracic, or saphenous veins.

In general, shorter catheters are less likely to cause thrombophlebitis. However, the tip of a short, stiff catheter can cause damage to the vessel wall as the patient moves, making this a poor choice for long-term catheterization. Typically, a 5-in.-long catheter is used in the jugular vein of an adult horse. For ponies or foals, a shorter catheter (2.5–3 in.)

may be appropriate. Long catheters are essential for monitoring central venous pressure (CVP). The tip of the catheter must extend into the right atrium. A pliable, long-term catheter measuring 30 cm can be used for this purpose in neonatal foals.

Method of Insertion and Number of Lumens

The two basic methods of catheter insertion used in equine medicine are over the -wire and over the needle. Over-the-needle catheters, in which the metal stylet passes through the catheter, are generally faster to insert and may be more appropriate in situations in which intravenous access is needed quickly. Over-the-wire catheters are more complicated to insert but allow placement of more flexible, longer catheters, which are less thrombogenic and can be maintained for a longer duration. This technique is appropriate for placement in veins other than the jugular as the guide wire aides in placement. Over-the-wire catheters are also available as double-lumen catheters. Double-lumen catheters have two ports and two lumens, which open into the vein at different sites. This allows for the simultaneous administration of fluids that are not compatible when combined in solution, such as calcium borogluconate and sodium bicarbonate. They are ideal for the administration of total parenteral nutrition (TPN) because they allow dedication of a port to TPN, which helps minimize contamination of the line. This type of catheter is convenient for blood sampling without interrupting fluid administration.

Catheter Placement

Catheter placement is a skill that can become quite easy with practice and is essential for all technicians. It is extremely helpful to practice the techniques before applying them to a live horse. They can be practiced with rubber tubing secured to a board to mimic the vein. Used or expired catheters can be saved for this purpose. This is particularly helpful for the over-the-wire technique, which requires multiple steps.

Preparation

After selection of an appropriate catheter and site for placement, preparation for placement of any

Table 11.5. Materials needed to place an intravenous catheter.

- Catheter.
- Clippers (with a #40 surgical blade).
- Surgical scrub solution (chlorhexidine- or iodine-based scrub) and alcohol on sterile 4 × 4 gauze.
- Sterile rinse or spray of alcohol or chlorhexidine solution.
- Nonsterile examination gloves for those scrubbing.
- A syringe of 1 to 2 ml of 2% lidocaine with a small bore (22- or 25-gauge) needle for a local skin block over the vein.
- Sterile gloves for those placing the catheter.
- Extension set of appropriate bore.
- Injection caps.
- Heparinized saline flush.
- #15 scalpel blade for making a stab incision in the skin (occasionally necessary for larger bore catheters like 12- or 10-gauge).
- A convenient and clean location to open the catheter.
- Suture and/or superglue to secure the catheter.
- Bandage material, if needed, including a sterile wound dressing, a sterile 4 × 4 to place over the catheter site and Elastikon to wrap the site.

catheter should begin with laying out all necessary materials in an organized and easily accessible manner. It is helpful to have these materials prepared ahead of time so that they are available immediately in an emergency. Regardless of the type of catheter being placed, the materials required are listed in Table 11.5.

Once all materials are gathered, the patient should be restrained adequately to allow for safe aseptic placement of the catheter. The level of restraint will vary depending on the patient. Most adult horses tolerate placement of jugular catheters with minimal physical restraint and no local anesthesia. Young horses may require chemical and physical restraint and the use of lidocaine is strongly recommended. Having adequate restraint and control of the patient is vital to placing the catheter aseptically and to ensuring the safety of personnel and patient.

Placement of an Over-the-Needle Catheter in the Jugular Vein

Step 1: Aseptic preparation of the site.

Strict aseptic technique should be used when placing intravenous catheters. The person preparing the site should wear gloves to avoid contamination of the site with bacteria from their skin. An area approximately 4 in. wide by 6 in. long over the site should be clipped. For jugular placement, the site should be at the junction of the cranial and middle third of the neck. Once the area is clipped, the area should be scrubbed using standard aseptic technique to provide 5 minutes of contact time. If a lidocaine block is used, this should be performed before the last scrub. When scrubbing is complete, the area can be rinsed with alcohol. Removing all scrub from the surrounding area can help prevent skin scalding.

Step 2: Insertion of the catheter.

The person placing the catheter (the operator) can open their sterile gloves and open the catheter on to the sterile field. To maintain sterility, care should be taken to only hold the hub of the catheter. It is crucial to hold the hub of the catheter and stylet together to ensure that they are moved as a unit to avoid the stylet piercing the end of the catheter. To allow for rapid detection of a flashback once the catheter is placed, an assistant can flush the catheter with heparinized saline, and the operator can maintain the saline in the catheter by occluding the top of the catheter with their finger. To place the catheter, the operator can hold off the vein with their nondominant hand. If this hand is outside the aseptically prepared area, it will now be considered contaminated and should not touch the catheter. To aide in accurate placement, hold off the vein until the fill is obvious. The vein may fill slowly in severely dehydrated patients. The catheter should be advanced through the skin and into the vein at a 45-degree angle, with the bevel toward the operator and in the direction of the heart. Because of the thickness of the skin, it is usually easier to first concentrate on puncturing the skin, then redirecting as needed to enter the vein. When the vein is entered, there is a decrease in resistance and a flashback of blood in the hub. Once a flashback is seen, the angle of the catheter should be decreased such that the catheter is more parallel with the vein and the catheter should then be advanced another few centimeters to ensure it is well seated in the vein. The stylet can then be held in place by the nondominant hand and the catheter slid down the stylet by the dominant, noncontaminated hand. When the catheter has been advanced completely, the stylet can be removed and the extension set attached. The catheter should then be checked for patency and flushed.

Step 3: Securing the catheter.

The catheter is then secured using suture (typically 2-0) on a straight, cutting, needle. Skin or superglue can be used but can cause damage to the skin and make repositioning impossible. Care should be taken not to kink the catheter while securing it. Wrapping the catheter is usually only necessary in young horses or those that rub their catheters. Although wrapping may help keep the site clean, it can also make it more difficult to inspect. Therefore, it is crucial that wraps be lifted to allow for daily inspection. It is also important that the catheter not be wrapped too tightly because this can cause edema to accumulate in the head and may restrict the airways. This is particularly a concern with Elastikon because it has a tendency to shrink when wet.

Placement of an Over-the-Wire Catheter in the Jugular Vein of a Neonatal Foal
Step 1: Aseptic preparation of the site.

The procedure is the same as step 1 for an over-the-needle catheter. The use of a lidocaine block is always indicated in foals because they tend to be more reactive, and this can result in a break in sterility. When placing an over-the-wire catheter in a neonatal foal for central venous pressure measurements, the site can be determined by measuring from the thoracic inlet to the insertion site. Jugular vein catheterization is most easily accomplished with three people and the foal restrained in lateral recumbency on a padded mat. By straddling the foal's front legs, the operator can help restrain the foal and have good access to the jugular vein. A second person can straddle the foal's hind legs and be available to pass materials to the operator. The third person can restrain and position the foal's head and hold off the jugular vein, allowing the operator to keep both hands sterile.

Step 2: Insertion of the catheter.

After the operator applies sterile gloves, an assistant can open the catheter kit by using sterile technique and hold the tray from the bottom or place it on a flat, stable, and easily reachable surface. If the catheter is to be used for the sterile collection of blood for culture, it should not be flushed before insertion. To prepare the catheter for insertion, the wire should be retracted into the introducer to straighten it. Because both hands must be kept sterile for this procedure, the vein can be held off in the clipped area or by an assistant well below the clipped area. The metal stylet is then inserted into the vein as described for placement of an over-the-needle catheter. It is important that the stylet is well seated in the vein to prevent accidentally coming out of the vein while the wire is passed. The stylet is then stabilized with the clean, nondominant hand, while the wire and introducer are picked up with the dominant hand and inserted in the hub of the stylet. The wire is then passed through the stylet and into the vein. This can be accomplished rapidly by stabilizing the stylet and introducer with the nondominant hand while sliding the plastic cover of the wire back to expose a small segment of wire with the dominant hand and then advancing this segment into the vein. The wire should advance easily with minimal resistance. Throughout this procedure, it is crucial to always have one hand holding the wire to prevent it from being dragged into the vein by blood flow. Once the end of the wire is free from the plastic cover, the wire is held with one hand while the introducer and stylet are backed out of the vein until wire is exposed between the stylet and the skin. This portion of wire is then grasped and the stylet and introducer are removed, taking care that the free end of the wire does not touch the horse's skin. The skin dilator is then threaded onto the wire and advanced to the hub to ensure it is in the vein, while holding the end of the wire. This dilator enlarges the opening in the skin and the wall of the vein to accommodate the catheter' it is normal to have tension at the skin as the dilator is forced through. The dilator is then backed out of the vein and removed, again keeping one hand on the wire at all times. Removal of the dilator will result in some bleeding at the site. Finally, the operator grasps the catheter by the hub and tip and threads it over the wire until the wire can be grasped at the hub. The catheter is then fully advanced into the vein down the wire. The wire can then be pulled by a steady motion while stabilizing the catheter hub at the insertion. The operator can then attach an extension and flush the catheter.

Step 3: Secure the catheter.

The catheter can be secured with suture and wrapped, if desired, as previously described. With recumbent foals, wrapping the catheter site may help prevent tension on the catheter while moving the foal or assisting it to stand.

Placement of Catheters in Other Locations

Over-the-wire or over-the-needle catheters can be used in the cephalic or saphenous veins of the limbs, whereas the over-the-wire is typically used for the lateral thoracic vein. These catheters should be placed with the flow of blood (i.e. with the tip toward the heart). If an over-the-wire catheter is used, the entire length may not be required. Regardless of the type of catheter, catheters on the limbs are more likely to clot due to gravity. Flushing with heparinized saline frequently or administering continuous fluids can prevent the catheter from clotting.

Catheter Monitoring and Maintenance

Intravenous catheters are easy to maintain if taken care of and monitored closely. They should be flushed with approximately 10 ml of heparinized saline solution every 6 hours to maintain patency (smaller volumes are appropriate for foals). The insertion site should be monitored at least once daily for any swelling, purulent discharge at the insertion, heat, or kinking of the catheter. The vein should also be held off below the catheter and palpated while distended and evaluated for even filling. If the vein appears compromised or more resistance is experienced when flushing the catheter, the catheter may need to be replaced. Horses that are developing thrombophlebitis may become febrile. Therefore, consider the catheter as a possible reason for an unexplained fever and consider replacing it even if the site palpates normally. The goal of monitoring is to catch problems early so that they do not develop into severe complications.

Administration of Medications

All medications that will be administered in a hospital set or dispensed from an ambulatory practice should be appropriately labeled. Each medication should be labeled with the drug name; drug concentration; the dosage rate; the dosage, route, and frequency of administration; patient name; veterinarian; and the expiration date of the drug. Additional instructions such as "refrigeration" should be included when appropriate. Medication in an unmarked syringe should never be administered. Premade labels for common drugs from antibiotics to sedatives are easy to obtain and improve the safety of administering medication in a busy practice. Medications can be given intravenously, intramuscularly, subcutaneously, orally, or through a subpalpebral lavage (SPL) for the treatment of eye problems.

Intravenous Medications

Most medications given intravenously in a hospital setting are administered through an intravenous catheter. Medications that are to be injected are clear to light yellow. An opaque (white) substance should never be injected into the vein. The only exception to this rule is TPN. Some drugs are incompatible, and they form a white or cloudy precipitant when mixed together. If this occurs, the injection should be immediately stopped and the line cleared.

Before administering a medication, the technician should double check the dose and the medical chart to make certain it is correct for the patient. The catheter caps should be wiped with alcohol before injecting through the port. If the catheter cap is damaged it should be replaced. It is advisable to stand on the side of the horse in which the catheter is inserted to observe the flow of drug through the extension set. If the catheter has any heat or swelling around the entrance to the vein, the clinician

should be notified and a note made on the examination sheet. The catheter should be flushed with saline before administration of the medication. After the drug has been given, the catheter should be flushed with heparinized saline to keep it from clotting.

If the catheter will not flush easily the fluid should not be forced through it. Catheters can develop blood clots inside the lumen, and if the clot is pushed into the vein, it can cause complications. If there is a change in the horse's behavior when flushing medications through the catheter, the process should stop immediately. Perivascular drug administration is possible if the catheter has a leak. It is also possible to place the catheter into the carotid artery by mistake. When medications are given in the carotid artery, the horse may pace compulsively, shake their head vigorously, or have a seizure.

Intravenous injections are best given in the cranial one-third of the neck. The horse should always be appropriately restrained, preferably held instead of tied. An 18- or 20-gauge needle is inserted up to the hub and should be felt just under the skin within the vein. This is a good method to avoid accidental injection into the carotid artery, which lies directly beneath the jugular vein. Once the needle is positioned in the vein, it can be confirmed by observing a flash of dark blood in the syringe. The medication should be administered slowly. If the horse moves during administration of the medication, the needle placement should be rechecked to ensure it is still seated in the vein.

Intramuscular and Subcutaneous Injections

Intramuscular injections are routinely administered in the muscles of the neck, pectoral area, or semimembranous or semitendinous muscles. For intramuscular injections an 18- or 20-gauge 1 1/2-in. needle should be used in an adult and a 20-gauge 1-in. needle should be used for a foal. Restraint of the horse or foal is important for safe administration of a vaccine or medication. The needle should be inserted and the syringe attached. It is critical to check that the needle is not in a vessel by aspirating before pushing the medication through the needle. If blood is obtained during aspiration, the needle should be repositioned and the process repeated. If the volume to be given is larger than 20 ml, the medication should be administered in more than one location. The location of all intramuscular injections should be recorded in the medical record and the muscle groups should be rotated when multiple doses are necessary. If heat or swelling occur in an area of an intramuscular injection site, evaluation by a veterinarian is prudent. The area may represent a minor site of inflammation or a severe bacterial infection.

Subcutaneous injections are rarely used in equine medicine. A 20- to 22-gauge needle is placed just under the skin in front of the shoulder. Only small volumes of medications are administered via this route. Heat pain or swelling should be evaluated for an infectious process.

Oral Medications
Oral medications are common in equine practice. The medication may come prepared in a paste form and easy to administer in the corner of the horse's mouth. The horse should not have hay or other feed in the mouth before administration of oral medications. If the medication is in a tablet form, it must be crushed and mixed with water and syrup first. Molasses should be avoided because it contains elevated levels of potassium, and it may interfere with drug absorption. The medications should not be made up too far in advance because the stability of the drug may change once it is mixed. Medications such as metronidazole are not palatable, and some horses will stop eating when given these antimicrobials. Rinsing the horse's mouth out with water after they swallow the medication may improve their appetite.

How to Use a Subpalpebral Lavage
Severe ocular injuries or infections warrant the placement of a SPL to administer frequent medications directly into the eye. The foot plate is located under the eyelid and the tubing is sutured to the skin. The tubing extends along the mane to the port located at the withers (Figure 11.14). The injection port should be changed daily to minimize contamination. The volume of medication administered can vary from 0.1 to 0.5 ml. This small amount of fluid

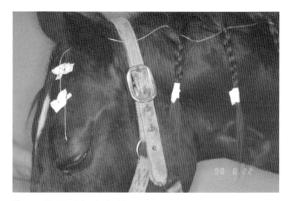

Figure 11.14. Subpalpebral lavage. Courtesy of Dr. Dennis Brooks.

is slowly pushed through the tubing followed by 3 to 5 ml of air. The horse should be observed to blink, or there should be evidence of when the liquid medication reaches the eye. At least 5 minutes is necessary between administration of each drug to allow for absorption of the medication into the eye. Rewarding the horse with a carrot after eye treatment can help make the treatment a positive experience for the horse.

Administration of Oral and Intravenous Fluids

Intravenous fluids are indicated for cardiovascular resuscitation in dehydrated patients, to replace ongoing losses from gastric reflux or diarrhea, and to provide maintenance fluid requirements in horses or foals that are unable or unwilling to drink adequate amounts of liquids. The type of fluid chosen, the route of administration (oral or intravenous), and the method of delivery (bolus or constant rate infusion) is dictated by the severity of the disease.

Calculation of Fluid Requirements
The first step in determining the fluid requirement for a sick patient is to assess the level of dehydration. Clinical signs of dehydration include an elevated HR, dry mucous membranes, prolonged capillary refill time, cool extremities, and weak pulses. Poor skin tugor and sunken eyes can be

Table 11.6. Assessment of dehydration in horses.

Clinical sign	Mild (4–6%)	Moderate (7–9%)	Severe (>10%)
Capillary refill time	1–2 seconds	2–4 seconds	>4 seconds
Mucous membranes	Fair	Tacky	Dry
Skin tent	2–3 seconds	3–5 seconds	>5 seconds
PCV (%)[a]	40–50	50–65	>65
TP (g/dl)[b]	6.5–7.5	7.5–8.5	>8.5

[a]Elevation in PCV without an elevation in TP may suggest splenic contraction from excitement or pain.
[b]TP can appear normal in dehydrated horses with severe protein loss.
PCV, packed cell volume; TP, total protein.

additional signs of dehydration. Evaluation of these parameters can predict the percent dehydration (Table 11.6).

The second step is to consider the maintenance fluid requirements based on body weight. The maintenance fluid requirement for and an adult horse is 50 ml/kg/day. The maintenance fluid rate for a neonatal foal (less than 30 days of age) is 75 to 100 ml/kg/day.

To determine the fluid therapy requirement of a sick patient, the maintenance fluid quantity is added to the amount of fluid needed to correct dehydration. To correct dehydration the following formula is used:

Calculation of total fluid deficit
[Body weight (kg)] × [% of dehydration]
= Total fluid deficit (L)

To calculate daily fluid requirement the following formula is used:

The last component to consider in developing a fluid therapy plan is to estimate the quantity of ongoing fluid losses from diarrhea or gastrointestinal reflux. Add all three together and this is the total fluid requirement per day (Table 11.7).

Calculation of maintenance fluid requirement
[Body weight (kg)] × [maintenance requirement (ml/kg/day)]
= Daily requirement (ml/day)

Oral (Enteral) Fluid Therapy
Administration of balanced, nonsterile fluids enterally can be an effective way to replace deficits

Table 11.7. Example: Calculation of fluid requirements.

Adult horse weighing 450 kg
Estimated to be 7% dehydrated
Fluid deficit = 450 kg × (.07) = 31.5 L
Maintenance = 450 kg × 50 ml/kg/day = 22,500 ml or 22.5 L/day
Total fluid requirement = 31.5 L + 22.5 L = 54 L/day

and is substantially more affordable than sterile fluids for intravenous administration. There is some evidence that enteral fluids may be superior to intravenous fluids (parenteral) at rehydrating colonic contents and therefore may be more appropriate for the treatment of large colon impactions. The disadvantage of enteral fluids is the inability to administer adequately large volumes rapidly in cases of severe dehydration. Enteral fluids are also inappropriate in cases with gastric reflux.

Enteral fluids can be given via a small indwelling nasogastric tube or periodically through a regular stomach tube. It is safest to use a funnel and gravity flow to prevent overfilling of the stomach. The capacity of the equine stomach is 8 to 10 L. Fluid should exit the stomach in 20 to 30 minutes when motility is normal. Administration of 6 to 8 L (2 gallons) of water by nasogastric tube every 4 to 6 hours is a reasonable method to treat mild dehydration in horses.

Administration of fluids via nasogastric tube that are isotonic or hypertonic (less than 800 mOsm/

L) can be given without causing a shift in the extracellular fluid into the gastrointestinal tract. Commercially available electrolyte solutions are available or a mixture (Table 11.8) can be made using table salt (NaCl), lite salt (KCl), and baking soda (NaHCO$_3$). Free choice electrolyte water is advocated in horses with electrolyte deficits, such as horses with enterocolitis; however, water should be available for drinking simultaneously.

When developing a fluid plan for a foal, it is important to remember that milk counts as part of the daily fluid requirements. The amount of milk being supplemented or an estimate of the amount the foal ingests from nursing should be considered when formulating a fluid plan.

There are many oral treatments administered through a nasogastric tube that target impaction of feed or sand. The most common fluid used in horses with colic is mineral oil (4 L). Mineral oil lubricates ingesta but does not treat dehydration. Other treatments include psyllium, magnesium sulfate (Epson salts), and dioctyl sodium sulfosuccinate (DSS; 10–20 mg/kg). Psyllium (16 oz in 8 L water) is a bulk laxative that is commonly used for treatment of sand colic. Magnesium sulfate (0.5–1 g/kg in 8 L water) is a cathartic laxative used in treatment of large colon or cecal impactions. DSS (4–8 oz in 8 L water) is irritant laxative that is used for treatment of impactions. Dehydration should be corrected before using laxatives, which can exacerbate dehydration.

Intravenous Fluid Therapy

The most rapid method to expand circulating blood volume is administration of intravenous fluid therapy. It is indicated in horses suffering from endotoxic or hypovolemic shock. Treatment of hypovolemic shock in a 450-kg horse can range from 30 to 50 L. Half of the calculated fluid deficit should be administered in 1 to 2 hours. The remainder of the deficit, plus maintenance and ongoing losses should be evenly divided over the next 12 to 24 hours. This can be administered at a constant rate infusion, or in 5- to 10-L bolus infusions. Large volumes of fluids can be administered rapidly by using 10-gauge or 12-gauge jugular catheter, two 14-gauge jugular catheters, a pressure bag, or a fluid pump. Large catheters and fluid given under

Table 11.8. Oral electrolyte therapy for a 500-kg horse.

	Impaction	Anorexia	Diarrhea	Supplement
Dehydration[a]	5%	6%	7%	—
H$_2$O deficit (L)	25	30	35	—
Na deficit (mEq)[a]	1,000	1,000	2,000	—
K deficit (mEq)[a]	800	2,100	800	—
HCO$_3$ deficit (mEq)[a]	—	—	1,000	—
Solutions	—	—	—	—
Water (L)	7	7	7	8
NaCl (tbsp)	3.6	1	1.8	2.6
KCL tbsp	3.8	5	1.9	1.8
NaHCO$_3$ (tbsp)	—	1.3	2.6	—
Osmolality (mOsm/L)	523	453	397	372
Total Na (mEq)	1,020	510	986	748
Total K (mEq)	804	1,072	402	375
Total HCO$_3$ (mEq)	—	238	476	

[a]These values are examples of horses with the described problem.

HCO$_3$, bicarbonate; K, potassium; KCl, potassium chloride; Na, sodium; NaCl, sodium chloride; NaHCO$_3$, sodium bicarbonate.

significant pressure increases the incidence of venous thrombosis.

Type of Fluids

There are two overall classifications of intravenous fluids: crystalloids and colloids. Crystalloids can be divided into replacement solutions and maintenance solutions. These fluids vary by the amount of electrolytes and the osmolality of the solution. Isotonic fluids, such as Ringer's, lactated Ringer's, Plasmalyte A, or Normosol-R, are commonly used to replace large volume deficits. Hypertonic (7.2%) saline solution is quite useful in treatment of hypovolemia because it will increase CO by shifting intracellular fluid to the extracellular space. The dose is 4 to 6 ml/kg over 10 to 20 minutes and must be followed by two to three times maintenance isotonic fluids. Normal saline (0.9%) is acceptable for replacement of fluid deficits but should not be used for maintenance fluid therapy because it can result in hypernatremia, hyperchloremia, and acidosis.

Colloids are indicated when the total protein and albumin are substantially decreased (less than 5 g/dl and 2.0 g/dl, respectively). The most frequent use of colloids is for treatment of enterocolitis. Hetastach a synthetic colloid is administered at 10 to 20 ml/kg. Fresh frozen plasma is commercially available and used frequently in horses with substantial protein loss.

Electrolytes and Acid-Base Balance

Clinical signs of electrolyte and acid-base imbalance can be mild, such as depression seen with acidosis or weakness associated with hypokalemia. Obvious electrolyte disturbances such as synchronous diaphragmatic flutter ("thumps") are caused by hypocalcemia. Moderate to severely dehydrated horses should have their electrolytes and acid-base balance (pH) monitored throughout the duration of fluid therapy.

Potassium is an intracellular ion that is often low in horses with anorexia, gastrointestinal reflux, or enterocolitis. Evaluation of serum potassium is not an accurate reflection of total body potassium because the majority of potassium resides within the cell not the blood. If serum potassium is low in the presence of acidosis, the total body deficit is likely to be severe. Hypokalemia is routinely treated with 0.02 to 0.08 mEq/kg/L KCl. The average horse would receive 20 to 40 mEq/L KCl. The maximum rate of potassium administration should not exceed 0.5 mEq/kg/hour to avoid the risk of arrhythmias.

Common clinical signs associated with hypocalcemia consist of muscle fasciculations, tachycardia, ileus, and synchronous diaphragmatic flutter. Hypocalcemia can be treated with 23% calcium gluconate (100–500 ml in 10 L in an adult).

Metabolic acidosis occurs in horses with diarrhea. Bicarbonate supplementation is indicated when the blood pH is less than 7.2 or the bicarbonate (HCO_3^-) is less than 15 mEq/L. The amount needed to correct acidosis can be calculated or if laboratory data is unavailable, an estimate of 1 to 2 mEq/kg is suitable. Excessive bicarbonate therapy can result in hypernatremia and hyperosmolality. Half of the deficit should be given over 1 to 2 hours and the remainder over 12 to 24 hours. Bicarbonate and calcium should not be mixed because they will form a precipitate. To calculate the bicarbonate deficit use the following formula:

Calculation of bicarbonate deficit
Bicarbonate deficit (mEq) = [24 − Patient's HCO_3^-] × [body weight (kg)] × [0.3]

Special Fluid Considerations for Neonates

Disorders of glucose metabolism are frequently observed in the neonatal foal. Hypoglycemia is the most common, and if severe enough, it can lead to irreversible cell damage. Causes of hypoglycemia include sepsis, shock, prematurity, asphyxia, hypothermia, and a decrease in nursing due to a systemic disorder. Clinical signs are vague but may include weakness, lethargy, collapse, and if severe enough, seizures. Treatment in the neonatal foal includes administration of a glucose solution, usually 5% to 10% at a rate of 4 to 8 mg/kg/minute. Older foals require less glucose supplementation (1%–2% glucose solution at foal's maintenance rate). Continuous infusion of glucose is preferred. Glucose containing fluids should not be used for resuscitation (bolus) fluid therapy. Frequent monitoring (every 2 to 6 hours) of glucose levels should be performed with a glucometer. The presence of glucose in the urine is an indication of excessive glucose administration. Hyperglycemia may result from sepsis, stress, or excessive administration of glucose. Treatment includes decreasing the amount of glucose administered or administration of insulin.

Hyperkalemia is seen in foals with uroperitoneum, volume depletion, renal disease, or acidosis. Excess potassium may result in hypotension and cardiac arrhythmias. Treatment of hyperkalemia involves avoiding fluids containing potassium and administration of fluids containing glucose to facilitate the movement of potassium into the cell. Sodium bicarbonate infusion will also lower potassium by driving it into the cell.

Too rapid administration of intravenous fluids in neonates can overload the vascular system and dilute the colloid osmotic pressure, resulting in edema formation. Many normal foals can tolerate rapid fluid infusion, but the more immature and compromised individuals may have difficulty eliminating any excess fluid. Clinically this can be seen as subcutaneous edema or respiratory compromise associated with pulmonary edema. Because continued losses frequently are difficult to quantitate, continued reevaluation of the patient's hydration status is critical throughout the duration of fluid administration. Aggressive correction of sodium imbalances may result in neurological signs due to the brain's inability to adapt to the changes in osmolality. Too rapid administration of calcium will result in cardiac arrhythmias. Excessive potassium administration will also have an adverse affect on the heart. During fluid treatment, electrolytes values and metabolic status should also be reassessed frequently.

Administration of Plasma and Blood

All blood products should be administered using a blood administration set (either high flow or regular) with an in-line filter to filter out blood clots (Figure 11.15). It may be necessary to change filters every few liters to maintain adequate flow rates. Blood should be warmed to room temperature if it has been frozen or chilled. Plasma should be thawed in water that is no warmer than about 100° F to avoid denaturing of plasma proteins.

All transfusions should be started slowly (about 1 ml/kg/hour) and the recipient should be monitored closely for signs of a reaction. The temperature, pulse, and respiration should be taken and recorded before starting the transfusion and then at frequent intervals throughout the transfusion, particularly before the rate is increased. The horse should also be observed closely for the development of urticaria (hives) or muscle fasciculations.

The rate of administration depends on the condition being treated. In general, if the component

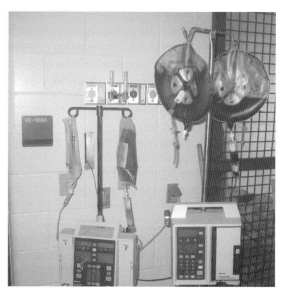

Figure 11.15. Both plasma and blood require a filtered administration set.
Courtesy of Dr. Laura Javsicas.

being given is also needed for volume expansion, as with whole blood for acute hemorrhage or plasma for acute colitis, faster rates are appropriate. For acute hemorrhage, a high-flow administration set with a pressure bulb attached can be used. Placing two catheters allows for simultaneous administration of crystalloid fluids for volume expansion and blood. After approximately 500 ml of blood has been given with no sign of a transfusion reaction, the remaining volume can be given rapidly. For cases in which rapid administration is not required, the blood or plasma can be administered using a regular blood transfer set at slower rates. The use of an infusion pumps aides in accurate rate control.

Transfusion Reactions and Complications
Transfusion reactions are possible, even if the donor and recipient are cross-matched and blood is typed beforehand. Signs of a reaction include tachycardia, tachypnea, dyspnea, fever, sweating, urticaria, anaphylactic shock, collapse, and sudden death. If signs of reaction occur, the need for transfusion often has to be weighed against the risk of further reaction. Depending on the severity of the reaction, the transfusion should immediately be slowed down or stopped while the horse is assessed. If urticaria occurs, an antihistamine (diphenhydramine at 0.5 mg/kg intravenously) can be given. Fever can be treated with anti-inflammatory agents such as flunixin. If fluid overload is suspected due to crackles on thoracic auscultation or peripheral edema, the transfusion should be slowed down and a diuretic (furosemide) can be given. Anaphylaxis requires prompt therapy with epinephrine, diphenhydramine, and dexamethasone.

Acute hypocalcemia can occur during a transfusion because the anticoagulant works by binding calcium to prevent clotting. If possible, the ionized calcium should be measured during or after the transfusion. If calcium supplementation is needed, it must be given through a separate catheter than the blood to prevent reversal of the anticoagulant and clotting.

There is also a risk of transmitting blood-borne illnesses via transfusions. Horses with a known history should be chosen as donors and all established donors should be tested for equine infectious anemia (EIA) and equine viral arteritis (EVA) and routinely vaccinated.

Administration of Parenteral Nutrition

Parenteral (intravenous) nutrition is required in patients that are unable or unwilling to take in adequate nutrients enterally (orally). This may include foals with diarrhea, hypoxic damage to the gastrointestinal tract, or gastroduodenal ulcer disease and adults with anterior enteritis, postoperative ileus, hyperlipidemia, or dysphagia. The three basic nutritional components that can be administered intravenously are glucose, in the form of dextrose; protein, as amino acids; and fat, as triglycerides. Partial parenteral nutrition (PPN) is typically used to refer to administration of dextrose or amino acids, whereas TPN refers to administration of all three components, dextrose, amino acids, and triglycerides. Trace minerals, vitamins, and electrolytes are sometimes added depending on the needs of the patient. The formulation administered is determined by the problem being treated. The use of triglycerides is contraindicated in horses that have hypertriglyceridemia or liver disease because the levels of fat in the blood are already elevated in the liver is not capable of processing triglycerides.

The key to safe administration of parenteral nutrition lies in understanding that just as these components provide nutrients to the patient, they can provide nutrients to bacteria and therefore must be handled with utmost attention to preventing contamination and infection (Table 11.9).

Administration of parenteral nutrition should be started slowly and increased gradually to allow the body time to adjust metabolically to processing of the nutrients. Due to the relatively low rates required and need for accurate administration, it is generally better to administer TPN using an infusion pump. If administration is too rapid, hyperglycemia, from dextrose administration, and hypertriglyceridemia, from fat administration, can occur. The rate of TPN to be administered is

Table 11.9. Guidelines for administration of total parenteral nutrition.

Solutions should be made under a laminar flow hood.

The bags should be refrigerated until administration.

Once opened the total parenteral nutrition (TPN) should be used within 24 hours.

All fluid lines should be changed every 24 hours.

Catheters should be inspected frequently for evidence of thrombophlebitis.

Ideally, a double-lumen catheter should be used and a port dedicated to administration of TPN.

determined by the caloric goal to be reached. Healthy neonatal foals ingest 100 to 150 kcal/kg/day. Depending on the disease process, foals may have clinically higher or lower requirements. Typically, TPN is used to provide up to 100 kcal/kg/day. Adults have much lower caloric requirements, approximately 32 to 35 kcal/kg/day. A typical goal for TPN supplementation would be 20 kcal/kg/day.

When initiating TPN therapy, start at a rate that is one-fourth of the target rate. The blood glucose is then checked every 4 to 6 hours. If the patient is normoglycemic, the rate can be increased by up to one-fourth of the target rate until the target rate is achieved. If the patient is hyperglycemic, the rate can be maintained and the glucose rechecked in a few hours, or insulin therapy can be initiated.

In general, adults are less likely to become hyperglycemic than neonates, particularly septic foals. Insulin resistance or intolerance is common in septic foals, and these foals are more likely to require exogenous insulin therapy or to only tolerate lower rated of TPN. Once the target rate is achieved and the patient is normoglycemic, the glucose can be checked less frequently, every 8 to 12 hours. In patients receiving TPN (containing fat), the triglyceride levels should also be monitored every few days.

When parenteral therapy is stopped, patients should be weaned off slowly to avoid hypoglycemia. Typically the parenteral solution is gradually decreased while the enteral intake is gradually increased. Decreasing the rate by one-fourth every 4 to 6 hours is generally safe.

Management of the Recumbent Horse

Management of the recumbent horse is time consuming and requires two to three people to be safe. Horses become recumbent from damage to the brain or spinal cord from traumatic injury or diseases such as equine protozoal myeloencephalitis, equine herpesvirus, and eastern equine encephalomyelitis. Horses that can not stand require intensive nursing care to maintain a good quality of life. Because of their large body mass they can not tolerate lying on one side for a more than 4 to 6 hours. The horse is at risk to damage their muscles, skin, eyes, and limbs from struggling to rise. Recumbent horses need to be turned frequently and when possible placed on padding to minimize trauma to the muscles and skin. Head padding is appropriate to protect the skull and eyes. Leg bandages can minimize trauma to the distal limbs.

When feeding horses that are recumbent they should be forced to maintain sternal recumbency when eating and drinking to minimize aspiration of feed into the lungs. Recumbent horses may need to have a urinary catheter placed to monitor urine production. The rectum may need to be manually evacuated to assist the horse to defecate. The use of a sling is appropriate for horses that are weak but still have enough strength to stand and need help to rise (Figure 11.16).

Critical Care Monitoring

Monitoring of the critically ill patient should begin with a thorough physical examination. Blood work abnormalities and more advanced equipment may be used to further characterize the disease process and monitor response to therapy. The goal of monitoring in critical care medicine is the early detection of metabolic or physiologic derangements. Early recognition of these derangements will allow prompt medical intervention and hopefully contribute to improving survival. Selection of monitoring aids should be based on reliability, availability, cost, and the value of information gained by their use. Once selected, these measurements should be obtained at regular intervals because trends and temporal changes are more

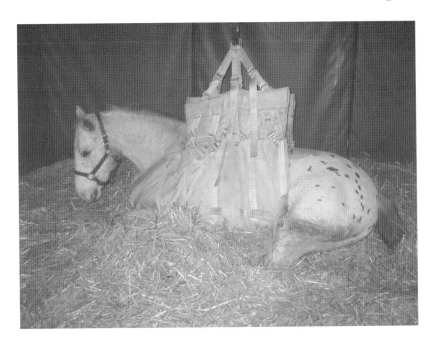

Figure 11.16. Use of a sling in a recumbent horse.
Courtesy of Dr. Dana Zimmel.

important than individual measurements at a given point in time.

Bacterial sepsis and hypoxic-ischemic encephalopathy are the leading causes of morbidity and mortality in neonatal foals. Foals affected with these diseases commonly have compromised cardiovascular and respiratory systems and require intensive monitoring. In adult horses, severe gastrointestinal and renal diseases can result in significant cardiovascular compromise, pH, and electrolyte derangements while severe pneumonia causes respiratory compromise. This text reviews indications, usefulness, and limitations of common monitoring practices in critically ill veterinary patients. Although clinical examples relate more specifically to foals, the principles discussed below can be applied to adult horses as well (Table 11.10).

Monitoring Respiratory Function

Arterial Blood Gas Analysis

Arterial blood gas (ABG) samples are most commonly obtained from the dorsal metatarsal artery in equine neonates. Other sites available include the median, brachial, or femoral arteries. In adult horses, the transverse facial artery is most commonly used. The site of puncture should be prepared with an antiseptic. A small bleb of lidocaine placed subcutaneously or application of lidocaine cream may decrease motion in response to sample collection. In foals with cold extremities due to vasoconstriction, placing warm, moistened gauze over the artery can help make the artery more easily palpable. The blood should be collected in a syringe coated with heparin and kept anaerobic and on ice. After evacuation of air bubbles, the sample should be sealed with a rubber stopper. A sample may be stored on ice for approximately 1.5 to 2 hours. Presence of room air in the sample will result in an artificially increased partial pressure of oxygen in arterial blood (PaO_2), decreased partial pressure of carbon dioxide in the blood ($PaCO_2$), and more alkaline pH. A number of portable clinical analyzers are available. ABG analysis is essential in for evaluating respiratory function in critically ill neonates and adults.

Parameter	Neonatal Foal	Adult	Units
PaO$_2$	40–50[a], 65–90[b]	80–100	mm Hg
SaO$_2$	95–100	95–100	%
PaCO$_2$	40–50	40–45	mm Hg
PetCO$_2$	35–40	35–40	mm Hg
ABP (systolic/diastolic)	80–120/65–90	125–165/85–120	mm Hg
ABP (mean)	70–95	110–130	mm Hg
Central venous pressure	3–12	7–18	cm H$_2$O
Cardiac index	170–190[a]	72–81	ml/kg/minute
Lactate	4–6,[a] 1–3[c]	<2.0	mmol/L
COP	17–19	20–30	mm Hg

Table 11.10. Selected normal values for critical care monitoring.

[a]At birth.
[b]four hours of age.
[c]twelve–twenty-four hours of age.
ABP, arterial blood pressure; COP, colloid osmotic pressure; PaCO$_2$, partial pressure of carbon dioxide in the blood; PaO$_2$, partial pressure of oxygen in the blood; PetCO$_2$, end-tidal partial pressure of carbon dioxide; SaO$_2$, oxygen saturation in the blood.

The PaO$_2$ is a reflection of the capability of the lungs to oxygenate the blood. This measurement is independent of hemoglobin (Hb) concentrations. Normally about 97% of the oxygen transported from the lungs to the tissues is carried in combination with hemoglobin. The remaining 3% is carried in the dissolved state in the water of plasma and cells. Values of PaO$_2$ between 60 and 80 mm Hg indicate hypoxemia and correlate with an arterial saturation (SaO$_2$) of 90% to 95%. PaO$_2$ of 50 to 60 mm Hg corresponds to a SaO$_2$ of approximately 90%. Hypoxemia (low PaO$_2$) does not necessarily result in hypoxia (poor tissue oxygenation). Therefore, hypoxemia alone is not necessarily an indication for oxygen supplementation. Similarly, oxygen supplementation does not always result in an increase in tissue oxygen availability. The lack of improvement in systemic oxygen transport during oxygen inhalation is explained by the tendency of oxygen to reduce systemic blood flow by causing vasoconstriction and decreasing CO.

Newborn foals in lateral recumbency have a PaO$_2$ of 40 to 50 mm Hg immediately after birth. PaO$_2$ increases progressively to approximately 65 to 90 mm Hg by 4 hours of age. Position of the foal can dramatically alter blood gas interpretation. PaO$_2$ is approximately 10 mm Hg lower in lateral recumbency than in standing position. Hypoxemia is a common finding in critically ill neonatal foals. Severe hypoxemia in a critically ill foal may warrant intranasal insufflation with humidified oxygen. Supplemental oxygen in foals should be considered in the following situations:

- Severe hypoxemia in foals older that 12 to 24 hours of age (PaO$_2$ < 55 mm Hg or SaO$_2$ < 90%) because it may promote pulmonary hypertension in neonates.
- Mild hypoxemia with evidence of tissue dysoxia such as high lactate, increased oxygen extraction ratio, or decreased oxygen uptake (see Hemodynamic Monitoring on page 294).

The PaO$_2$ in the standing adult horse should be 80 to 95 mm Hg. Hypoxemia in adult horses most often occurs due to infectious pneumonia and heaves. Supplemental oxygen in adult horses should be considered when the PaO$_2$ is 60 to 80 mm Hg or SaO$_2$ 90% to 95%.

As blood flows through the lungs, the carbon dioxide (CO_2) produced by the tissues is exhaled. Therefore, PaCO$_2$ is a measure of ventilatory status. Excess CO_2 stimulates part if the brain that controls breathing, the respiratory center. As a result, CO_2 is the main drive for ventilation. Changes in PaO_2 have no significant direct effect on the respiratory center. However, changes in arterial oxygen can be detected by peripheral chemoreceptors in the carotid artery and aorta. These chemoreceptors in turn transmit signals to the respiratory center of the brain to help regulate respiratory activity. The effect of oxygen on stimulation of peripheral chemoreceptors is particularly pronounced at PaO_2 less than 60 mm Hg.

$PaCO_2$ is approximately 40 to 50 mm Hg in newborn foals in lateral recumbency. $PaCO_2$ is also affected by positioning with values 3 to 5 mm Hg higher in laterally recumbent foals. Venous PCO_2 is usually 3 to 6 mm Hg higher than arterial PCO_2 and reflects tissue metabolism in addition to ventilatory status. Hypoventilation causes an increase in $PaCO_2$, whereas hyperventilation causes a decrease. Changes in $PaCO_2$ can cause changes in the blood pH. Values greater than 65 to 75 mm Hg may warrant mechanical ventilation or chemical stimulation of ventilation with doxapram, particularly if blood pH is affected. It must be emphasized that CO_2 diffuses about twenty times better than oxygen across the respiratory membrane. As a result, mild lung pathology is more likely to cause a decrease in PaO_2, hypoxemia, than an increase in $PaCO_2$, hypercapnea. Causes of hypoxemia with a normal $PaCO_2$ include decreased inspired oxygen (rare), right-to-left shunting of blood, diffusion impairment, or ventilation/perfusion (V/Q) mismatching. Hypoxemia with markedly increased $PaCO_2$ indicates hypoventilation and defines respiratory failure. Foals with hypoxic ischemic encephalopathy commonly have a low PaO_2 and high $PaCO_2$ as a result of the inability of their brain to increase ventilation in response to increased CO_2. These foals are typically comatose, and they have a low respiratory rate. In contrast, foals with hypoxemia and high $PaCO_2$ as a result of lung pathology tend to have a high respiratory rate and increased respiratory effort.

Pulse Oximetry

Pulse oximetry is a noninvasive method to assess the patient's need for oxygen. Pulse oximeters estimate SaO_2 by evaluating the absorption of light at two different frequencies. At SaO_2 above 70%, saturation recorded by pulse oximeters is accurate. SaO_2 from ABG is not a measured variable but rather is derived from an equation, and this derived parameter has been shown to be much less accurate than measurement provided by pulse oximetry. The use of pulse oximetry allows a considerable reduction in the frequency of arterial sampling for blood gas analysis. Frequent monitoring of SaO_2 via oximetry coupled to once or twice daily ABG monitoring is typically recommended.

A variety of probes are available for use in different locations. The best sites are those that have minimal pigment or hair, and include the tongue, lip, ear, rectum and a clipped fold of skin on the flank (Figure 11.17). The probe should be held in place gently to avoid constricting the underlying blood vessels. As with any hemodynamic monitoring device, the SaO_2 reading should only be recorded when the pulse measured by the monitor matches the HR auscultated.

Capnography

Capnography is measuring the concentration of CO_2 in respiratory gases. The most common use of this technique is during mechanical ventilation. Infrared CO_2 detectors can be used to measure the CO_2 in exhaled air, known as the end-tidal CO_2. Normally, the difference between the arterial and end-tidal partial pressure of carbon dioxide (PCO_2, called the $PaCO_2$-$PetCO_2$ gradient, is less than 5 mm Hg. However, when gas exchange in the lungs is impaired, $PetCO_2$ decreases relative to $PaCO_2$, so that the gradient increases. An increased $PaCO_2$-$PetCO_2$ gradient suggests an increase in dead-space ventilation (i.e., areas of lung that are ventilated but not properly perfused). Virtually any pulmonary or systemic disorder where CO is reduced will produce an increased $PaCO_2$-$PetCO_2$ gradient. Thus, in foals with cardiopulmonary disease an ABG is necessary at the onset to determine the gradient. End-tidal CO_2 can then be monitored continuously. Changes in $PetCO_2$ should be equivalent to changes in $PaCO_2$ as long as gas

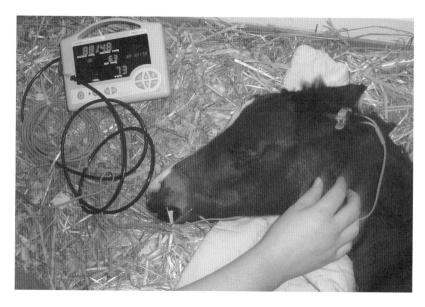

Figure 11.17. Use of pulse oximetry in a foal.
Courtesy of Dr. Steeve Gigère.

exchange remains constant. Just like pulse oximetry reduces the need for PaO_2 monitoring, capnometry reduces the need for frequent $PaCO_2$ measurements. However, ABG must be done periodically to ensure that the $PaCO_2$-$PetCO_2$ gradient has not changed.

Because a decrease in CO will decrease $PetCO_2$, capnometry can be used to monitor trends in CO during volume resuscitation in hypovolemic shock and during cardiopulmonary resuscitation. Capnometry is also an easy way to ensure correct endotracheal tube placement as the CO_2 in the trachea should be about 40 mm Hg, while it is 0 in the esophagus.

Imaging Techniques
Ultrasonography and radiography are useful to detect the presence and assess the severity of lung pathology. The normal aerated lung parenchyma is not penetrated by the ultrasound beam, rendering only the pleura and superficial lung surface available for study. Deep lung pathology with overlying aerated lung would therefore not be detected ultrasonographically. Radiographs are superior to

ultrasound for evaluation the deep pulmonary parenchyma. However, ultrasonography offers a considerable advantage over radiographs in the study of the pleural surfaces and space. A small amount of pleural effusion that would otherwise be missed clinically or on radiographs can be detected. Endoscopy is useful when upper airway obstruction is the suspected cause of respiratory difficulties.

Hemodynamic Monitoring
The ultimate goal of hemodynamic monitoring is to ensure adequate oxygen delivery to tissues in an attempt to maintain normal organ function.

Arterial Blood Pressure
Arterial blood pressure monitoring is routine practice in equine neonatal intensive care units, allowing recognition of some cardiovascular derangements and titration of therapy with intravenous fluids, vasopressors (medications that increase blood pressure), and inotropic agents (medications that increase cardiac

contractility). Mean arterial pressure (MAP), rather than systolic or diastolic pressure, is the true driving pressure for systemic blood flow and organ perfusion. In addition, the MAP is less likely to change because the pressure waveform moves distally (from the aorta to a peripheral artery). As a result, MAP is superior to systolic or diastolic pressure for arterial pressure monitoring. Arterial blood pressure can be measured by direct and indirect methods. Direct monitoring via cannulation of a peripheral artery is accurate and provides a continuous display of blood pressure results. However, the difficulty in maintaining an arterial catheter in nonanesthetized foals makes direct blood pressure measurement less practical for routine monitoring. Indirect methods of measuring blood pressure include manometric measurement and Doppler and oscillometric methods. Oscillometric techniques offer the advantage of providing systolic, diastolic, and mean arterial pressures whereas other indirect methods do not provide MAP.

Several automated oscillometric blood pressure devices are currently available for use in human or veterinary medicine. Most of these monitors provide a reasonable assessment of MAP in foals. Sites of cuff placement that have been recommended for indirect blood pressure measurement in foals include the coccygeal, dorsal metatarsal, or median arteries (Figure 11.18). Adequate sites for cuff placement depend on the type of monitor used. In general, cuff placement over the coccygeal artery results in more accurate results and is also the most common site used in adults. The metatarsal artery is a reasonable alternative. The cuff width should be approximately 40% of the diameter of the appendage. Cuffs that are too wide or tight cause falsely low indirect blood pressure readings, whereas cuffs that too loose or narrow cause falsely high readings. Indirect blood pressure readings will also be influenced by the level of the cuff relative to the position of the heart. Cuffs placed below the heart level result in falsely elevated blood pressure, whereas cuffs placed above heart level

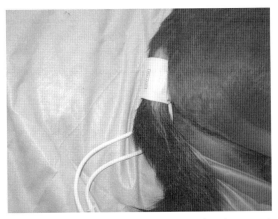

Figure 11.18. Indirect blood pressure measurement from the coccygeal artery.
Courtesy of Dr. Steeve Giguère.

result in an artificially decreased blood pressure. It is therefore important to obtain subsequent indirect blood pressure measurements with the animal in the same position. This is particularly important when the cuff is placed over the metatarsal or median arteries in foals because the level of the cuff relative to the heart will vary greatly whether the foal is standing or in lateral recumbency. In adult horses, maintaining a consistent head position between readings is vital because the MAP can vary up to 20 mm Hg with changes in head position.

Normal blood pressure varies with age, size, and breed, as well as, technique used. A MAP of 70 to 95 mm Hg in neonatal foals and 110 to 130 mm Hg in adult horses is considered normal. A minimum MAP of approximately 60 to 65 mm Hg is vital to adequate cerebral, renal, and coronary blood flow. Increasing the MAP to 75 or 85 mm Hg does not provide additional advantages on systemic oxygen metabolism, skin microcirculatory blood flow, urine output, and splanchnic perfusion compared with 65 mm Hg. As a result, cardiovascular support with vasopressor drugs in foals is typically initiated when MAP readings fall below this critical level of 60 to 65 mm Hg. A low MAP in an adult horse is usually a result of hypovolemia and indicates the need for aggressive fluid treatment.

Blood Pressure Versus Blood Flow
Blood flow and blood pressure are distinct physical entities. MAP is the product of CO and systemic vascular resistance (SVR), which is the resistance to blood flow through the vessels:

24 is the normal bicarbonate level in the blood
Obtain the patient's bicarbonate level from the blood gas
Use 0.3 for adults or 0.5 for neonates, which represents the percent body weight that is extracellular fluid

How to calculate mean arterial pressure
$MAP = CO \times SVR$

When vascular resistance is abnormal due to constriction or dilation of the vessels, the arterial pressure is not a reliable index of arterial flow. Blood flow rather than blood pressure is the driving force for tissue perfusion and measurement of CO is required for calculation of global oxygen delivery and consumption. Because measurement of CO is currently considered impractical for routine use in foals, arterial blood pressure is commonly used as an indicator of blood flow.

Cardiac Output
CO is the best available parameter to assess overall cardiovascular function. CO is the product of stroke volume (SV) and HR.

How to calculate cardiac output
$CO = SV \times HR$

Measurement of CO, along with blood Hb concentration and oxygen saturation of Hb, also allows calculation of global tissue oxygen delivery and consumption. CO monitoring is valuable in critically ill or anesthetized neonatal foals. Accurate measurement of this parameter

leads to a better detection and understanding of cardiovascular derangements and aids in optimal titration of fluid therapy and inotropic or vasopressor agents. Because measurement of CO has traditionally been considered impractical for routine use in foals, arterial blood pressure is commonly used as an indicator of blood flow. As previously explained, arterial pressure is a poor indicator of blood flow in situations when vascular resistance is altered. SVR is often altered during sepsis, therefore limiting the usefulness of blood pressure as an indicator of blood flow in critically ill neonatal foals. An echocardiographic technique has been described that allows a reliable and noninvasive means of monitoring CO in foals. Because CO varies considerably with the size of the foal, it is usually converted to cardiac index (CI). The CI is equal to the CO divided by body weight. Normal CI in clinically healthy 1-day-old foals restrained in lateral recumbency is 180 ± 10 ml/kg/minute and increases to 222 ± 22 ml/kg/minute by day 14. Determining CO in the standing adult horse is more challenging but can be done using Doppler studies, lithium dilution, thermodilution, or other techniques. Normal CI in standing adult horses is 72 to 81 ml/kg/minute.

Lactate
Blood lactate is a marker of perfusion of blood and oxygen delivery to tissues. When oxygen supplies are adequate, glucose is metabolized using aerobic metabolism. When oxygen delivery does not match metabolic requirements, anaerobic metabolism is performed, and a portion of the glucose metabolism is diverted to lactate production. Therefore, an increase in lactate can be used as evidence of impaired tissue oxygenation relative to demand. Causes of hyperlactatemia include hypoxemia, hypotension, low oxygen content (due to anemia), and hypermetabolic states (due to increased muscle activity including seizure or sepsis). Postpartum foals have immediate lactate concentrations of 4.9 ± 1 mmol/L. These values decrease rapidly within 12 to 24

hours. Normal foals older than 12 hours of age have lactate concentrations less than 3.0 mmol/L with most foals having less than 2.0 mmol/L. Blood lactate should be measured immediately after collection unless placed into tubes containing fluoride that inhibit in vitro erythrocyte production of lactate.

Unfortunately, anaerobic metabolism is not the only source of increased blood lactate concentration. Other causes of high lactate include liver failure (decreased clearance), severe metabolic alkalosis and hyperglycemia (stimulates anaerobic metabolism), thiamine deficiency, catecholamines surges, and endotoxemia.

Central Venous Pressure
CVP is the intraluminal pressure within the intrathoracic cranial vena cava or right atrium. It is an estimate of preload and right ventricular filling pressure and is determined by the CO and venous return. CVP decreases with hypovolemia and increases with iatrogenic fluid overload and right-sided heart failure. Central catheters can easily be placed in neonatal foals. Although central catheters can be placed in adults, a regular catheter can also be used to measure trends in the pressure in the jugular vein. The value of the jugular vein pressure will be lower than the CVP but changes in this value should correlate with changes in the CVP. Normal CVP is 3 to 12 cm H_2O in neonatal foals and 5 to 15 H_2O in adults. CVP can be used to guide fluid replacement in patients with hypovolemia. It is extremely valuable in patients at risk for fluid overload, such as neonates and any patient with impaired renal function. As with arterial blood pressure, trends in CVP are more informative than single measurements. Serial or continuous monitoring is useful in determining the end point of fluid resuscitation.

CVP can be measured intermittently using a water monometer. A saline-filled extension set is attached to the catheter and to a three-way stop cock. The water monometer and a saline filled syringe are attached to the stopcock. The monometer should then be positioned such that the baseline (0) is at the level of the right atrium, using the point of the shoulder as a landmark. The line should then

be closed to the monometer and opened to the syringe, and the line to the patient should be flushed. The line to the patient should then be closed and the manometer should be flushed. To obtain a measurement, the three-way should be turned so that the patient line is open to the manometer. The fluid column in the monometer will then fall to the level of the CVP. To obtain accurate, consistent readings, it is important that the horses head remain in a neutral position during monitoring and that all air bubbles be flushed from the lines.

The CVP can also be measured using a pressure transducer and electronic monitor, which also allows for continuous monitoring. The monitor is first zeroed to the environment and then the patient line is opened to obtain a recording. In this case, the transducer is held level with the point of the shoulder.

Urine Output
Urine output is a good indicator of renal blood flow. Therefore, it can be used as a marker of organ perfusion and fluid balance. Hypovolemia, inadequate perfusion, hypotension, and renal disease may all result in decreased urine output. Urine production should be monitored at least subjectively in all sick horses. USG is often used as an indicator of adequate hydration in neonatal foals. A normal foal nursing voluntarily will consume 15% to 25% of its body weight in milk to maintain caloric requirements. To eliminate excess fluid, normal foals have hyposthenuric urine (USG 1.001–1.015). Therefore, in the absence of renal disease, a low USG indicates adequate voluntary milk intake. Urine output of recumbent foals can be monitored semi-quantitatively through the use of absorbent pads. These can be weighed to estimate the volume of urine produced. In foals with severe hemodynamic disturbances, urine output can be monitored quantitatively through the use of a urinary catheter attached a collection bag. Normal foals nursing voluntarily produce urine at a rate of 4 to 8 ml/kg/ hour. However, urine production in critically ill foals should be more a reflection of fluid balance. Urine output that is less than 66% of the amount of

fluid intake is a source for concern. Reduced urine output may reflect prerenal (i.e., hypovolemia or hypotension), renal, or postrenal (i.e., uroperitoneum or obstruction of the catheter or urethra) causes.

Electrocardiography

Indications for electrocardiogram (ECG) monitoring in neonatal foals and adult horses include the presence of dysrhythmias, marked electrolyte abnormalities (e.g., hyperkalemia), and therapy with vasopressor or inotropic agents. Continuous, real-time, monitoring can be achieved using telemetry-based recording systems and is appropriate for monitoring of critical cases and for exercise tests. A Holter monitor can be used to identify infrequent dysrhythmic events, for evaluation of drug therapy, and are indicated in horses with a history of syncope or an arrhythmia with no detectable arrhythmias at rest or during exercise. For both systems, the positive electrode is placed over the left apex of the heart (fourth intercostal space), and the negative electrode is placed in the left saddle area, just behind the withers. The electrodes can be secured using a surcingle.

Colloid Oncotic Pressure

The plasma colloid osmotic, or oncotic, pressure (COP) is the pressure generated by the osmolarity of plasma proteins that are unable to cross capillary membranes. These proteins attract water and therefore help maintain the intravascular volume. Albumin is the largest determinant of oncotic pressure, making up 80% to 90% of the COP. Thus, in diseases causing hypoalbuminemia, such as protein losing enteropathy or nephropathy, the COP will be decrease, resulting in peripheral edema. Serial monitoring of the total protein and albumin levels is adequate to monitor the response to natural colloid therapy, plasma or whole blood because these values correlate with the COP. However, synthetic colloid fluids, such as hydroxyethylstarch (Hetastarch) and dextran, do not change protein measurements. Therefore, direct colloid osmometry using a colloid osmometer is indicated to monitor the response to synthetic colloid therapy. A COP measurement of less than 15 mm Hg, a total protein of less than 3.0 g/dl, or an albumin of less than 1.5 g/dl is considered an indication of the need for treatment with colloids.

Additional Monitoring

Body Weight

Serial body weight is a good estimate of fluid balance in horses of all ages and nutritional status in foals. Healthy neonatal foals should gain an average of 1.6 kg/day if adequate caloric requirements are met. Foals in neonatal intensive care units should be weighed daily. Plotting the growth curve over a period of days is more accurate than just comparing two values obtained on subsequent days.

Laboratory Data

Measurement of serum electrolytes, packed cell volume, total protein, blood urea nitrogen, and creatinine concentrations are essential in critically ill foals. Interpretation of laboratory data is covered in Chapter 8.

References and Further Reading

Smith, B. P. 2001. *Large Animal Internal Medicine*. 3rd ed. St. Louis: Mosby.

Davis, H. 2004. Intravenous access. *Proceedings of the Northeast Veterinary Conference*, Retrieved from the Veterinary Information Network web site: www.vin.com/Members/Proceedings/Proceedings.plx?CID=nevc2004&PID=pr06925&O=VIN.

Furr, M. 2002. Intravenous nutrition in horses: Clinical applications. *Proceedings of the ACVIM Annual Forum*, Dallas, Texas, May 29–June 1, 2002.

Hardy, J. 2006. Monitoring the equine patient: Pulse oximetry and more. *Proceedings of the International Veterinary Emergency and Critical Care Symposium*, San Antonio, September 17–21, 2006.

Lester, G. 2002. Fluid therapy in the horse with colic. *Proceedings of the ACVIM Annual Forum*, Dallas, Texas, May 29–June 1, 2002.

Madigan, J. 2002. Fluid and electrolyte balance. *Proceedings of the Western Veterinary Conference*, Las Vegas, February 11–14, 2002.

Magdesin, K. G. 2002. Monitoring techniques. *Proceedings of the ACVIM Annual Forum*, Dallas, Texas, May 29–June 1, 2002.

Monnet, E. 2002. Cardiovascular monitoring. In *The veterinary ICU book,* ed. W. Wingfield and M. Raffe, 266–280. Jackson, WY: Teton New Media.

Stashak, T. 1987. *Adams' lameness in the horses*. 4th ed. Philadelphia: Lea & Febiger.

Walesby, H. A., and J. M. Blackmer. 2003. How to use the transverse facial venous sinus as an alternative location for blood collection in the horse. *Proceedings of the Forty-ninth Annual Convention of the American Association of Equine Practitioners, New Orleans, November 21–25, 2003.*

CHAPTER 12

Technical Procedures

DeeAnn Wilfong and Bryan Waldridge

Nasogastric Intubation

Common Indications

Nasogastric (NG) intubation can be used to deliver fluids and medications, relieve an esophageal obstruction ("choke"), and is indicated in the diagnosis and treatment of colic. Regardless of intended use of the NG tube, the technique for placement is the same. The equipment needed is an appropriately sized nasogastric tube, a bucket filled with a premeasured amount of warm water, and either a 400-ml dose syringe or standard bilge pump (Figure 12.1).

Procedure

The NG tube should be immersed in warm water until it becomes more flexible. Water can be an adequate lubricant; however, many practitioners choose to use an additional water-based lubricant on the distal end of the tube to ease placement. The horse should be restrained appropriately with injectable sedation, but it is suggested to have a twitch available. Standing to the left side of the patient, place the right hand on the horse's nose, and using the thumb, move the alar fold of the nostril dorsally. Using the left hand to guide the NG tube ventrally and medially into the nasal passage, taking care to avoid the middle meatus and lateral meatus, the tube should be advanced firmly but not forced. If resistance is encountered, partially with-

draw the tube, reposition and try to advance it or remove the tube completely and try using the other nostril. At the larynx, time the patient's swallow reflex to expedite the tube passing through the larynx and into the esophagus. Blowing into the tube or gently bumping the epiglottis is thought to trigger the swallow reflex in resistant patients. Once it is thought that the tube is in the esophagus, placement must be checked before any medications or water is delivered. A correctly placed NG tube can be seen or felt passing down the esophagus on the left side of the neck. Blowing into the tube from this point on can help to advance the tube through the cardia and into the stomach. The NG tube placement should again be assessed before anything is put through the tube. Suction on the end of the tube should yield negative pressure, breaths should not be felt from the end of the tube (not always reliable), and gastric contents or gas can be smelled from the end of the tube. After placement is confirmed, the stomach should be checked for reflux, which can occur spontaneously or can require lavage. The normal horse may have 1 to 2 L gastric reflux present in the stomach. If no reflux is found, then medications and fluids can be delivered. If reflux is present, it should be removed by creating a siphon with the tube and using measured amounts of water (Figure 12.2). Using the dose syringe or bilge pump to create a siphon, 1 to 2 L water should be pumped through the tube. The NG tube can be lowered into a bucket and the water with reflux will run out until the siphon is broken. The process

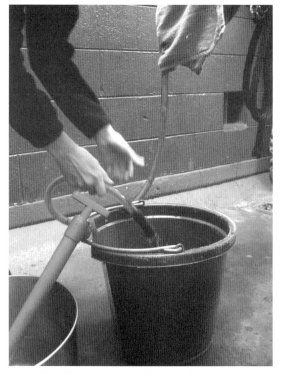

Figure 12.1. Bilge pump being used to reflux a horse.

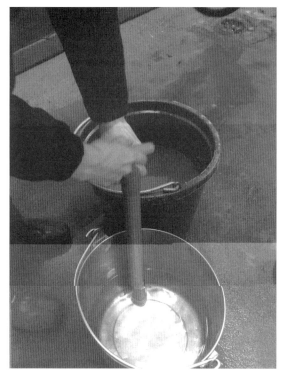

Figure 12.2. Creating a siphon.

should be repeated until the water runs clear and reflux is no longer seen. Before removing a tube, lower it to be sure there isn't excessive pressure on the stomach. To remove the NG tube, pinch or clamp it off, and placing a hand on the horse's nose, pull the tube in one fluid motion.

Complications

The most common complication is epistaxis. Although this should be monitored, it is usually of little concern. If this occurs during NG tube placement, pull and rinse the tube out, and try again using the other nostril. There is a chance of mucosal irritation in the nostril and the esophagus, which can be minimized with the use of lubricants and a gentle technique. If esophageal erosion or injury is suspected, the tube should be removed and the area can be endoscopically examined. Aspiration pneu-

monia from a NG tube placed in the trachea can be a fatal complication, especially when large volumes of fluids are administered. This is a completely avoidable complication as long as correct placement of the NG tube is assessed.

Abdominocentesis

Common Indications for the Procedure

Abdominocentesis collects peritoneal fluid for evaluation of gastrointestinal disease. Abdominocentesis is commonly performed in horses with colic, weight loss, or diarrhea.

Procedure

This procedure is performed aseptically and consists of placing a needle or teat cannula into the abdomen and withdrawing a sample of fluid from the peritoneal cavity. The area for sampling is slightly to the right of ventral midline (to avoid hitting the spleen that is on the left side) and approximately 5 cm caudal to the xiphoid. This is the most dependent point of the abdomen, allowing for greater sampling success. Abdominal ultrasound is helpful in locating pockets of fluid but is not necessary.

The area should be clipped and aseptically prepared (see Chapter 10 for aseptic techniques). Use of adequate restraint is vital not only for a successful procedure but also for the safety of the veterinarian doing the procedure. Once the area is clean, care should be taken to glove and maintain asepsis during the procedure. An 18- or 20-gauge 1 1/2-in. needle is adequate, but a longer needle may be needed in obese animals. Foal intestinal walls are thin, and it is recommended not to use needles but rather a smaller diameter teat cannula (Figure 12.3). The needle is placed through the skin and the linea alba. If fluid is not seen, a second needle is often placed to release negative pressure. The needle is rotated to free the bevel from any tissue it is against, or a syringe is used to carefully aspirate a sample.

Alternatively a teat cannula can be used. The area should be aseptically prepped and a subcutaneous bleb of local anesthetic placed at the intended site. A #15 blade is used to make a stab incision through

the skin and subcutaneous tissue. The teat cannula tip can be pressed through a gauze sponge to decrease blood contamination. The teat cannula is inserted into the incision and pushed through the linea alba (Figure 12.4).

Once peritoneal fluid is obtained, it should be collected by free catch directly into an ethylenediaminetetraacetic acid (EDTA) collection tube and a red top collection tube. Normal peritoneal fluid is pale yellow and clear with a white cell count less than 5,000 cells/μl, total protein of less than 2.0 g/dl, and a specific gravity of 1.005 mg/dl. Common cytologic findings are 40% to 80% neutrophils and 20% to 80% mononuclear cells. Abnormal findings vary by the condition present. Yellow to white with increased turbidity results from large numbers of white cells as in inflammation or infection, and red to brown with increased turbidity results from ischemia or necrosis of the intestine.

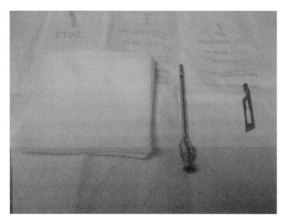

Figure 12.3. Fenestrated teat cannula and 15 blade.

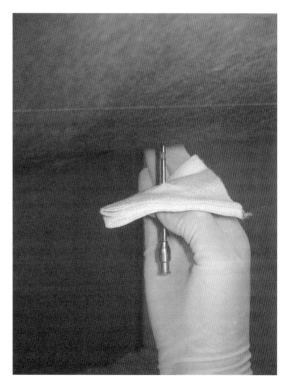

Figure 12.4. Use of a teat cannula for abdominocentesis.

Plant or feed material in the sample results from gastric or intestinal rupture. When frank blood is sampled, the abdominocentesis sample should be compared with the peripheral packed cell volume (PCV); if it is higher in the abdominal sample, it is likely the spleen was entered during the procedure. This is helpful to differentiate the samples when hemoabdomen is suspected.

Complications

Complications include enterocentesis, which can contaminate the sample with feed material, or splenic aspiration, which can contaminate the sample with blood. Local cellulitis or abscess formation at the sample site (usually from breaks in sterile technique) is rare. Occasionally, abdominocentesis in foals will result in a small amount of omentum exiting the sample site.

Rebreathing Examination

The rebreathing examination should be part of the routine physical examination of most patients examined for respiratory disease. The objective of a rebreathing examination is to make the horse take a deep breath. This is accomplished by placing a bag over the horse's nose to raise the inspired carbon dioxide CO_2 and the partial pressure of carbon dioxide in the blood (PCO_2) concentrations, which will stimulate respiration and increase the effort and rate of respiration. This allows better auscultation of subtle or quiet lung sounds.

Equipment and Supplies

To perform a rebreathing examination all that is needed is a large plastic bag (such as a clean garbage bag) or a rectal sleeve (if the patient is small). One person should hold the horse and the bag while another person performs the examination.

Procedure

The bag is fitted around the horse's muzzle fairly snugly and the edges are tucked underneath the

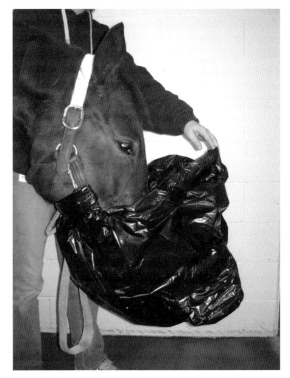

Figure 12.5. Rebreathing examination.

halter (Figure 12.5). Enough room should be left in the bag so that the horse can easily breathe without the bag interfering with its nostrils. Some horses may be too fractious to allow a bag over their nose. In this case, the nostrils may be occluded by pressing over the alar folds and preventing airflow. This technique is also useful for small horses and foals.

The bag is held in place for 1 to 2 minutes or until the horse begins to breathe deeply. The examiner should begin listening to the horse's lung fields as soon as rebreathing begins and continue to listen until respiratory rate and effort return to normal after the bag has been removed. It is important to listen to both sides of the thorax and the trachea.

The normal horse may require only four to six breaths after removal of the rebreathing bag to return to normal respiration. Abnormal sounds include crackles, wheezes, or pleural friction rubs. Normal horses should not cough during or after the procedure.

Procedure Complications

Rebreathing examination is contraindicated for any horse that has signs of obvious dyspnea or respiratory compromise at rest. Some horses resent nasal occlusion or the presence of the bag on their nose. The examiner and assistant should be wary of avoidance behaviors. Horses with respiratory disease may cough, sometimes profusely, during a rebreathing examination. Horses with pleuritis or pleuropneumonia may become more painful with increased respiratory effort.

Bronchoalveolar Lavage

Common Indications for the Procedure

Bronchoalveolar lavage (BAL) is indicated for the diagnosis of diffuse, noninfectious pulmonary disease. Lung disease must be assumed to be diffuse when performing BAL because only a localized, relatively small area of one lung will be sampled. Most commonly, BAL is used to diagnose pulmonary pathology that may be causing poor performance such as recurrent airway obstruction or heaves, inflammatory airway disease, or exercise-induced pulmonary hemorrhage (EIPH). Samples obtained using BAL are not suitable for culture because the BAL catheter or gastroscope is contaminated as it passed through the nasopharynx and trachea. In the case of suspected fungal pneumonia, a pure, heavy growth of fungi from a BAL sample can support the diagnosis of fungal infection.

Equipment and Supplies

BAL can be performed with either a commercially available BAL catheter (normally around 30 French diameter and 240–300 cm in length) or a standard 3-m gastroscope (Figure 12.6). The BAL catheter or gastroscope needs to be clean but not necessarily sterile.

Horses are sedated with detomidine (0.01–0.02 mg/kg intravenously) or xylazine (0.5 mg/kg intravenously). The addition of butorphanol (0.02–0.04 mg/kg intravenously) is recommended to

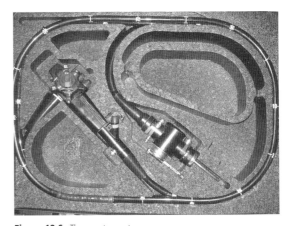

Figure 12.6. Three-meter gastroscope.

reduce coughing and provide additional sedation. Some horses will require a twitch for additional restraint while passing the BAL catheter or gastroscope. Most clinicians use between 180 and 300 ml of sterile isotonic saline to perform the lavage. The saline can be prepared into 60-ml syringes to instill sequentially. The first 60-ml syringe to be administered should contain 30 ml of sterile 2% lidocaine or mepivacaine, which will serve as a local anesthetic. After aspiration of BAL fluid, it can be placed into plain glass or plastic tubes or a sterile 120-ml specimen cup for processing.

Procedure

The horse is sedated with an α_2-agonist and butorphanol as previously described. BAL can be performed when the horse shows signs of sedation and begins to drop its head. A nose twitch is applied as needed. The BAL catheter is advanced through a nostril as for an NG tube. BAL catheters are generally quite soft and flexible, therefore keeping the horse's head and neck extended will facilitate passage into the trachea. The catheter is passed until it can be felt to wedge in a distal bronchus. The cuff on the BAL catheter is then gently inflated. If a 3-m gastroscope is used, it is passed as previously described. The advantages of using a 3-m gastroscope are that any mucous or hemorrhage in the airways can be easily observed

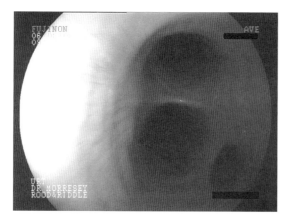

Figure 12.7. Gastroscope wedged in distal brochus.

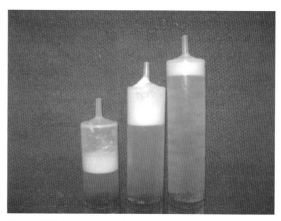

Figure 12.8. Bronchoalveolar lavage samples containing surfactant.

and recorded or followed to the affected areas of the lung.

The syringe containing local anesthetic and saline is injected first. This syringe should be kept ready as the catheter or gastroscope is passed. Some horses will cough vigorously during BAL and injection of local anesthetic before wedging into a distal bronchus can reduce the cough reflex. Most horses quickly become more comfortable following injection of local anesthetic. If using a 3-m gastroscope, lavage fluid is injected through the instrument portal of the endoscope. Once wedged into a distal bronchus, the remaining syringes of isotonic saline are quickly injected (Figure 12.7).

As soon as the final syringe has been injected, suction is applied to the syringe, and the BAL fluid is aspirated. The previous syringes are then used to aspirate as much of the saline as possible, generally greater than 50% of the total volume injected. A diagnostic BAL will appear foamy with pulmonary surfactant. The first aspirated syringe usually does not contain as much surfactant as the others, due to aspirating the remaining saline in the channel of the gastroscope or BAL catheter (Figure 12.8). If using a BAL catheter, the cuff is then deflated and the tube removed. The 3-m gastroscope can be removed immediately and any sections of the trachea and distal airways can be re-examined if desired.

Samples are then transferred to 10- to 15-ml glass or plastic tubes. First filtering BAL fluid through a 4 × 4 sponge into a specimen cup to remove surfactant and any feed material that may have been aspirated when the horse coughs during the procedure is preferred.

Tubes are spun for 5 minutes at about 3,000 rpm. Most of the supernatant is removed and the cell pellet is resuspended. A small drop of this placed and smeared onto a glass slide. Slides are allowed to air-dry completely and then stained and read or mailed to the pathologist.

Normal Bronchoalveolar Lavage Fluid

The vast majority of cells normally observed in BAL fluid should be macrophages and lymphocytes (Figure 12.9). Neutrophils should account for less than 5% of leukocytes observed. There should be minimal to no mucus present. Occasional eosinophils and mast cells (<2%) may also be observed.

Procedure Complications

Some horses with more inflamed or reactive airways can cough very vigorously during the procedure. This is usually reduced by the administration of butorphanol and injecting the syringe with local anesthetic as the catheter or gastroscope enters the distal bronchi. If the gastroscope or BAL catheter

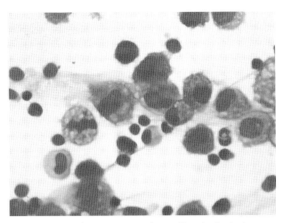

Figure 12.9. Cytologic appearance of normal bronchoalveolar lavage fluid. Note that the majority of cells are macrophages or lymphocytes. Courtesy Dr. Elizabeth Welles, Auburn University, AL.

Table 12.1. Supplies needed to perform a transtracheal wash.

- Clippers.
- Sterile scrub.
- Lidocaine.
- Sedation.
- Sterile 4 × 4 gauze.
- Sterile gloves.
- Antibiotic ointment.
- Elasticon.
- #15 scalpel blade.
- Transtracheal wash kit (stylet, cannula, and catheter).
- Sterile saline.
- Ethylenediaminetetraacetic acid tube.
- Bacterial transport media.

does not adequately wedge and seal into a distal bronchus, then the BAL sample will be non-diagnostic (not foamy with surfactant). This can be prevented using the gastroscope by ensuring that the gastroscope is aimed into the lumen of the bronchus and not stuck against the mucosa or at a bronchial branch point.

Occasionally, there is some mild bronchial hemorrhage due to coughing or local irritation from the BAL catheter or gastroscope. This is sometimes visualized if using an endoscope. or the BAL sample may be slightly blood tinged in a horse without a previous history of EIPH. If iatrogenic hemorrhage is suspected, the slides should be carefully inspected for free erythrocytes rather than hemosiderophages. However, horses that have had a recent episode of EIPH may have both erythrocytes and hemosiderophages present. A neutrophilic infiltration of the bronchus sampled may persist for at least 48 hours after BAL.

Bronchoalveolar catheters are quite flexible and may be inadvertently passed or coughed into the oropharynx. This may result in severe damage of the BAL catheter. If the oropharynx is sampled or severely contaminates the BAL tube, then squamous epithelial cells, feed material, and numerous types of bacteria will be observed cytologically.

Transtracheal Wash (Transtracheal Aspiration)

Common Indications for the Procedure

Transtracheal wash (TTW) is indicated whenever infectious (bacterial or fungal) pneumonia is suspected. TTW provides a mixed sample from the entire lower respiratory tract. The procedure is performed aseptically, which decreases the possibility of contamination with upper respiratory, nasopharyngeal, or skin flora.

Equipment and Supplies

Supplies that are needed are listed in Table 12.1. Horses are sedated with detomidine (0.01–0.02 mg/kg intravenously) or xylazine (0.5 mg/kg intravenously). Butorphanol (0.02–0.04 mg/kg intravenously) can also be administered to reduce coughing and provide additional sedation. Diazepam (0.1 mg/kg intravenously) may be substituted for xylazine in foals. Some horses will require a twitch for additional restraint. Commercially prepared TTW kits contain a stylet, blunt-ended open cannula, and catheter (Figure 12.10). The technician will need to prepare two syringes containing 20 to 60 ml of sterile isotonic saline, provide sterile gloves, and obtain a culture transport vial and EDTA tube for a cytology sample. Some clinicians prefer to

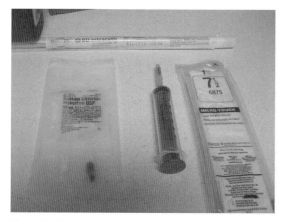

Figure 12.10. Commercially prepared transtracheal wash catheter.

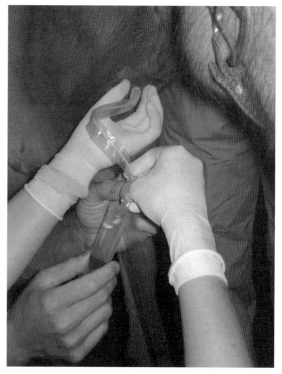

Figure 12.11. Advancing the transtracheal wash catheter through the lumen.

make a small incision in the skin using a #15 scalpel blade.

Procedure

The horse is sedated as previously described. Most clinicians choose to perform TTW near the juncture of the cranial and middle one-third of the neck in an area where the trachea and tracheal rings are easily palpable. In large horses, the TTW should be performed as distally as possible on the neck where the trachea and tracheal rings are still easily identified.

The desired area is clipped (generally a 5-cm square is sufficient) and aseptically prepared. Once the TTW site is clean, a bleb of 2 to 3 ml of 2% lidocaine is injected subcutaneously. It is important to inject sufficient volume that the TTW site can be identified.

A small stab incision can be made through the skin using a #15 scalpel blade if desired. The TTW stylet and cannula are positioned perpendicular to the horse's trachea and skin. The tracheal rings should be carefully palpated and the stylet should enter between two tracheal rings. It is advised that the trachea be identified and securely held by the clinician's "off" hand to avoid hitting the carotid artery or jugular vein. The cannula and stylet are

advanced and pushed between the tracheal rings into the lumen of the trachea. Penetration between the tracheal rings can take some effort and the clinician should feel or hear air flow as the tracheal lumen is entered. It is important to maintain proper positioning of the stylet and cannula as they are advanced. Excessive cranial to caudal or abaxial movement of the stylet and cannula should be avoided.

Once the tracheal lumen has been entered, the stylet is removed and the cannula is pointed somewhat distally in the trachea. The TTW catheter is then advanced to most of its length through the cannula (Figure 12.11). Horses will often cough during this part of the procedure.

Then, 20 to 50 ml sterile isotonic saline is injected through the cannula. Steady, gentle aspiration should then be applied to the syringe to aspirate tracheal contents. The catheter should be slowly

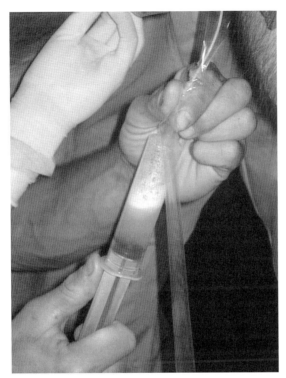

Figure 12.12. Aspirating sample before withdrawing the catheter.

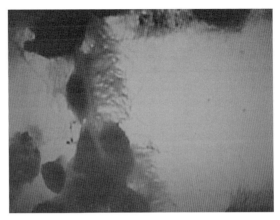

Figure 12.13. Cytologic examination of a transtracheal wash obtained from a normal horse. Most of the cells present are ciliated, columnar respiratory epithelial cells.

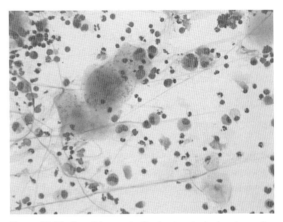

Figure 12.14. Bacterial contamination in a transtracheal wash sample. Courtesy Dr. Elizabeth Welles, Auburn University, AL.

withdrawn at the same time. As much fluid as possible should be aspirated from the trachea before the catheter is withdrawn (Figure 12.12). The majority of the saline will pool near the thoracic inlet. Extremely thick or inspissated secretions can be difficult to aspirate. Additional saline may need to be injected if secretions are extremely thick or no fluid can be aspirated.

Once the TTW catheter has been completely withdrawn, the cannula is removed. Aspirated fluid is then aseptically transferred to bacterial transport vials and the remainder is injected into a sterile EDTA tube for cytologic examination. Injecting 2 to 3 ml of an aqueous broad-spectrum antibiotic, such as gentamicin, subcutaneously around the TTW site is preferred. The TTW site can be lightly wrapped with 4-in elastic tape over a 4 × 4 sponge and antibiotic ointment. The wrap can be removed the following morning.

Evaluation of Transtracheal Wash Fluid

Normal cytology in a noninfected TTW sample is composed of ciliated columnar respiratory epithelial cells (Figure 12.13), macrophages, and lymphocytes (Figure 12.14). There should be no bacteria present. Pigmented fungi are often observed, but they do not indicate fungal pneumonia because most fungal hyphae observed are inhaled contaminants from hay or stall bedding.

If significant numbers (>5% of leukocytes observed) of nondegenerate neutrophils are present, then the horse may be affected with recurrent airway obstruction or heaves. Horses with heaves may or may not have concurrent respiratory tract infection.

Procedure Complications

Subcutaneous emphysema, especially localized to the site of TTW, is fairly common. Some horses can develop extensive subcutaneous emphysema, particularly if they have impedance of airflow at end-expiration. Subcutaneous emphysema is usually minimized by wrapping the TTW site overnight.

There is a chance that the TTW site can develop mild cellulitis if bacteria invade the subcutaneous tissues. It is important to remove the TTW catheter before the cannula to avoid tracking bacteria through the site. Most abscesses secondary to TTW are relatively small and localized. However, some can become quite large and require surgical drainage. This problem can be prevented or minimized by wrapping the site at the time of the procedure. If cellulitis occurs, the area can covered with an osmotic sweat or dimethyl sulfoxide ointment.

If the horse coughs excessively during the procedure or the TTW catheter is inadvertently fed up the trachea toward the mouth, then the sample will be contaminated with oropharyngeal contents. This is readily recognized cytologically by the presence of squamous epithelial cells, feed material, and numerous types of bacteria. If this occurs, then the TTW must be repeated. Waiting approximately 24 hours for oropharyngeal contamination to clear and then repeating TTW is recommended.

Some horses may cough up small amounts of blood for a few minutes after TTW. Hemoptysis is usually mild and self-limiting.

It is possible to inadvertently pass the TTW catheter into the subcutaneous tissue. If this occurs, then only fibroblasts will be observed cytologically.

Due to the proximity of the trachea to the carotid arteries and jugular veins, these blood vessels can be traumatized or punctured during TTW. Local manual compression over the vessel, application of osmotic sweat, and careful wrapping with appropriate pressure usually reduce resultant swelling.

Localized infection or chondritis of the tracheal rings is relatively uncommon. Cartilage problems can be prevented by appropriately placing the stylet and cannula between tracheal rings and limiting excessive movement of the stylet and cannula during TTW.

Occasionally the TTW catheter may break off or be cut, especially if the procedure is performed using only a large-gauge needle to enter the trachea. Usually the horse will cough up the catheter fragment in 20 to 30 minutes without any complications. The horse can be put in an unbedded stall to facilitate finding the fragment. Alternatively, it can be removed with an endoscope, but this is seldom necessary unless the horse fails to cough out the fragment.

Whole Blood Transfusion

Common Indications

The most common indications for whole blood transfusion are acute hemorrhage from trauma, elective surgery complications, hemorrhage following parturition, red maple toxicity, and neonatal isoerythrolysis. Clinical signs of anemia can include tachycardia, tachypnea, weakness, mucous membrane pallor, weak peripheral pulse, and colic. Whole blood transfusions are meant to support the patient because the benefits obtained are short lived. Transfused cells typically only survive in circulation 2 to 4 days, and whole blood transfusion is a means to stabilize the patient until the bone marrow can respond to the crisis by increasing erythrocyte production.

Although there is no set PCV value to indicate when to transfuse, when paired with clinical signs, PCV values can be an effective and fast way to monitor anemia. It is important to remember that due to splenic contraction, PCV values can transiently be normal or high. The measured PCV values can lag behind the patient's true anemia by 12 to 24 hours. A good rule of thumb for determining when to transfuse is if the PCV value is less than or equal to 12% for acute blood loss. Elevations in blood lactate levels can indicate poor oxygenation and perfusion of tissues and further support the decision to perform a transfusion.

Cross-matching

Once it is determined that a transfusion is needed, a cross-match can be performed between the patient and possible donors. Cross-matching is composed of two parts: the major cross-match and the minor cross-match. The major cross-match combines recipient serum with donor erythrocytes, and the minor cross-match combines recipient erythrocytes with donor serum. Both sides must test compatible for a true match.

Equine alloantibodies actually act more as hemolysins than agglutinins and when possible, hemolysin testing should be conducted. This requires a referral laboratory as an exogenous complement (pooled rabbit serum), and specialized handling of the sample is needed, making it difficult for the equine practitioner.

A simple agglutination test is both inexpensive and the most often used test for crossmatch compatibility. For this test, take an EDTA blood tube from both the patient and possible donors. Spin the samples for 3 minutes (can vary by centrifuge) and pipette the concentrated erythrocytes into separate test tubes. Mix a small amount of saline in with the cells and centrifuge the samples again for 3 minutes. Remove the saline from the packed cells, add fresh saline, and mix the samples gently, again suspending the erythrocytes. Centrifuge for 3 minutes and repeat the process until cells have been washed a minimum of three times (Figure 12.15). During the washing process, spin down the EDTA tubes of both the patient and the donor. Once cell-washing process is complete, label new test tubes as major and minor cross-matches, being careful to label the tubes properly with the correct donor names. To major match test tubes add 6 to 10 Gtts of washed donor erythrocytes and 6 to 10 Gtts of patient serum from the spun down EDTA tube. To minor

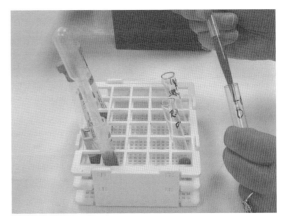

Figure 12.15. Washing erythrocytes.

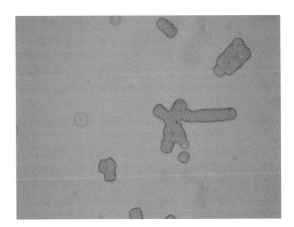

Figure 12.16. Normal rouleaux.

match test tubes add 6 to 10 Gtts of patient washed erythrocytes and 6 to 10 Gtts of donor serum. Gently mix both tubes; although a trained eye can detect agglutination immediately, it is advantageous to evaluate the sample using a microscope. Place 1 Gtt of both samples onto a clean slide, labeling major and minor cross-matches, and cover both samples with a coverslip and read under microscope. Compatible samples will show only normal rouleaux (Figure 12.16). Single erythrocytes, although an incompatible sample, will show large clumps (agglutinations) of red cells

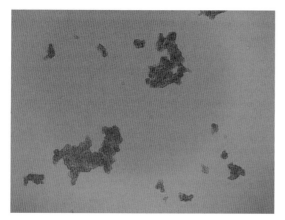

Figure 12.17. Incompatibility agglutination.

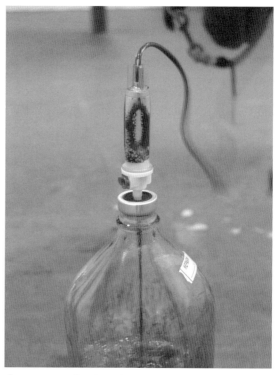

Figure 12.18. Pulling donor blood into an evacuated container.

(Figure 12.17); even though rouleaux will still be observed, there will be decreased amounts of single erythrocytes.

If no compatible donor is found, then it is possible to wash large volumes of donor erythrocytes, rendering it safe for transfusion. This can be time consuming and will likely incur additional expenses because specialized equipment is needed; but this may be the only option in some cases. In some areas it is possible to contract with a local human blood bank to have equine erythrocytes washed.

Collecting Blood from the Donor

Once a donor is selected from the cross-match, a Temperature, Pulse, Respiration (TPR) and Packed Cell Volume/Total Protein (PCV/TP) should be performed. It is easiest to sedate the donor when no assistant is available to help with the collection. The horse can then be placed in stocks and the jugular vein is aseptically prepared. Place local block of 1 ml 2% lidocaine over the catheter site and sterilely place a 14-guage temporary intravenous catheter. Suture the catheter in place to stabilize it during the procedure. Direct connect a primary basic set and insert set into a prepared 2-L evacuated blood container or blood bags (Figure 12.18).

Evacuated containers pull blood quickly and save time as opposed to blood bags. Each bottle should contain an anticoagulant. The preferred anticoagulant is 2.5% to 4.0 % acid-citrate-dextrose (ACD). Add nine parts blood to one part ACD. For example, 200 ml of ACD should be added to a 2-L blood collection bottle. Be careful not to lose the suction in the bottle when added the ACD. Glass evacuated containers are contraindicated if platelets are needed because the platelets will stick to the glass. If a platelet transfusion is required, the blood should be collected in plastic blood bags.

Gently agitate the bottle or bag while it is filling to mix the anticoagulant with the blood. After all containers are filled, flush and pull the donor intravenous catheter. The donor should be monitored for any signs of discomfort or colic. If the blood was removed quickly from the donor for a life-threatening emergency, the donor may display mild signs of colic. If this occurs, the donor should receive intravenous replacement fluids and a dose of flunixin. Most donors do fine and require no additional care.

The amount of blood to be transfused is approximately 15 ml/kg for an average adult horse (500 kg). A healthy horse can safely donate 6 to 8 L every 30 days. Donors are given alfalfa and sweet feed following blood collection. There should be at least 30 days or greater between blood collection from the same horse.

Administering Blood to the Patient

Whole blood transfusion is typically begun immediately on the patient. Additional units should be refrigerated, agitated every 15 to 30 minutes, and brought to room temperature when needed. Attach a blood set with an in-line filter to the bottle, and a pressure bulb is connected to the line to assist with administration (Figure 12.19). Pressure bulbs are useful to be keep a constant rate of infusion, but they should not be used to overpressurize or bolus blood products. The blood set is attached to the patient's intravenous catheter and run at a rate of 0.1 ml/kg for 5 to 10 minutes, monitoring the patient's heart rate and respiratory rate every 5 minutes. If the patient is handling the transfusion well, the rate can be increased to 20 to 30 ml/kg/hour and patient monitoring continues throughout the transfusion.

Donor Selection

Blood transfusions in horses are more difficult than humans because a "universal donor" does not exist. Horses have more than 400,000 possible blood types. Horses with the red cell antigens Aa and Qa should be avoided because these blood types have the highest incidence of reactions.

All potential blood donors should be blood typed. Ideally a donor should be an adult gelding weighing 450 kg or more, healthy (including a normal PCV and blood proteins) with a complete vaccina-

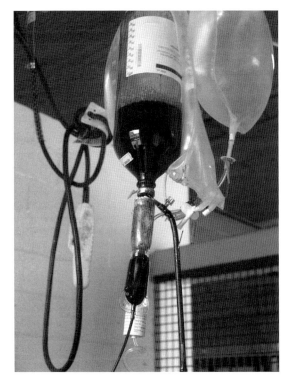

Figure 12.19. Whole blood administration.

tion history, negative for equine infectious anemia (EIA), never been transfused, has a good temperament, healthy bilateral jugular veins, be Aa and Qa alloantigen negative, and lack antibodies against Aa and Qa. The practice's needs determine what kind of a donor is required, where a donor is found, and how many may be secured for transfusion services.

Complications

Transfusion reactions can vary from mild (slight increase in heart rate or respiratory rate) to severe (sudden collapse). Signs of reaction can include piloerection, restlessness, urticaria, tachypnea, tachycardia, muscle fasciculations, trembling, and sweating. For most reactions, decreasing the rate of transfusion or stopping it will alleviate the symptoms and further medical treatment isn't required. In case of a serious reaction, flunixin meglumine 1.1 mg/kg intravenously can be given. Severe reactions may require prednisolone sodium succinate and/or epinephrine.

Urinary Catheterization

Common Indications

Urinary catheters are most often used to collect uncontaminated urine samples but can also be used to check the integrity of a bladder and to allow postoperative patients to urinate freely.

Procedure

Due to the sterility of the bladder, precautions must be taken to maintain sepsis while passing the catheter. Equipment includes a sterile urinary catheter, sedation, 60-ml catheter tip syringe, sterile gloves, and sterile lubricant. The procedure for passing the catheter is different depending on the sex of the horse.

Males
Sedation not only calms the patient but will also facilitate penile drop. The penis should be scrubbed with an antiseptic solution and rinsed. Wearing sterile gloves, grasp the penis with one hand and gently advanced the lubricated catheter. The urethral sphincter may cause some resistance but administering 60 ml air or 10 ml lidocaine can aid passage into the bladder, approximately 60 cm. Urine may not flow freely, so a catheter-tipped syringe can be used to gently aspirate urine.

Females
Sedation is not always needed to catheterize mares, but it will facilitate the procedure. The tail can be wrapped and tied or held by an assistant. The perineum should be cleaned with an antiseptic solution and rinsed. Wearing sterile gloves, locate the urethral opening on the floor of the vagina and using a finger as a guide, gently guide the lubricated catheter into the urethra. The bladder is

approximately 5 to 10 cm^2 and the urine may not flow freely without gentle aspiration.

Complications

The most common complications are urethra irritation, or if sepsis isn't maintained, infection of the bladder.

Arthrocentesis

Common Indications for Procedure

Arthrocentesis is defined as the insertion of a needle into a joint space for the purpose of removing joint fluid for diagnostic purposes as in the case of septic arthritis. This procedure can also be used as a diagnostic or therapeutic modality if an anesthetic or medication is injected into the joint during the procedure. Strict asepsis is a necessity during intra-articular, intrathecal (insertion of a needle into a synovial sheath), or intrabursal (insertion of a needle into a synovial bursa) injection or aspiration.

Procedure

Aseptic preparation of the site is a necessity and is described elsewhere. Clipping of the hair over the site is often controversial as owners do not want to have visible evidence of diagnostic or therapeutic measures (Table 12.2). The rationale for clipping should be carefully discussed with them, and the final decision to proceed without hair removal should remain in the hands of the clinician. Horses which have recently been clipped during winter months and horses with short summer hair coats may present with less need for clipping of the site. Following aseptic preparation and the donning of sterile gloves, synovial fluid from joints, sheaths and bursae may be collected for synovial fluid analysis, cytology, and culture, or anesthetic solutions or medications may be injected for diagnostic or therapeutic procedures. Sterility and the compatibility of these solutions with synovial fluid are imperative and should include consideration of acid-base balance (pH) and solubility. Solutions

Table 12.2. Supplies needed to perform arthrocentesis.

- Scrub (povidone iodine or chlorhexidine).
- Compatible bactericidal solution.
- Sterile water.
- Isopropyl alcohol.
- Gauze sponges.
- Sterile gauze sponge.
- Sterile gloves.
- Appropriate syringes and needles.
- Ethylenediaminetetraacetic acid tubes.
- Culture media (aerobic and anaerobic).
- Microscopic slides.
- Sterile anesthetic solutions.
- Injectable antibiotics.

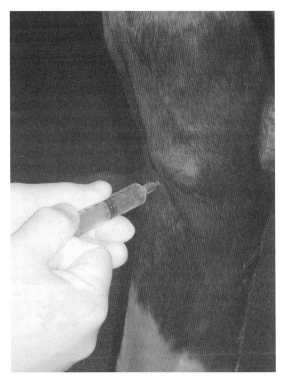

Figure 12.21. Arthrocentesis.

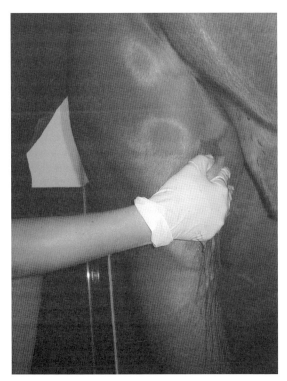

Figure 12.20. Aseptic preparation of site.

rather than suspensions are preferred to avoid precipitants within the synovial structures.

Diagnostic anesthetic solutions and many therapeutic medications are combined with compatible injectable antibiotics for injection.

Following completion of the procedure, the site should be protected from contamination for several hours, if possible, to permit the puncture site to seal. Administration of systemic analgesic/anti-inflammatory medications after completion of the procedure may be indicated and beneficial in preventing postinjection flares, especially involving the large synovial joints (tarso crural and femoropatellar) and specific joints, which seem predisposed to inflammatory response (distal interphalangeal).

Anatomical Sites

Access to the majority of the appendicular articulations is possible and individual description is beyond the scope of this manual. Individual preferences at each site vary, and the technician is well advised to familiarize himself or herself with the particular approach preferred by the clinician. Injection of the dorsal cervical articular facets, facilitated by ultrasound guidance, for both therapeutic and diagnostic procedures may also be accomplished. Adherence to aseptic technique and familiarity with anatomical landmarks make this technique a valuable addition to one's clinical skills that may be used with reasonable risk.

References and Further Reading

Becht, J. L., and B. J. Gordon. 1987. Blood and plasma therapy. In *Current Therapy in Equine Medicine*, ed. N. E. Robinson. Vol. 2:317–21. Philadelphia: W. B. Saunders.

Collatos, C. 1997. Blood and blood component therapy. In *Current Therapy in Equine Medicine*, ed. N. E. Robinson. Vol. 4:290–92. Philadelphia: W. B. Saunders.

———. 1999. Blood and blood component therapy. In *Manual of Equine Medicine and Surgery*, ed. P. T. Colahan, J. N. Moore, and I. G. Mayhew, 42–44. St. Louis: Mosby.

Divers, T. J. Adult ICU. 2003. In: *Clinical Techniques in Equine Practice*, ed. J. A. Orsini and T. J. Divers. Vol. 2:141–3. Philadelphia: W. B. Saunders.

Divers, T. J. 2000. Liver failure; Hemolytic anemia. In *Manual of Equine Emergencies*, ed. J. A. Orsini and T. J. Divers. 2nd ed., 326–38. Philadelphia: W. B. Saunders.

Gonzales, G. 2001. How to establish an equine blood donor protocol. *Proc Am Assoc Equine Pract* 47:326–38

Gaughan, E. M. 2006. *Evaluating horses with colic. Proceedings, The Latin American Veterinary Conference TLAVC*, Lima, Peru, September 29–October 2, 2006.

Malikides, N., D. Hodgson, and R. Rose. 2000. Whole blood transfusion. In *Manual of Equine Practice*, ed. R. J. Rose and D. R. Hodgson. 2nd ed., 458–59. Philadelphia: W. B. Saunders.

McIlwraith, C. W. and G. W. Trotter. 1996. *Joint Disease in the Horse*. Philadelphia: W. B. Saunders.

Moyer, W., J. Schumacher, and J. Schumacher. 2007. *A Guide to Equine Joint Injection and Regional Anesthesia*. Yardley, PA, Veterinary Learning Systems.

Orsini, J. A., and T. J. Divers. 2003. *Manual of Equine Emergencies*. 2nd ed. Philadelphia: W. B. Saunders.

Pasquini, C. S. Pasquini, and P. Woods. *Guide to Equine Clinics*. 3rd ed. Pilot Point, TX: SUDZ Publishing.

Radostits, O. M., C. C. Gay, K. W. Hinchcliff, and P. D. Constable. 2007. *Veterinary Medicine*. 10th ed. Philadelphia, W. B. Saunders.

Rose, R. J., and D. R. Hodgson. 2000. *Manual of Equine Practice*, 2nd ed. Philadelphia: W. B. Saunders Co.

Ross, M. W., and S. J. Dyson. 2003. *Diagnosis and Management of Lameness in the Horse*. Philadelphia: W. B. Saunders.

Rush, B., and T. Mair. 2004. *Equine Respiratory Diseases*, Oxford: Blackwell Publishers.

Schaer, B. D., and J. A. Orsini. 2008. Urinary tract catheterization. In *Equine Emergencies: Treatment and Procedures*, ed. J. A. Orsini and T. J. Divers. 3rd ed., 473–77. St. Louis: Saunders.

Slovis, N. 2001. How to approach whole blood transfusions in horses. *Proc Am Assoc Equine Pract* 47: 266–69

Waldridge, B. M., and E. G. Welles. 2006. How to perform a bronchoalveolar lavage using a three-meter gastroscope. Proceedings of the Fifty-Second Annual Convention of the *American Association of Equine Practitioners*, San Antonio, Texas, December 2–6, 2006.

Westermann, C. M., T. T. Laan, R. A. van Nieuwstadt, S. Bull, and J. Fink-Gremmels. Effects of antitussive agents administered before bronchoalveolar lavage in horses. *Am J Vet Res* 66:1420–24.

Diagnostic Procedures

Katherine Garrett and Midge Leitch

Regional Analgesia and Anesthesia

Regional analgesia and anesthesia, including both perineural and intra-articular injection, are commonly used in equine practice. Understanding the sites of injection of anesthetic agent will aid technicians in site preparation. Some of the more common techniques are reviewed in this chapter; however, it should be noted that there are many techniques in use by veterinarians, and technicians are well advised to familiarize themselves with the preferences of the clinician whom they are assisting. Techniques for injection of the forelimb may be applied to analogous nerves and joints in the hind limb unless otherwise indicated.

There are two major categories of regional anesthesia: perineural, which involves the deposition of anesthetic solution in close proximity to a nerve, thus desensitizing the structures it innervates, and intrasynovial in which anesthetic is injected directly into synovial structures.

Anesthetic Options

The three most common local anesthetics used in equine practice are lidocaine, Mepivicaine, and bupivacaine. These drugs bind to the sodium channels in neurons, preventing depolarization and nerve impulse generation and transmission. Lidocaine has the most rapid time of onset (5–15 minutes) and the shortest duration of action (60 minutes). It is frequently used for short procedures because of its quick onset and low cost. Mepivicaine has a slightly longer time of onset but a longer duration of action (2–3 hours). Bupivacaine has an even longer time of onset (>10 minutes) and duration (3–5 hours), making it useful for situations in which longer-lasting anesthesia is required.

Patient Preparation

Proper site preparation aids in reducing the chances of local cellulitis or septic arthritis secondary to injection of anesthetic agents. Regional nerve blocks should be performed on a clean site. Clipping may reduce the need for extensive scrubs; however, the resultant evidence of diagnostics or therapy may not be acceptable to some clients. Recent work has shown that three 30-second scrubs of povidone iodine are sufficient to achieve an aseptic skin site in areas lacking hair. For intra-articular blocks, aseptic preparation of the site is the standard of practice and should include a 3- to 5-minute scrub with povidone iodine or chlorhexidine scrub followed by an alcohol rinse. Care should be taken to scrub and rinse from clean areas to dirty areas to decrease recontamination of a clean area. Sterile gloves must be worn for intra-articular injections and may be preferred for regional injections if inadequate facilities are available to permit adequate hand cleansing.

Safety

As with any procedure, safety should be the primary concern. Selecting the smallest gauge needle suitable for the site is the first step in minimizing patient discomfort. Horses may respond unpredictably to both the needle stick and the injection of the anesthetic. The individual handling the horse is responsible for the safety of everyone involved and should have his or her attention entirely focused on the horse and the people around it. Minimizing the number of people and the activity level in the room can help to reduce anxiety on the part of the horse. The handler should always be on the same side of the horse as the person performing the procedure.

Additional restraint may be necessary at the time the injection is performed. This may come in the form of a lip twitch, a lip chain, a shoulder twitch, intravenous sedation, or a combination of these techniques. Often distraction, such as offering a horse feed or tapping on its forehead while the injection is being made, can provide adequate restraint and this approach should be considered first. If xylazine is used as a sedative, a side effect known as xylazine aggression must be anticipated, and the handler should always grip the halter to avoid being bitten.

The person performing the block should make sure the handler is prepared for the placement of the needle and should take care to perform the block as efficiently as possible to minimize the time that the horse is subjected to intensive restraint. He or she should also take care in selecting where to stand for the procedure. Standing directly in front of or behind the horse should be avoided so as to decrease the risk of being struck at or kicked. When performing procedures on the hind limb, it is often best to stand as close to the horse's body as possible so that if the horse does kick and make contact, the power of the impact will be reduced.

Perineural Anesthesia

Palmar or Plantar Digital Perineural Analgesia
This block will anesthetize the medial and lateral palmar digital nerves that innervate the navicular bone and bursa, the distal sesamoidean ligaments, the distal portions of the superficial and deep digital flexor tendons, the digital cushion, the corium of the frog and the sole, the palmar or plantar third and solar surface of the third phalanx, as well as, part or all of the distal interphalangeal joint. It is important to perform this block as far distally as possible; however, despite efforts to limit the distribution of this nerve block, the dorsal portion of the hoof and the proximal interphalangeal joint may also be desensitized. Migration of the anesthetic solution, especially if larger quantities are used, can result in desensitization of the majority of the pastern region and extend to the level of the fetlock joint.

The nerves can be palpated as they course distally along the pastern palmar or plantar to the digital vein and artery and then continue deep to the collateral cartilages of the hoof (Figure 13.1). Needle selection is likely to include 5/8-in. 25- or 27-gauge or 1-in. 20- or 22-guage needle. Controversy exists over the optimal amount of anesthetic

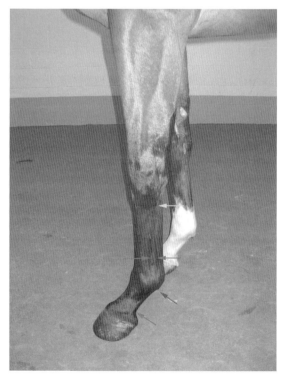

Figure 13.1. Injection sites for perineural anesthesia. *Red arrow:* palmar digital. *Blue arrow:* abaxial sesamoid. *Green arrows:* low four-point suspensory. *Yellow arrow:* high four-point/high suspensory.

to be delivered, but generally ranges from 0.5 to 1.5 ml delivered to each nerve. Many clinicians will perform this block with the leg held off the ground; facing the front of the horse's front limb, the leg is held curled against one's body with the hoof held in the free hand.

Clinicians also differ in their opinions as to the interval between injection of anesthetic agent and reevaluation of the lameness, with intervals ranging from 5 to 15 minutes. Before reevaluating the lameness, skin sensation can be checked at the heels to determine if the block has been successful. Assessing skin sensation at the dorsal aspect of the coronary band determines if the dorsal branches were inadvertently anesthetized as well. Some clinicians will also evaluate the results at multiple time intervals following injection.

The dorsal structures of the hoof can also be anesthetized from this location. After performing the block as described, the needle is redirected dorsally parallel to the ground, just proximal to the coronary band, to a subcutaneous position without exiting the skin. This avoids the need for another needle stick. An additional 1 to 1.5 ml of anesthetic is delivered on both the medial and lateral sides followed by gentle massage of the anesthetic bleb to ensure wider distribution.

Abaxial Sesamoid Perineural Analgesia

The medial and lateral palmar or plantar digital nerves can be anesthetized at this more proximal location, where they are easily palpable along the abaxial aspects of the sesamoids, resulting in desensitization of the majority of the pastern, the foot, as well as, the fetlock region. This includes the first, second, and third phalanges, the proximal and distal interphalangeal joints, the laminae of the hoof, the distal sesamoidean ligaments, the extensor branches of the suspensory ligament, the distal deep and superficial digital flexor tendons, the distal common digital extensor tendon, and portions of the fetlock joint.

The bundle containing the digital vein, artery, and nerve can be palpated over the abaxial aspect of the sesamoid (see Fig. 13.1). The nerve is the most palmar or plantar structure in the bundle.

Needle selection is similar to that described for the palmar digital nerve and 1 to 3 ml of local anesthetic is delivered both medially and laterally. Repeat lameness examination is usually performed 15 minutes after injection. This block is often performed with the leg held off the ground by the clinician in the same manner as described for the previous block.

Low Four Point or Low Ring or Low Palmar Perineural Analgesia

This block will desensitize structures distal to and including the fetlock joint by blocking the medial and lateral palmar and palmar-metacarpal nerves (see Fig. 13.1). Needle selection for these nerve blocks remains the same as previously described, and the palmar metacarpal nerves are anesthetized at the distal end of the medial and lateral splint bones. Because the nerves lie deep to the splint bones, it is important to inject the anesthetic deeper than the subcutaneous level.

The palmar nerves are blocked with 3 ml of anesthetic delivered subcutaneously medially and laterally between the suspensory ligament and the deep digital flexor tendon. This is done at the same level as or slightly proximally to the distal aspect of the splint bone to avoid penetration of the digital sheath. Some clinicians will block the medial and lateral palmar nerves with one injection by using a 1.5-in. needle, penetrating the skin on the lateral side of the leg, depositing anesthetic agent at this site, and then advancing the needle between the suspensory ligament and the deep digital flexor tendon to the medial aspect of the limb, where additional anesthetic is injected. The dorsal branch of the ulnar nerve may be blocked by depositing a bleb of anesthetic along the lateral edge of the digital extensor tendon just proximal to the fetlock joint. Selective desensitization of the deeper structures of the fetlock joint, such as the condyles of MCII (cannon bone) may be accomplished by blocking only the palmar metacarpal nerves. It is important to remember that anesthetic agent readily diffuses within soft tissue and so larger areas may be desensitized than intended.

High Four Point or High Ring or High Palmar Perineural Analgesia

The palmar and palmar metacarpal nerves can also be anesthetized at a level just distal to the carpus resulting in desensitization of the majority of the metacarpal region. The medial and lateral palmar metacarpal nerves lie on the palmar aspect of the third metacarpal bone axial to the second and fourth metacarpal bones (see Fig. 13.1) and may be blocked using a 1- or 1.5-in. 20- or 22-gauge needle. The palmar nerves run on the dorsal and abaxial surface of the deep digital flexor tendon and are blocked using a 5/8-in. 25- or 27-gauge needle or 1-in. 20- or 22-gauge needle. Inadvertent injection of the middle carpal or carpometacarpal joint makes aseptic preparation of this site all the more important. The dorsal portion of the metacarpal region will not be desensitized unless a dorsal ring block is performed subcutaneously at this level as well.

Personal preference may include holding the limb during injection, and for this site the leg is usually grasped while the clinician faces the same direction as the horse and holds the leg at the level of the fetlock with the free hand.

Suspensory Origin Infiltration

This is a diffusion block that acts via local infiltration of the area of the proximal suspensory ligament at its origin on the proximal palmar metacarpus to desensitize this region (see Fig. 13.1). In the forelimb, a 1- or 1.5-in. 20-gauge needle is inserted axial to the head of the lateral splint bone, and 5 to 10 ml of local anesthetic is injected. Some clinicians prefer to inject from the medial side as well. The injection site in the hind limb is similar and in both cases, individual preference may dictate holding the leg off the ground during injection, in a fashion similar to that described for the high palmar block. Hind leg restraint by the clinician is usually accomplished by holding the limb in a similar position to that for applying hoof testers. In the hind limb, some clinicians may choose to insert the needle only on the lateral side of the limb and inject 10 ml of anesthetic in that location. Inadvertent entry into the distal carpal or tarsal joints and subsequent anesthesia of these structures is not uncommon.

Intra-articular Anesthesia

Distal Interphalangeal Joint

The distal interphalangeal (coffin) joint lies just distal to the coronary band. Intra-articular anesthesia of this joint may result in anesthesia of the navicular bursa even when repeat lameness examination quickly follows injection. Diffusion of anesthetic agent out of the joint capsule through the injection site can result in desensitization of significant portions of the foot, including the sole. Considerable controversy exists over the optimal time to wait between injection and follow-up lameness evaluation and what structures may be blocked at what time points.

The coffin joint may be entered on the dorsal aspect of the limb approximately 1 cm medial or lateral of midline and 0.5 cm proximal to the coronary band. A 1- or 1.5-in. 20- or 22-gauge needle is directed distally and axially, and 8 to 10 ml of local anesthetic is injected. After the needle is withdrawn, pressure should be applied to the injection site because anesthetic has a tendency to leak out after injection. An alternative injection technique is to insert a 1-in. 20- or 22-gauge needle parallel to the ground at the level of the coronary band on midline. This will penetrate the proximal dorsal pouch of the coffin joint. A third site of injection is dorsal to the dorsal border of the collateral cartilage using a 1- to 1.5-in 22-gauge needle.

Metacarpophalangeal Joint

The metacarpophalangeal (fetlock) joint may be accessed at multiple sites, the most popular of which is along the proximal border of the collateral ligament of the lateral proximal sesamoid bone, with the leg in flexion, between the palmar aspect of MCIII and the dorsal margin of the sesamoid bone. Alternatively the dorsal pouch may be entered in a distal and axial direction at the level of the epicondyle of the third metacarpal bone along the lateral or medial borders of the common digital extensor tendon. Care must be taken to avoid damage to the articular cartilage, especially that of the prominent sagittal ridge of MCIII. The palmar pouch is bordered by the palmar aspect of the distal third metacarpal bone, the distal aspect of the fourth metacarpal bone, and the dorsal aspect of the lateral sesamoid bone. Injection through this site is frequently complicated by hemorrhage from the rich vascular bed associated with the proximal aspect of the joint capsule in this region. Injection into either of the more palmar sites has the advantage of being performed with the limb held in flexion, thus minimizing the likelihood of having the horse suddenly jerk its foot off the ground as the needle is inserted. Regardless of the technique used, a 1-, 20-, or 22-gauge needle is used to instill approximately 10 ml of anesthetic into the joint.

Carpal Joints

These joints maybe entered from either the dorsal or the palmarolateral aspect. It is unnecessary to inject the carpometacarpal joint separately as it communicates with the middle carpal joint. A 1-in. 20- or 22-gauge needle may be used to deliver approximately 10 ml of anesthetic to each joint. The dorsal site for injection of either joint is located immediately lateral or medial to the common digital extensor tendon. Injection is performed with the leg held off the ground and the joints in a flexed position, allowing the dorsal aspect of the joints to open up to avoid damage to the articular cartilage. The antebrachial or radial carpal joint is injected in the palpable depression between the distal radius and the proximal row of carpal bones, and the middle carpal joint is injected between the proximal and distal row of carpal bones. The needle is directed in a caudal direction perpendicular to the skin.

The palmarolateral approach is performed with the horse standing on the leg. The radial carpal joint site is bordered by the distal caudal aspect of the radius and the proximal border of the ulnar carpal bone. The middle carpal joint injection site is bordered by the proximal palmar aspect of the fourth carpal bone and the distal palmar aspect of the ulnar carpal bone. The injection sites may be confirmed by flexing the carpus, locating the specified joint, following the joint in a palmar direction, and then flexing and extending the carpus while palpating the joint space. The needle is directed parallel to the ground in a medial and slightly dorsal direction for both joints.

Tarsal Joints

The tibiotarsal or tarso crural joint is one of the largest and most accessible joints in the horse. It communicates with the proximal intertarsal joint. There are a number of locations at which the joint may be penetrated. The most common location is located dorsomedially between the medial malleolus of the tibia and the saphenous vein. A 1-in. 20-gauge needle is used to deliver 20 ml of anesthetic.

The distal intertarsal and tarsometatarsal joints do communicate in some horses, but they should be injected separately to ensure that anesthesia is delivered to both joints. The distal intertarsal joint can be injected on the dorsomedial aspect of the limb. The cunean tendon is followed distally and medially until a depression is felt along its distal border at the junction of the second, third, and central tarsal bones. If there is extensive new bone formation involving either of the distal tarsal joints, injection into them may be difficult. The tarsometatarsal joint may be entered on the plantarolateral aspect of the joint at the head of the fourth metatarsal (splint) bone is palpated and a depression is identified just proximal to it. Needle selection will be clinician driven.

Stifle Joints

Communication between the medial femorotibial and the femoropatellar joints is not uncommon, but it is not present in all horses. To be certain that the entire stifle is anesthetized, all three compartments should be injected separately. Large volumes of local anesthetic are used (15–20 ml) in the femorotibial compartments and 30 to 50 ml in the femoropatellar joint. Special care should be taken when injecting the stifle joint because horses may respond unpredictably.

The medial femorotibial compartment can be entered through a palpable depression between the medial patellar ligament and the medial collateral ligament. The lateral femorotibial compartment is entered between the long digital extensor tendon and the lateral collateral ligament. The femoropatellar joint may be entered between the medial and middle patellar ligament in the more proximal aspect of the pouch or, with the limb in a resting, non–weight-bearing position, on the medial aspect of the leg between the distal border of the patella and the proximal rim of the medial trochlear ridge of the femur.

Radiography

Radiography is a mainstay of equine imaging. Portable equipment is relatively inexpensive and easy to use in an ambulatory practice.

Image Formation and Equipment

To produce a radiographic image, it is necessary to have a source of x-irradiation and a detector to receive the x-rays and convert them to an image. X-ray generators come in a variety of styles (Figures 13.2 and 13.3). Small, lower power portable units are available for ambulatory use, and large, more powerful units are often used in a clinic. A smaller unit is generally sufficient to radiograph the extremities and the head, but a more powerful unit is required to produce diagnostic-quality images of the spine, thorax, abdomen, and proximal extremities of adult horses. The x-ray beam can be restricted in its shape by the use of a collimator, which changes the width and height of the beam and thus helps to eliminated backscatter.

Detector plates come in variety of styles. In traditional film-screen radiography, the x-ray photons impact a cassette. A radiographic cassette is made of fluorescent intensifying screens between which lies a sheet of radiographic film coated with a gelatin emulsion containing silver. The fluorescence resulting from the collision of the x-ray photons and the intensifying screens results in a flash of light that causes the silver to precipitate. The x-rays themselves also cause some precipitation of silver, but to a much smaller degree than does the fluorescence. The greater the number of x-rays that strike a region of the intensifying screen, the greater the amount of light produced, the greater the amount of silver precipitated, and the darker the region of the radiographic image. This silver precipitate turns black after film processing, during which it is fixed to the film and any remaining nonprecipitated silver is washed off. Regular cleaning of the cassettes and screens is mandatory to prevent artifacts and poor image acquisition.

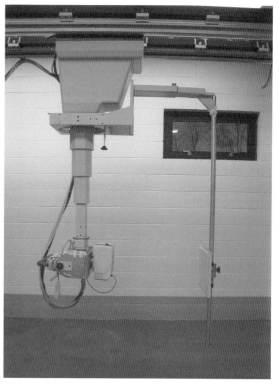

Figure 13.3. Ceiling-mounted x-ray generator. A grid and detector holder can be attached at a set focal film distance to radiograph the proximal extremities, axial skeleton, thorax, and abdomen.

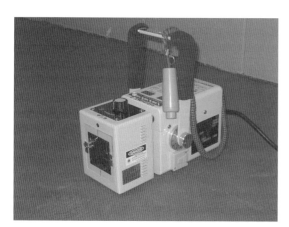

Figure 13.2. Portable x-ray generator.

Computed radiography (CR) uses a phosphorescent screen called an image plate (IP) housed in a cassette to capture the energy of the x-ray photons (Figure 13.4). When the photons impact the phosphorescent screen, electrons in the screen are excited. The number of electrons excited is proportional to the number of x-ray photons reaching the screen. The IP is then loaded into a reader, where a laser reads the information about the number and location of excited electrons which is then converted to digital information. The IP is erased and can be used again. The data from the IP is processed by a computer and shades of black, white, and grey are assigned to each pixel in the resultant image using body region-specific algorithms. If an IP is not processed soon after acquisition, the image begins to degrade, limiting its use in ambulatory practice. The image can be digitally manipulated using additional software.

Direct (digital) radiography (DR) uses a different type of detector called a flat panel (Figure 13.5). These detectors are directly connected to a computer via a fiber optic cable. The x-ray photons impact either a semiconducting or scintillation/photodiode layer. These materials convert the energy from the x-ray photons to electrical energy. This electrical energy is then transferred to the computer via the fiber optic cable where it is digitized and processed in the same manner as in CR. Calibration of the detector at weekly intervals is strongly recommended to avoid progressive development of artifacts within the images it produces.

The major difference between CR and DR is that CR uses an intermediate step in which the information is transferred temporarily to the IP before being read and digitized. In DR, the information is acquired digitally without an intermediate step.

X-irradiation occurs at a specific section of the electromagnetic spectrum. This type of radiation has sufficient energy to pass through tissue, making it useful in diagnostic imaging. When directed at a body part, x-rays can either pass through the body part or be attenuated by the tissue. Attenuation is caused by absorption or scattering of the x-ray beam by the tissue. Attenuated x-rays will not impact the detector, but x-rays that pass through the tissue impact the detector and contribute to image formation. Different types of tissue attenuate the x-rays to a different degree thus resulting in the different appearance of bone versus soft tissue in radiographic images.

Tissue that attenuates the x-ray beam to a large degree, resulting in fewer x-rays' reaching the

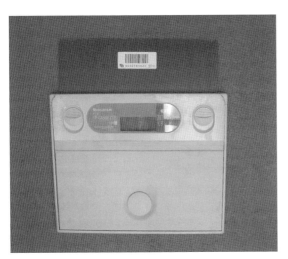

Figure 13.4. Computed radiography detector plate. The image plate has been partially removed from the protective cover.

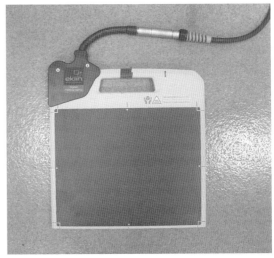

Figure 13.5. Digital radiography detector plate. The fiber-optic cable connected to the computer is seen at the top of the figure.

detector, is said to be radiopaque and appears whiter. Tissue that attenuates the x-ray beam to a lesser degree is said to be more radiolucent and appears blacker. Given the same tissue thickness, tissue opacity in order from most radiolucent to most radiopaque begins with air, fat, soft tissue, bone, and ends with metal.

Production of Images

There are many excellent descriptions of radiographic views used in equine radiography, and the reader is referred to these publications. However, some general principles of image production will be discussed. Clinician preference will determine the particular positioning for each view. Consistent positioning is vital for reproducible results and to avoid repeat exposures.

The horse should stand quietly, in a balanced position during the examination. The area to be examined should be clean and dry to prevent artifacts in the radiographic image. Horses may require chemical or physical restraint to stand quietly and to ensure the safety of the personnel performing the examination. This is particularly true when examining hindlimbs and sensitive areas such as the stifle or head. The horse handler should be aware of the safety of other personnel working around the horse. Common sense and experience should always guide decisions about restraint.

Radiographic markers identifying the limb being examined should be placed on the lateral aspect of the image or on the dorsal, cranial, or rostral aspect of the image should the lateral profile be unavailable (such as in a lateral to medial view).

Generally, the detector should be placed perpendicular to the x-ray beam, although there are some views in which this is not the case. The radiographic detector should be placed against the skin (or as close to it as possible) to reduce magnification artifacts from increased subject-film distance. It should be held steady to reduce blurring in the resultant image. The x-ray generator should be positioned at the appropriate focal film distance and the collimator should be set to expose only the area of the detector, or in some cases, only

the specific body part being imaged. This reduces scatter radiation and exposure to personnel. The exposure should be made when the patient and detector are properly positioned and motionless.

Radiographic images are generally named based on the path traveled by the x-ray beam. The path is described in reference to the dorsal/cranial, palmar (plantar)/caudal, lateral, and medial aspects of the body. For example, to produce the image in Figure 13.6, the beam traveled from the lateral aspect to the medial aspect of the metacarpophalangeal joint, resulting in a lateral to medial view. If the x-ray beam is directed in a proximal to distal direction (instead of traveling level to the ground in the horizontal plane), this is referred to as elevation. In Figure 13.7, the x-ray beam traveled from the dorsal to the palmar aspect of the metacarpophalangeal joint. The beam was also elevated 20 degrees from the horizontal plane and the detector was placed perpendicular to the x-ray beam. Oblique

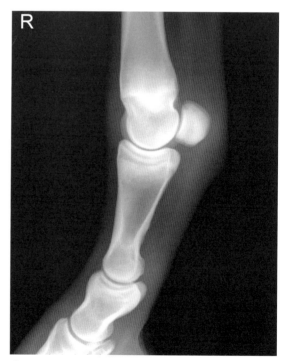

Figure 13.6. Lateral-medial radiographic image of the metacarpophalangeal joint.

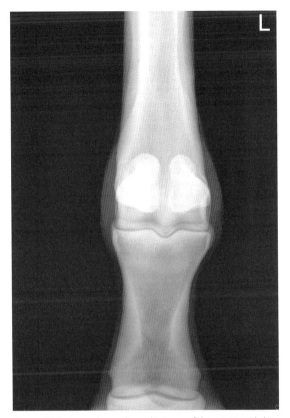

Figure 13.7. Dorsopalmar radiographic image of the metacarpophalangeal joint with 20 degrees of elevation.

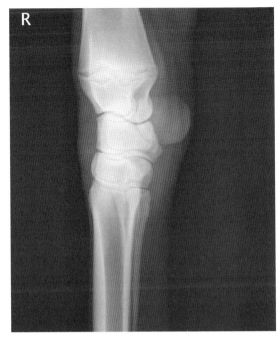

Figure 13.8. Oblique radiographic image of the carpal joints. The radiographic beam originated 15 degrees dorsal to the medial plane.

radiographic views will necessitate directing the x-ray beam in directions between the planes described above. The direction of the beam in these directions is called angulation. In Figure 13.8, the x-ray beam originated at a location 15 degrees dorsal to the medial plane and passed from the dorsomedial aspect to the palmarolateral aspect of the carpus.

Descriptive naming of oblique radiographic images of the equine extremities may vary, but most commonly the path of the radiographic beam from generator to plate is utilized. Consider the image seen in Figure 13.8. To produce this image, the radiographic beam travels from the dorsomedial aspect of the carpus to the plate positioned on the palmarolateral aspect of the carpus, so it would be referred to as a dorsomedial-

palmarolateral oblique view. Whichever convention is chosen, it is important to remain consistent to avoid confusion and in symmetrical joints, such as the fetlock; it is necessary to know which convention is being employed to differentiate medial from lateral.

A customized technique chart is a necessity for each generator and detector combination. In conventional radiography, the amount of contrast is adjusted by changing the relative contributions of the voltage, measured in peak kilovolts (kVp), current, measured in milliamperes (mA), and exposure time, measured in seconds (s). The kVp contributes to the energy (penetrating power) of the x-rays produced. The mA determines the amount of x-rays produced. The contributions of the current and time are often combined in a value known as mAs because they both play a role in the number of x-rays produced. For high-contrast radiographic images, a relatively low kV setting is used and a relatively high mA setting is used. The opposite is used for lower contrast images. To keep overall film exposure similar, but to change contrast, kVp is changed by 15% and mA is changed in the opposite direction by a factor of two. In CR and DR, the amount of contrast is also affected by the algorithms applied by the computer after data acquisition.

When radiographic images of thick body parts are produced, a large amount of scatter radiation is produced. This scatter radiation can result in reduced image quality because x-ray photons will impact the detector after having been scattered resulting in loss of definition of anatomy. A grid can be used to eliminate some of the scatter and resultant decrease in image contrast and quality. A grid consists of rows of thin lead bars. It is placed between the skin and the detector. If x-ray photons travel straight from the generator to the detector, they will pass straight between the lead bars and impact the detector. If a photon is scattered within the patient, it will enter the grid at an angle and be absorbed by the lead bars instead of impacting the detector. However, because fewer x-rays reach the detector, higher exposure factors are necessary. The x-ray beam must also be lined up correctly with the grid to avoid artifacts.

For radiography of the axial skeleton, abdomen, and thorax, a stand should be used to hold the detector to prevent detector motion and reduce radiation exposure of personnel. Some stands can be fixed to the x-ray generator to ensure the proper focal film distance (see Fig. 13.3). Others are placed next to the horse. Stands can also be built to accommodate grid and detector together.

Safety

Any personnel who may be exposed to ionizing radiation should wear appropriate monitoring equipment, including radiation badges and rings. The readings generated by the monitoring equipment should be reviewed and appropriate measures for reducing exposure should be taken as necessary.

The number of people in the room at the time of the radiographic exposure should be kept to the minimum needed to allow the procedure to be performed safely and correctly. Individuals who are in the room at the time of the radiographic exposure should wear lead gowns and lead thyroid collars. If the detector must be handheld, whenever possible, distance between the detector and the person holding it should be maximized by uses of a holding device (Figure 13.9). The person holding the detec-

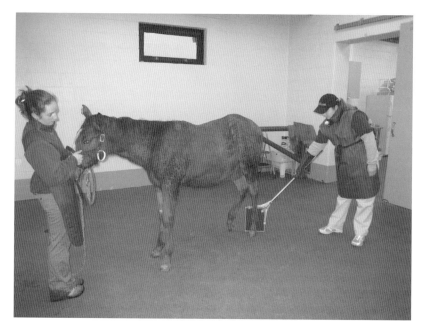

Figure 13.9. Radiation safety. The distance between the person holding the detector and the primary x-ray beam is increased with the use of a detector holder. Lead gowns, gloves, and thyroid protectors are worn, as are radiation monitors.

tor or holding device must wear lead gloves or mittens to further decrease exposure. At no time should personnel be in the path of the primary beam of x-rays and proper collimation should always be used.

Use of Radiography in Equine Practice

Contrast Radiography

Iodinated contrast materials, which appear radiopaque on radiographic images (similar opacity to metal), can be used to obtain additional information. Contrast material can be administered orally or rectally to assess passage through the gastrointestinal tract, as in gastric outflow disorders or atresia coli. It can also be introduced into wounds or fistulas to determine the path of the tract and in the imaging of the spinal cord (myelogram), urinary bladder (cystogram), and urethra (urethrogram).

Recent Improvements

DR not only results in a higher quality image than conventional radiography but also allows the veterinarian t to achieve a preliminary diagnosis while still at the farm. This is particularly advantageous in an emergency situation when the results of the radiograph may significantly impact therapy. The cervical spine, thorax, and upper extremities can be difficult to radiograph with standard cassettes, but with the advent of portable DR, images of these regions may be produced on an ambulatory basis in some situations.

Ultrasound

Ultrasonography provides excellent visualization of many soft tissue structures. Its usefulness in breeding management and evaluation of tendon and ligament injuries has become the standard of practice.

Image Formation

Diagnostic ultrasound uses acoustic (sound) waves produced in pulses by vibrating piezoelectric crystals in a transducer and transmitted into the body through a contact gel. As the waves pass through tissues, they will either penetrate into deeper tissues or be attenuated. Attenuation occurs in three different ways. The acoustic waves can be absorbed (energy converted to heat), scattered in directions away from the transducer, or reflected back toward the transducer to contribute to image formation.

Medical ultrasound uses the difference in acoustic impedance between tissues to reflect waves back toward the transducer. Acoustic impedance is an innate property of tissue, determined by the density of the tissue and the speed with which sound travels through the tissue. When acoustic waves encounter a junction between tissues with different acoustic impedances, some waves are reflected back toward the transducer, and others continue to travel through to deeper structures. More waves are reflected at the junction of tissues with a large difference in their acoustic impedances than at the junction of tissues with a small difference in acoustic impedance. Many of the soft tissues in the body, such as water, fat, muscle, and internal organs, have similar acoustic impedances so some acoustic waves will be reflected back to the transducer and some will penetrate deeper into the tissues.

Air has a low acoustic impedance and bone has a high acoustic impedance as compared to soft tissues. Because of these large differences, nearly all of the acoustic waves will be reflected back toward the transducer with few waves able to penetrate more deeply at the junction of air or bone with soft tissues. This results in a strong echo returning to the transducer from this interface and the absence of echoes from deeper structures. In a practical sense, this means that ultrasound waves cannot "see through" bone or air.

The reflected acoustic waves are received by the ultrasound transducer. These waves are then processed to create an image that is displayed on the screen of the ultrasound machine. The image consists of a two-dimensional map made from the received echoes. For a given location on the image, the amplitude of the returning wave determines the brightness. The location of the origin of the wave along the transducer head determines the position along the horizontal axis. The location along the vertical axis (depth of the echo) is calculated from the known speed of ultrasound waves traveling through soft tissue and the time elapsed between when the echo is transmitted and when echo is received.

Production of Images

In a simple sense, an ultrasound machine consists of a monitor on which to display an image, a transducer to produce and receive acoustic waves, and a computer to process the data and control the transducer.

Transducers

Diagnostic ultrasound is generally performed with frequencies ranging from 2 to 13 MHz. Higher frequencies produce higher resolution but have a shallower depth of penetration because these acoustic waves are absorbed by the tissues more than waves of lower frequencies. Lower frequency waves are able to penetrate more deeply but do not provide high resolution. In a practical sense, this means that lower frequencies are used to be able to image deeper body structures, such as abdominal organs. However, the resolution will be relatively low. For more superficial structures, such as tendons, a higher frequency should be used to provide enhanced resolution. Generally, the highest frequency transducer with adequate penetration power for the structure of interest should be used to optimize resolution.

For deep structures (>10 cm deep), such as abdominal organs, deep thoracic structures ,and deep musculoskeletal structures, frequencies of 2 to 5 MHz are typically used. More superficial musculoskeletal and thoracic structures (<5–10 cm deep) can be imaged with 7.5 to 12 MHz frequencies. Transrectal reproductive ultrasound is typically performed with 5 to 7.5 MHz frequencies. Some transducers produce acoustic waves at only one frequency; others can produce acoustic waves over a set range of frequencies and the operator can select the operating frequency to optimize penetration or resolution.

Transducers may be of a linear or sector design. In a linear transducer, multiple crystals are arranged in straight line along the probe head. A rectangular image results from the sequential production of acoustic waves by the crystals along the transducer head. Curvilinear transducers have the crystals arranged in a curved line and produce a wedge-shaped image but are otherwise identical to traditional linear transducers.

Sector transducers produce a wedge-shaped image using a different mechanism than curvilinear transducers. The crystals in a sector transducer are rotated instead of fired sequentially. Annular transducers also produce a wedge-shaped image. Phased-array transducers have many crystals that produce acoustic waves in carefully timed groups. They also produce a wedge-shaped image.

Transducer design can also be customized for specific applications. Transrectal transducers have a slim design and can be held in a cupped hand. T-shaped linear probes permit examination of a longer section of the body part of interest such as tendon or ligament and are easily stabilized in the operator's hand. Small microconvex linear probes have a small footprint with a small cutaneous window, but allow fanning of the beam to assess a wider area. This is particularly useful in situations such as thoracic ultrasonography in which a microconvex probe can fit easily in the intercostal spaces. Sector and annular transducers also have a smaller footprint than linear transducers, as well as, increased depth of penetration.

Imaging Parameters

There are many parameters that can be adjusted by the operator. A few of the more common parameters will be described, but this is not an exhaustive description of all of the ways in which an ultrasound image can be optimized or adjusted.

Specific terminology is used to describe an ultrasound image. Areas of the image that appear black are said to be anechoic because no echoes were returned from that body region. If area A of an image appears brighter than area B, area A is said to be hyperechoic as compared to area B and area B is hypoechoic as compared to area A. Regions in the image close to the transducer are in the near-field and regions far from the transducer are in the far-field.

The gain control determines how much all returning echoes are amplified and therefore how bright the entire image appears. The time-gain compensation control allows the gain at various depths of the image to be fine-tuned. Echoes reflected from deep within the tissue will have smaller amplitudes than echoes reflected from more superficial structures due to increased attenuation. Without correction, this would result in an image that was very bright for superficial structures but very dark for deep structures. Correction allows echoes from deeper structures to be amplified and echoes from more superficial structures to be dampened, producing an image of uniform brightness to be displayed.

The power controls the energy of the echoes produced by the transmitter. Increasing the energy of produced echoes will also increase the amplitude of the returning echoes, resulting in a brighter image. However, this can introduce artifacts into the resultant image, so amplifying the returning echoes by increasing the gain instead will improve image quality.

The reject control determines the minimum echo amplitude used to construct the image. Echoes with amplitudes lower than this limit will not be included in the image. This allows faint echoes from background noise to be eliminated. Changing the dynamic range alters the range and contrast of shades of grey that will be used to form the image.

The depth control alters the displayed depth of the image. It should be set deep enough to create an image that contains the anatomy of interest and enough surrounding anatomy to provide context for anatomy and comparisons of echogenicity between tissues. However, it should not be set so deep that small abnormalities are missed. The focal zone of the ultrasound beam can also be adjusted to provide increased resolution at a particular depth.

Frame rate describes the number of frames, or images, displayed in each second. Slower frame rates will result in increased resolution. This is useful when imaging nonmoving structures. However, for examinations in real-time of moving organs, such as the heart, high frame rates are necessary to accurately depict motion and function.

There are two modes of ultrasound used most often in equine practice. Brightness mode (B-mode) is a two-dimensional map of the location and strength of returning echoes in the plane of the transducer. It is used to obtain anatomic information about the location and structure of tissues. Motion mode (M-mode) displays how one thin slice of tissue moves over time. M-mode is used in cardiac examinations to examine heart wall contraction.

Doppler ultrasonography allows assessment of direction and velocity of blood flow. It is used most often in cardiac ultrasonography. Using pulse-wave Doppler, the flow data can be evaluated as velocity as a function of time. With color flow Doppler, blood flow within the heart can be seen. Flow toward the transducer is represented by shades of red and flow away from the transducer is represented by shades of blue.

Patient Preparation

Production of high-quality images is dependent on careful patient preparation. It is crucial to eliminate as much air as possible between the transducer and the surface of the patient to maximize the number of acoustic waves transmitted to the patient. This can most easily be achieved by clipping the hair in the area to be examined. The surface of the skin should be cleaned with isopropyl alcohol or warm water to remove dirt. Acoustic coupling gel should then be applied to the transducer and the patient, further improving acoustic wave transmission by eliminating air between the transducer and the skin. In some situations, the patient cannot be clipped. In this case, the hair should be soaked with alcohol or warm water and the probe can be applied with or without coupling gel. The probe should be moved only in the direction of hair growth to minimize trapping of air underneath the hair and subsequent reduction in image quality.

Chemical or physical restraint may be required for an ultrasound examination. The most important consideration is the safety of the operator and the horse handler. Evaluation of certain body parts, such as the distal hind limb, necessitate that the operator position himself or herself in a vulnerable position. In these situations, an experienced, attentive handler is necessary, but additional restraint should be considered. Ultrasound equipment is often expensive and must be positioned in close proximity to the patient, so precautions should be taken to safeguard the ultrasound machine as well. The horse must also stand quietly to allow a thorough evaluation to be performed.

Use of Ultrasound in Equine Practice

Abdominal ultrasonography provides useful information about the location (nephrosplenic entrapment of bowel) and character (gastric dilatation) of abdominal organs in assessment of colic, colitis, pregnancy, urinary tract, liver disease, and unthriftiness. Evaluation of intestinal motility, wall thickness, and diameter are also valuable, as is assessment of peritoneal fluid. Abnormal parenchymal structure of the liver, kidney, and spleen can be assessed, and ultrasound-guided biopsies are possible. Abnormal abdominal masses may also be identified. In foals and other horses with abdominal pain who are not candidates for rectal palpation, ultrasonographic imaging of the abdominal viscera provides an important piece of information when formulating a diagnosis.

Transrectal ultrasonography is often used in reproductive management of broodmares. Follicle diameter can be measured and the cervix and uterus can be evaluated to optimize time of breeding relative to ovulation. Pregnancy can be diagnosed, and twin pregnancies can be managed at an earlier stage than with transrectal palpation alone. Mares with uterine abnormalities, such as cysts or uterine fluid accumulation, can be diagnosed and monitored. Information about the health of the fetus and placenta can be obtained.

Thoracic and cardiac ultrasonography permits assessment of lung surface and heart anatomy and function. The presence and character of excess pleural fluid, pathology on the surface of the lung, such as abscess formation, lung consolidation, and pleural thickening, can be evaluated. Structure and function of the heart, including assessment of valvular disorders, septal defects, and congenital abnormalities is possible with ultrasonography.

Ultrasonographic evaluation of tendons, ligaments, synovial structures, and bone surfaces can provide information about the fiber pattern of tendons and ligaments, septic and nonseptic joint inflammation and can be more sensitive to small changes in bone contour at the origin or insertion of ligaments than radiography. Evaluation of some pelvic areas and contours of the scapula or hip joint may be better achieved in the standing horse with ultrasonography than with radiography. Synovio centesis of structures covered by soft tissues, such as the shoulder, hip, cervical facet joints, or bicipital bursa, can be aided with ultrasound guidance.

Increased exposure to and experience with ultrasound will result in improved skills and diagnostic use. In addition to the uses previously described, ultrasound examination can be used to assess a variety of additional structures such as the eyes, superficial masses, wounds, vascular structures, and lymph nodes.

Nuclear Scintigraphy

Nuclear scintigraphy provides us with a screening tool that can locate areas of increased metabolic activity in soft tissue or bone associated with a site of inflammation or trauma. The horse is injected with a radionuclide that is absorbed in increased amounts in regions of the body undergoing remodeling processes. Using a special gamma camera, any areas of increased uptake can be identified and pursued further with other diagnostic techniques. It does involve specialized equipment and some additional safety measures, so its use is limited to the clinic setting (Figure 13.10).

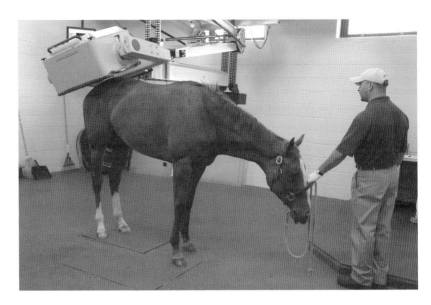

Figure 13.10. Horse undergoing nuclear scintigraphic examination.

Image Formation

A technetium isotope (Tc-99m) is the most commonly used radionuclide in equine scintigraphy. It can be coupled to other molecules to target specific organ systems, resulting in a compound called a *radiopharmaceutical*. In the horse, the musculoskeletal system is the most common system examined. In this case, Tc-99m is coupled to a diphosphonate salt. The diphosphonate salt will bind to a compound (hydroxyapatite) in bone. The binding is proportional to the blood flow to and bone metabolism of the area, so areas of increased metabolism will have increased binding of the radiopharmaceutical. The Tc-99m will emit gamma radiation from this bound location, which is detected and localized with a gamma camera. The resultant image is a map showing the anatomical locations and amount of gamma radiation from each location. Increased gamma radiation indicates increased metabolism of the bone and blood flow in that area.

Nuclear scintigraphy, like radiography, takes advantage of the properties of electromagnetic radiation to form an image. Nuclear scintigraphy uses gamma rays instead of x-rays, but both types of radiation have enough energy to penetrate body tissues and be detectable afterward. The gamma rays or photons escaping from the Tc-99m in the body are detected by a gamma camera. The gamma camera is made of multiple parts. The photons first interact with a scintillation crystal made of sodium iodide and thallium. When the photons interact with the scintillation crystal, a flash of light is released. The back of the scintillation crystal is coated with optical grease, allowing the flash of light to be transmitted through the optical grease to photomultiplier tubes, which turn the light energy into electrical energy. The electrical energy generated by the photomultiplier tube is proportional to the intensity of the light it receives. This electrical energy is then converted to a digital signal that is processed by a computer to form an image.

Each flash of light generated by the scintillation crystal will be transmitted to multiple neighboring photomultiplier tubes. However, the intensity of the light received by each tube (and the strength of the electrical current generated from that location) will be inversely proportional to the distance between the flash and the photomultiplier tube. The photomultiplier tubes closest to the original flash of light will generate a stronger electric current than those further away. A computer analyzes the strength of the signals from the photomultiplier tubes and calculates the position of the photon-scintillation crystal interaction.

Ideally, all gamma rays leaving the body would travel in a straight line from the point of emission from the radionuclide to the point of detection in the camera. This would result in an image showing amounts of gamma radiation coming from each location accurately. Unfortunately, the gamma rays do not all travel in a straight path. They may interact with other atoms as they exit the body. Some of these interactions, called *Compton interactions*, lead to the photons being deflected in a new direction with less energy. If the spatial information from this photon were included in the image, it would provide misleading information because the direction of entry into the camera is not the same as the direction of origin. If Compton interaction has occurred, the energy in the scattered photon will be less than the energy from a photon, which has not interacted with any atoms. Therefore, the intensity of the light flash (and electrical current generated) when a Compton scattered photon interacts with the scintillation crystal will be smaller than a non-interacting photon. Using this information, the computer is able to determine which photons have been scattered from Compton interactions (lower energy) and which have traveled in a straight path (known amount of energy for a specific radionuclide). The energy window of the gamma camera can be set to a narrow window to only include information from photons received with a specific energy range, so scattered photons with less energy can be excluded from contributing to image formation.

Even if all the gamma rays leaving the body did travel in a straight line, the scintillation crystal would still be impacted by photons originating from all parts of the body in all directions. A collimator is used to collect only the photons exiting the body that travel perpendicular to the camera. The collimator is attached to the front of the camera. It consists of a sheet of lead with small holes perpendicular to the camera. If a photon is traveling perpendicular to the camera, it enters the hole

and travels straight through to the scintillation crystal. If the photon enters a hole at an angle, instead of traveling straight through the hole, it will impact the wall of the hole and be absorbed by the lead. As a result, an anatomically accurate image of gamma ray origin can be generated.

Gamma Camera Care and Maintenance

Calibrating the gamma camera to the known amount of energy emitted by a specific radionuclide is done via a process known as "peaking." A pure sample of the radionuclide is used to tune the camera to its specific gamma ray energy. A peak-shaped graph of the gamma ray emissions from the radionuclide allows the operator to center the window of allowable energies (energy window) over the energy value from the specific radionuclide used (photopeak). This will result in exclusion of radiation from other sources and from scattered gamma rays in image formation.

The functionality of the photomultiplier tubes must also be checked periodically. Because not all photomultiplier tubes create the same electrical energy when exposed to a given amount of light, computations must be done within the computer to compensate for these small differences to provide a uniform image that accurately reflects the amount of gamma radiation emitted. Creating the data for these computations is called a *uniformity flood*. Other factors that may affect the crystal and therefore image quality are rapid changes in temperature and physical trauma, so the room should be kept at a constant temperature and the camera should be protected from damage.

Safety

Nuclear scintigraphy involves the use of electromagnetic radiation, so appropriate safety measures should be taken. Radiation dosimetry badges and rings should be worn by all personnel. A dedicated, locked room should be used for storage of radiopharmaceuticals and used syringes, needles, and personal protective equipment. Protective flexible gloves must be worn at all times when handling the radiopharmaceutical to provide protection from direct contamination. Radiopharmaceuticals should be stored inside leaded shields, protected from spills, and lead syringe covers should be used when injecting patients. All areas involved in nuclear scintigraphy (e.g., storage room, scan room, stalls, barn aisle) should be monitored routinely using a radiation detector.

Tc-99m is excreted in the urine, so horses should remain in a dedicated stall until the radioactivity has decayed to an acceptable level. If the stall is cleaned, any bedding should be isolated until the radioactivity has decayed, as should any syringes, needles, or personal protective equipment used in the examination. Local regulations vary, so all appropriate precautions should be taken. If the stall must be entered, gloves and protective footwear should be worn. If the horse urinates outside of the stall a purpose-designed cleanser for radioactive waste should be used to clean up the urine if the urine cannot be contained within a bucket.

Examination

Patient Preparation

An appropriate dose of radiopharmaceutical based on body weight should be calculated for each patient, taking into consideration that older horses require a higher dose than young, actively growing horses because of their slower rate of bone remodeling and resultant decreased binding to hydroxyapatite in bone. Cold ambient temperatures will reduce blood flow to the distal limbs, resulting in reduced radiopharmaceutical binding; heated stalls and leg wraps can be used to improve blood flow to the distal limb during cold weather.

Perivascular injection of radiopharmaceutical can be quite irritating, so the use of an intravenous catheter is recommended. After injection of radiopharmaceutical, the horse's feet should be covered with sturdy tape. This is done in case the horse urinates between injection and examination because Tc-99m is excreted in the urine. If the feet are not

covered, they could become contaminated with urine, resulting in artifactual appearance of increased radiopharmaceutical uptake in the foot region. The tape should be removed and stored with other contaminated waste before the horse is examined.

Because the radiopharmaceutical is excreted in the urine, increased uptake will be seen in the kidneys and bladder because the kidneys filter the blood and the increased gamma radiation may interfere with image acquisition and interpretation of the caudal spine, pelvis, and proximal hind limbs. A diuretic can be administered to facilitate urination and bladder emptying if necessary.

It is important to have the horse stand still to produce high-quality images. An excellent horse handler can greatly facilitate an efficient examination. Most, if not all, horses require appropriate chemical sedation during the examination; care to avoid excess sedation will help to decrease the likelihood of ataxia and swaying. If horses are afraid of the camera, covering the ipsilateral eye may help to improve cooperation.

Image Acquisition

Acquisition and processing software are variable, but there are some common principles. Images can be obtained either by collecting data over a set amount of time or until a set number of gamma rays have been received by the gamma camera (counts). After the data has been collected, the image is stored and the next region can be examined.

Scintigraphic images may be generated in either static or dynamic mode. In static mode, the camera will record data for a set time or for a set number of counts. All data will be collected and analyzed to form one image. This mode is useful in areas of the body where mild, involuntary motion (swaying) of the horse is not a problem as higher resolution images can be obtained with this mode.

In dynamic mode, the camera collects a set number of frames over time. These frames will exist as multiple images that can then be processed in different ways. For some examinations concerned with change over time, the frames can be evaluated in a sequence. Alternatively, the frames can be used to correct motion during acquisition. This is done with software that analyzes the frames to determine where motion has occurred. These frames are then discarded from a final calculation, which combines the frames to produce a final static image. The disadvantage of a dynamic acquisition is that lower resolutions must often be used to employ motion correction software. However, in areas of the body where horse movement is a problem (proximal limbs and axial skeleton), the advantage of motion correction usually outweighs the decrease in resolution. It is important to note that motion correction is meant to correct small amounts of motion. If the operator observes large amounts of motion, the resultant image is usually of poor quality, and the acquisition of that image should be repeated.

Images should be acquired in the same order for every examination. This will prevent views from being forgotten and will allow for a more efficient examination by reducing positioning time. When acquiring images of the limbs, a lead blocker should be placed between the limb(s) being imaged and the contralateral limb (in the case of lateral views) or between the forelimbs and hind limbs (for dorsal or palmar or plantar views). This will prevent radiation from other limbs from being detected by the gamma camera and decreasing image quality.

Because the strength of the gamma radiation decreases exponentially as the distance from the source increases, it is vital to position the gamma camera as close to the anatomy to be imaged as possible. Failure to do so will lead to low counts or increased scan time and blurry images. Consistent, symmetrical positioning is also important because the left and right sides of the body are often compared to find areas of subtle increased uptake.

There are three phases used in Tc-99m equine scintigraphy. Not all phases will be used in every examination. The vascular phase shows the distribution of the Tc-99m within the blood supply and lasts for approximately 90 seconds immediately after injection, so only one or two images can generally be acquired. The soft tissue (pool) phase shows the movement of the Tc-99m in extracellular fluid from 2 to 20 minutes after injection. This window of time also limits the number of images that can be acquired because movement of Tc-99m into bone starts at approximately 10 minutes after injection. The bone phase shows the localization of the Tc-99m to the bony skeleton, where it is bound to hydroxyapatite via the diphosphonate salt and occurs maximally 2.5 to 4 hours after injection.

Use of Nuclear Scintigraphy in Equine Practice

Nuclear scintigraphy permits imaging of an entire horse and can be useful in instances in which lameness is subtle or difficult to eliminate with regional or intra-articular analgesia, so long as the lack of specificity of uptake is considered as is the failure of uptake in regions that may be of clinical significance. Increased uptake of radionuclide requires increased blood flow and metabolism of bone. These two conditions appear both at sites of injury and in anatomic regions that are clinically normal, such as the cartilaginous caps of the dorsal spinous processes of the withers and in young horses' growth plates (physes). Examination immediately following an injury may be negative for 3 or 4 days until increased bone metabolism has begun.

Stress fractures or remodeling of the humerus, radius, tibia, metatarsal condyles, and ilial wing are excellent examples of lesions which are well depicted by nuclear scintigraphy. Subtle areas of bone remodeling such as the attachments of ligaments (e.g., suspensory, sacroiliac, or collateral) are less consistent in isotope uptake and so can be missed if scintigraphy alone is selected.

Thermography

Thermography uses a thermal camera to map the surface temperature of the body. The camera detects heat in the form of infrared radiation. The image is displayed in real time, with different colors representing different relative temperatures. Comparing surface temperatures allows assessment of local blood flow to identify areas of potential inflammation.

Computed Tomography

One of the newer diagnostic imaging modalities used in equine medicine is computed tomography (CT). CT is a cross-sectional imaging technique that allows images of extremely thin slices of tissue to be generated and examined without superimposition of neighboring tissues. This makes CT a sensitive modality and allows much more precise localization of lesions. It produces a series of high-detail images that can be reconstructed into a three-dimensional representation. CT is particularly useful for bony detail such as in the sinus cavities of the horse.

Image Formation

Although it may not appear to be the case, CT bears many similarities to radiographic imaging. CT involves producing radiographic images of the same thin slice of tissue from multiple angles and then using a computer to combine these images to give a complete representation of the slice contents. The process is then repeated for the adjacent slice of tissue. The process of image formation in CT is the same as the process in radiography: x-ray production by a generator, x-ray attenuation in tissue, and x-ray interaction with a detector.

The x-ray generator produces a thin beam of x-rays that are directed across the patient. A detector positioned on the other side of the patient receives the x-rays. X-rays that have passed through the body will be attenuated to different degrees, depending on the tissues through which they have passed. The generator rotates around the patient, so one anatomic area is imaged from different angles. A detector receives the x-rays and converts the x-ray energy to electrical energy. A computer receives the data in the form of electrical energy and generates a two-dimensional representation created from the attenuation information gained from multiple angles. Based on the amount of attenuation in different structures, each pixel in the image is assigned a numerical value. This value is represented by a shade of grey on the image.

As in radiography, the brightness of a structure depends on how many x-rays are attenuated as they pass through. Brightness in CT images is measured quantitatively in Hounsfield units (HU). This is a scale based on air being assigned a value of −1,000 HU, water a value of 0 HU, and bone a value of +1,000 HU. Other tissues are assigned values relative to this scale based upon their attenuation of x-rays.

Equipment

No CT scanner designed specifically for horses exists, so scanners designed for use in humans have been adapted specifically with regard to table design (Figure 13.11). A CT scanner is a cylindrical structure with a gantry or the hole in the center of the doughnut into which the body part to be imaged is placed. The periphery of the cylinder houses the x-ray generator and the detectors.

Conventional CT scanners acquire the data for each slice separately by moving the patient slightly forward in the gantry after each acquisition cycle during which the x-ray generator rotates about the patient. This process is repeated until the scan is complete.

Spiral (also known as helical) CT scanners acquire data continuously. The x-ray generator is continually on and the generator rotates around the patient as the patient table moves continuously. A helical or spiral set of data is acquired as a volume rather

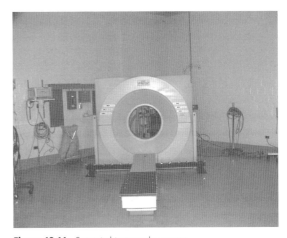

Figure 13.11. Computed tomography scanner.
Image courtesy of Dr. J. Brett Woodie.

than a disc-shaped set of data acquired as individual slices. Spiral CT scanners are faster than conventional scanners and have improved reconstruction capabilities. Some spiral CT scanners (known as multidetector spiral CT scanners) are able to acquire larger amounts of data with each rotation of the x-ray generator. Multiple rows of detectors are used, allowing a wider x-ray beam to be used, and multiple slices are acquired simultaneously. These scanners are faster than traditional spiral CT scanners and allow for thinner slices and superior reconstructions.

CT images are acquired in the axial plane. However, the images can be reformatted into any other plane, and three-dimensional reconstructions can be generated with the use of specialized software. This allows multiplanar evaluation of the anatomy. The brightness and contrast of the image can also be manipulated after acquisition by changing window and level settings. This allows for a wide range of tissue types to be evaluated by using different window and level settings.

Iodinated contrast material can be used in CT imaging. The contrast material causes an increase in the attenuation of x-rays. The contrast material is administered intravenously and thus allows detection of pathology by identifying patterns of abnormal blood flow. Alternatively, intra-articular contrast can be administered to outline structures more effectively. The images generated before and after contrast administration are also compared to detect abnormal locations of contrast.

Patient Preparation

Adult patients must be positioned in dorsal or lateral recumbency on a specialized table to be accommodated within the gantry of the machine. Foals may also be examined in sternal recumbency. The patient must also remain motionless during the examination to prevent blurring of the images and damage to the equipment. As a result of these factors, CT examination for horses requires general anesthesia and all of the accompanying preparation. This technique provides high-detail images of one specific area, so it is important that the ana-

tomic site of the problem be pinpointed precisely because it is often impractical or impossible to image the entire body.

Safety

CT scanners use x-rays, so the same precautions should be taken as with radiography if personnel are present in the room. However, because horses undergoing CT examination are under general anesthesia and immobilized, it is possible and recommended that no one be in the room when scanning is taking place. The scanner is controlled from an adjacent room. Anesthesia personnel can monitor the patient from a window in the control room, using binoculars to see the monitors if necessary. This is often a feasible situation because of the short scan times associated with CT imaging.

Use of Computed Tomography in Equine Practice

CT allows multiplanar imaging of structures otherwise difficult or impossible to image with conventional imaging techniques. CT has superior three-dimensional reformatting capabilities and short scan times as compared to magnetic resonance imaging (MRI). When examining injury to bony structures, such as the sinus cavities, the stylohyoid apparatus, the calvarium, or fracture sites, it is often preferable to MRI. It is extremely useful for presurgical imaging of complex fractures and sinus problems. The horse can be anesthetized, examined using CT, and then be prepped for surgery during the same anesthetic episode. The reformatting capabilities allow more complete surgical planning and improved treatment. The increased spatial resolution is particularly useful when evaluating bony abnormalities.

Availability of CT is limited to referral hospitals because of the need for general anesthesia and specialized equipment. The diameter of the gantry also limits the anatomical areas that can be evaluated.

Magnetic Resonance Imaging

MRI is a three-dimensional imaging technique that uses a strong external magnetic field in combination with changing magnetic gradients to create various types of cross-sectional images. It is similar to CT in the sense that thin-slice, high-detail, cross-sectional images are created. MRI provides superior soft tissue and bone detail and is considered the gold standard in many cases.

Image Formation

Magnetic field strength is measured in Tesla (T). The strength of the magnetic field varies between types of magnets, but it is typically between 0.25 T and 1.5 T for most magnets currently in routine equine clinical use. Magnets for clinical use in humans can be a strong as 3 T, and there are much stronger magnets used for research applications. As a point of comparison, the earth's magnetic field ranges between 0.00003 T and 0.0006 T.

Application of the strong magnetic field causes protons within the body to orient themselves with relation to the magnetic field, which permits further manipulation of their orientation when radio waves are intermittently applied. Different tissues return to their normal state at different times and in different ways as the radiofrequency pulses (RF) are discontinued. These influences allow us to gain more information about the tissues in which they are found, such as changes in anatomical structure or molecular composition in the case of fluid accumulation with edema.

The images that result from an MRI examination are thin cross sections through a specific body part. These cross sections are typically between 2 mm and 4 mm thick. Unlike with CT imaging, the orientation of the slices obtained during each pulse sequence can be selected by the operator. Each set of cross sections is set up in a specific orientation to the body part being examined. For example, to image the metacarpophalangeal joint, three different orientations are typically used. Coronal (dorsal) images slice from the front to the back of the joint (providing a "front view"), sagittal images slice from the left side to the right side of the joint (providing a "side view"), and axial (transverse) images slice from the top to the bottom of the joint (providing cross sections along the long axis of the limb). The resulting sets of images will consist of a large number of orthogonal slices through the fetlock in each direction.

For each series of slices, the operator must choose the orientation of the slices, as well as, the type of pulse sequence used. A typical MRI examination will consist of many series, each with a different combination of orientation and pulse sequence. A complete examination produces hundreds of individual images to be reviewed and usually takes between 1 and 2 hours to complete. Some series are acquired in a way that permits reconstruction in multiple planes or in three dimensions.

Equipment

The main magnetic field can be generated in a variety of ways. Permanent magnets are used in lower field systems (<0.4 T). These magnetic fields are generated by using ferromagnetic materials of the same type as in everyday magnets. Stronger magnetic fields are produced using superconducting electromagnets. These magnets use liquid helium to cool the electromagnetic coils and reduce the resistance, allowing much stronger magnetic fields to be generated. Liquid helium is expensive and requires periodic replenishment but is necessary to efficiently generate the stronger magnetic fields in clinical use. The room must be shielded to prevent any external radio frequency pulses (e.g., radio signals, cellular phone transmission) from entering the room and introducing artifacts. Copper sheeting is usually used for this purpose.

There are two major groups of MRI systems in use for horses: high field magnets with strengths greater than or equal to 1.0T, which are closed bore construction and require the horse to be under general anesthesia (Figure 13.12) and positioned either in lateral or dorsal recumbency on a nonferromagnetic padded table with the body part of

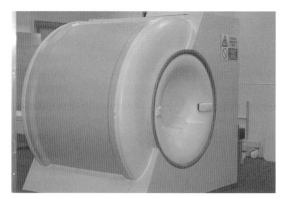

Figure 13.12. High-field magnetic resonance imaging scanner. This scanner was designed for humans but has been repurposed for equine use.

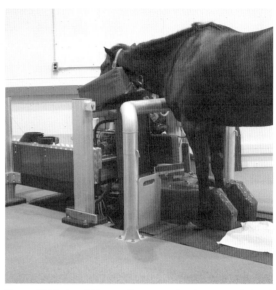

Figure 13.13. Low-field magnetic resonance imaging scanner designed for horses.

interest pushed into the bore. Foals that are small enough can be scanned using a human table in several positions.

The other group consists of magnets that have been specifically designed for horses (Figure 13.13). The low-field magnets have strength in the 0.25 T range but are open bone and can be positioned about a body part; some require general anesthesia and some only sedation. The images produced with these weaker magnets require longer scan times to obtain and are of lower resolution. Motion artifact in studies obtained on standing horses can significantly reduce image quality.

The isocenter of a magnet describes the location of the center of the magnetic field and is usually located in the center of the magnet bore. Examinations are limited to regions that can fit into the bore of the magnet to be positioned at or near the isocenter. Depending on the type of magnet, this requires that either the horse be pushed into the center of the magnet bore or that the magnet be positioned around the region of interest. These limits will vary between magnets based on their construction.

Intravenous or intra-articular contrast can also be used in MRI. Gadolinium compounds are typically used that allow assessment of abnormal patterns of blood flow or delineation of anatomic structures, similar to the use of contrast in CT imaging.

Safety

Most safety hazards associated with MRI are related to the introduction of ferromagnetic objects into a strong magnetic field as opposed to the existence of the magnetic field itself. There are no known adverse effects of MRI at field strengths currently used in equine clinical imaging. Any object that is magnetic (e.g., scissors, oxygen tanks, IV poles, scalpel blades) will be attracted to the magnet thus all the equipment in the room must be non-magnetic or MRI compatible, including the anesthesia equipment. The strength of the magnetic field increases exponentially as the distance to the magnet decreases. In practical terms, this means that the pull of the magnet on any ferromagnetic object becomes quickly stronger as the object approaches the magnet, and this is especially important in relation to the stronger magnets.

The strong magnetic field can also affect internal implants and is especially dangerous for people with cardiac pacemakers who should never enter an MRI room because of the potential for serious cardiac arrhythmias that can result from the effect of the magnetic field on the pacemaker. Metal shards in the cornea can also be affected by the magnet and can move within the cornea, causing ocular damage.

The changing magnetic gradients produced by high-field magnets can be quite loud. Any personnel who remain in the scan room during the examination should wear protective equipment to prevent hearing damage.

Patient Preparation

Horseshoes should be removed before the examination to eliminate the risk of potential magnetic attraction. If the foot or pastern region is to be examined, radiographic images of the foot should be obtained to ensure that all nail fragments and as much residual rust is removed as possible because these will both cause artifacts in the images.

For images requiring general anesthesia, appropriate preparations should be carried out. After induction to anesthesia but before entering the scan room, any metal objects (such as halters) should be removed from the horse. A specialized, nonferromagnetic table must be used to support the horse during the examination. After the horse is positioned in the bore of the magnet, it must remain completely motionless during image acquisition to prevent blurring of the image.

Because MRI examinations typically take between 1 and 2 hours, urinary catheterization or some other means of urine collection is recommended to protect the equipment from contamination with fluid.

Use of Magnetic Resonance Imaging in Equine Practice

Because an MRI examination of one region takes between 1 and 2 hours, it is extremely important for the region of interest be localized as specifically as possible because it is not feasible to examine an entire limb. MRI has proven particularly useful in areas that are not amenable to examination using other diagnostic imaging modalities, such as the equine foot. Navicular disease has long been classified as a group of clinical signs and typical responses to diagnostic local anesthesia. With the use of MRI,

the diversity of problems associated with this syndrome has been considerably better defined to include tendonitis of the deep digital flexor tendon, inflammation or sclerosis of the navicular bone itself or inflammation of the supporting ligaments of the navicular bone. The optimal treatment for each of these problems is not the same, so more specific diagnosis now leads to more specific treatment.

Identifying specific cause of lameness at earlier stages is possible with MRI: cartilage and subchondral bone damage have been demonstrated. The character and location of sinus disease can be defined much more accurately than with radiographic images, aiding in surgical planning. Imaging of the brain is essentially impossible without MRI or CT because the brain is a soft tissue structure encased in a bony housing, and ultrasound waves are unable to penetrate the bone while radiography is insensitive to soft tissue problems. MRI has also assisted in the diagnosis of masses, hemorrhage, and inflammation in the brain.

References and Further Reading

Bassage II, L. H., and M. W. Ross. 2003. Diagnostic analgesia. In *Diagnosis and Management of Lameness in the Horse*, ed., M. W. Ross and S. J. Dyson, 93–124. Philadelphia: W. B. Saunders.

Brant, W. E. 2007. Diagnostic imaging methods. In *Fundamentals of Diagnostic Radiology*, 3rd ed., ed. W. E. Brant and C. A. Helms, 3–25. Philadelphia: Lippincott Williams and Wilkins.

Bushberg, J. T., and E. M. Leidholdt Jr. 2003. Radiation protection. In *Diagnostic Nuclear Medicine*, 4th ed., ed. M. P. Sandler, R. E. Coleman, J. A. Patton, F. J. Wackers, and A. Gottschalk, 133–63. Philadelphia: Lippincott Williams & Wilkins.

Butler, J. A., C. M. Colles, S. J. Dyson, S. Kold, and P. Poulos. 2000. *Clinical Radiology of the Horse*, 2nd ed. Boston: Blackwell Publishers.

Day, T. K., and R. T. Skarda. 1991. The pharmacology of local anesthetics. *Vet Clin North Am Equine Pract* 7:489–500.

Dyson, S. J., R. C. Pilsworth, A. R. Twardlock, and M. J. Martinelli. 2003. *Equine Scintigraphy.* Newmarket, England: Equine Veterinary Journal.

Ferrell, E. A., P. R. Gavin, R. L. Tucker, D. C. Sellon, and M. T. Hines. 2002. Magnetic resonance for evaluation of neurologic disease in 12 horses. *Vet Radiol Ultrasound* 43:510–16.

Hague, B. A., C. M. Honnas, R. B. Simpson, and J. G. Peloso. 1997. Evaluation of skin bacterial flora before and after aseptic preparation of clipped and nonclipped arthrocentesis sites in horses. *Vet Surg* 26:121–25.

Kraft, S. L., and P. Gavin. 2001. Physical principles and technical considerations for equine computed tomography and magnetic resonance imaging. *Vet Clin North Am Equine Pract* 17:115–30, vii.

Grainger, R. G., D. Allison, A. Adam, and A. K. Dixon. 2001. *Grainger & Allison's Diagnostic Radiology: A Textbook of Medical Imaging*, vol 1. 4th ed. London: Churchill Livingston.

Novelline, R. A. 2004. *Squire's Fundamentals of Radiology*, 6th ed. Cambridge: Harvard Univeristy Press.

Nyland, T. G., J. S. Mattoon, and E. R. Wisner. 1995. Physical principles, instrumentation, and safety of diagnostic ultrasound. In *Veterinary Diagnostic Ultrasound*, ed. T. G. Nyland and J. S. Matton, 3–18. Philadelphia: W. B. Saunders.

Percuoco, R. Plain radiographic imaging. 2005. In *Clinical Imaging*, 2nd ed., ed. D. M. Marchiori, 3–42. St. Louis: Mosby.

Rantanen, N. W., and A. O. McKinnon. 1998. *Equine Diagnostic Ultrasonography*. Baltimore: Williams & Wilkins.

Puchalski, S. M. 2007. Computed tomography in equine practice. *Equine Vet Educ* 19:207–9.

Reef, V. B. 1998. *Equine Diagnostic Ultrasound*. Philadelphia: W. B. Saunders Company.

Stashak, T. S. 2002. Examination for lameness. In *Adams' Lameness in Horses*, 5th ed., ed. T. S. Stashak, 113–83. Philadelphia: Lippincott Williams & Wilkins.

Thrall, D. E. 1994. *Textbook of Veterinary Diagnostic Radiology*, 2nd ed. Philadelphia: W. B. Saunders.

Weissleder, R., J, Wittenberg, M. Harisinghani M. 2007. *Primer of Diagnostic Imaging*, 4th ed. Philadelphia: Mosby.

Westbrook, C., C. K. Roth, and J. Talbot. 1998. *MRI in Practice*, 3rd ed. Boston: Blackwell Publishers.

Widmer, W. R. 2008. Acquisition hardware for digital imaging. *Vet Radiol Ultrasound* 49: S2–S8.

Zubrod, C. J., K. D. Farnsworth, and J. L. Oaks. 2004. Evaluation of arthrocentesis site bacterial flora before and after 4 methods of preparation in horses with and without evidence of skin contamination. *Vet Surg* 33:525–30.

CHAPTER 14

Common Equine Medical Emergencies

Michael Porter

Colic

Colic is defined as abdominal pain in the horse. Colic represents the most common and important medical problem of domesticated horses. There are four basic mechanisms that cause abdominal pain: gas distension of a viscus, pulling on the root of the mesentery, ischemia, and inflammation of the gastrointestinal (GI) tract.

Clinical Signs of Colic

Clinical signs of colic in the horse can be subtle, such as anorexia, depression, or decreased manure output. Obvious symptoms of colic include pawing, flank watching, repeated posturing to urinate ("parking out"), prolonged recumbency, rolling, flehmen response, and abdominal distension (Figure 14.1). Clinical signs of colic usually reflect a problem within the GI tract. There are horses that display symptoms of colic when the pain is originating from outside the abdominal cavity. For instance, a horse with pleural pneumonia can have significant thoracic pain that will mimic symptoms of colic. A horse that has severe foot pain associated with laminitis may be recumbent for excessive periods of time and be mistaken to have colic. Rarely neurologic diseases, such as rabies, may cause colic behavior.

Specific Types of Colic

The most common causes of abdominal pain in the horse are gas distension, impaction, or spasmodic colic. These conditions usually respond to pain management and correction of dehydration. There are a variety of lesions that can cause colic in the horse. A complete review of colic can be found in other texts. The major problems can be categorized by location within the GI tract (Table 14.1).

Colic associated with the stomach could include gastric impactions, gastric ulcerations, and rarely, gastritis (Figure 14.2). Any cause of pain within the GI tract can result in ileus. Ileus is the lack of intestinal peristalsis. The intestine is no longer motile, and a large quantity of fluid may accumulate within the stomach. A distended stomach can cause severe pain even though another problem may be the primary cause of the colic episode. Horses are unable to vomit, putting them at risk of gastric rupture from excessive fluid accumulation. For this reason every colic evaluation should include passage of a nasogastric tube to check for gastric reflux. If net gastric reflux is present, it must be determined if the reflux is the result of a primary problem with the small intestine or secondary to ileus of the GI tract. If the small intestine is blocked with a feed impaction or twisted as in a small

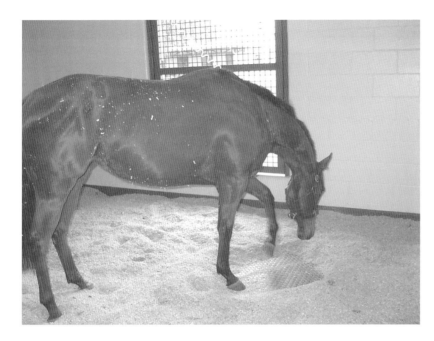

Figure 14.1. Horse with colic. Courtesy Dr. Chris Sanchez.

intestine volvulus, fluid will accumulate proximal to the obstruction.

Horses with a large colon lesion, such as a large colon volvulus, may appear bloated. A rectal examination can determine if the abdominal distension is caused by gas or an impaction of the large colon. Abnormal placement of the colon can determine if a colonic displacement is present.

Other sources of abdominal pain outside of the GI tract include generalized peritonitis, urogenital tract obstruction, and liver disease. Causes of colic associated with these organs include cholelithiasis, hepatic abscessation, nephroliths, and urinary bladder calculi.

Diagnosis of Colic

Clinical evaluation of horses with colic involves a complete history, physical examination, passage of a nasogastric tube, and a rectal examination. Recur-

rent or severe pain indicates the horse may need intensive nursing care and advanced diagnostic evaluation.

History

Collection of an accurate and thorough history is the first step toward determining the cause for the colic behavior. The history can determine the urgency with which to start therapy. Important questions are:

1. How painful is the horse?
2. What has been the horse's activity the past 24 hours?
3. How long has the horse been demonstrating signs of colic?
4. Does the horse have a fever?
5. Does the horse appear bloated?
6. Is the horse passing feces? Any diarrhea?
7. What is the horse's deworming history?
8. When was the horse's teeth last floated?
9. What does the horse eat? Any recent changes?

Table 14.1. Common lesions in horses with colic.

Stomach	Cecum/colon
Gastric ulceration	Cecal impaction
Gastric impaction	Pelvic flexure impaction
Gastritis	Small colon impaction
Neoplasia	Enterolith
	Right dorsal displacement
Small intestine	Left dorsal displacement
Duodenitis-proximal jejunitis	Large colon volvulus
Ileal impaction	Ceco-colic intussception
Strangulating volvulus	Colitis
Strangulating lipoma	Parasites
Intusseption	
Inflammatory bowel disease	
Epiploic foramen entrapment	
Mesenteric rent	
Thromboembolic	
Ascarid impaction	

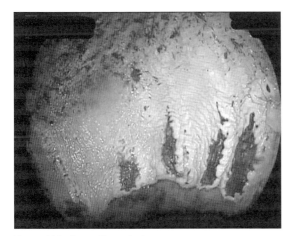

Figure 14.2. Horse with gastric ulcers.
Courtesy Dr. Michael Porter.

Physical Examination

The initial physical examination should include heart rate, respiratory rate, capillary refill time (CRT), mucous membrane color, rectal temperature, GI motility, assessment of hydration, and a evaluation of the horse's pain level. There is no other single physical examination parameter that provides as much information as the heart rate. An elevated heart rate (tachycardia) may be caused by pain, excitement, dehydration, severe blood loss, heart failure, or endotoxemia. The heart rate should be ausculted for 15 to 30 seconds to calculate the beats per minute (bpm). A slight elevation in heart rate (48–55 bpm) may imply mild pain. An elevated heart rate (90–120 bpm) suggests a serious medical condition. *The urgency with which to respond and treat a horse with colic is positively correlated with the degree of tachycardia.* Irrespective of the cause a horse with a heart rate greater than 60 bpm should receive aggressive medical care. In addition to tachycardia, a prolonged CRT (>2 seconds) is indicative of significant systemic disruption. Common causes of a prolonged CRT include hypovolemia, dehydration, endotoxemia, and sepsis. A CRT of greater than 4 seconds suggests impending cardiovascular collapse. The normal mucous membrane color is pink. Dark pink or red mucous membranes can indicate severe dehydration and endotoxemia. Elevation in respiratory rate (tachypnea) may indicate pain, pyrexia, respiratory disease, and excitement. Compared to tachycardia, tachypnea is not as consistent an indicator of pain. A painful horse with significant tachypnea that does not show any obvious GI disruption should be evaluated for respiratory disease. An elevated rectal temperature indicates an inflammatory or infectious process. Occasionally a fever may indicate hyperthermia secondary to physical activity or anhidrosis (non-sweater). The most common causes of colic in horses with a fever are peritonitis, enteritis, or colitis. GI motility can be described as either being present or absent. The absence of gut sounds is significantly more important than the intensity, frequency, or loudness of gut sounds.

Passage of a nasogastric tube and a rectal examination are commonly performed when evaluating a horse with colic. The goal of the rectal examination is to determine if there is gas distension, an impaction, or abnormal placement of the intestine. In a normal horse, the small intestine cannot be palpated because it is located in the cranial abdomen. If small intestine is felt on a rectal examination it is considered a significant finding. In addition, palpation of tight bands of the large colon can indicate a displacement or volvulus. It is important to understand that a rectal examination may not determine the diagnosis. The veterinarian can only palpate the caudle one-third of the abdomen potentially missing a problem. For this reason, the rectal examination provides additional information on the possible cause of colic but may not provide the exact diagnosis. If the horse is painful or the colic episode is prolonged, advanced diagnostics performed are a complete blood count, chemistry panel, venous blood gas, abdominocentesis, and abdominal ultrasound.

The purpose of a complete blood count is to monitor for anemia and to determine if severe infection or inflammation is present. Horses with a heavy parasite load or that have internal bleeding may be anemic. Horses with colitis or enteritis often have a low white blood cell count. These parameters can help differentiate the type of colic.

The goal of performing a chemistry panel is to evaluate electrolytes and renal and liver function. Electrolytes are often deranged if the horse has colitis. Lactating mares may develop low calcium that can cause colic. Renal evaluation is important as dehydration is a common component to colic. The use of hypotensive medications and nonsteroidal anti-inflammatories are common to control pain in horses with colic. These medications can adversely affect the kidneys, further justifying the use of fluids in horses with colic.

A venous blood gas is critical for horses with severe abdominal pain. The purpose of performing a venous blood gas is to evaluate the acid-base status of the horse. Profoundly dehydrated horses will suffer from severe lactic acidosis. This test can immediately evaluate the patient's status and allow for quick and aggressive treatment.

An abdominocentesis is used to evaluate the free fluid in the abdomen. It can determine if the bowel is ischemic by the change in color from yellow to red. Strangulation of intestine will result in an elevated white blood cell count and total protein in the abdominal fluid. This test will help narrow the diagnosis (Figure 14.3).

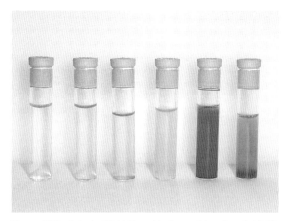

Figure 14.3. Abdominal fluid. Normal is clear to light yellow. Red fluid represents increased red blood cells from ischemic bowel or blood contamination during the procedure.
Courtesy Dr. Michael Porter.

Abdominal ultrasound is another tool used to evaluate the abdomen. This diagnostic test is helpful to investigate the abdomen that can not be reached by rectal palpation. The goal of abdominal ultrasound is to look for evidence of thickening of the intestine that occurs from inflammatory diseases (colitis) or edema from strangulating lesions. The kidney, liver, and spleen can be visualized and ruled out as a potential cause of colic.

Treatment of Colic

The treatment for horses with colic includes pain management and correcting dehydration. In severe cases of colic, treatment for endotoxemia and surgery may be warranted. The first basic principle for pain management includes decompression of a distended viscus, which relieves pain and promotes motility. Gastric distention is the most common cause of distension and is easily relieved by passage of a nasogastric tube. Gastric rupture can occur despite the presence of an indwelling stomach tube unless frequent siphoning is performed. Walking horses for short periods of time (15–30 minutes) can help eliminate mild gas discomfort. Excessive walking is contraindicated because it worsens dehydration and exhausts the horse.

Common drugs used for pain management include nonsteroidal anti-inflammatory drugs (NSAIDs), α_2-agonists (e.g., xylazine, detomidine, and romifidine), and opiates (butorphanol). Flunixin meglumine is the current drug of choice for treatment of colic in horses. When flunixin is administered intravenously, the time of onset of action is approximately 20 minutes but can be up to 2 hours. The duration of action is 8 to 12 hours. When given intramuscularly, the time of onset of pain relief is prolonged and the level of analgesia does not appear to be clinically the same. One treatment of flunixin is typically all that is needed for most episodes of colic. Recurrent signs of colic, such as lying down, stretching out and flank watching, *after* administration of flunixin indicate that a more serious problem may be present. Persistent elevation in the heart rate and respiratory rate provides subtle clues that additional diagnostics and therapy is warranted. Most horses with surgical lesions will become painful despite administration of flunixin; however, the clinical signs may be muted compared to the initial display of pain. NSAIDs should not be administered more often than every 8 to 12 hours. Excessive administration of NSAIDs may result in GI ulceration or renal disease and can mask ongoing signs of colic. In addition to NSAIDs, an antispasmodic drug called Buscapan is commonly used to treat horses with colic.

For immediate relief of severe abdominal pain, α_2-adrenergic agonists provide excellent analgesia, sedation, and muscle relaxation. These drugs provide more potent analgesia, and the onset of action is more rapid compared to NSAIDs. Xylazine has a short duration of action (20–60 minutes), which is preferred for the initial examination. Detomidine is 100 times more potent than xylazine and lasts 40 to 120 minutes. The major side effects of α_2-adrenergic agonists are transient hypertension followed by hypotension, bradycardia, and ileus. When several doses are administered to control pain, it is prudent to monitor vital signs frequently and provide fluid therapy for cardiovascular support. The hypotension and ileus effects last longer than the sedation and analgesia effects. Using the lowest dose necessary to control pain and

combining α_2-adrenergic agonists with opioids can minimize ileus and hypotension.

Assessment of the patient's hydration status is relatively subjective; however, it can be precise enough to predict the appropriate fluid therapy. A horse that is greater than 12% dehydrated is typically in cardiovascular collapse and may be near death. In contrast a horse that is less than 5% dehydrated may have a normal heart rate and show no signs of distress. Determining how dehydrated the patient is depends on hear rate, CRT, skin tenting, and known fluid losses (e.g., diarrhea, gastric reflux). A significantly elevated heart rate along with a prolonged CRT is highly suggestive of 7% to 10% dehydration, whereas a mild increase in heart rate and a normal CRT may only indicate 5% dehydration. Identifying significant fluid losses such as those in exhausted horses (endurance athletes) or horses with diarrhea or gastric reflux is critical for predicting the level of dehydration. Mild dehydration is treated with oral fluids. Severe dehydration requires intravenous fluids. Additional treatments may be administered through the nasogastric tube, such as mineral oil for treatment of impactions.

Most horses with colic can be treated with pain medication and fluid therapy. A small percentage of horses will develop surgical lesions. The prognosis for survival from colic surgery depends on the specific lesion and the duration of the colic. The age and physical condition of the horse will impact the prognosis. The most common complications from colic surgery are incisional infections, abdominal adhesions, and endotoxemia.

The key to successful treatment of colic is early intervention. Investigation of the cause of colic should include evaluation of the feed and management on the farm. A good deworming program, regular dental care, and exercise are the best practices to prevent colic in the horse.

Exhausted Horse Syndrome

Dehydrated patients are at risk for developing signs of colic due to the loss of essential electrolytes and minerals. Normal gut motility is dependent on a multitude of factors, especially serum levels of calcium. During extended strenuous work, horses tend to lose significant amounts of calcium plus sodium. The most common example is the endurance horse that has completed 35, 55, or 100 miles of competition over a 12- to 24-hour period. These horses often lose >10% of body weight during the competition and tend to become depleted of calcium, electrolytes, and total body water. This often results in a decline in GI motility or ileus. Ileus is one component of the "exhausted horse syndrome." On initial examination these horses will be depressed, painful (colic), and may be experiencing diaphragmatic flutter (thumps). These patients are critically ill and need aggressive intravenous fluid therapy plus constant decompression of the stomach.

Rhabdomyolysis

Exertional rhabdomyolysis or "tying up" is a disease causing severe pain associated with muscle cramping and breakdown of muscle tissue. The common clinical signs are a stiff or stilted gait. Some horses may refuse to move. The horses will have elevated heart rates and may sweat profusely from pain. The breakdown of muscle pigment can result in renal failure, and the urine will be dark red in color (Figure 14.4). This syndrome can occur in athletic

horses during a long competition, racehorses, or an unfit horse ridden extremely hard. Careful palpation of the gluteal, semimembranous, and semitendinous areas identifies firm painful muscle tissue. The early identification of horses that are tying up is critical for proper treatment. These patients are at risk of developing fatal renal failure if not treated properly. The treatment plan includes analgesia, aggressive fluid therapy, and monitoring renal function.

Choke

Choke is a common medical emergency in equine practice. In humans "choke" refers to obstruction of the airway. In horses choke is an obstruction of the esophagus. The most common causes of esophageal obstruction are hay, pellets, cubes, and foreign bodies, such as apples or potatoes (Figure 14.5). Choke occurs when a horse rapidly eats pellets without adequate chewing. Most obstructions occur proximally in the esophagus. Rarely the obstruction may be at the thoracic inlet. Less common precipitating causes of choke include esophageal diverticulum, intramural esophageal cyst, tumor, abscess, or stricture from prior esophageal injury.

Clinical signs of choke include distress, head extension, salivation, and nasal discharge

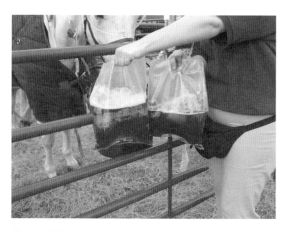

Figure 14.4. Urine from an endurance horse that is dehydrated and "tying up." The red color of the urine is due to myoglobin. Courtesy Dr. Michael Porter.

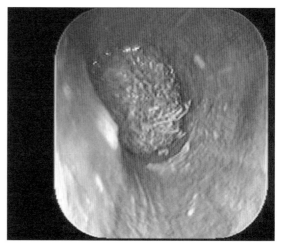

Figure 14.5. Endoscopic view of esophageal choke. Courtesy Dr. Guy Lester.

containing feed particles. If the horse has been choked for several hours, they can be depressed and dehydrated. Occasionally the obstruction in the esophagus is palpated externally. Secondary complications from choke include aspiration pneumonia (fever, abnormal lung auscultation) or esophageal rupture (with or without subcutaneous emphysema and crepitus).

Diagnosis is based on history and clinical signs and is confirmed by failure to pass a stomach tube. Endoscopy or radiography (plain and contrast) is helpful in identifying feed type and if underlying anatomic disease is present.

Treatment is successful in horses that have been choked for less than 48 hours, assuming there are no underlying anatomical defects. Sedation with xylazine will aid in restraint and cause the head to be lowered, reducing the risk of aspiration. Gentle passage of a stomach tube and lubrication with warm water will resolve most cases. If conservative lavage does not alleviate the choke, it is best to treat the horse for 12 to 24 hours with intravenous fluid therapy, NSAIDs, antibiotics, and mild sedation to keep the head low and reduce the risk of aspiration pneumonia. Most horse with choke will resolve with this treatment. The last option is to remove the obstruction surgically, but this increases the risk of esophageal stricture and fistula formation. If the esophageal mucosa is damaged then healing may reduce the size of the lumen, predisposing the horse to repeated episodes of choke.

Prevention

If the horse is an aggressive eater and "bolts" the feed, placing large stones in the feed tub will discourage this behavior. Evaluation of the teeth should always be considered in cases of choke. A painful tooth or irregular grinding surface may be the cause of the inadequately chewed hay bolus. Feeding hay cubes soaked in water can minimize the incidence of choke.

Lacerations

Soft tissue lacerations may represent the second most common equine emergency. Successful man-

Table 14.2. Management of lacerations.

1. Lavage the wound with copious cold water (low pressure).
   - Wash for 20 to 30 minutes.
   - Remove the hair along the borders of the laceration with clippers.
2. Disinfect the wound with gentle scrubbing.
   - Use dilute chlorhexidine or Betadine solution.
3. Primary closure:
   - For multiple level closure, use monofilament absorbable suture.
   - For skin closure, use monofilament nonabsorbable suture or staples.
4. Secondary closure:
   - Daily wound management.
   - Topical medication plus bandaging.
   - Proud flesh management.
5. Wound bandaging:
   - Wet-to-dry bandages.
   - Change bandages daily.

agement of lacerations depends on accurate assessment of the injury, thorough cleaning of the affected area, appropriate treatment of the wound, and follow-up care (Table 14.2).

Assessment of Wounds

Assessment of a laceration involves determining the age of the wound, what caused the laceration, and how much tissue damage has occurred. It may be necessary to sedate the horse to thoroughly examine the wound. It can be difficult determine when a laceration occurred unless it was witnessed. An approximate time frame can be calculated based on when was the last time the horse was seen without the injury. This information is important when determining if primary closure of a laceration is reasonable. Primary closure is defined as the closure of a lesion using sutures or staples. Suturing a wound greater than 24 hours old is unlikely to heal well due to excessive contamination. If the laceration is not properly cleaned before closure, it may still result in dehiscence (Figure 14.6). An injury caused by wood as opposed to metal is going to be more difficult to thoroughly clean and may result in future surgical explorations to remove splinters left behind.

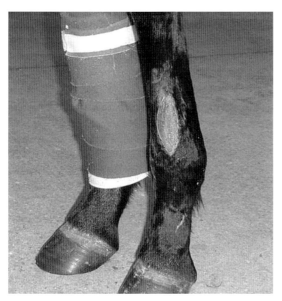

Figure 14.6. Laceration of a horse's leg. The wound will heal by secondary intention.
Courtesy of Dr. Dana Zimmel.

Cleaning Wounds

The most critical part of managing a laceration is thoroughly lavaging the wound immediately after it is discovered. Lavaging of the wound can be accomplished with cold water from a water hose under low pressure. An added benefit of cold water therapy is that it can provide pain relief from the injury. If the wound is near a joint or tendon sheath, sterile fluids should be used to clean the area. After thoroughly lavaging the wound with water the laceration may be gently cleaned with a dilute disinfectant such as chlorhexidine or betadine. Rubbing alcohol is not recommended or is any product that contains ethyl alcohol. Hydrogen peroxide is a good solution to clean a puncture wound of the foot. Hydrogen peroxide should not be applied to lacerations of the skin because it will cause the hair to grow back white, leaving an obvious scar. Gentle scrubbing of the laceration surface should cause slight bleeding. If the tissues are not bleeding, they may require surgical debridement back to more vital tissues before closure.

Compared to lacerations, puncture wounds should not be closed regardless of when they occurred. Puncture wounds created by another animal's bite tend to be highly contaminated with bacteria and will become abscesses if the puncture site is closed. More time should be spent cleansing the puncture wounds with dilute antibacterial solution. After thoroughly lavaging the puncture wound sterile packing material can be introduced and replaced daily.

In addition to determining what caused the wound, deciding what tissues are involved will impact the treatment plan. Any laceration that is near an articular surface or a tendon sheath requires careful examination to determine if the joint or tendon sheath has been penetrated. It is not uncommon for simple lacerations to become infected and subsequently seed underlying joint spaces with bacterial contamination. A laceration should be examined for any damage to surrounding structures such as veins, arteries, nerves, tendons, and ligaments.

Treatment of Wounds

Closure of lacerations can be accomplished with primary closure or via secondary intention. Adequate primary closure involves bringing the tissue edges together such that the skin layer is under minimal tension. In some cases the wound or laceration is too wide for primary closure and the injury heals via second intention (Figure 14.7). Primary closure often requires closing the deep layers independent of the skin layer and reducing the tension by undermining the tissue edges. Any suture that is below the skin layer should be a monofilament, absorbable suture. Material used for skin closure should be monofilament, nonabsorbable, or stainless steel staples. If there is excessive tension on the skin closure, it is likely that the skin closure will fail or result in scar formation.

After deciding how to close the wound the next step is to determine what kind of bandage will enhance the likelihood of a successful outcome. Important concepts to consider include what type

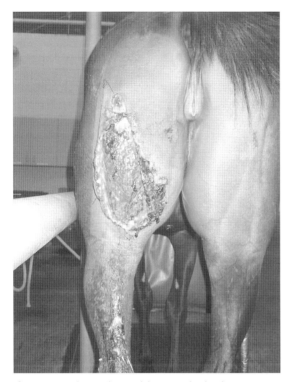

Figure 14.7. A large wide wound that cannot be closed via primary closure.
Courtesy of Dr. Michael Porter.

of bandaging material, proper placement of bandage material, and how often to change the bandage. The basic idea is to provide a bandage that will be a wick or "wet-to-dry" bandage. These types of bandages will absorb the discharge and keep the wound site clean and dry. To achieve a wet-to-dry bandage, adequate layers of material are necessary. A perfect example of a wicking bandage is a human diaper. Diapers come in a variety of sizes, shapes, and absorptive capabilities. Alternatively bandages with several layers of absorptive material can be created using stacks of 4 × 4 sponges, laparotomy sponges, or multiple layers of sheet cotton. A second advantage to using wet-to-dry bandages is that they tend to provide significant padding, which reduces the likelihood of applying a bandage that is too tight. Waterproof material may be ideal for the final layer (outside layer) to prevent contamina-

tion from the environment. Care must be taken using waterproof material because these materials typically do not stretch or expand.

Proper application and management of the bandage is of utmost importance. The bandage needs to be on tight enough to prevent it from moving out of position and help reduce tissue edema. If the bandage is too tight, venous return, or more importantly, arterial supply may be compromised resulting in decreased blood flow to the limb and tissue death. The amount of inflammation underneath the bandage may either increase or decrease significantly from day to day; hence, it is critical that bandages be changed daily to keep the wound clean and make sure that the bandages are properly applied. If the bandages become too loose, inappropriate pressure can injure the limb. Application of even padding and thickness of wraps is critical to avoid creating a "bandage bow" or worse an ischemic limb.

The final step in management of lacerations is formulating a systemic treatment plan. It is recommended to treat horses with lacerations or wounds with NSAIDs for several days to reduce pain and inflammation. Antibiotic therapy may be indicated for some injuries. If the wound is directly over or near a joint surface or a tendon sheath the horse should be treated with systemic antibiotic therapy. Too often these types of wounds are only managed topically for several days until the wound scabs over. If the tissue deep to the surface continues to harbor bacteria the septic process may work itself into nearby articular surfaces. As a result, the horse suddenly becomes severely lame from a septic joint. Treatment of a septic joint can be expensive and the prognosis for athletic performance can be poor. Despite aggressive medical and surgical treatment of septic injuries the horse may remain chronically painful and euthanasia may be necessary.

Bandages for Emergencies

Bandages are used to stop bleeding, apply medication to wounds, protect incisions, keep a wound clean, and minimize edema. There are several types of bandage material available that can be applied to a variety of conditions. Most bandages are composed of three layers. The most common bandages used in equine practices are standing bandages, Robert Jones (RJ) bandages, and foot bandages.

Standing bandages are used for a variety of practical purposes. A thick fleece, quilt, or sheet cotton is applied to the limb in a counterclockwise direction on the left legs and a clockwise direction on the right legs. The quilt should be smooth and no wrinkles should be present. The quilt is secured with a standing bandage or vet wrap applied in a spiral fashion overlapping half of the previous wrap. Even tension is applied over the entire limb to minimize the risk of damaging the tendons. There should always be a portion of the quilt exposed above and below the application of the vet wrap to ensure equal pressure is disturbed under the bandage (Figure 14.8).

A RJ bandage is a multilayer bandage that can be applied to any portion of the limb from the hoof to the elbow or stifle. It is most commonly used when a horse has a fracture or major soft tissue injury. Usually the bandage is composed of heavy cotton, brown gauze, and vet wrap (Figure 14.9). A modified RJ can use sheet cotton instead of heavy roll cotton, making the bandage lighter. This maybe more appropriate for horses with severe cellulitis and edema of the limbs.

A foot bandage is commonly used in equine practice when a horse has a puncture wound to the foot, foot abscess, or a hoof injury. Thick sheet cotton or a diaper can be used for the first layer. Brown gauze is applied in a figure-eight pattern around the hoof (Figure 14.10). Vet wrap is applied over the brown gauze in a similar fashion. To make the bandage impervious to water, a duct tape patch is applied over the bottom of the bandage.

Splints are used to help stabilize a fracture of the distal limb. They can be made from a variety of materials such as wood and PVC pipe. There is a metal splint designed primarily for use on a front leg called a Kimzey Leg Saver Splint. The same company does make a special metal splint for the hind limb. The Kimzey splint is best used for severe injuries on the racetrack including fractures of the

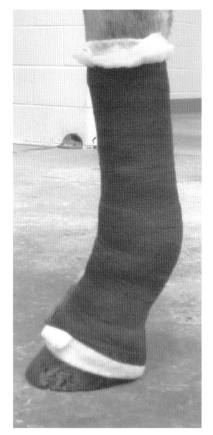

Figure 14.8. Standing bandage. Courtesy of Dr. Dana Zimmel.

sesamoids, fractures of the long and short pastern bones, fractures of the cannon bone, and failure of the suspensory ligament system.

Sudden Non–Weight-Bearing Lameness

A classic equine emergency call is for a horse that was normal yesterday and is now non–weight-bearing lame on a single leg. This type of lameness has been described as "three-legged lame," "fracture lame," or "5 out of 5 lame." There are several likely causes for such sudden, severe lameness that include a subsolar foot abscess, a fracture, infected joint, infected tendon sheath, or acute laminitis. The most common cause of sudden lameness is subsolar foot abscess. Foot abscesses develop

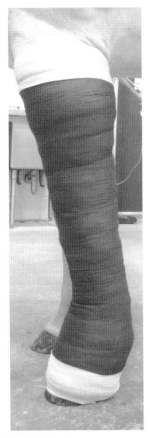

Figure 14.9. Robert Jones bandage.
Courtesy of Dr. Dana Zimmel.

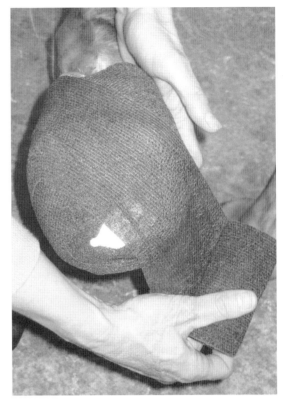

Figure 14.10. Foot bandage.
Courtesy of Dr. Dana Zimmel.

secondary to trauma to the foot (sole bruise), improperly placed shoe nails, and chronic laminitis. As a result of hemorrhage (bruising) or the accumulation of purulent debris, severe pressure develops within the hoof capsule resulting in crippling lameness. Until the pressure is relieved by the expulsion of the purulent debris the horse will remain non–weight-bearing lame on that limb. Horses with a hoof abscess can have an elevated heart rate and refuse to place any weight on the affected limb. They may be hypersensitive to touch along the entire limb and have edema surrounding the pastern, fetlock, and distal canon bone of that limb. An important physical examination finding is the detection of "bounding" digital pulses.

Digital pulses can be detected in normal horses and correspond the arterial supply to the foot at the level of the fetlock or pastern. During periods of significant inflammation of the foot, these pulses become more readily detected and can be described as bounding. Confirmation of the foot's involvement may only need application of pressure along the sole with fingers or hoof testers. In some cases, a peripheral nerve block may be required to confirm the location of pain and allow examination of the foot. Diagnostic radiology of the foot is an effective way to diagnose subsolar abscessation. If the horse is shod, the shoes should be removed since the nails or the shoe itself may be contributing to or be the source of pain. The abscess may erupt along the sole-hoof wall margin or in drainage along the coronary band (Figure 4.11). Those abscesses that erupt along the sole hoof wall

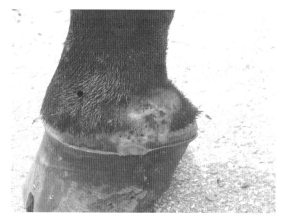

Figure 14.11. Foot abscess rupture at the coronary band of a horse (gravel).
Courtesy of Dr. Michael Porter.

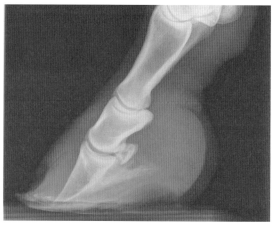

Figure 14.12. Radiograph of a horse's foot with significant ventral rotation of the coffin bone due to chronic laminitis.
Courtesy of Dr. Michael Porter.

margin typically resolve quicker and the process may be hastened by soaking the feet in warm Epson salt solution for 20 to 30 minutes per day. A variety of products are available to "pack" the foot that help in softening the sole and hastening abscess drainage. The veterinarian may choose to carefully explore the sole for the presence of a subsolar abscess with a hoof knife. If a draining tract is identified, the tract is followed to expose the deep pocket of purulent debris. Due to the significant pain and inflammation these patients benefit from NSAIDs treatment until the abscess has resolved. Once drainage is established most horses return to full soundness within a short period of time. If the abscess has drained and the horse remains lame or becomes lamer, additional diagnostics such as radiographs are indicated. Depending on the size of the subsolar abscess, a specialized shoe called a hospital plate may be necessary to keep the draining tract clean and reduce sole contact with the ground.

Occasionally sudden lameness is due to a fractured bone. The third phalanx or coffin bone is the most likely structure to be fractured. The second phalanx (short pastern bone) and the first phalanx (long pastern bone) may also be fractured resulting in sudden lameness. Care must be taken when

evaluating a possible fracture because anesthesia of the distal limb may result in a *nondisplaced* fracture becoming a catastrophic *displaced* fracture. Accurate diagnosis of a fracture requires diagnostic radiographs. Once the diagnosis has been confirmed consultation with a surgeon and farrier is indicated.

There is an increasing population of older horses that are overweight and suffer from recurrent episodes of laminitis. Laminitis also known as "founder" can be defined as inflammation and damage of the sensitive laminae of the hooves. The cause of the laminitis is multifactorial and in these patients it is believed to be associated with a state of insulin resistance and subsequent inability to properly manage blood sugar levels. This medical condition has been termed *metabolic syndrome*. Regardless of the initial cause, once the first episode of laminitis has occurred these horses are predisposed to subsequent laminitic episodes and the development of subsolar abscesses. Managing these patients requires diagnostic radiographs, therapeutic shoeing, and serum biochemical analysis (Figure 14.12). Regardless of the cause for the sudden non–weight-bearing lameness there are several important steps to follow as highlighted in Table 14.3.

Table 14.3. How to manage acute non–weight-bearing lameness.

1. Limit the horse's activity to a heavily bedded stall. Deep sand is the most ideal bedding to provide foot support.
2. Provide nonsteroidal anti-inflammatory drug therapy. The most common drug used for lameness is phenylbutazone. Follow recommended dose.
3. Remove the shoes from the affected limb and the contralateral limb.
4. Perform diagnostic radiographs of the feet.
5. If an abscess is suspected or diagnosed, the foot will benefit from frequent soaks in Epson salt solutions and application of a clean bandage.
6. Reduce caloric intake of pelleted feed by 50%.

Ophthalmologic Emergencies

Any injury to the eye should be treated as an emergency. Eye injuries may include trauma to the soft tissue surrounding the eye, including the eye lids, skin, and bony orbit. More severe cases may involve trauma to the cornea (Figure 14.13). Inflammation of the cornea or internal components of the eye (anterior uveitis) may result in diffuse edema of the cornea (Figure 14.14).

Clinical signs of an eye injury are blepharospasm, tearing, pupil constriction, or conjunctivitis. All of these clinical signs indicate that the patient is in pain. The initial examination of the eye requires adequate sedation of the patient and peripheral nerve blocks of the muscles controlling eye movement and eyelid tone. The eye lid margins should be examined for lacerations that will require careful suturing. The eye should be lavaged thoroughly with eye wash to remove any debris or foreign particles that may be trapped below the eyelids or the nictitating membrane (third eyelid). The cornea should be stained with a fluorescein stain. Any excess stain should be lavaged with eye wash and the eye examined with a powerful light source. The slightest amount of green uptake is consistent with a corneal ulcer and requires aggressive management. A comprehensive list of ophthalmic diagnostics can be found in Chapter 11.

The most common eye injury is a corneal ulcer. Treatment of corneal ulcers involves topical antibiotics, topical anticollagenese solution (serum), topical atropine, systemic NSAIDs, and possibly

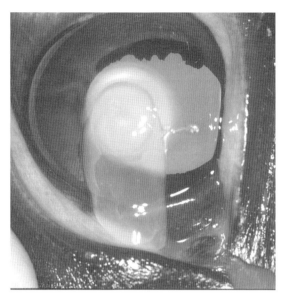

Figure 14.13. Rupture of the cornea due to severe corneal ulcer. Courtesy of Dr. Michael Porter.

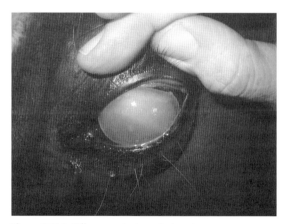

Figure 14.14. Diffuse corneal edema of a horse's eye. Courtesy of Dr. Michael Porter.

topical antifungals. The topical therapy should be administered three to six times per day until the eye stains negative. A subpalpebral lavage system can be inserted to allow for frequent medication of the eye. A small corneal ulcer may heal in 3 to 5 days. Severe infections, such as fungal keratitis, can require intensive treatments every 1 to 2 hours to preserve the eye.

A cloudy or opaque eye may be caused by glaucoma, anterior uveitis, stromal abscess, hyphema, or hypopyon. Although these ocular maladies may not stain positive for corneal ulceration, they are serious issues that require topical and systemic medication. In general, ophthalmologic emergencies should be considered quite serious, and the eye needs to be examined quickly by an experienced veterinarian.

References and Further Reading

Barnett, K. C., S. M. Crispin, J. D. Lavach, and A. G. Matthews. 1995. *Equine Ophthalmology*. Italy: Mosby-Wolfe.

Nixon, A. J. 1996. *Equine Fracture Repair*. Philadelphia: W. B. Saunders.

Orsini, J. A, and T. J. Divers. 2003. *Manual of Equine Emergencies*, 2nd ed. Philadelphia: Elsevier.

White, N. A. 1990. *The Equine Acute Abdomen*. Philadelphia: Lea & Febiger.

Equine Office Procedures

Deborah Reeder

The purpose of this chapter is to point out the differences one can encounter when working in or managing an equine office or practice. Basic descriptions of regulatory bodies are included as is a review of various practice types and their needs, including forms, staff, inventory management, scheduling of appointments, import and export regulations, differences in financial management, marketing and client communication, and education.

Regulations and Definitions

The practice of veterinary medicine is governed by a different veterinary practice act in each state. Each state has a Veterinary State Board that oversees and regulations regarding the practice of veterinary medicine. The American Association of Veterinary State Boards (AAVSB) is the national body that assists in administrating state boards. The American Veterinary Medical Association (AVMA) is the national association representing veterinarians, regardless of practice discipline. The AVMA has developed a model practice act that provides an example of what should be included and legislated and is available at www.avma.org/issues/policy/mvpa.asp. The practice of veterinary medicine is described in the AVMA Model Practice Act as:

"Practice of veterinary medicine" means:

a. To diagnose, treat, correct, change, alleviate, or prevent animal disease, illness, pain, deformity, defect, injury, or other physical, dental, or mental conditions by any method or mode, including:
   i. the prescription, dispensing, administration, or application of any drug, medicine, biologic, apparatus, anesthetic, or other therapeutic or diagnostic substance or medical or surgical technique, or
   ii. the use of complementary, alternative, and integrative therapies, or
   iii. the use of any manual or mechanical procedure for reproductive management, or
   iv. the rendering of advice or recommendation by any means including telephonic and other electronic communications with regard to any of the above.
b. To represent, directly or indirectly, publicly or privately, an ability and willingness to do an act described in subsection 19(a).
c. To use any title, words, abbreviation, or letters in a manner or under circumstances that induce the belief that the person using them is qualified to do any act described in subsection. (AVMA)

There are several terms used to describe the veterinary technician and assistant. The definition of a veterinary technician is defined in the AVMA Model Practice Act as: a graduate of a 2- or 3-year accredited program in veterinary technology. A veterinary technologist is a graduate of a 4-year accredited program in veterinary technology. A credentialed veterinary technician or technologist is a veterinary technician or veterinary technologist who is validly and currently registered, certified, or licensed by the Board. The Model Practice Act defines the practice of veterinary technology as:

a. To perform patient care or other services that require a technical understanding of veterinary medicine on the basis of written or oral instruction of a veterinarian, excluding diagnosing, prognosing, surgery, or prescribing drugs, medicine, or appliances.
b. To represent, directly or indirectly, publicly or privately, an ability and willingness to do an act described in subsection 20(a).
c. To use any title, words, abbreviation, or letters in a manner or under circumstances that induce the belief that the person using them is qualified to do any act described in subsection.

It is important to note that there is a difference between a credentialed veterinary technician and an assistant. Most credentialed veterinary technicians have gone through an AVMA-accredited program (usually 2–4 years) in veterinary technology and have passed the Veterinary Technology National Examination. They then receive a designation based on their individual state that can be licensed veterinary technician (LVT), registered veterinary technician (RVT), certified veterinary technician (CVT), or animal health technician (AHT). The role of a veterinary technician and assistant is defined by individual state law.

There are other important national regulatory bodies that govern how a veterinary practice is operated: the U.S. Department of Agriculture (USDA), which oversees the labeling of drugs, the inspection and movement of animals, and performs laboratory tests to assure the safety and health of animals; the Drug Enforcement Administration (DEA), which regulates how and which drugs are used in a veterinary practice; and the Radiation Safety Board, which ensures that the practice is using radiation equipment safely and staff is properly protected and educated. All of these regulatory bodies help to define how a veterinary practice is managed and which procedures need to be followed.

Every aspect of management of personnel is affected by or controlled by some form of law. There are laws regarding what you can and cannot ask on an employment interview, laws allowing for military and pregnancy leaves of absence, job protection, time off, exempt and non-exempt, employment at will, contract employees, hiring, and firing. Some of the regulatory agencies or laws you may deal with are:

The Immigration Reform and Control Act: requires employers to verify eligibility for employment in the United States;

Fair Labor Standards Act (FSLA): addresses minimum wage requirements, exempt and non-exempt, and independent contractors; (It is important to note here that the credentialed veterinary technician is considered a professional and by law [FLSA] falls under the category of non-exempt, meaning they are to be paid on an hourly basis unless they are in a supervisory role. Be sure to check with your state's Department of Labor for specifics.)

Equal Employment Opportunity Commission (EEOC): enforces laws regarding sexual harassment, pregnancy discrimination, Americans with disabilities, and age discrimination;

Family and Medical Leave Act (FMLA): entitles employees to leave for the birth of their child, care of a dependant for serious health reasons, or for a personal health condition;

Occupational Safety and Health Administration (OSHA): requires a place of employment to be free of recognized hazards and issues minimum safety standards to be met. It is a good practice to initiate OSHA procedures, identify potential problem areas, and seek their advice as to how to best to correct them. Material Safety Data Sheets should be accessible for all drugs and supplies. Eye wash stations should be installed wherever appropriate.

Workers Compensation, Unemployment Insurance, Pensions, and Employee Benefits are also benefits that all equine practices must provide regulated by both state and federal. Appropriate posters, warnings, and notices should be displayed at the practice headquarters.

Variations of Types of Equine Practice

Equine practices can be placed roughly in four categories or profiles:

1. Referral hospital.
2. Primary clinic.
3. Ambulatory/specialty.
4. Mixed practice.

The referral hospital has multiple doctors and usually includes boarded specialists in areas such as surgery, internal medicine, and reproduction. Internships and residencies are often offered. This type of practice could also be in the university setting. The referral practice may have a primary case load of its own but also receive other cases, which the primary care practice refers for a second opinion, or to provide additional care, which the primary practice decides is beyond its scope. An excellent working relationship between the primary and referral practices is essential if quality patient care is to be provided. The referral practice may designate centers of expertise within its scope, such as surgery, lameness, internal medicine, ambulatory, reproduction, or rehabilitation. A referral center may have the resources and the staff to offer the latest medical technology, such as digital imaging, magnetic resonance imaging (MRI), and scintigraphy, as well as specialized rehabilitation equipment including swimming pools, an Aqua Tread, or hyperbaric oxygen treatment (HBOT). The referral hospital may employ a practice administrator, as well as an office manager to supervise defined areas, such as data entry, front office reception, billing, human resources, and accounting. They may employ seasonal help, experience high turnover in staff, offer externships, and have a large and varied clientele and case load. Satellite facilities at different locations to support various venues, such as sport horse competitions or racing, may be a feature of such a large practice. The challenges with the operation of a referral hospital can be multiple and difficult.

The basic equine clinic will usually have fewer doctors (some of whom may have specialty training) and limited support staff and facilities for hospitalization of patients. The diagnostic and therapeutic modalities, which the practice offers, may be less extensive. The staff need is reduced but may include an office manager. Staff will often combine duties and are likely to be noted for their long service and loyalty. This practice may or may not offer 24-hour emergency coverage or intensive care for critical patients.

The ambulatory practice may consist of any number of veterinarians who practice "out of their trucks"; there is usually a central location where all supplies are stored, a pharmacy is maintained, and data entry and billing is done. This practice type may also apply to a specialist who travels to patients and provides a specific service, such as an ophthalmologist. Office and technical work are performed by limited staff whose duties often extend into both areas, and it is not unusual for the veterinarian to travel solo, do his or her own scheduling and billing, and rely on his or her clients to provide assistance in handling patients. The challenge for the practice staff can be time management with the "8-hour day" an unlikely common occurrence. Referral of patients for specialty or intensive care is not unusual.

The last profile involves a mixed practice that provides veterinary care for a variety of species, which may include horses and other large and small animal species. The type and levels of service offered may vary from species to species, and challenges for the staff may become more complex because as a result. However, there are advantages associated with the ability to provide the convenience of multiple services and there are usually resources available to promote growth.

The Equine Client and Communications

Communication is the key factor in the success of any service business. Veterinary medicine is no exception, and the clients' interactions with the practice can be the most important factor in the success or failure of a practice. There may be daily communications with the backyard owner of a single horse, multiple owners of a million dollar racing Thoroughbreds, buyers, sellers, agents, referring veterinarians, barn managers, trainers, riders, an insurance company, the USDA, or a farrier.

All these instances require correctness of information and professionalism, and some may require compassion as well.

Complete and correct messages delivered in a timely fashion to the appropriate person with prompt follow-up will go a long way toward reassuring clients that their requests are being well handled. Confidentiality when dealing with client information is an absolute necessity, which if not strictly adhered to, can result in loss of a client or practice reputation, at the minimum, or a lawsuit attacking profession ethics. Consistent and timely communication between staff is a challenge that must be met if the practice is to run smoothly.

Office managers must take into consideration differences in staff capabilities and work to provide the most cohesive team possible. Staff responsibilities include reception, inventory control, equipment maintenance, veterinary assistance, and animal husbandry for clinic patients. Policy and procedure manuals, which include job descriptions, are vital for the effective operation of a practice and may be compiled in an employee handbook.

The Receptionist Role and Appointments

The receptionist plays a key role in an equine practice and is the individual responsible for creating the first impression of the practice to clients and practice service providers alike. The ability to ask the right questions, obtain accurate and complete information, maintain a calm atmosphere, prioritize the information and forward it to the appropriate person(s) with the appropriate sense of urgency, and make appointments are not talents within every person's resources. Assembling everything needed to complete an appointment in an equine practice can be a challenge. Familiarity with each doctor's preferences and likely procedure require-

ments, including time, is a daunting task in itself. Familiarity with the time and scheduling requirements of different procedures takes practice, so that both the practice and individual veterinarian schedules mesh in an efficient fashion. Failing to provide adequate time for diagnostic modalities when scheduling a prepurchase examination can result in serious client and staff dissatisfaction. Organizing multitasking of compatible procedures with adequate assistance can maximize the productivity of a veterinarian. Recognizing the unpredictability of lameness examinations, whose diagnoses can range from a hoof abscess to a shoulder lameness with obvious significant time differentials, or providing for the client who shows up with multiple horses for a single horse appointment or who, when the veterinarian shows up for the farm call, greets him with "While you are here," requires a cheerful dedication to the success of the practice. Creative solutions for these problems, rather than unhappy complaining, are the key characteristic of the effective equine support staff. Every practice is different, so preparing for these scheduling snafus in advance with doctor and support staff participation is the most effective way to devise a means of smooth solutions.

Scheduling ambulatory veterinarians in a multiperson practice can be a difficult time management issue, and appointment calendars must be current and readily available at all times. Some ambulatory practices schedule their appointments by geographical area; some adhere to client preferences. Providing correct and complete client/patient information is a staff responsibility that can determine the success or failure of a busy day of calls. Correct telephone numbers and accurate directions (Mapquest, or some other mapping service, can make all the difference in timely completion of a day's work), in addition to complete service requests, packaged medications to be dropped off during a call, and a well-stocked vehicle, at a minimum, are standards to be adhered to. Courtesy calls to clients with expected arrival times are appreciated and are a must if the veterinarian is delayed. Software that includes a scheduling module is beginning to replace the appointment book, allowing access by staff and veterinarians alike from office, home, and vehicle.

The information should be gathered when making an appointment includes the name of the owner (or trainer or agent responsible), contact numbers, the name and description of the horse, the location of/directions to the barn/animal, and the reason for the call (emergency or elective). Additional information should include medical history, if appropriate, include breeding history, vaccinations, recent therapy, and any other pertinent information as it relates to the nature of the call. Explanation of the payment plan of the practice should be handled by the staff, including collection of credit card information and billing policy.

Admission of Patients

Admittance forms should collect the remaining information necessary to complete a medical record. A method of payment should be in place, as should a signed authorization for diagnostic procedures, treatment including surgery, contact information for insurance companies, and in the case of a hospital, a drop off form for that conveys feeding information, vices, equipment or medication provided by the client, and an estimate of cost of services with a duplicate for the client. Accurate and complete communications with the client detailing proposed procedures can create a sense of security in the client. When the client is not present at the time of admission, it is even more important that prompt communication of this information be achieved. The client or agent for the client must sign a release form at the time of admission authorizing diagnostic and therapeutic procedures, especially if general anesthesia and surgery are anticipated. Transmission of such forms to an absent client by fax will allow the acquisition of a valid client signature, which a deficiency of e-mail communications.

An estimate for a procedure, treatment, or surgery is an excellent form of communication and prevents owner surprise at the time of billing. Discussing several options with estimated price ranges will facilitate owner understanding, and the signed copy of the estimate can become a part of the medical record. Daily discussion of the additional charges will permit the client to stay abreast of costs while deciding on what diagnostics and therapeutics can be underwritten and will facilitate collection.

Emergency cases admitted to a clinic must receive appropriate lifesaving treatment, even if owners are unavailable. Telephonic permission for treatment or euthanasia must be witnessed by a third party at the clinic and recorded in the medical record with signatures of the witnesses.

Make your practices policies fully known to all clientele, trainers, and facility managers. A new client packet including appropriate policy statements is an excellent means of communicating this information at the time of initial contact.

If the patient has been referred by another veterinarian, then prompt professional communication between veterinarians is absolutely essential as diagnosis and treatment progress and before discharge. This is the cornerstone of current and future successful relationships. A thank you letter for the referral along with a summary of the case and the discharge instructions is an appropriate gesture. Referral hospitals run a risk of "generating" new clients from referrals, and this practice can destroy otherwise productive and profitable referral relationships. A referral hospital should accept a referred patient for diagnosis or treatment and then discharge it to the referring veterinarian.

Medical Records

Accurate medical records, completed in a timely fashion, are a legal necessity and the only protection against successful malpractice litigation. The challenges associated with obtaining and recording this information must be met. At the same time, when horses change owners or are presented for prepurchase examination, absolute confidentiality of information must be maintained and cannot be included in the medical record or communicated to a second owner or potential buyer without the express written permission of the original owner.

It is important to note that the physical images (e.g., radiographs, ultrasound images, or bone scan images) are the property of the practice that created them. The information contained in these images is the property of the client who paid for them to be made. Release of this information requires a signed release from that client. Absolute adherence to this law is essential. The length of time that patient records, including imaging, must be maintained by a practice, regardless of the status of the patient, varies from state to state; however, a minimum of 10 years provides a good rule of thumb.

Discharge

The attending veterinarian or his or her designated colleague should sign the discharge form and provide the client with a thorough explanation, oral and written, of the horse's condition, including instructions for immediate posthospitalization treatment and care. The client should be informed as to the estimated day and time for discharge and the statement and payment plan explained by the appropriate member of the hospital staff. Immediate medication required, with accurate instructions including route, dose, and frequency of administration, should also be supplied. Long-term medication needs should be provided by the referring veterinarian unless he or she requests otherwise. Reexamination appointments should be in consultation with the referring veterinarian. Before a horse is discharged, a checklist should be made to ensure that the records are complete. Specific arrangements must be made for patients that are not discharged during regular hours so that an attendant from the clinic is present and prepared to contact clinic staff if circumstances should so dictate.

Inventory Management

Inventory management is one of the largest expenses in an equine practice, as well as, the greatest sources of lost income. Successful management of inventory must address the following challenges:

1. Multiple locations for drugs and supplies: pharmacy, sterilizing, anesthesia carts, outer examination areas, trucks, farms, and satellite facilities.

2. Absence of a designated inventory manager leading to disorganized ordering, failure of accurate recording of receivables, and updating of price lists.
3. Unrestricted access to drugs and supplies accompanied by an ineffective record system resulting in little accountability. With emergency practices, access to the pharmacy needs to be 24/7.

Solutions to successful inventory management include designation of a one or more, if necessary, inventory manager(s) responsible for physical inventory of supplies and drugs (especially with regard to expiration dates), purchase, and reconciliation of orders. Limiting availability of individual doctor's "favorite" medications, maintaining an inventory budget (inventory can account for 18%–23% of a practice expenses), consulting with distributors to develop good notification policies regarding specials, while resisting overstocking related to specials are all practices that will help to maintain orderly inventory management. Bar codes have become a popular means of inventory control, especially when combined with coded pharmacy and central supply entry so that checking out supplies is expedited. Staffing of the supply room on a 24-hour basis is cost prohibitive in most circumstances.

Itemized check sheets of all supplies kept in ancillary areas (e.g., ambulatory vehicles, the satellite offices) along with photos of the various drawers or shelves will facilitate inventory and restocking. Recording items used or dispensed will serve as a duplicate reference for inventory control and billing. Veterinary management software can provide current information about inventory so long as the program has been accurately entered including type and concentrations of preparations. One way to help with turnaround time of inventory is to place new items received behind current stock.

Material Safety Data Sheets should be accessible for all drugs and supplies.

Logs

A controlled substance log is a legal requirement for any practice that uses such medications and should be reconciled on a weekly basis. Legal storage of controlled substances requires that they be maintained in locked containers, which are permanently attached to the wall or floor to prevent their being carried off. This includes all trucks, satellite facilities, and surgery examination rooms. This is a potential area for severe fines and a great place for a good technician to step in and prevent a legal disaster.

Radiation licensing and safety requires regular evaluation of both mobile and stationary generators, as well as proof of dosimetry records for all individuals exposed to radiation. This will include veterinarians, technicians, and assistants, as well as, barn staff who may be in contact with horses following scintigraphic examinations. Appropriate safety equipment, including lead aprons, gloves, and thyroid collars must be maintained in functional condition and their use is required.

Radiation safety is extremely important for staff to enforce. The use of cassette holders that distance technicians for the x-ray beam are highly recommended. Those taking x-rays need to be conscious of the x-ray beam, its direction, the focus area, and possible scatter. All required signage should be posted in the clinic and staff should be aware of open examination areas where there are multiple appointments, clients with children, and the potential for others to be around when x-rays are being taken. Digital radiography has the potential to increase radiation exposure because of the ease with which films can be repeated.

Additional logs that may facilitate equipment use and maintenance records could include anesthesia, surgery, and imaging modalities (MRI, computed tomography, ultrasound, and scintigraphy).

Drug logs that document inappropriate reactions can be of assistance when reporting these reactions is required. These logs should include the date, patient name, owner name, procedure, drugs used (i.e., amount, administered when, by whom and route), and the doctor's name.

Import and Export

Another regulatory area that is critical to successful client service is an accurate understanding of export and import regulations. As these regulations, which

cover not only live animals but also the importation of animal products such as serum, plasma, and urine, are subject to frequent change, assistance from importing or exporting agencies is highly recommended. International transport of horses is highly regulated and appropriate documents should be provided by the shipping agency with instructions for correct completion. Knowledge of laboratory testing and vaccination requirements well in advance of travel is imperative so that all constituencies are satisfied. National identification papers or Federation Equestre International (FEI) passports are frequently a requirement for international travel and require weeks to obtain so advance planning is a necessity.

Here is an example of the regulations if you are shipping a horse from the United States to Canada:

"All horses destined for Canada for breeding purposes must return negative samplings for EIA by Coggins test within 60 days and piroplasmosis within 30 days. Prior to export horses must undergo quarantine for 30 days, unless they are on a show or race circuit. Mares and stallions over 2 years of age must undergo special CEM testing with negative results within 40 days: this involves three separate swabs taken within ten days of export."

There are three equine quarantine locations in the United States: Newburg, NY; Miami, FL; and Los Angeles, CA. Horses arriving for entry into the United States from anywhere outside the United States, with the exception of Canada, must be quarantined on arrival at one of these facilities and must be accompanied by an International Health Certificate, endorsed by the Ministry of Agriculture of the Country of Origin of the Animal. The horse must arrive into the United States with no visible signs of communicable disease, skin rashes, or infections of any kind. All horses arriving in the United States are subjected to a quarantine period during which they must test negative to the following diseases, before they are eligible for entry into the United States: dourine, glanders, piroplasmosis (equi and caballi) and equine infectious anemia (EIA). The samples must be tested at the USDA lab in Ames,

Iowa. Any horse testing positive to any one of these diseases may be refused entry into the United States unless suitable treatment arrangements can be made for some of these diseases. The owner, at his expense, will have to make arrangements for accepted treatment or organize export of the horse to the country of origin, if possible, or agree to have the USDA euthanize the animal. The normal quarantine period is between 24 and 72 hours, pending the results of the blood tests. However, the USDA charges a minimum of $810.00 for a 3-day stay regardless of when the horses are released within that time frame. After the minimum 3-day stay, should a horse be held in quarantine, the charge is $195.00 per day from days 4 through 7 and $166.00 per day after that.

Clients must be required to make their own arrangements for shipping, including directly contacting the shipping agency of their choice. Advice from the veterinarian must be carefully worded so as to avoid any suggestion of warranty of the arrangements. The client should be informed that they should request that the shipping agent then contact the veterinarian directly to ensure that appropriate measures are undertaken and forms filled out correctly in a timely manner. The veterinarian should insist that the shipping agent provide appropriate health papers, correctly marked for the country of destination, and written directions as to the completion of these papers and the necessary vaccination and testing to be performed, including the appropriate time frame for this work. Financial arrangements for shipping, exclusive of veterinary charges, must be arranged between the client and shipping agent.

Procedure notes on the acquisition of samples (serum or plasma), testing lab, times required for testing, contact information are well advised and should be kept updated with current laboratory and practice charges for specific tests. Clients are well advised to run preimportation tests before exportation of horses so as to ensure against shipping a horse out of the country with a positive test. However, it is strongly recommended that the shipping agent be contacted for every horse traveling internationally so that no mistakes are made in the provision of travel papers. Maintaining good contacts with shipping agents who can provide accurate advice is imperative regardless of whether they are the agency selected by the client.

Common Forms used in an Equine Practice

A Coggins form is used to submit a sample for testing for EIA, which ordinarily requires approximately 24 hours (Agar method) or 1 hour if it is an enzyme-linked immunosorbent assay (ELISA) test once the sample has been received at the testing laboratory. ELISA tests are not always acceptable, and original copies of the Coggins test are required in some instances (i.e., Florida border). Laboratories in many locations, including private equine clinics, are certified to perform Coggins tests.

A health certificate is issued by a veterinarian accredited by the USDA before interstate travel for any reason. Accreditation by the USDA requires an active veterinary license and certification by the area USDA office. The USDA accreditation number is required on all Coggins tests and health certificates. Please note that interns and new associates may not have USDA accreditation.

Most laboratories use laboratory-specific submission forms. The National Veterinary Services Laboratories (NVSL) has laboratories in two locations: Ames, Iowa, and the Foreign Animal Disease Diagnostic Laboratory (FADDL) at Plum Island, New York. Diagnostic test services range from importation testing to specific pathogen testing during suspected disease outbreaks. A partial list of diseases for which the NVSL provides testing includes equine encephalomyelitis, equine herpesvirus, EIA, equine influenza, and acariasis or equine viral arteritis.

Billing and Data Entry

Many equine practices have two billing methods that accommodate both payment at the time of service or monthly statements, which detail the charges for that time period. Some practices leave a copy of the invoice for the client at the time of the stable call and then follow up with a statement at the end of the month. Software programs are becoming more sophisticated by allowing direct charging for procedures and medications, which assists in capturing all client expenses. Invoices must be clearly composed because they often provide the only written communication to clients of services performed. Encouraging payment at the time of services will reduce accounts receivable and constitutes an excellent use of technician initiative if practice policy supports this effort. Credit card or check payment can be arranged in advance with clients who may not be present at the time of service.

Accounts receivable requires an ability to discuss financial matters with clients in a calm, but forceful fashion. A collection letter is usually the first contact with clients whose accounts are overdue and is sent as a gentle reminder at 15 days after the payment is late, or in other words at 45 days following the initial end of the month statement. The next letter is usually sent out at 60 days along with a phone call, followed by another at 90 days. Many large equine practices employ the services of a collection agency or have a full-time staff member assigned to this task.

Accounting and Budgets

Although technicians are unlikely to be involved in the accounting practices for their employers, attention to minimizing waste, keeping inventory at an efficient minimum, and ensuring that drug and medical supplies pricing is kept current, while keeping expenses at a minimum, is always appreciated.

Client Education

Clinic Web sites have become a great resource for clients, and they a wonderful means of communication for practices. The American Association of Equine Practitioners (AAEP) provides pamphlets on a multitude of subjects and most of the pharmaceutical companies offer information on products, anatomy, and physiology, as well as general horse wellness and care. The equine technician and assistant have a wonderful opportunity to educate the equine client and build a trusting relationship. This is not only an area that can be a practice builder and potential income producer but also an area where a technician or assistant can shine, create a niche and develop expert knowledge in areas such as nutrition, senior care, or foal care. Your practice can host client education seminars and demonstrations. You can leave information pamphlets with an invoice, send out newsletters, post an informative article on your Web site, or send information about an education Web site in a mass client e-mail.

The Internet is a source of vast amounts of information, most of which is anecdotal and unedited. Providing clients with reliable sources is much appreciated by them and helps to protect the veterinarians from being blindsided by client questions about unheard of or untested products. Any assistance that the technician or assistant can provide in the area of client education is sure to be an appreciated practice builder.

References and Further Reading

American Veterinary Medical Association Web site: www.avma.org.

Catanzaro, T. E. 1997. *Building the Successful Veterinary Practice.* vol. 1. Ames, IA: Iowa State Press.

Coumbe, K. 2001. *Equine Veterinary Nursing Manual.* Ames, IA: Blackwell Publishing.

Heinke, M. L. 2001, *Practice Made Perfect: A Guide to Veterinary Practice Management.* Lakewood, CO: American Animal Hospital Association Press.

Heinke, M. L., and H. Nyland. 2007. *Equine Vet Manage J* 3: 32–37

Mersant International, LLC, Horse Shipping Web site: www.mersant.com/horse_shipping.

Shilcock, M., and G. Stutchfield. 2003. *Veterinary Practice Management: A Practical Guide.* Philadelphia: W. B. Saunders.

Steingold, F. S. 2002. *The Employer's Legal Handbook.* 5th ed. Berkeley: NOLO Legal Press.

United States Department of Agriculture Web site: www.usda.gov.

United States Department of Agriculture, Animal and Plant Health Inspection Service (APHIS) Web site: www.aphis.usda.gov/.

HORSE INFORMATION

Has ESMS seen this horse before? (*circle one*) _____ yes _____ no

Registered Name: _____ Nickname: _____

Age: _____ Breed: _____

Sex: (*circle one*) Mare Stallion Gelding   Color: _____

Tattoo/MicroChip ID # _____

   NOTE: ESMS policy requires every horse hospitalized more than two days or scheduled for
   surgery be microchipped for security & medical practice reasons.
   _____ I authorize ESMS to microchip   _____ I do not authorize ESMS to microchip
            this horse.   this horse, and I am aware of the
                                                               ramifications.

Primary Complaint: _____

Is this horse insured? (*circle one*)   _____ yes _____ no

   Insurance Agency: _____ Telephone: _____

REFERRING VETERINARIAN

Name: _____ Telephone: _____

OWNER(S) INFORMATION (*party responsible for bill*)

Name(s): _____

Address: _____
               street/city/state/zip

Telephone (*home*): _____ (*mobile*): _____

            (*work*): _____ (*bam or ohter*): _____

Driver's License # _____ State _____ SS# _____

TRAINER INFORMATION

Name: _____

Address: _____
               street/city/state/zip

Telephone (*home*): _____ (*mobile*): _____

            (*work*): _____ (*bam or ohter*): _____

IMPORTANT-REVERSE MUST BE READ, COMPLETED & SIGNED BEFORE ANY SERVICES ARE PERFORMED

AUTHORIZATION AND CONSENT FOR TREATMENT

I am the owner or authorized agent of the horse named on the reverse of this consent, am responsible for it, and have the authority to execute this consent for EQUINE SPORTS MEDICINE & SURGERY, INC. ("ESMS") to render services. I understand that during the performance of the foregoing procedure(s) or operation(s), unforeseen conditions may be revealed that necessitate an extension or addition of the foregoing procedure(s), as are necessary and desirable in the exercise of the attending veterinarian's professional judgment. In the process of correcting my animal's primary problem or in the treatment or correction of conditions during a hospital stay, the use of anesthetics and/or other medications, and the performance of surgical or therapeutic procedures deemed advisable by the clinician in charge is authorized by me. I understand that hospital support personnel will be employed as deemed necessary by the veterinarian. I have been advised as to the nature of the precedure(s) or opration(s) and the risks involved. I realize that results cannot be guaranteed, and I agree to release ESMS and its employees from any liability associated with the above-described animal.

_____
Authorized Signature

Payment is expected when services are rendered, or, in the event of hospitalization, upon the time of the horse's release.

PAYMENT METHOD (*circle one*):   **VISA**   **MASTERCARD**   **DISCOVER**   **CHECK**   **DEBIT**   **CASH**

All sums remaining unpaid after thirty (30) days from the invoice date shall accrue interest at the highest rate allowable under the Texas Law. A collection fee will be assessed to any account 90 days past due.

Please check one of the following:

_____ I hereby authorize ESMS to charge my credit card account for any payment due or for any delinquent status.

_____ I will be paying by check any payment due or for any delinquent status.

_____ I will be completing a credit application and agree to set payment plan for any charges and to fulfill payment of any delinquent charge status.

_____ Please bill the owner/party responsible for bill. All charges are due in full thirty (30) days from the date of invoice/statement. I am the authorized agent and the owner has authorized these charges. I understand that , if the charges are not paid. I can be held liable for the charges incurred.

I have read and understand this authorization and consent, and have completed all information requested. I hereby agree that, in the event of default in the payment of any amount due, and, if this account is placed in the hands of an agency or attorney for collection or legal action, to pay any additional charges incurredd by ESMS, including agency, attorney fees & court costs, and any other reasonable fees assessed, permitted by laws governing these transactions.

_____   Date: _____
Signature of Legal Owner/Authorized Agent

_____
Print Name

On today's date, this horse was released in stable condition from the hospital into my care.
_____   Date: _____
Signature of Legal Owner/Authorized Agent

_____
Print Name

Case #:

Accession #: _____

Owner: _____

INITIAL ESTIMATE OF CHARGES FOR HOSPITALIZED PATIENT

Prepared by: _____   Admission Date: _____
                    Clinician

                                                                    Estimate/Range

Initial Exam ☐   Routine ☐   Emergency ☐ $ _____

Hospitalization: _____ per day _____ number of days $ _____

Laboratory: $ _____
    Data Base _____   Histopathology _____
    Clin Path _____   Cytology _____
    Microbiology _____   Other _____
    Parasitology _____

Radiology: $ _____
    Survey Exams _____   Special Exams _____

Diagnostic Procedures: $ _____
    Endoscopy _____   Ultrasound _____
    Biopsy _____   Other _____
    Aspirate _____

Anesthesia: $ _____
    Sedation _____   Local _____   General _____

Surgery: $ _____
    Materials/ _____   Professional _____
    Supplies _____   Services _____
    Implants _____   Other _____

Therapeutics: $ _____
    Vaccinations _____   Transfusions _____
    In-Hospital Treatments _____   Deworning _____
    Materials _____

Pharmacy: $ _____
    Hospital Medications _____   Materials _____
    Discharge medications _____

Other: _____ $ _____

_____

Contingencies/Comments

              Total Estimate/Range $ _____

  Understanding that the practice of medicine and surgery is not an exact science, I acknowledge that no guarantees have been made to me regarding the results of examination or treatment of this animal at this hospital. I understand that if further services are required for this animal (for the same or other condition), additional expenses will occur. Do not allow the total bill to exceed $ _____ without my authorization. I have read and understand the above statement have received a copy of this estimate.

Owner (Agent): _____   Date: _____

HOSPITAL CARE AND FEE ESTIMATE: Fetlock Arthroscopic Surgery

SERVICES/PROCEDURE	ESTIMATE

Clinical Pathology: .... $_____
      Blood Analysis Required for Joint Fluid Analysis Or Preoperative Evaluation,

Anesthesia: .... $_____
      Sedation, Injection/Inhalation, Fluids, Medications, Intraoperative Electronic/ Direct Monitoring, Anesthetist

Surgery Fee:... $_____
      Surgeon and Assistants Fees, Surgical Procedure

Suite Fee:.. $_____
Preparation of Patient, Surgical Supplies, Surgery Suite and Recovey Rm

Medications (NSAIDs, Antibiotics etc).. $_____

Bandages, (Including Bandage Changes).................................. $_____

Hospitalization_____days at_____perday.. $_____
      Includes Daily Physical Exam and Assessment

Miscellaneous Fees.. $_____

Follow-up Examination:.. $_____
      Suture Removal, Recheek, Lab, X-rays, Bandage Change, Call Chg

ESTIMATE TOTAL.. $_____

Payment Policy: Payment in full is expected at discharge or upon completion of procedure(s), or service. Payment may be made by Visa, MasterCard, Check or Cash. If credit is necessary, arrangements must be made prior to initiation of service and a credit application must be completed. A depossit may be required.

I understand that is an **ESTIMATE** of the total charges based on the best information currently available and is not a guarantee of charges. Complications may occur which cannot be anticipated and are not included in above estimate and it is my responsibility to stay in communication with the attending veterinarian and be advised of any changes / updates in charges.

_____ Date: _____

SURGICAL CONSENT FORM

Owners Name: **Name of Animal:**

Address: Species:

                                     Breed:

                                     Sex:

                                     Color:

- I am the owner or agent for the owner of the above-described animal and have the authority to execute this consent.
- I hereby consent and authorize the performance of the following procedure(s) of operation(s):

  _____

- I understand that during the performance of the foregoing procedures(s) or operation(s), unforeseen conditions may be revealed that necessitate an extension of the foregoing procedure(s) or operation(s) or different procedure(s) or operation(s) than those set forth above. Therefore, I hereby consent to and authorize the performance of such procedure(s) or operation(s) as are necessary and desirable in the exercise of the veterinarian's professional judgment.
- I also authorize the use of appropriate anesthetics, and other medications, and I understand that hospital support personel will be employed as deemed necessary by the veterinarian.
- I have been advised as to the nature of the procedure(s) or operation(s) and the risks involved. I realize that results cannot be guaranteed.

Estimate of Cost

The estimated fee for surgery is $_____. *The total estimated cost of surgery, hospitalization, and/or treatment is* $_____. You may request an itemization of this amount if desired. This estimate may not be the actual amount of the total charge in the event of complications or if additional treatment is required. A deposit of $_____is required and the balance of the fee for services rendered shall be due and payable upon completion of the case. Any sums, not timely paid, shall bear interest at the rate of 18% per annum and shall be payable in Dallas County, Texas.

I have read and understand this authorization and consent.

_____   _____
        Date   Signature of Owner or Agent

                                                _____

                                                Witness to Above Signature

GENERAL PROCEDURE SHEET

DOCTOR:_____   DATE:_____

OWNER:_____   TRAINER:_____

PATIENT:_____   T_____ P_____ R_____

ANESTHESIA
___ Ace _____ cc
___ Dormosedan _____ cc
___ Rompum _____ cc
___ Torb _____ cc

___ _____ _____ cc

___ _____ _____ cc

BANDAGES
___ Apply bandage $ _____
___ Change Bandage
___ Sweat

___ _____

___ _____

DENTAL
___ Float Teeth

___ _____

___ _____

DEWORMING
___ Eqvalan Paste
___ Eqvalan Sol
___ Ivermectin
___ Panacur Paste
___ Quest Paste
___ Tube Deworm

___ _____

EXAMINATIONS
___ Colic
___ Endoscope
___ Exam Wound
___ Examination
___ Lameness Exam
___ Neuro
___ Opthamalic
___ Otoscopic
___ Palpation Rectal
___ Physical
___ Postmortem
___ Re-Check
___ Respiratory
___ Ultrasound

___ _____

___ _____

INJECTIONS
___ Bute _____ cc
___ Bananine _____ cc

___ _____ _____ cc

___ _____ _____ cc

___ _____ _____ cc

JOINT INDECTIONS
___ Arthrocentesis
___ Carpal-IC (R/L)
___ Carpal-RC (R/L)
___ Coffin (FR, FL, HR, HL)
___ Elbow (R/L)
___ Fetlock (FR, FL, HR, HL)
___ Hamstring (R/L)
___ Hock Distal Intertarsal (R/L)
___ Hock Tarsometatarsal (R/L)
___ Hock Tibiotarsal (R/L)
___ Pastern (FR, FL, HR, HL)
___ Shin (FR, FL, HR, HL)
___ Splint (Lateral/Medial) (R/L)
___ Stifle (R/L)
___ Suspensory Ligament (R/L)
___ Tendon Sheath (FR, FL, HR, HL)

___ w/Carbocaine
___ w/Celestone
___ w/Celestone & HA
___ w/Celestone & Legend
___ w/Celestone & Vetalog
___ w/Depo & HA
___ w/Depo-Medol
___ w/Hyaluronic Acid
___ w/HyVisc
___ w/HyVisc & Vetalog
___ w/Legend
___ w/Vetalog
___ w/Vetalog & Depo

___ _____

___ _____

LABORATORY
___ Allergy Profile
___ Biopsy
___ Brucellosis
___ CBC
___ Coggins (AGID/ELISA/INTER)
___ Culture/Sensitivity
___ Cytology
___ Electrolyte
___ Fibrinogen
___ Granulosa Cell Tumor
___ Joint Fluid
___ Progesterone
___ Protozoal
___ Rhodococcus
___ Serum Chemistry
___ Spinal Tap
___ T4/T3
___ Urinalysis

___ _____

___ _____

RADIOLOGY ( ) DIGITAL ( ) CONV
___ Carpus (R/L) (X_____)
___ Cranium (X_____)
___ Elbow (R/L) (X_____)
___ Fetlook (FR, FL, HR, HL) (X_____)
___ Foot (FR, FL, HR, HL) (X_____)
___ Hock (R/L) (X_____)
___ Jaw (R/L) (X_____)
___ Max. Sinus (X_____)
___ Navioular (FR, FL, HR, HL) (X_____)
___ Neck (X_____)
___ Pastern (FR, FL, HR, HL) (X_____)
___ Pelvis (X_____)
___ PPE (16/32 views)
___ PPE-Ray
___ Radius (R/L) (X_____)
___ Shin (FR, FL, HR, HL) (X_____)
___ Shoulder (R/L) (X_____)
___ Splint (FR, FL, HR, HL) (X_____)
___ Stifle (R/L) (X_____)
___ Tendon (R/L) (X_____)
___ Thorax (R/L) (X_____)
___ Tibia (R/L) (X_____)
___ Withers (R/L) (X_____)

___ _____

___ _____

SERVICES

___ _____

___ _____

___ _____

___ _____

___ _____

VACCINATIONS

___ _____

___ _____

___ _____

DISPENSED

___ _____

___ _____

DISCOUNT

___ _____

DISCHARGE INSTRUCTIONS

DISCHARGE DATE:_____

DEAR MR(S) _____

THE CARE OF _____ IS AGAIN IN YOUR HANDS. CONSCIENTIONSLY FOLLOWING THE DIRECTIONS GIVEN BY YOUR VETERINARIAN CAN SIGNIFICANTLY CONTRIBUTE TO RECOVERY AND REDUCE CONVALESCENT TIME. FAILURE TO FOLLOW THESE DIRECTIONS MAY NEGATE PRECEDING EFFORTS.

CLINCIAL DIAGNOSIS:_____

FEEDING: ☐ NORMAL DIET ☐ SPECIAL_____

EXERCISE: ☐ NONE ALLOWED ☐ UNLIMITED ☐ SPECIAL_____

MEDICATION: ☐ NONE DISPENSED ☐ PRESCRIPTION ☐ MEDICATION DISPENSED

Medication	Size or mg/cc	Amount Dispensed	Instructions
1.			
2.			
3.			

RETURN TO HOSPITAL:　　☐ NOT REQUIRED　　　　　☐ REQUIRED IN_____ DAYS
　　　　　　　　　　　　☐ PLEASE REPORT IN_____ DAYS AS TO YOUR ANIMAL'S PROGRESS.

RETURN TO REFERRING VETERINARIAN FOR:　　☐ SUTURE REMOVAL IN_____ DAYS
　　　　　　　　　　　☐ CHECK UP IN_____ DAYS ☐ RE-EVALUATIONWHEN?_____

ADDITIONAL INSTRUCTIONS:_____

_____

_____

_____

_____

IN THE EVENT OF ANY UNUSUAL DEVELOPEMENTS, PLEASE CONTACT OUR OFFICE OR YOUR REFERRING VETERINARIAN.

Index